SURGEONS AND SOMETHING MORE

THE HISTORY OF SURGERY AT THE UNIVERSITY OF PENNSYLVANIA

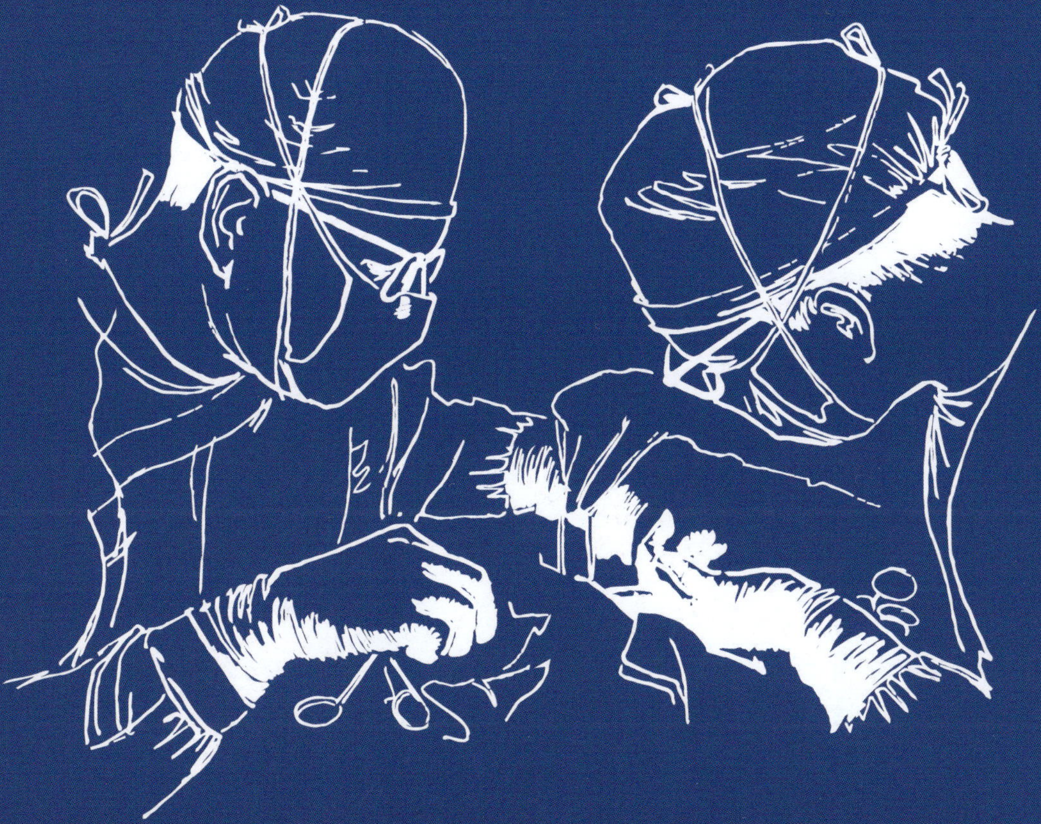

CLYDE F. BARKER & ELIZABETH D. BARKER

American Philosophical Society Press
Philadelphia

For Dode

and

for the residents, for maintaining the department's traditions and excellence.

"Research is essentially intellectual play, to be equated with organized sport and imbued with competitive spirit."

Macfarlane Burnet

"In research, look for the unexpected finding."

Peter Medawar

"Treasure your exceptions . . . [They] are like the rough brickwork of a growing building which tells there is more to come and shows where the next construction is to be."

William Bateson

Published by
The American Philosophical Society Press
Philadelphia, Pennsylvania 19106-3387

www.amphilsoc.org

Printed in the United States of America on acid-free paper
10 9 8 7 6 5 4 3 2 1

Library of Congress Cataloging-in-Publication Data
Hardcover ISBN: 978-16061-8020-4

About the Authors' Image Credit (with dog): Fred G. Barker, photographer

Author Headshots Credit: Kevin Peragine, photographer

Cover Image Credit: This line drawing is used with the permission of the University of Pennsylvania Archives and Records Center. The drawing of two surgeons appeared in the 1966 *Scope*, School of Medicine Yearbook on page 85.

Back Cover Image Credit: Hospital of the University of Pennsylvania with new Pavilion building on the left. Courtesy of Daniel Burke Photography.

Contents

Acknowledgments

To Ron DeMatteo, for his encouragement and support, for suggesting we turn the newsletter into a book, and for writing the afterword. To Ron Fairman, who has been too kind in his chapter on me, for reviewing other sections, and helping in many other ways. To Dan Dempsey, a wise sounding board for reviews and advice. To Bennett Lorber and Scott Jones, for helpful reviews of the manuscript. To Colonel Jeremy Cannon, for his perspective on surgeon soldiers. To Mike Acker, for his assessment of Penn Surgery's role in cardiac surgery's miracles. To Ali Naji, for his recollections of the early transplant program. To Hank Edmunds, the department's academic star. To Mory Ziegler, for his profile of C. Everett Koop and for starting islet transplantation. To Jim Markmann, the past and future leader of transplantation. To Linton Whitaker, for the new field he started and his history of Penn plastic surgery. To Alan Wein, the department's most persistently decorated surgeon, for his history of Penn urology. To Mike Fitts, Bill's son, for his observation that historical lineage is the soul of our department. To Noel Williams, for providing news of current events. To Annie Ravdin, for personal stories of her grandfather, who started Penn Surgery's modern scientific department. To Beth Fisher, for information about her father, Bernard Fisher. To Richard Pryor, for the biography of his brother, John. To Richard Davis, for insights on Henry Keep from his novel, *Yours, D3*. To Jim Mullen, for his insights about the department's faults and greatness. To John Daly and Jeff Drebin, for bringing new blood to the department. To Jon Morris, Laura Huth, and their division of surgical education, for providing information on the accomplishments of Penn residency graduates. To Aron Wahrman, for sharing stories from his library of treasures. To the shade of Rupert Billingham, for his guidance. To Deb Rose, for her encouragement. To Pete Atherton, for his archives. To Tim Horning and Jim Duffin of the University of Pennsylvania Archives, for their generous time tracking down photographs. To our family, for critiquing drafts of the book and cautioning us from being too frank—Fred, Marilyn, Bill, Diana, John, Gwen, Katherine, George, Rebecca, Erik, Chase, and Allison. To Lori Martinsek, our book producer, for her patience, guidance, and advice, and to her team, Becky Taylor, Aldo Rosas, and Jason Pankoke, for their editorial and design work. To Kenny Chumbley, for his image credits research. To Peter Dougherty, director of the APS Press, for his wise counsel. To our friend Bob Hauser, APS Executive Officer, who, with his publications committee, agreed to publish the book. And to Robin Noel, Penn's talented graphic artist, without whose image archives, endless efforts, and patience the book would not have been possible.

Introduction

Penn Surgery was born in the tumultuous years leading up to the American Revolution. Medicine was in a sorry state. Surgeons were limited to bloodletting, setting fractured bones, and amputations. As the next two and a half centuries went by, the new nation experienced a dozen wars, four presidential assassinations, several worldwide epidemics, and the expansion of US territory nine times over. This book describes how Penn surgeons participated in these events and the concomitant, slow, and painful medical advances, such as anesthesia, antisepsis, heart surgery, X-rays, organ transplantation, cancer chemotherapy, IV nutrition, and gene therapy. It is the story of how surgery and medical science evolved to their present, still imperfect forms.

So far, there have been nineteen Penn Surgery department chairmen. Biographical sketches of these leaders show how they were responsible for much of the progress and some of the setbacks of the department. Timelines integrate their experience with the school's history and other medical events of the period.

Attention has also been given to the historical lineage of the department's leaders, that is, who trained whom and who trained the next generation. The obsession surgeons have with this is especially strong at Penn and is an underlying theme of the book.

Contributions of other surgeons, some of whom were as or more important, are also detailed. For example, Julian Johnson was hated by the residents but was perhaps their most effective teacher as well as a pioneer in thoracic surgery. Others were at Penn only for a short time as part of their residency or career. For example, Bernie Fisher, Ravdin's Hospital of the University of Pennsylvania (HUP) resident for only two years, pioneered clinical trials that not only revolutionized treatment of cancer but also are the foundation of what we now call evidence-based medicine; or John Gibbon, the Jefferson surgeon who, with his wife, Mary, conducted at Penn much of their work on the heart-lung machine.

In the beginning, the department was comprised of a single individual—the professor—whose teaching was limited to formal lectures delivered to the assembled student body of several hundred. Later, the faculty roster included a few junior members who functioned more or less as apprentices to the chairman. Only in the last seventy-five years, since it was mandated by the American Board of Surgery, has there been anything like a formal training program in surgery. Because much of the impact of the department since then has been through its trainees, the substantial contributions of these Penn surgeons have been included, such as TPN and pediatric, plastic, and endovascular surgery.

My personal experience in the department as an intern, resident, and faculty member now extends back sixty-five years. Conversations with my older brother—a Penn student, intern, and Ravdin resident—extends my memory fifteen years further. Thus much of the history as far back as the early 1940s is based on personal and family recollections, experiences, and stories, as well as contemporary accounts.

Several sections were written at my request by other faculty members or Penn surgeons, such as pediatric surgeon Mory Ziegler's section on C. Everett Koop and Linton Whitaker's section on plastic surgery. Ronald Fairman agreed to write the chapter on my chairmanship since I could hardly be expected to be objective. Ron DeMatteo's afterword attempts to put the history in perspective and predict the future.

CHAPTER 1

Feuding Founders Poison the Atmosphere of America's First Medical School

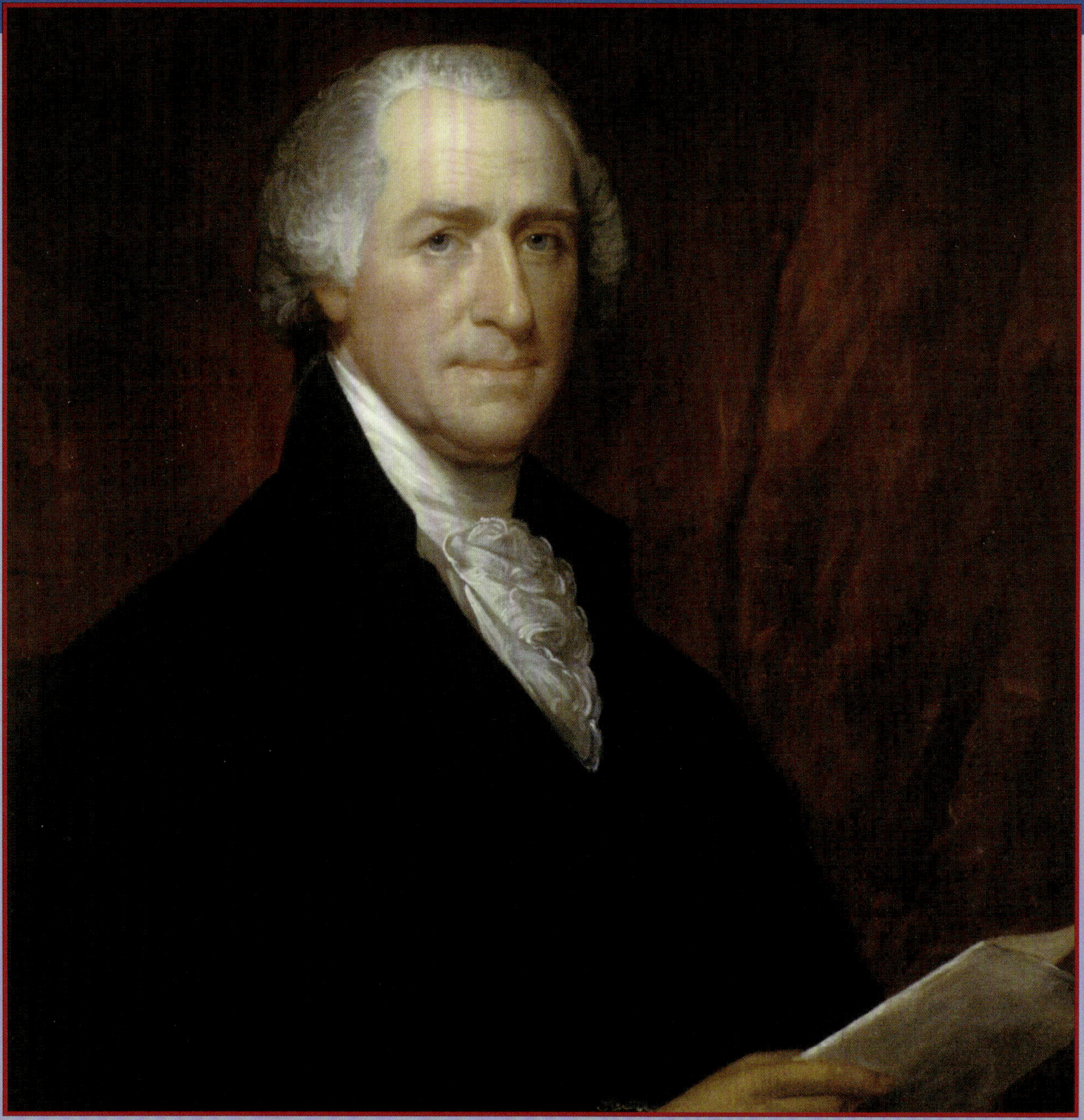

William Shippen Jr.

William Shippen Jr. (1736–1808)

Professor of Surgery, Anatomy, and Midwifery (1765–1805)

John Morgan and Benjamin Rush

Until the last half of the eighteenth century, there was no Department of Surgery, or even a medical school, in America. The colonists were consumed with establishing the necessities of life and not with education, culture, or medicine. With few exceptions, America's doctors had been educated by apprenticeships, if at all. Those with any formal medical education had acquired it abroad. There was no system of licensing or accreditation, so anyone could call himself a doctor and practice medicine. There were no hospitals, no specialists, no anesthesia, no understanding of antisepsis or asepsis, and thus no abdominal or thoracic surgery. Medicine could not have been an especially satisfying or lucrative field. Many doctors had part-time jobs as farmers, shopkeepers, politicians, and soldiers. When the Revolutionary War began in 1775, almost half of all doctors enlisted in the Continental Army, many serving as combatants.

Until 1765, there are no American medical schools. Medical training is by apprenticeship, if at all

During the mid-18th century, the only formal medical training is abroad

Philadelphia is the political and cultural center of the country

At the mid-point of the eighteenth century, the colonies had become well-enough established for wealthy Americans to send their sons abroad to be educated, some of them in medicine. For several reasons, the University of Edinburgh was a natural choice for American medical students. First of all, English was spoken there. Second, Oxford and Cambridge, which might otherwise have been more attractive to Americans, were available only to those of the Anglican religion. Because facilities for study of anatomy and clinical medicine were better in London, many Americans also spent time there. A pattern evolved that was followed in the education of most of the young colonials who were destined to become the leaders in US medicine. After college in America, they usually served an apprenticeship of several years with a local medical practitioner. Those who could afford it then traveled to Europe (usually London) where they studied anatomy at William Hunter's famous school of anatomy. They acquired exposure to clinical medicine by "walking the wards" of the great London hospitals and exposure to surgery by watching operations by established surgeons. After this practical training in

1754
Shippen graduates from Princeton then serves as apprentice to his physician father

1765
Philadelphia is site of America's first medical school

London, they would complete their education by attending a university, usually Edinburgh, to obtain an MD degree.

The best known Americans to follow this pattern were three young Philadelphians: William Shippen, John Morgan, and Benjamin Rush. In 1765, Morgan and Shippen founded America's first medical school at the College of Philadelphia—which subsequently became the University of Pennsylvania. At that time, with a population of 30,000, Philadelphia was, except for London and Edinburgh, the largest English-speaking city in the British Empire. It was the political and cultural center of Colonial America. Of Philadelphia's thirty doctors, most had been educated only by apprenticeships. John Redman was one of only a few who had gone abroad for an MD degree. He became the most important preceptor of Philadelphia medicine's future leaders.

The Philadelphia story is interesting not only because its medical school was the first, but because we know a great deal about the three main founders: Morgan, Shippen, and Rush. In fact, since they all had some undesirable characteristics, we know almost more about them than we would like. Their story was played out against the tumultuous background of the American Revolutionary War in which all three of our stars had important and controversial roles. At the University of Pennsylvania, these founders are now so venerated that the usual telling of their story is censored—inspirational, but less compelling than the truth. Nothing is to be gained by demonizing the founders of our school, but their story becomes much more interesting if we don't gloss over the crucial parts played by selfishness, jealousy, plagiarism, betrayal, hatred, fraud, graft, treason, failure, and despair. In addition, of course, there were substantial amounts of bravery, sacrifice, loyalty, and success.

William Shippen Jr. (1736–1808)

The story of our Department of Surgery begins in 1765, with the opening of America's first medical school, the College of Philadelphia, and the appointment of Shippen as its Professor of Anatomy, Surgery, and Midwifery. The history of Shippen's career cannot be understood if we leave out the roles played by the school's other founders: his bitter enemies, John Morgan and Benjamin Rush. Their three lives were so intertwined that to tell about one and not the other two makes the story meaningless.

Our first protagonist, William Shippen, was from a socially prominent Philadelphia family,[1] one with connections to the elite families of other colonies, the Lees and Washingtons of Virginia and the Adamses of Massachusetts. Among Shippen's forebears were the governor and the mayor. He grew up in the city's largest house where important visitors like Washington and Jefferson were often entertained. Young Shippen, after graduating first in his class from the College of New Jersey (now

Princeton), spent the next several years as an apprentice to his father, a socially and professionally prominent Philadelphia physician.[2] In 1758, Shippen went to London where he was taken under the wing of his family friend, Benjamin Franklin. For two years, Shippen attended the anatomy lectures of William Hunter, studied midwifery with London's expert, Colin MacKenzie, walked the wards of St. Thomas, St. Bartholomew, and Guy's, and watched operations by Percival Potts and other great surgeons.[3] For eight months he lived in John Hunter's house. John Hunter, William's brother, is considered the father of experimental surgery. Shippen wrote in his diary that he talked and dissected "anatomically" with Mr. Hunter—sometimes late into the night.[4] During this period, Shippen worked hard and applied himself effectively to his studies. Since his mentors were the world's experts, he could hardly avoid becoming an extremely well-prepared young physician.

1758–1760
In London, Shippen lives with and studies anatomy and surgery with John Hunter

1761
Shippen gets MD from University of Edinburgh

William Hunter's school of anatomy

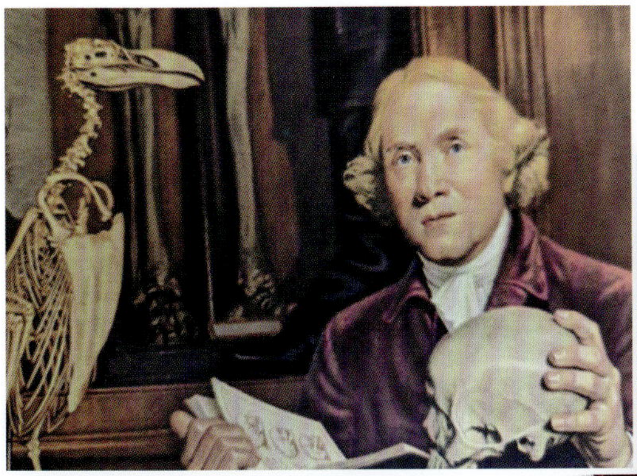

John Hunter

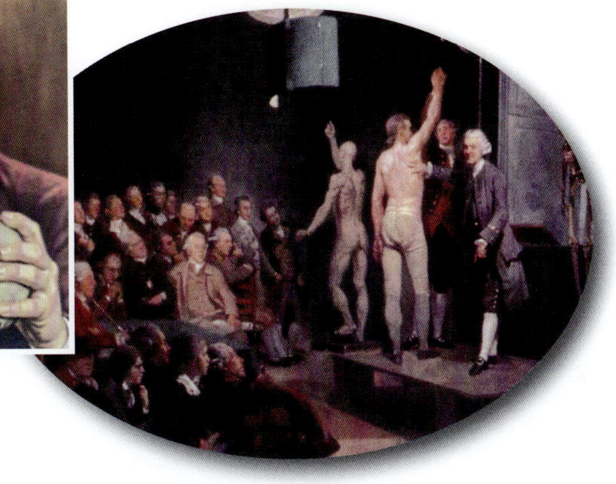

But William Shippen was never inclined to spend all of his time working.[5] While in London, he attended meetings of the Royal Society with Benjamin Franklin, learned to play the flute, went to the theater to see Garrick play Macbeth, and dined with Samuel Johnson and his biographer Boswell. In 1760, carrying letters of introduction from Franklin, he went off to Edinburgh where he obtained his MD degree. Then Franklin arranged for him to travel in France (even though at that time England and France were at war). He also married Alice Lee, a girl from Virginia, who had traveled to London to pursue her earlier relationship with Benjamin Franklin's son, William.[6] To the extent that after two and a half centuries we can characterize Shippen's persona, he was talented, socially ambitious, and personable—perhaps to a fault—and throughout his life well-liked by everyone (with the important exception of his colleagues John Morgan and Benjamin Rush).

A central feature of our story is that shortly before returning home, Shippen met in London with John Morgan, another Philadelphian who

1762
In London, Shippen and Morgan discuss founding a medical school in America

1762
Shippen returns to Philadelphia and lectures on anatomy, surgery, and midwifery

was studying anatomy with the Hunters. They made a pact that when both were back in Philadelphia, they would join forces to start a medical school.[7]

In 1762, Shippen returned to Philadelphia and at the State House (now known as Independence Hall) began to teach courses in anatomy, surgery, and midwifery. In America, his was the first formal course in any medical subject.[8] Shippen assumed that his lectures were the prelude to the medical school curriculum he and John Morgan would collaborate to develop as soon as Morgan finished his education and returned to Philadelphia. Unfortunately, this was not to be. Indeed, when Morgan returned in 1765, a medical school was started, but in such a way that the two founders, rather than collaborators, became lifelong enemies. Two and one-half centuries later, though, it is rarely mentioned at Penn Medicine that there are still remnants of the dispute between these former friends.

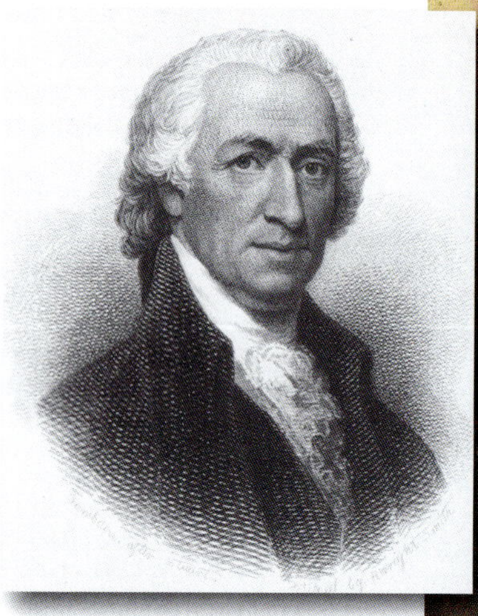

William Shippen Jr.

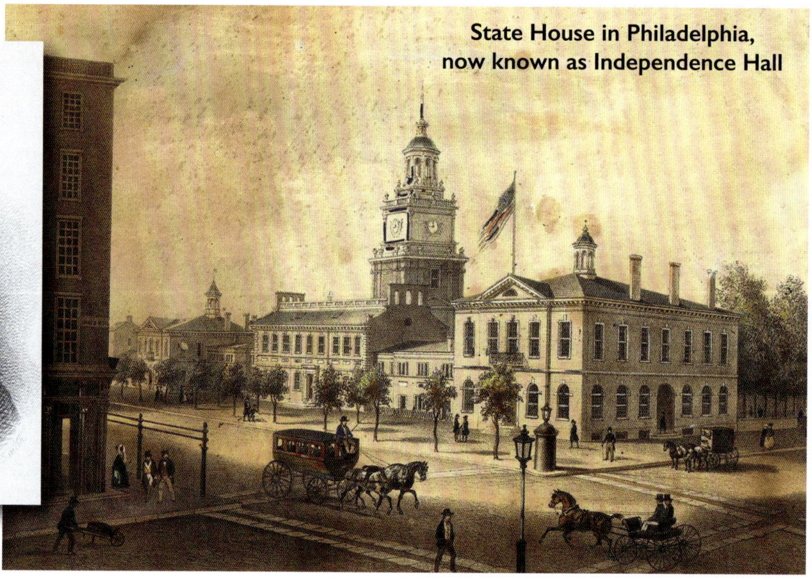

State House in Philadelphia, now known as Independence Hall

John Morgan (1735–1789)

Our second young star, John Morgan, was the son of a Welsh immigrant, who had become a prosperous Philadelphia shopkeeper. At age fifteen, Morgan was apprenticed to Dr. John Redman. Over the next decade, in addition to six years with Redman, he obtained his BA from the College of Philadelphia (University of Pennsylvania) as a member of its first graduating class. He next served with distinction as an army surgeon on the western frontier of the French and Indian War. It is said that he was a talented operating surgeon. Then in 1760, he traveled to London where he studied anatomy with William Hunter and walked the wards at St. Thomas Hospital. Like Shippen, he lived briefly in John Hunter's house. The two young Philadelphians were said to have been friends as schoolmates in Philadelphia. They resumed their friendship in London. On one occasion, they double-dated in attending the coronation of George III.[9] With Franklin, his friend Dr. Fothergill, and others, they openly discussed their plan to collaborate in founding an American medical school.[10] Morgan's friends later admitted they were not sure this was his intent.

After the London experience, Morgan went to Edinburgh for his MD as had Shippen two years before. As a student in Edinburgh, Morgan was a great academic and social success. It appears to have been his ambition to acquire as credentials as many memberships in scientific and other societies as possible. He was elected a member of the Royal Medical Society and, remarkably for a student, was made a Freeman of the City of Edinburgh. After graduating with his MD in 1763, Morgan spent the next year touring Europe with his friend, James Boswell. In Paris, he applied unsuccessfully to become a member of the French Academy of Surgeons by presenting as his own work the corrosion method of demonstrating the internal blood vessels of organs, a technique he had learned from the brothers William and John Hunter. The Hunters were incensed when they learned of this, especially since they believed Morgan's thesis at Edinburgh on the formation of pus had failed to acknowledge that it was based on John Hunter's ideas and experiments.[11] In Rome, the twenty-eight-year-old Morgan had an audience with the Pope and arranged to have his portrait painted. At Padua, he visited with Giovanni Morgagni and in Ferney with Voltaire.[12] During his passage home to America, though his qualifications were really limited to his ambitious personality and his MD thesis, he was elected a member of the Royal Society. Benjamin Franklin paid his initiation fee.[13]

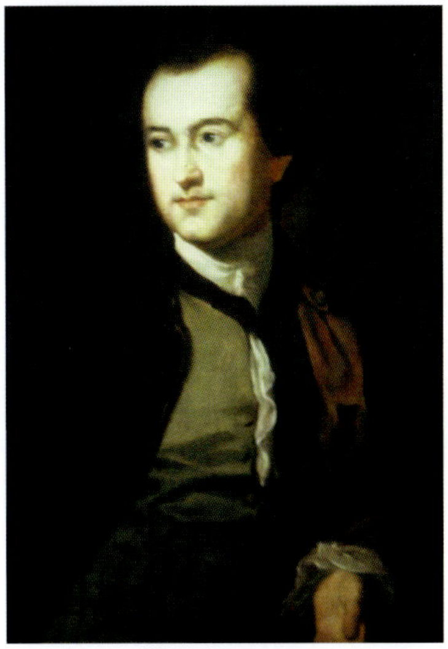

John Morgan

On Morgan's return to Philadelphia in 1765, he totally reneged on the commitment he and Shippen had made in London to work jointly in establishing a medical school. Within days of his return to Philadelphia, while purposely avoiding any contact with Shippen, Morgan presented to the university trustees his independent plan to organize a school of medicine.[14] He asked to be recognized as the sole founder of the school and its first professor of medicine. Greatly impressed with his plan, the trustees agreed. Morgan was not about to share the credit for founding the school with Shippen, but it was necessary for the school to offer a course in anatomy. So several months later, Morgan acknowledged that Shippen was qualified to teach anatomy. The trustees then appointed him professor of anatomy, surgery, and midwifery.[15] Shippen was not likely ever to forget what he interpreted as Morgan's treachery.

1750–1756
Morgan is apprentice to Dr. John Redman

1757
Morgan receives BA from College of Philadelphia

1757–1760
Morgan serves as surgeon in French and Indian War

1760–1762
In London, Morgan studies with John and William Hunter

1763
Morgan receives MD from University of Edinburgh

1763–1764
Morgan travels in Europe

1765
Returning to Philadelphia, Morgan presents to Trustees his independent plan for a medical school, making an enemy of Shippen

1765
Morgan disparages surgery, making enemies of many doctors who practice surgery

1765
Trustees accept Morgan's plan. The medical school is founded

1765
Morgan appointed professor of medicine

1765
Because the school needs to teach anatomy, Shippen is appointed professor of anatomy, surgery, and midwifery

The reason for Morgan's betrayal of Shippen will never be known, but it could hardly have been accidental. Nor was the insult confined to Shippen as an individual. Morgan claimed for himself higher status than Philadelphia's established medical practitioners. He condemned the apprenticeship system as "lame and insufficient," thereby alienating the many well-established, politically powerful apprenticeship-trained doctors, such as Shippen's father, who was also a university trustee.[16] Furthermore, Morgan specifically disparaged surgery as an "unintellectual, mechanical act, repugnant to sensitive men" and appropriate only for those trained by apprenticeships. The enmity of the school's founders would poison the air at the school until they died. Its fallout would blight both of their careers and, as sides were taken by their colleagues, would divide the faculty for decades. Even today, surgeons search for evidence of weaknesses in Morgan as a medical man, while in telling the same story, internists focus their criticism on surgeons like Shippen.

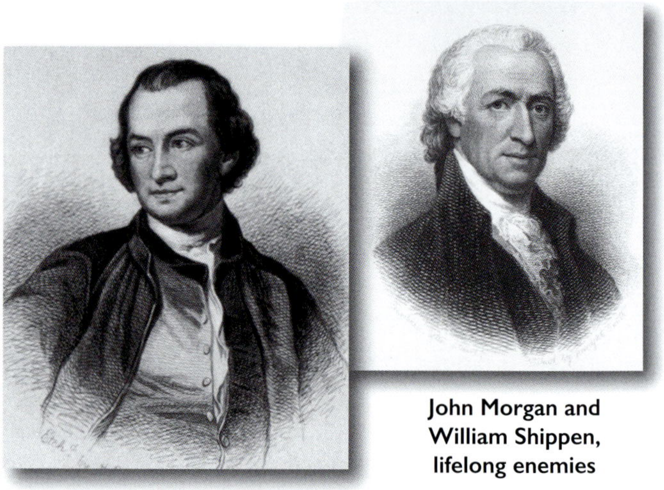

John Morgan and William Shippen, lifelong enemies

Morgan's plan for the new school was extensive, ambitious, and detailed, though totally impractical for the time.[17] It was to be part of the university and for admission, required education in Latin, Greek, and the liberal arts. Its extensive curriculum was modeled after that of the University of Edinburgh. It was 100 years ahead of its time, and at the fledgling university, it would take even longer than that to accomplish anything like it. However, the trustees were impressed not only with the plan but also with Morgan's many memberships and honors. With great enthusiasm, they endorsed Morgan's plan and elected him professor of the theory and practice of medicine. Morgan also asserted that, as an exalted field, medicine should be separated from the "low drudgery of surgery" and from the sale of drugs. Morgan's plan called for professorships in all the "usual disciplines" including physics, chemistry, materia medica, botany, and so forth. Not mentioned were professorships in surgery and midwifery (coincidentally, Shippen's areas of greatest interest and expertise). Morgan's denigration of apprenticeships and of surgery proved to be extremely unwise since it not only insulted his former friend Shippen, but also made enemies of Shippen's powerful family and friends.[18] In addition, it antagonized the many established physicians of older generations whose livelihood depended on their practice of medicine, surgery, and the sale of drugs. Morgan could have used the support of these powerful individuals later when he and Shippen fought over leadership positions in the medical department of the Continental Army.

Despite the poisonous feud of its founders, the medical school quickly became very successful. Students flocked to the new school, which would allow them to become doctors without having to travel to Europe. Morgan's personal reputation grew as he lectured in the medical school, allowing him to build a large practice. He was soon not only Philadelphia's most prominent physician, but also one of its most famous and recognizable citizens. It was said that people would run to catch sight of him as he walked down the street.[19] He was easily recognized since he was a dapper dresser and was the first American to carry an umbrella to shield him from the sun. He seemed to have everything going for him. He could not have realized his life was about to turn sour. According to his biographer, Whit Bell of the American Philosophical Society, "Morgan comes to us across the centuries as something of a dandy, an extremely ambitious, proud, and jealous young man more respected than loved."

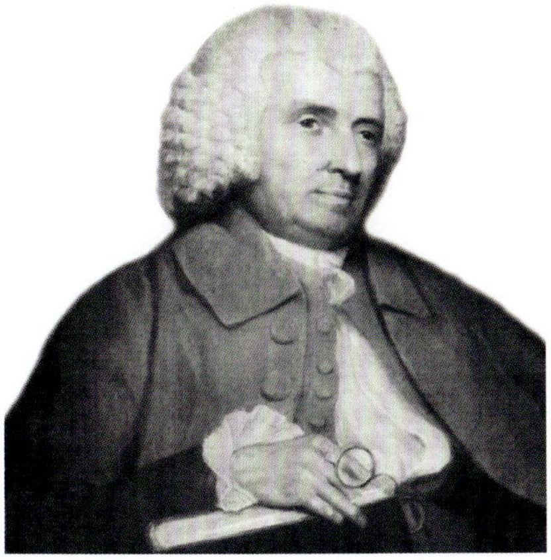

John Morgan

1765–1775
Medical school is successful

1775–1783
Revolutionary War

1775
Morgan appointed surgeon general

In 1775, while feelings of patriotism and American independence were on the rise in Philadelphia, Morgan made another mistake. He wrote a treatise on the advantages of colonialism. Despite this and further indications of his loyalist leanings even after the revolution began, Morgan's exalted reputation led to his appointment as surgeon general of Washington's Continental Army.[20] Then, for the first time in his life, he was unsuccessful. It may have been that his personality and administrative skills were ill-suited for this position, or at the time this job may simply have been impossible. The Army's medical care was totally disorganized.[21] Each regiment had its own independent surgeon, and most of them resisted Morgan's efforts at unification or standardization of policies. Supplies, such as medicine, dressings, blankets, and surgical instruments, were scarce, contributing to the suffering and death of soldiers. Morgan's appeals to Congress and General Washington for help were largely ignored. The many American casualties sustained early in the war as Washington lost battle after battle, combined with a smallpox epidemic, soon hospitalized fully 25 percent of the soldiers. Morgan was doing his best, and one wonders if anyone else could have been more successful under the circumstances. However, it didn't help that Morgan's temperament included neither tact nor patience. His whining over lack of support was not appreciated by Washington and Congress. Thus, Morgan was increasingly blamed for the disorganized medical system and bad outcomes. Shippen and his powerful friends

1777
Morgan is fired as surgeon general, succeeded by William Shippen

1777–1778
British occupation of Philadelphia

1779
Morgan appeals and is exonerated but not restored as surgeon general

1779
Because of political criticism, College of Philadelphia loses its charter, closes, and is replaced by University of the State of Pennsylvania. Charter of College of Philadelphia is restored in 1789

1780
Shippen is court-martialed as surgeon general

1781
Shippen narrowly wins court-martial but resigns in disgrace as surgeon general

and relatives (including some in Congress) were happy to intensify the criticism. No one came to Morgan's defense, so he was abruptly fired without a hearing.[22] Ironically, it was his rival, Shippen, who was chosen to replace him as surgeon general.

Embittered over the perceived unfairness of his dismissal and blaming Shippen for undermining him, Morgan devoted most of his time for the next two years to petitioning Congress for a hearing. In criticizing Shippen's performance as his successor as surgeon general, Morgan then enlisted the support of his powerful friend and colleague, Benjamin Rush. Since conditions in the Army hospitals were not improving under Shippen, this became quite effective. Eventually, Morgan was given a hearing by Congress and was officially vindicated of any wrongdoing.[23] However, he was not reinstated, and Shippen remained surgeon general.

Morgan and Rush then turned their full attention to a vicious personal attack on Shippen, lodging charges of malpractice and misconduct. Shippen, during this time, continued to enjoy his customary comfortable lifestyle and spent little time caring for wounded soldiers or even visiting to comfort them in the miserable surroundings of the wartime hospitals. Even more serious accusations were that Shippen was selling for his own profit wine, sugar, and other army supplies that were badly needed by the soldiers.[24] What followed was indeed a sorry scene: Morgan, at considerable expense and discomfort, traveled on horseback around the country to collect testimony to support his charges against Shippen. Meanwhile Shippen, affecting unconcern, tried to ignore the evidence against him. Since the evidence was considerable, eventually Shippen was arrested, court-martialed, and put on trial. It may have helped him that during the trial, he entertained some of the jurors in his fancy house. Although the vote was close, the always amiable, socially popular and politically powerful Shippen was acquitted. The findings of the court-martial were sent to Congress, which confirmed the not-guilty verdict but at the same time labeled Shippen's speculating and selling army hospital stores as "highly improper and justly reprehensible."[25] His reputation badly tarnished, Shippen resigned four months later.

The dispute of these cofounders of Penn's medical school did not cease as they returned to civilian life. Instead, they continued to snipe at each other, Morgan reiterating endlessly the charges of Shippen's fraud and Shippen raising the question of Morgan's patriotism, pointing out that during the British occupation of Philadelphia, Morgan had been seen openly mingling with and walking arm-in-arm with British officers.[26] Eventually, the public tired of their wrangling. An editorial in the newspaper put an end to the public aspects of it by publishing a blank form, suggesting that they both use it so that they need not bother to compose new accusations.[27] This form said, "Know all men by these presents that I (JM or WS) do announce, attest, and declare that my fel-

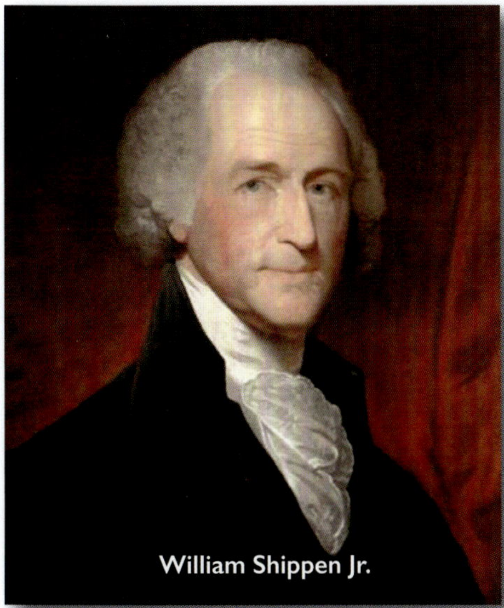
William Shippen Jr.

low citizen (WS or JM) is a rogue, rascal, villain, thief, scoundrel; that he is a Tory, traitor, conspirator: that he is a backbiter, slanderer and liar; that he is a mean, dirty, stinking, sniveling, sneaking, pimping, pocket picking d—d son of a bitch."

Morgan had been broken by this dispute and never recovered. Although he returned to the practice of medicine in Philadelphia, he never returned to teaching at the medical school, refusing to participate in any faculty of which Shippen was a member.[28] In 1789, at the age of fifty-four, John Morgan died in relative poverty and obscurity. Benjamin Rush, his former colleague, when called to attend him, found him dead "in a small hovel surrounded by books and papers." Rush said, "The man who once filled half the world with his name now had scarcely friends enough left to bury him."[29]

The amiable William Shippen resumed his social activities, practice, lectures, and professorship in the medical school, teaching anatomy, surgery, and midwifery for another twenty years. His personality, senior status, and eloquence combined to make him one of the most honored and popular faculty. Among his accomplishments during this time was the founding of the country's first maternity hospital, revolutionizing the nation's obstetrical practices.

In his personal life, Shippen was not so fortunate.[30] His favorite son, a promising young lawyer, died early, and he forced his daughter into an unhappy marriage. During his final illness at age seventy-two, he called in his old enemy, Benjamin Rush. Rush later said:

> He had talents, but which from disuse became weak . . . but with the stock of knowledge he acquired when young he maintained some rank in his profession, especially as a teacher of anatomy, in which he was eloquent . . . He lived chiefly in convivial company, in which he was always a welcome and agreeable member. His chief pleasure consisted in the enjoyments of the table. To these, and to young company he retained an attachment.[31]

The implication and innuendo of the last remark were reinforced by a critique registered in the diary of his young niece who wrote, "the doctor is so fond of kissing; he really would be much more agreeable if he were less fond."[32]

1781–1789
Shippen–Morgan feud continues. Morgan never returns to medical school faculty or teaching

1789
Death of Morgan

1789–1791
Two rival medical schools exist in Philadelphia

Shippen returns to teaching and social activities until death in 1808

1760
Rush receives BA from Princeton

1761–1766
Rush apprentices with Dr. John Redman

1768
Rush receives MD from University of Edinburgh

1768
Rush returns to Philadelphia, appointed chairman of chemistry at the medical school of College of Philadelphia

1776
Rush signs Declaration of Independence

Benjamin Rush (1745–1813)

The third young star of the Philadelphia school, Benjamin Rush, has been labeled "The American Hippocrates." No doubt, he was the most famous American doctor of his day but also the most controversial. Perhaps only Benjamin Franklin, in the early United States, was more versatile in his interests and expertise. The extravagant claim has even been made that next to Washington, Franklin, Jefferson, and Adams, Rush may have been the most important American of his time. But even Rush's heroism is ambiguous. Born near Philadelphia a decade after Morgan and Shippen, Rush followed the usual pattern of education. After graduating from Princeton, he served an apprenticeship with John Redman and then went to Edinburgh where he was a great success. Remarkably, for a student, he attained the status of Burgess and Guild Brother of the City. Influential beyond his years, the young Rush recruited John Witherspoon, a Scottish minister, to come to America to succeed Rush's uncle as president of Princeton.[33] After obtaining his MD degree in Edinburgh, Rush went to London to attend lectures and dissect with William Hunter. His friendship with Benjamin Franklin was an entry to the city's social scene. One night, in Sir Joshua Reynold's house, he sat at dinner with Samuel Johnson and Oliver Goldsmith.[34]

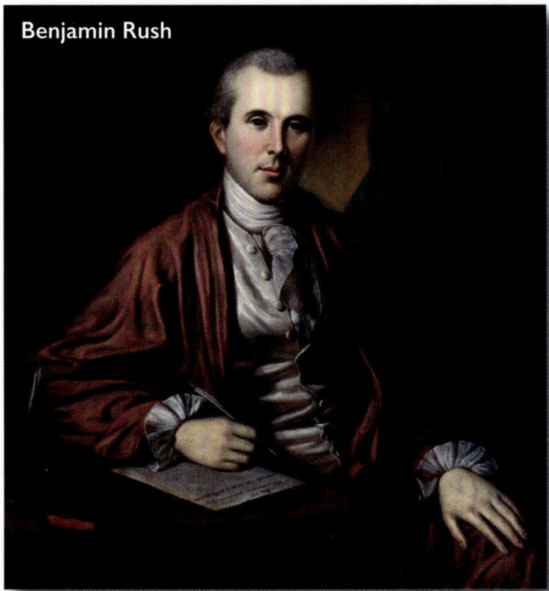

When he returned to Philadelphia, the twenty-four-year-old Rush was at once appointed professor of chemistry, becoming the fourth faculty member of the new medical school. Unlike Morgan and Shippen who wrote little, Rush became a prolific writer on medical and many other topics. In addition, his broad interests and scholarship led to widespread recognition. However, his contemporaries, friends and foes alike, also noted that he was impetuous, hot-headed, ambitious, dogmatic, and unable to separate his professional from his political and religious loyalties. From the beginning, Rush hated the Shippens.

In 1775, as anti-British sentiments peaked, Rush, quite the opposite of his loyalist-sympathizing friend John Morgan, became one of the most active and widely recognized proponents of American independence.[35] When war broke out, he was elected to Congress and was a prominent signer of the Declaration of Independence.[36] In 1777, he became surgeon

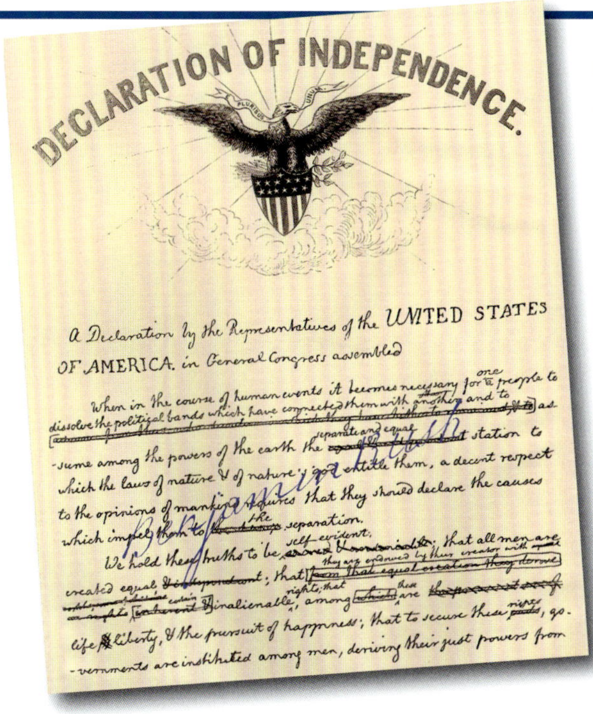
DECLARATION OF INDEPENDENCE.

a Declaration by the Representatives of the UNITED STATES OF AMERICA, in General Congress assembled

When in the course of human events it becomes necessary for one people to dissolve the political bands which have connected them with another, and to assume among the powers of the earth the separate and equal station to which the laws of nature & of nature's god entitle them, a decent respect to the opinions of mankind requires that they should declare the causes which impel them to the separation.

We hold these truths to be self-evident; that all men are created equal; that they are endowed by their creator with certain unalienable rights; that among these are life, liberty, & the pursuit of happiness; that to secure these rights, governments are instituted among men, deriving their just powers from

general of the Middle Department of the Army. He soon became critical of the inefficiency of the medical department and the poor care given the wounded soldiers. In public forum and private letters to John Adams and others, he criticized Shippen, who by then had replaced John Morgan as surgeon general. Rush's influence was a major factor in provoking Shippen's court martial.

Soon, Rush's criticism extended beyond Shippen and army medicine to Washington's leadership. Earlier, Rush had been Washington's friend and confidant. Indeed, Rush's military activities were not limited to the care of the wounded. He was with Washington in the planning and conduct of the general's famous crossing of the Delaware for his surprise attack on the British at Trenton, which was considered the turning point of the War.[37] Contributing importantly to the success of this crucial mission was a message Washington entrusted to Rush, which required him to ride all night and unescorted through sixty miles of enemy-occupied territory. Delivery of another message resulted in bringing reinforcements largely responsible for Washington's success in the crucial Battle of Princeton. But later, as Rush pondered Washington's defeats at Brandywine

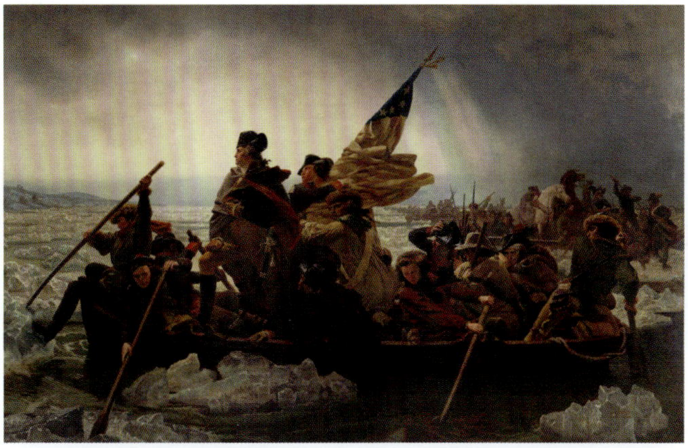
George Washington crossing the Delaware River—a boat missed by Rush.

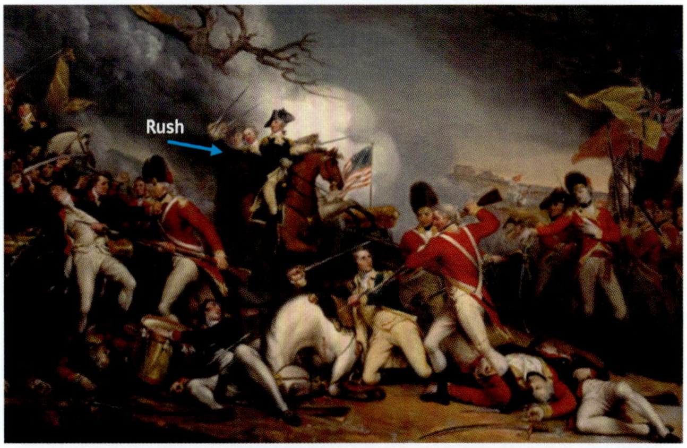

Rush brought crucial reinforcements to the Battle of Princeton

1777
Rush is appointed surgeon general of Middle Department of the Army

1777
Rush shown in painting with Washington at Battle of Princeton

1778
Rush criticizes Washington's leadership in letter to Patrick Henry

1778
Rush is allowed to resign as surgeon general

1791
Although controversial for his extreme belief in bloodletting for all diseases, he is appointed professor of medicine at Penn

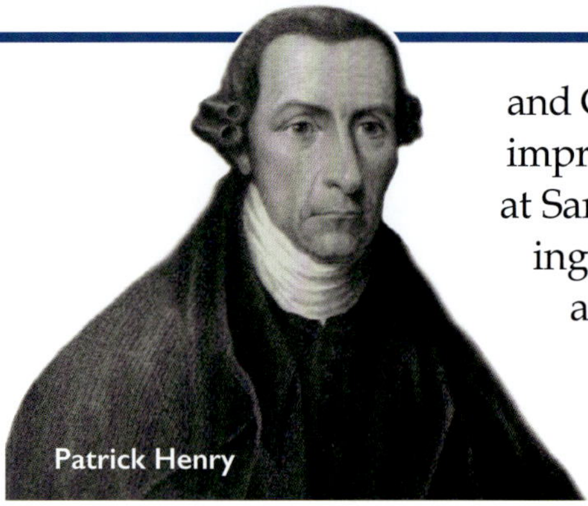

Patrick Henry

and Germantown, and compared these to the impressive victory of General Horatio Gates at Saratoga, Rush came to believe that Washington should be relieved of his command and replaced by Gates.[38] In an unsigned letter to his friend, Patrick Henry, the governor of Virginia, Rush communicated this recommendation. Henry shared the letter with Washington who easily recognized Rush's handwriting.[39] This was the end of Rush's military career and any political ambitions he may have had. Fortunately for Rush, Washington accused him only of disloyalty and not of treason. He was not court-martialed but was allowed to quietly resign his commission. Clinically depressed, he spent some months in seclusion in Princeton before returning to Philadelphia and civilian medicine.[40]

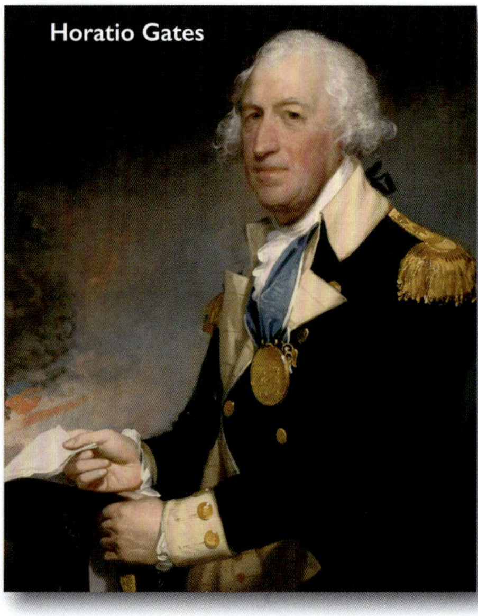

Horatio Gates

Although Rush's reputation was lastingly damaged by his quarrel with Washington, his image was considerably rehabilitated by his heroic performance during the yellow fever epidemic of 1793 that killed 4,000 to 5,000 (about 10 percent) of Philadelphia's citizens. Rather than leaving the city, as many physicians did, Rush worked tirelessly in care of the afflicted. Rush himself contracted the disease, and three of his five apprentices died from it. Rush believed that this disease and fevers of any source were caused by excessive excitability of the blood vessels. He thought that normal balance could be restored by depletion, that is, bleeding and purging.[41] His usual prescription was "10 and 10" (10 ounces of blood, 10 grains of jalap, a powerful laxative). Although in serial bleedings he sometimes removed as much as four-fifths of a patient's normal blood volume, he attributed

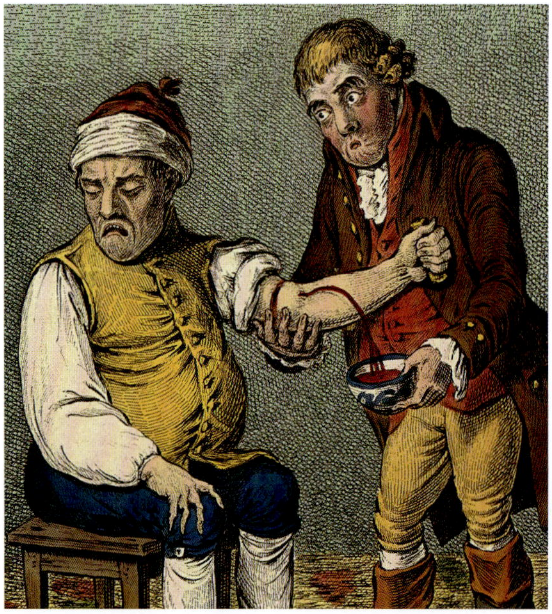

Bloodletting—Rush's universal treatment

failures of the treatment to insufficient bleeding and purging. Some of his patients got better, but many died. Many doctors disagreed with Rush's treatment. Rush could defend his position and combat his critics only by rhetoric. He kept no systematic records and offered no experimental proof. He was passionate, eloquent, and indignant in advocating his treatment. He wrote with fury and conviction and advocated the same treatment for other diseases as well as for yellow fever.[42] He claimed that the mercury he used as a purgative was the "Sampson of Medicine."[43] His critics agreed saying that with his mercury, Rush had killed more Americans than Sampson slew Philistines.

1799
Rush is accused of malpractice for excessive bleeding by journalist Cobbett. Rush sues Cobbett

1799
Death of Washington hastened by excessive bleeding

As additional yellow fever epidemics occurred in the next few years, the controversy and criticism over Rush's treatment increased. He now became unpopular for both political and professional reasons. He considered leaving Philadelphia for a faculty position at Columbia, but Alexander Hamilton, his political enemy, vetoed this. The final straw was an accusation that Rush's treatment was malpractice brought by the journalist William Cobbett whose newspapers, *The Porcupine* and *The Rush Light*, had led the criticism. Rush sued Cobbett for libel.[44]

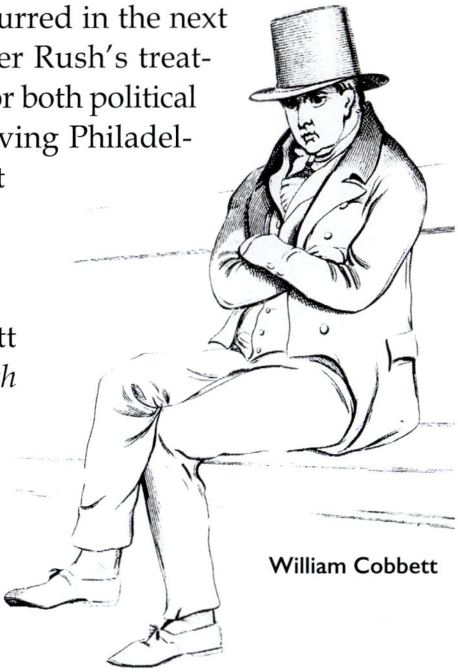
William Cobbett

Ironically, this libel trial and George Washington's final illness occurred simultaneously. The relatively robust sixty-eight-year-old former president of the United States was suffering from acute pharyngitis. He was attended to by two Edinburgh-trained physicians, both of whom were under the strong influence of Rush's reliance on bleeding and purging. Over a period of twenty-four hours, they removed nine pints of blood from Washington before he died.

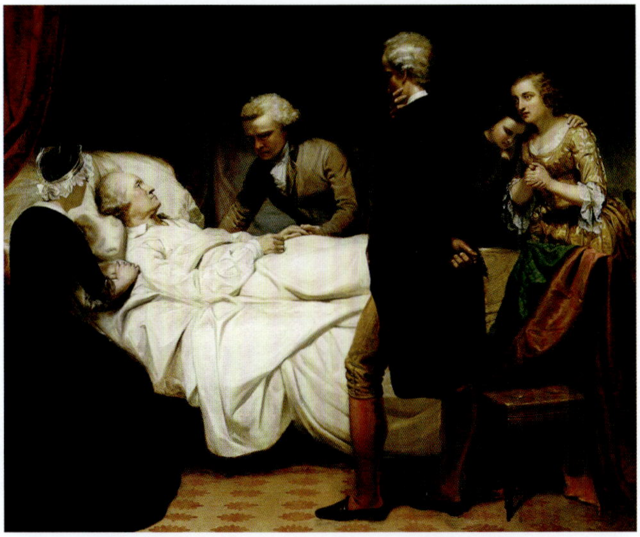
Exsanguination of George Washington (Bled of nine pints in twenty-four hours)

At almost the same time that Washington expired, the verdict of the libel trial was rendered in Rush's favor. He was awarded $5,000.[45] Nevertheless, the news of Washington's death and the details of the treatment by excessive bleeding spoiled this legal triumph and contributed to a growing condemnation by both

1813
Death of
Benjamin Rush

the medical and general community of bloodletting (and of Rush, as its greatest champion). As a result, Rush's practice dwindled to almost nothing. At the end of his life, he was rescued from the resultant financial distress by his appointment as treasurer of the US Mint by his friend, President John Adams.[46]

Today, Rush is remembered almost entirely for his praiseworthy social and humanitarian interests and advocacy. He was a foe of slavery (perhaps in part because he believed that leprosy was the cause of black skin). He was opposed to capital punishment and was an advocate of education of women and of free public schools. He was ahead of his time with the realization that mental disease was an illness, not demonic possession. Thus, he reformed treatment of the mentally ill, replacing cruelty with compassion. He wrote the first American textbook on psychiatry and is considered the father of this specialty. Despite the harm that came to many patients by Rush's stubborn reliance on bloodletting, his overall impact may have been positive. Others have said that with his theories, he sullied the reputation of American medicine for fifty years.

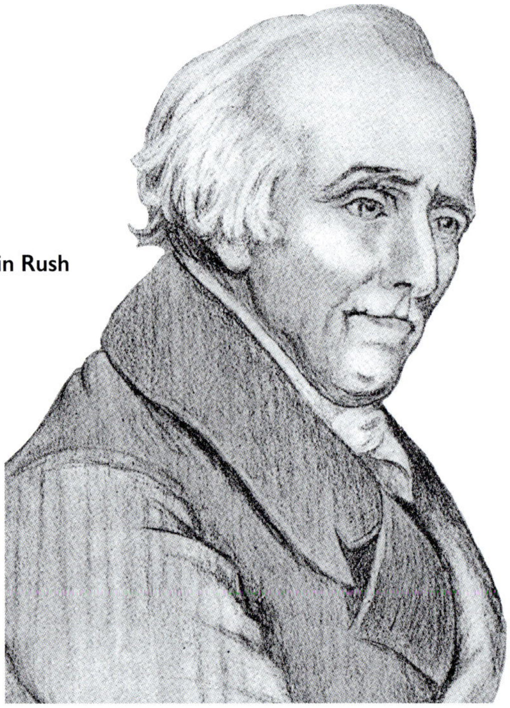

Benjamin Rush

Timeline of Events During the Career of William Shippen

1754	Shippen graduates from Princeton, becomes apprentice with his physician father.
1758–1762	Shippen studies anatomy and surgery in London with the Hunter brothers and midwifery with Colin Mackenzie.
1762	Shippen's MD from Edinburgh. Shippen and Morgan plan to collaborate in starting an American medical school.
1762	Shippen returns to Philadelphia and delivers America's first lectures on anatomy and surgery.
1763	Morgan gets MD from Edinburgh.
1765	Morgan returns to Philadelphia and, avoiding contact with Shippen, presents to the trustees his independent plan for a medical school. The Trustees accept. Shippen and Morgan become lifelong enemies.
1765	Medical school founded (College of Philadelphia). Morgan is appointed chairman of medicine. Shippen is appointed chairman of anatomy, surgery, and midwifery.
1765–1775	Medical school thrives for a decade.
1768	Adam Kuhn appointed chairman of botany and materia medica, thus completing first School of Medicine faculty.
1768	First medical diplomas are awarded by Penn School of Medicine.
1769	Benjamin Rush returns to Philadelphia from education in England and is appointed chairman of chemistry at the medical school; joins Morgan in a feud against William Shippen.
1775	John Jones, a New York surgeon, publishes America's first medical book: *Clean Concise Practical Remarks on the Treatment of Wounds and Fractures.* It is not a comprehensive surgical text. It is a useful handbook for military doctors.
1775–1783	Revolutionary War.
1775	In October, John Morgan appointed surgeon general.
1775–1780	In medical school, no lectures, no diplomas.
Sep 26, 1777–June 17, 1778	The British occupy Philadelphia.
1777	In January, John Morgan is fired as surgeon general.
1777	William Shippen appointed surgeon general on April 11.
1777	John Jones (called "Father of American Surgery" by some) moves to Philadelphia and practices surgery there until his death in 1791.
1778	Benjamin Rush sends letter to Patrick Henry, criticizing George Washington, ending Rush's political prospects.

1779	Pennsylvania legislature revokes the charter of the College of Philadelphia. The faculty and trustees are dismissed. The medical school closes.
1779	In June, Morgan is exonerated by Congress.
1779	A new board of trustees is appointed and a new medical school is formed (the University of the State of Pennsylvania) in November.
1780	Court-martial of William Shippen on March 14.
1780	Benedict Arnold's treason is discovered in September.
1781	Shippen is fired as surgeon general on January 3.
1788	The charter of the College of Philadelphia is restored on September 25.
1789–1791	Two rival medical schools exist in Philadelphia: the College of Philadelphia and the University of the State of Pennsylvania.
1789	Casper Wistar begins a thirty-year career on the faculty of the medical school. He is the first chairman of physiology (Institutes of Medicine).
1789	John Morgan dies.
1790	Benjamin Franklin dies.
1791	The two medical schools are merged and become the medical school of the University of Pennsylvania.
1792	Philip Syng Physick returns to Philadelphia after training in England with John Hunter and obtaining his MD in Edinburgh.
1793	The yellow fever epidemic kills 10 percent of Philadelphians, as Physick and Wistar assist Benjamin Rush in bleeding patients for cure.
1802–1831	Physick's research makes him famous.
1803	Expedition of Lewis and Clark after coaching on medical matters by Benjamin Rush and Caspar Wistar.
1805	Physick succeeds Shippen as chairman of surgery.
1808	Death of William Shippen.

Notes

[1] Corner, George W. *Two Centuries of Medicine: A History of the School of Medicine, University of Pennsylvania* (Philadelphia and Montreal: J.B. Lippincott Company, 1965) p. 6.

[2] Bell, Whitfield J. *Patriot-Improvers: Biographical Sketches of Members of the American Philosophical Society Volume Three 1767–1768* (American Philosophical Society, 2010) pp. 11–15.

[3] Corner, George W. *Two Centuries of Medicine: A History of the School of Medicine, University of Pennsylvania* (Philadelphia: J.B. Lippincott Company, 1965) pp. 6–7.

[4] Bell, Whitfield J. *Patriot-Improvers: Biographical Sketches of Members of the American Philosophical Society Volume Three 1767–1768* (American Philosophical Society, 2010) p.18.

[5] Ibid., p. 19.

[6] Ibid., p. 19.

[7] Corner, George W. *Two Centuries of Medicine: A History of the School of Medicine, University of Pennsylvania* (Philadelphia: J.B. Lippincott Company, 1965) p. 10. Carson, Joseph. *A History of the Medical Department of the University of Pennsylvania with Sketches of the Lives of Deceased Professors* (Philadelphia: Lindsay and Blakiston, 1869) p. 49.

[8] Corner, George W. *Two Centuries of Medicine: A History of the School of Medicine, University of Pennsylvania* (Philadelphia and Montreal: J.B. Lippincott Company, 1965) p. 13.

[9] Bell, Whitfield J. *John Morgan: Continental Doctor.* (University of Pennsylvania Press, 1965) p. 52, http://www.jstor.org/stable/j.ctv4v2xn6.

[10] Corner, George W. *Two Centuries of Medicine: A History of the School of Medicine,* University of Pennsylvania (Philadelphia and Montreal: J.B. Lippincott Company, 1965) p. 10. Bell, Whitfield J. *John Morgan: Continental Doctor*, p. 52.

[11] Corner, George W. *Two Centuries of Medicine: A History of the School of Medicine, University of Pennsylvania* (Philadelphia: J.B. Lippincott Company, 1965) p. 16.

[12] Bell, Whitfield J. *Patriot-Improvers: Biographical Sketches of Members of the American Philosophical Society Volume Three 1767–1768* (American Philosophical Society, 1997) p. 330.

[13] Bell, Whitfield J. *John Morgan: Continental Doctor* (University of Pennsylvania Press, 1965) p. 102.

[14] Ibid., p. 116.

[15] Ibid., p. 117.

[16] Corner, George W. *Two Centuries of Medicine: A History of the School of Medicine, University of Pennsylvania* (Philadelphia and Montreal: J.B. Lippincott Company, 1965) p. 22. Bell, Whitfield J. *Patriot-Improvers: Biographical Sketches of Members of the American Philosophical Society Volume Three 1767–1768* (American Philosophical Society, 1997) p. 331.

[17] Bell, Whitfield J. *John Morgan: Continental Doctor* (University of Pennsylvania Press, 1965) pp. 118–129.

[18] Cooper III, David Y. and Ledger, Marshall A. *Innovation and Tradition at the University of Pennsylvania School of Medicine, An Anecdotal Journey* (Philadelphia: University of Pennsylvania Press, 1990) p. 12.

[19] Bell, Whitfield J. *Patriot-Improvers: Biographical Sketches of Members of the American Philosophical Society Volume Three 1767–1768* (American Philosophical Society, 1997) p. 327.

[20] Ibid., p. 333.

[21] Ibid., p. 333.

[22] Corner, George W. *Two Centuries of Medicine: A History of the School of Medicine, University of Pennsylvania* (Philadelphia: J.B. Lippincott Company, 1965) p. 33. Bell, Whitfield J. *Patriot-Improvers: Biographical Sketches of Members of the American Philosophical Society Volume Three 1767–1768* (American Philosophical Society, 1997) p. 334.

[23] Bell, Whitfield J. *Patriot-Improvers: Biographical Sketches of Members of the American Philosophical Society Volume Three 1767–1768* (American Philosophical Society, 1997) p. 334.

[24] Ibid., p. 334.

[25] Corner, George W. *Two Centuries of Medicine: A History of the School of Medicine, University of Pennsylvania* (Philadelphia: J.B. Lippincott Company, 1965) p. 34. Bell, Whitfield J. *Patriot-Improvers: Biographical Sketches of Members of the American Philosophical Society Volume Three 1767–1768* (American Philosophical Society, 1997) p. 335.

[26] Bell, Whitfield J. *John Morgan: Continental Doctor* (University of Pennsylvania Press, 1965) p. 211.

[27] Bell, Whitfield J. *Patriot-Improvers: Biographical Sketches of Members of the American Philosophical Society Volume Three 1767–1768* (American Philosophical Society, 1997) p. 335.

[28] Ibid., p. 335.

[29] Rush, Benjamin. *The Autobiography of Benjamin Rush; his Travels through Life Together with his Commonplace Book for 1789–1813* (Westport, CT: Greenwood Press, 1970) p. 180.

[30] Bell, Whitfield J. *Patriot-Improvers: Biographical Sketches of Members of the American Philosophical Society Volume Three 1767–1768* (American Philosophical Society, 2010) p. 29.

[31] Ibid., p. 30.

[32] *Extracts from the Journals of Miss Sarah Eve*, p. 25. https://archive.org/stream/jstor-20084486/20084486_djvu.txt.

[33] Fried, Stephen. *Rush: Revolution, Madness, and Benjamin Rush, the Visionary Doctor Who Became a Founding Father* (New York: Crown, 2018) p. 54.

[34] Ibid., p. 60.

[35] Bell, Whitfield J. *Patriot-Improvers: Biographical Sketches of Members of the American Philosophical Society Volume Three 1767–1768* (American Philosophical Society, 1997) p. 454.

[36] Ibid., p. 457.

[37] Fried, Stephen. *Rush: Revolution, Madness, and Benjamin Rush, the Visionary Doctor Who Became a Founding Father* (New York: Crown, 2018) pp. 180–182.

[38] Bell, Whitfield J. *Patriot-Improvers: Biographical Sketches of Members of the American Philosophical Society Volume Three 1767–1768* (American Philosophical Society, 1997) p. 458.

[39] Ibid., p. 458.

[40] Ibid., p. 458.

[41] Ibid., p. 461.

[42] Ibid., p. 461.

[43] North, Robert A. Benjamin Rush, MD assassin or beloved healer? *Baylor University Proceedings* Vol 13 No 1 January 2000, pp. 45–49.

[44] Brodsky, Alyn. *Benjamin Rush, Patriot and Physician* (New York: Truman Talley Books, 2004) pp. 338–343.

[45] Fried, Stephen. *Rush: Revolution, Madness, and Benjamin Rush, the Visionary Doctor Who Became a Founding Father* (New York: Crown, 2018) p. 402.

[46] North, Robert A. Benjamin Rush, MD assassin or beloved healer? *Baylor University Proceedings*, Vol 13 TT, No 1 (January 2000) pp. 45–49.

CHAPTER 2

Interruption of Progress by Revolution and Plague

Caspar Wistar, John Jones, Benjamin Rush, and Yellow Fever

1770s
America's status as a British colony is debated

1775–1783
Revolutionary War

During the forty years of William Shippen's chairmanship, so much was going on in Philadelphia and even in Penn's department of surgery that the story of his life is inadequate even as a framework. An incomplete list of the important events of those decades includes:

1. The founding of America's first medical school. After a decade of success, the school is closed, the faculty dismissed, and a new school is opened. Then the original one reopens. Eventually the two rival schools are merged.
2. The War for American Independence, America's early losing battles, the British occupation of Philadelphia, treason committed by one of our best generals, and eventual victory.
3. The careers of three giants of American medicine, all probably greater than Shippen but now largely forgotten at Penn.
4. A plague more vicious than COVID-19 killed 10 percent of Philadelphians and drove half of the survivors from the city. Some say Philadelphia has never fully recovered.

The start of Penn's medical school and the bitter rivalry of its founders are reviewed in Chapter 1. Despite the poisoning of the school's atmosphere by the enmity between Morgan and Shippen, the first decade of the school was quite successful. Scores of young Philadelphians, eager to enhance their status with a degree in medicine, flocked to enroll in the new school. The school's young faculty were equally eager to participate.

Then revolution and war intervened. Even before the shooting began, there was bad blood between the wealthy, liberally inclined members of the school's faculty and the conservative citizens in other parts of the state. Many of the school's professors were suspected of being British sympathizers, including Provost William Smith, an admitted loyalist who actively opposed the revolution.[1] Indeed, many Philadelphians were quite satisfied with the relationship with England and would have been happy with only minor changes in governance to remain as colonists. For a long time, this included members of the school's faculty and even Benjamin Franklin.

While the British occupied Philadelphia in 1777–1778, Penn medicine's founder, the much-admired John Morgan, was observed to be on friendly terms with the British officers. William Shippen's cousin, Peggy, was married to the military commander of Philadelphia, Benedict Arnold. It was rumored that she was the mistress of British spy, John Andre, and the inspiration for the betrayal and desertion of her husband to the English side.

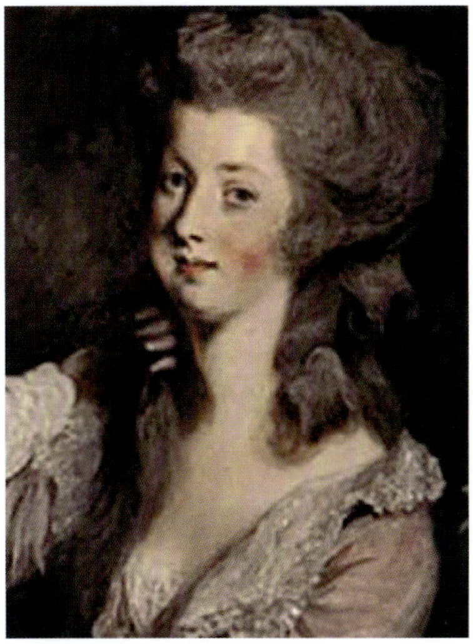
Peggy Shippen

1777–1778
British occupation of Philadelphia. Legendary accounts blame Peggy Shippen for Benedict Arnold's treason

1779–1791
America's first medical school is closed, a new one replaces it, and finally the two schools merge

The state legislature was comprised mainly of noncollege educated individuals more strongly committed to the revolutionary cause than to the academic mission of the College of Philadelphia or its medical department. In June 1779, the legislature revoked the charter of the College of Philadelphia and its School of Medicine. This resulted in the entire faculty of the school and its trustees being dismissed. In short, the medical school and the college were closed. Some of the activities of the medical school's faculty and classwork were not completely interrupted, but commencements and the awarding of diplomas ceased. In November 1779, a new board of trustees was appointed by the legislature and teaching restarted under the auspices of an institution now called the University of the State of Pennsylvania. The new school was largely funded by money from confiscation of the estates of the loyalists. Of the faculty of the original school, the College of Philadelphia, only William Shippen joined the faculty of the new school at first. Morgan and Rush declined appointments, saying they would join no faculty of which William Shippen was a member. Rush later recanted and joined the new faculty, but Morgan never did.

By 1788, the war had been over for five years, and much of the bitterness surrounding the revolution had dissipated. The charter of the College of Philadelphia was restored and its trustees and faculty rehired. The result was a curious situation. From 1789 to 1791, two rival medical schools competed, the College of Philadelphia and the University of the State of Pennsylvania.[2] Shippen was professor of anatomy, surgery, and midwifery in both, but most of the other departments of the two schools had separate faculties. Philadelphia didn't need two medical schools and lacked sufficient medical educators to staff them. Therefore in 1791, the logical outcome prevailed, and the two schools merged to form the University of Pennsylvania.

1777
Battle of Germantown. Wistar serves as nurse, is inspired to study medicine

1779
College of Philadelphia's medical school is closed and replaced by the medical school of the State of Pennsylvania

1786
After three years of study in Europe, Wistar gets MD from University of Edinburgh

1788
Wistar appointed chairman of chemistry

Caspar Wistar (1761–1818)

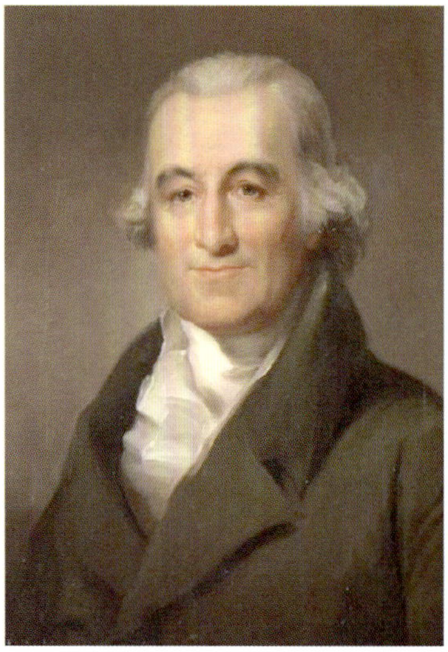

Caspar Wistar

Caspar Wistar is listed in the history of Philadelphia as one of the city's most important citizens, physicians, and paleontologists. Yet, though he was an important member of the Penn surgical faculty for seventeen years, he does not appear in the department's annals. This is an unfortunate oversight. Perhaps because he was more comfortable with medical practice than operative surgery, Wistar was not widely known as a surgeon, but he had extensive training and experience in surgery.

Born a Quaker in 1761 and educated in Philadelphia's Friends schools, his religion prevented him from enlisting as a soldier during the war for American independence. But at age sixteen, he volunteered as a nurse in 1777 at the Battle of Germantown. His experiences in caring for drastically ill or wounded patients inspired him to pursue a career in medicine.[3] At age eighteen, he commenced his medical studies under the physician John Redman. For a year, he was also the student of John Jones, a surgeon who was considered by some of his contemporaries to be the father of American surgery; by others as simply the world's best surgeon. In 1779, Wistar enrolled as a student in the medical department of the College of Philadelphia, which a few months later was closed and replaced by the University of the State of Pennsylvania, from which he received his bachelor of medicine degree in 1782. He then spent three years of study in England and Scotland. Before he was allowed to depart for this European tour, he had to secure a certificate testifying to his adherence to conduct as a Quaker. He had some difficulty with this since he had succumbed to the "scandalous and alarming temptation" of fighting in a duel.[4] While a student in Edinburgh, he was elected president of the Royal Medical Society and also president of the Society for Investigation of Natural History. His mentors in England included William Hunter and the best-known surgeons of the time, John Hunter and Percival Pott. In 1786, he obtained his MD from the University of Edinburgh.

Returning to Philadelphia, Wistar established a private practice that grew into one of the largest in the city. He was elected to the College of Physicians and served as a physician to the Philadelphia Dispensary. In 1788, he was appointed professor and chairman of chemistry in the medical school. After the merger of the College of Philadelphia with the University of the State of Pennsylvania to form the University of Pennsylvania in 1791, Wistar became adjunct professor of anatomy, surgery, and midwifery. In this role, he was the assistant of William Shippen for the next seventeen years until Shippen died. As Shippen aged, Wistar gave many of the surgery and anatomy lectures to the Penn medical students. In 1793, he joined the staff of Pennsylvania Hospital. There he again came under the influence of the famous surgeon, John Jones, who mentored him by standing with him at the operating table to help mature his surgical skills.[5] In spite of this, Wistar's pupil Charles Caldwell considered Wistar indecisive as a surgeon, writing that, "no sooner did he engage in an important operation . . . his hand became unsteady, and his mind at times perceptibly discomposed . . . did any unexpected event occur, even an unlooked-for jet of blood from an artery, the expedient, best calculated to remedy the evil seldom if ever, presented itself with promptness."[6] Thus it seems that the study of paleontology probably better suited Wistar's temperament than surgery.

1791
Philadelphia's two medical schools merge. Wistar is appointed adjunct professor of anatomy, surgery, and midwifery, serving for seventeen years in this role as Shippen's assistant

1793
Philadelphia is hit by the worst of a series of yellow fever epidemics. Wistar helps Benjamin Rush bleed patients and contracts the disease himself

1808–1818
Wistar is Chairman of Anatomy

In 1793, a terrible yellow fever epidemic hit Philadelphia. Wistar was one of a small number of doctors who did not flee the city, even though he believed the disease was contagious. Wistar contracted the disease as he accompanied his friend Benjamin Rush to evaluate bleeding as his method of treating infected patients. Wistar soon disagreed with Rush about the benefits of extensive bleeding and purging, and started advising milder treatments. Rush viewed this as a betrayal and was furious.[7] Wistar and Rush both wrote nasty pieces in the newspaper about their disagreement. Of course, neither of them knew what caused the disease.

In 1808, after William Shippen died, Wistar was appointed to the chair of anatomy at the medical school, an appointment which he retained until his death in 1818. Wistar was a popular teacher who enlivened his lectures with drawings and models that allowed the students to follow his demonstrations even from the back row of his large audience. Some of his teaching aids were life-sized anatomical models of dried or wax-injected human limbs and organs. Others were larger-than-life models, fashioned out of wood, carved by America's famous sculptor William Rush. Before his death, Wistar appointed William Horner, his assistant in anatomy, as a caretaker of these models. Horner enlarged the collection, and it was eventually donated to become the anatomical collection of the Wistar Institute, which was named after Caspar Wistar.[8]

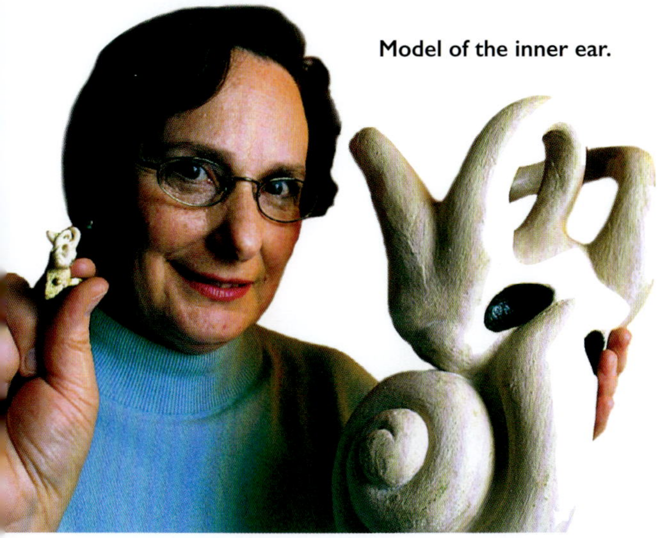

Model of the inner ear.

Wistar wrote the first textbook on anatomy to be published in the United States, titled

1811 and 1814
Caspar Wistar publishes *A System of Anatomy* for the use of students of medicine. This is the first anatomy textbook published in America

1815–1818
Wistar is President of American Philosophical Society

A System of Anatomy, in two volumes, in 1811 and 1814. It eventually went through nine editions. He was also well known for his breadth of knowledge in the humanities. He published a paper on what may have been the first dinosaur bones discovered in the United States. Another article was on the bones of the giant megalonyx that his close friend Thomas Jefferson had deposited with the American Philosophical Society. Jefferson thought it was a giant carnivore, such as a lion, a species he thought might still be living in the American West. Wistar correctly identified it as a less-exciting giant sloth. The Lewis and Clark expedition dispelled the possibility that either species had escaped extinction.[9] Wistar also collaborated in Jefferson's efforts to obtain the bones of a mastodon, and he studied many other specimens returned from the West by Lewis and Clark.

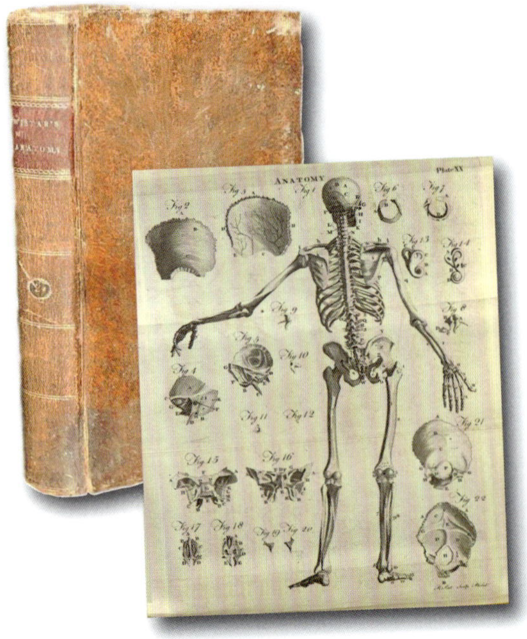

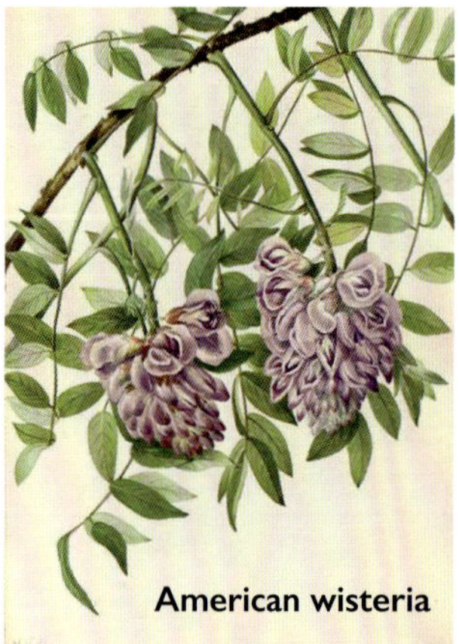
American wisteria

Wistar was very active in the American Philosophical Society and succeeded Thomas Jefferson as the president of the society. He was perhaps even better known at the time for his hospitality. At his home, he held weekly meetings of students, scientists, and often distinguished foreign visitors. These "Wistar parties" became so popular that after Wistar's death, they were continued by his friends for many decades.[10] Wistar lent his support to many progressive causes. He was a founder of the Society for Circulating the Benefit of Vaccination, and he belonged to the Humane Society and the Society for the Abolition of Slavery, of which he became the president in 1813. The plant genus *Wisteria* was named for him by botanist Thomas Nuttall.

John Jones (1729–1791)

John Jones was one of early America's greatest surgeons, perhaps the greatest.[11] Rush rated him as "without a rival in Surgery in the United States."[12] Although Jones was never a member of the Penn faculty, he deserves a prominent place in our department's annals. He was born and grew up in New York, but a significant part of his education and later years took place in Philadelphia. At Pennsylvania Hospital, he was an important surgical mentor of our surgery department's Caspar Wistar and a teacher of Penn medical students. Arguably valid is the claim made by many that Jones should be deemed the father of American surgery instead of Philadelphia's Philip Syng Physick. Support for this assertion was that Jones was appointed as the first professor of surgery at King's College when it opened in 1767. This was two years after William Shippen's first appointment at Penn, but Shippen's appointment was as a combined professor of anatomy, surgery, and midwifery. It was forty-one years before Penn appointed Philip Syng Physick as its first professor of surgery (surgery alone, without including anatomy and midwifery). Putting aside the somewhat unimportant arguments over timing and nomenclature, Physick and Jones were unquestionably both great surgeons.

1729
Birth of John Jones

1737–1740
In Philadelphia Jones is apprenticed to his cousin, Thomas Cadwalader

1751
Jones receives MD from University of Rheims

1767
Jones is cofounder of America's second medical school to open, King's College (Columbia). He is appointed professor of surgery

John Jones was born in 1729 in Long Island where his grandfather, a Welsh immigrant, and his father both practiced medicine. His early education was in private schools of New York, but he then spent three years in Philadelphia studying medicine as an apprentice to his cousin Thomas Cadwalader. Cadwalader, a Quaker, was himself a former apprentice of John Jones's father. John Jones later wrote that both in physic and morals, he "received the earliest and best lessons of my life from Dr. Cadwalader."[13]

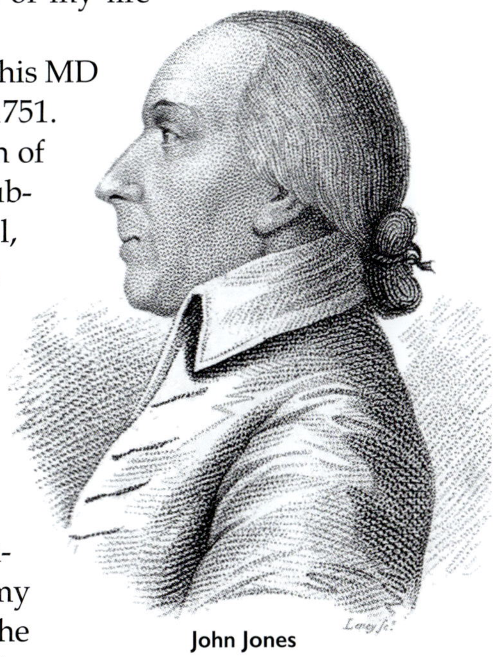
John Jones

Jones went to France where he obtained his MD degree from the University of Rheims in 1751. He later expanded his thesis on observation of wounds to become the first medical book published in America.[14] After medical school, Jones extended his medical education by a whirlwind tour of the major medical institutions of Europe. In Rouen, he learned about lithotomy from the famous Claude Nicholas Le Cat. At the Hotel-Dieu in Paris, he met Jean Lewis Petit and Henri Francoise. In Leyden, he visited Boerhaave's successor Siegfried Albinus. In London, he attended William Hunter's anatomy school, and at St. Bartholomew's Hospital, he developed a close friendship with one of the most accomplished surgeons of the time, Percival Pott, with whom he maintained a lifelong correspondence.

Returning to New York and applying what he had learned from Europe's famous lithotomist, Le Cat, he became the first American to perform this operation. Technically gifted, Jones could do this procedure in slightly more than a minute.

In 1755, he interrupted his surgical practice by volunteering for the New York Militia, which during the French and Indian War was sent

1775
Jones publishes America's first medical book

1776
British capture New York City. Jones enlists in Continental Army

1777–1791
Jones moves to Philadelphia and practices there until his death

north to protect Fort Edward. The French commander, Baron Dieskau, was wounded, and as a result of Jones's burgeoning reputation, the baron requested that Jones care for him.[15] This further enhanced Jones's reputation as one of the preeminent surgeons of the time.

Returning to New York in 1767, Jones joined with the New York physician, John Bard, to found America's second medical school at King's College (now Columbia). He was appointed professor and chair of surgery, thus becoming the first to hold this title in an American university.[16] In his inaugural lecture, he outlined his vision for the American surgeon. His strongly held view was that a surgeon must be first a physician and then something more. This was at variance with the European paradigm of surgeons as limited to a role as technicians.

In 1771, New York Hospital was chartered, and Jones went to Europe to raise funds for it. He renewed his acquaintance with Percival Pott and studied hospital design. Returning to New York, he played an important role in the design of the hospital, making sure there was adequate ventilation and sufficient space to avoid crowding of patients.

In 1775, shortly before the Revolutionary War began, Jones published a book titled, *Plain Concise Practical Remarks on the Treatment of Wounds and Fractures.* It included a badly needed section on hygiene and sanitation. Dedicated to his teacher, Thomas Cadwalader, it was the first medical book published in America. Rather than a comprehensive surgery textbook, it was more of a handbook, specifically intended for use by military surgeons in the coming war and found very useful for that purpose.[17]

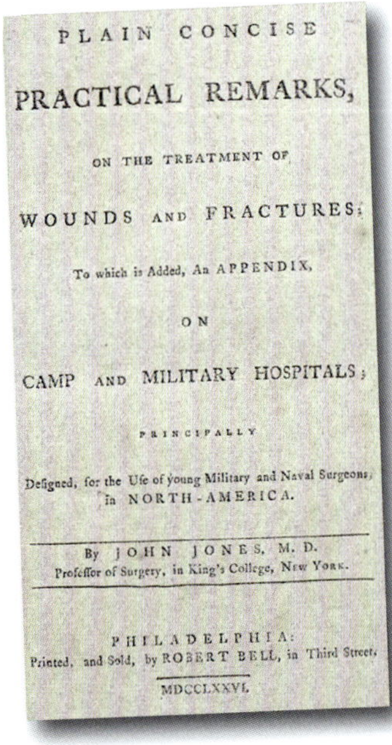
PLAIN CONCISE
PRACTICAL REMARKS,
ON THE TREATMENT OF
WOUNDS AND FRACTURES;
To which is Added, An APPENDIX,
ON
CAMP AND MILITARY HOSPITALS;
PRINCIPALLY
Defigned, for the Ufe of young Military and Naval Surgeons, in NORTH-AMERICA.
By JOHN JONES, M. D.
Profeffor of Surgery, in King's College, New York.
PHILADELPHIA:
Printed, and Sold, by ROBERT BELL, in Third Street,
MDCCLXXVI.

Jones was not a rabid revolutionist. For him, the separation from England was difficult since he had extensive ties with colleagues there. He condemned those extremists who boycotted Americans who did not promise to sign an oath to execute every action of the Continental Congress. However, he was a Whig and wished actively for American independence. Yet, like many colonists, he could have been satisfied with reconciliation and peace with England under appropriate conditions. But when New York City was captured by English troops in 1776, Jones had to take sides. Virtually all of the King's College medical faculty members were Tories and remained in New York. But Jones immediately left for Albany to enlist in the Continental Army as assistant surgeon and was soon promoted to surgeon of the 10th Massachusetts Regiment.[18] He was also active in revolutionary politics and was a member of the first session of the New York Senate.

In 1777, due to poor health and worsening of his chronic asthma condition, he was forced to leave Albany. He came to the recently liberated city of Philadelphia where he practiced for the remaining fourteen years of his life. He continued in the service of the Continental Army until 1781, when he resigned his commission and devoted himself to the practice of medicine in Philadelphia.[19] Because of his international reputation and his likable demeanor, he was immediately successful in his practice and popular with his colleagues.[20] He was invited to join the staff of the Philadelphia dispensary, Pennsylvania Hospital, and was elected vice president of the College of Physicians of Philadelphia.

1791
In caring for George Washington, Jones contracts infection and dies

Due to his fame and service to the country, Jones soon acquired prominent patients, notably Benjamin Franklin and George Washington. Jones was the physician who was called to attend Franklin during his final illness. Franklin's will specified that twenty guineas was to be "given to John Jones, his good friend and physician." In 1790, President George Washington contracted pneumonia and was attended by Jones. A year later, while Jones was again attending Washington for pneumonia, he contracted his own fatal infection. He died in 1791 at age sixty-one and was buried in the Arch Street Cemetery. All traces of this cemetery were erased during the yellow fever epidemic of 1793 when the cemetery was used for mass burials.

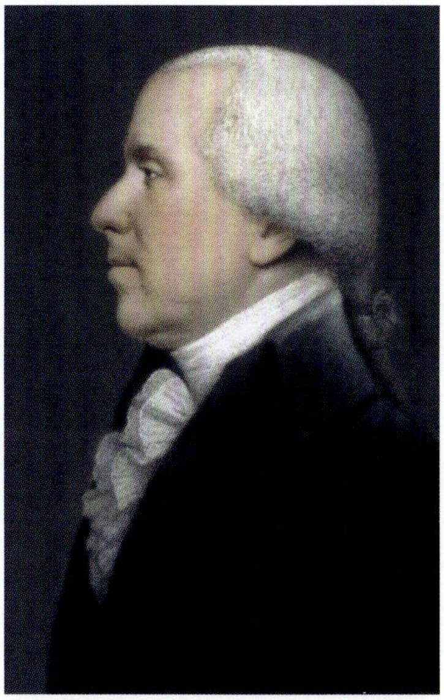
Benjamin Rush by Ellen Sharples

Benjamin Rush and Yellow Fever

Before the yellow fever epidemic in the spring of 1793, Philadelphia was the place to be. It was the center of the new country's postwar euphoria. The city was at the peak of its prestige. It was the new nation's capital. It was the largest and wealthiest city, the center of commerce, science, medicine, learning, and culture. It was positioned to be America's great city, its London, its Paris. And yet the city was dirty, there was no public sewage disposal or water supply, and dead animals were left to decay in the streets. An imported shipload of spoiled coffee had been left to rot on the wharf. No matter, the young people gathered in the streets to talk, drink, and otherwise carry on, provoking the city's Quaker elders to warn that the revelry, drinking, and dissipation were signs of moral decay.[21] They asked, was the city overconfident? Were things too good? Was retribution inevitable?

For the patriot Benjamin Rush, success of the revolution and separation from Britain were impossible dreams come true. And he saw winning the revolution as only the beginning. To him, it was a moral as

1793 (July)
Philadelphia is the nation's largest city, its cultural and economic center, and capital

1793 (August)
Suddenly citizens begin to sicken and die by the hundreds.

Benjamin Rush is convinced that yellow fever can be cured by bleeding and purging

1793 (September)
Philadelphia becomes a ghost town. Washington and Jefferson flee, the government collapses

well as a physical triumph. Winning independence indicated that America could do anything, that it could even overturn and overcome nature. He believed the new government and its people had proven themselves superior to Europe's. Americans must be fundamentally different, he thought, better and tougher. Even the diseases were different in America, and new treatments and cures would surely come about. Rush's practice was thriving. He was rich and famous. His lectures had made him the darling of the medical students. Everything was just great.

And then suddenly, overnight, the revelry ceased. As though by divine decree, citizens began to sicken and die, to collapse, vomit, bleed, and die like flies by the hundreds. For the next hundred days, the city was gripped by panic, terrorized by a mysterious, relentless, overwhelming plague.[22] It began with a mild headache and aching muscles. Nausea progressed rapidly to vomiting of blood. Hundreds of tiny hemorrhages appeared all over the body. The eyes and skin soon turned yellow and in a few hours or days, whatever the treatment, death usually followed. Dr. Rush identified it as yellow fever. The name itself deepened the panic. His diagnosis was disputed at first by other doctors and by merchants who feared the financial consequences of an epidemic.

For 100 years, no one would know what caused it. Rush believed it came from a miasma, evil air rising from a load of coffee overturned, abandoned, and left to rot on the dock. Others argued that the origin was not local, that it must have been brought by ships coming from the West Indies. Caspar Wistar accumulated evidence that it was contagious. Physicians of Philadelphia, the nation's finest, gathered at their prestigious College of Physicians to discuss the cause and craft a response. But they went away without an answer. Their best advice to the city's citizens was to flee. About 17,000, or one-third to one-half of the city's population of 40,000 citizens, followed this advice, somehow finding ways out, despite quarantines and roadblocks set up by surrounding cities and states to keep them out and prevent the spread of the disease.

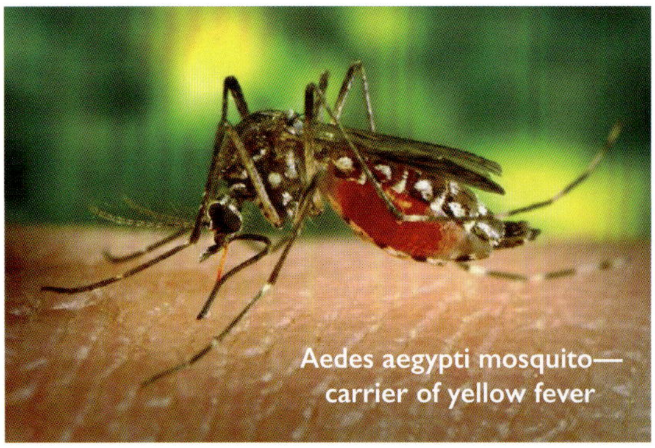
Aedes aegypti mosquito—carrier of yellow fever

Most people thought the disease contagious and kept to themselves. To hold off the mysterious plague, they started fires, burned gunpowder, and shot at it with their muskets.[23] But nothing helped. Parents deserted their sick children, and children abandoned their dying parents. Philadelphia became a ghost town, empty except for those rioting and looting or carrying out the mass burials of hundreds of victims daily. Soon the government of the nation's capital collapsed. President Washington and Vice President Jefferson left

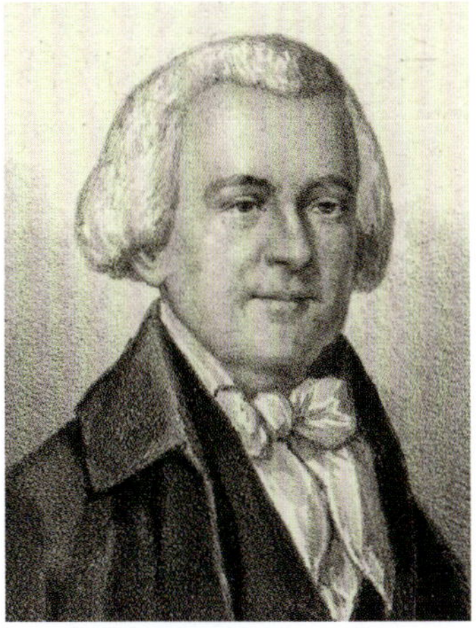

Mayor Matthew Clarkson

town. The mayor and a group of courageous citizens formed a committee to take charge, meeting daily to see what they might do to help the ill and dying.[24] Four thousand Philadelphians, one-tenth of the city's population, would die before it was over. It was probably the worst disaster ever faced by an American city. Some say Philadelphia has never recovered from it.

But then Dr. Rush stepped in. Some, including Dr. Rush himself, said he was able to save the city. Others say he only made it worse. Many doctors left town. Ten of them died, including three of Dr. Rush's five apprentices. But Rush refused to leave. Sleepless, hardly stopping to eat, he visited 100 patients a day, but he had no answer at first. He was on the point of giving up, but then Dr. Rush remembered something, a paper Benjamin Franklin had given him that was submitted to the American Philosophical Society fifty years before by a Virginia physician, John Mitchell. It described the successful treatment of six yellow fever victims in a 1744 epidemic in Virginia. Mitchell claimed that he had employed heavy purging and bleeding with success. He specified that this treatment should be employed, even in patients who were greatly weakened by their fever or by earlier bleedings. Rush tried it. It seemed to work.[25] His confidence in himself returned at once, and this was reflected in his relationship to patients and even in his posture and gait. It seemed to him that this was an epiphany sent by God for him to save his city. He wrote to his wife that he was overjoyed to find the answer.[26] He now redoubled his efforts. Two of the young Penn doctors helping him were Caspar Wistar and Philip Syng Physick. He continued to see hundreds of patients a day, purging them with huge doses of mercury-based laxatives, bleeding most of them, sometimes multiple times, and removing as much as a fifth of their blood volume. He claimed 90 percent success in patients he treated this way. Later, he said he had saved 6,000 Philadelphians from death. Some doctors were impressed with Rush's

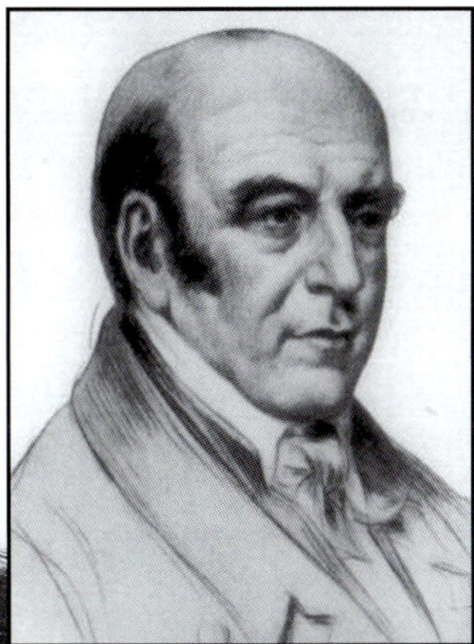

Stephen Girard

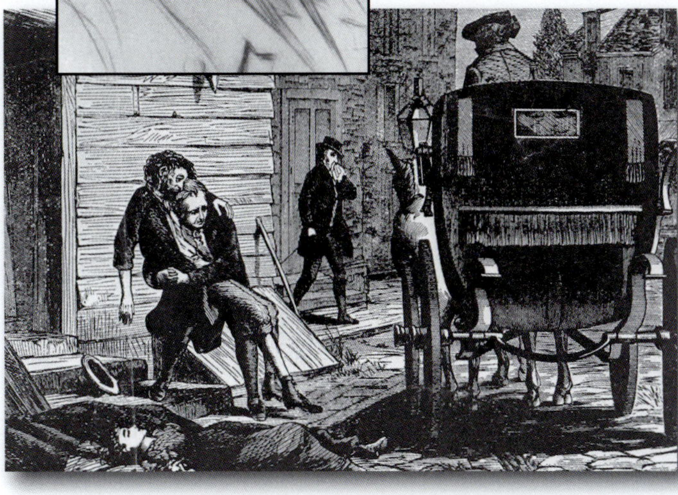

Stephen Girard takes a man infected with yellow fever to his Bush Hill hospital in his personal carriage.

1793 (October)
Mayor Clarkson forms a committee and takes charge

Rush is convinced he is saving the city. Other doctors are not convinced

Stephen Girard, Philadelphia's wealthiest citizen, helps during the yellow fever epidemic by transporting victims to his Bush Hill hospital

Most doctors dispute Rush's treatment

African-Americans are said to be immune but are not. Richard Allen and Absalom Jones of the Free African Society are heroes in volunteering care of victims

1793 (November)
With the first frost the plague is over after killing 10 percent of Philadelphians. Some say the city has never recovered

treatment and followed his advice. Most were not, and they criticized him severely.[27] Rush kept no records and could defend his treatment only by rhetoric. This dispute with members of the College of Physicians caused Rush, a founder of the college, to resign his membership.[28] If a patient thought he or she was too weak to be bled more and refused Rush's further treatment, he became angry and abandoned the patient. Thomas Jefferson and Alexander Hamilton avoided Rush's treatment and survived. Other doctors employed milder treatment, such as exposure to cold temperatures and Peruvian bark that contained quinine. Jefferson attempted to compare the results of Rush with those of others. He reported that 46 percent of Rush's patients died compared to only 33 percent of those treated without bleeding and purging by "non-mercurial" doctors. With the first frost, mosquito season ended. The hundred days of the 1793 epidemic were over. Some say Philadelphia has never recovered from it. But in the eyes of many, it had made Rush a hero. To others, he had become a killer. More than any of his many accomplishments, his lasting fame depends on his performance during this tragic period.

For forty years, Rush was the most popular teacher at the medical school, lecturing to at least 3,000 students over the years on his theory that yellow fever, in fact all fevers, had the same cause and therefore the same treatment—bloodletting. Rush believed this "American theory of disease" was the key to all subsequent advances in medicine and would ensure his eternal fame.[29] Instead, this widely circulated view sullied the reputation of American medicine for fifty years.

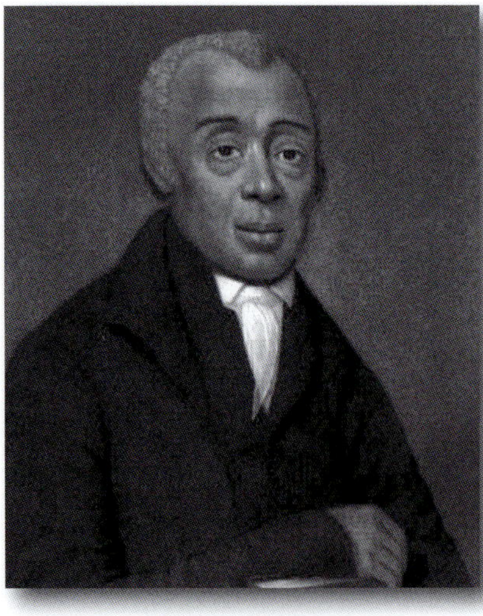

Richard Allen

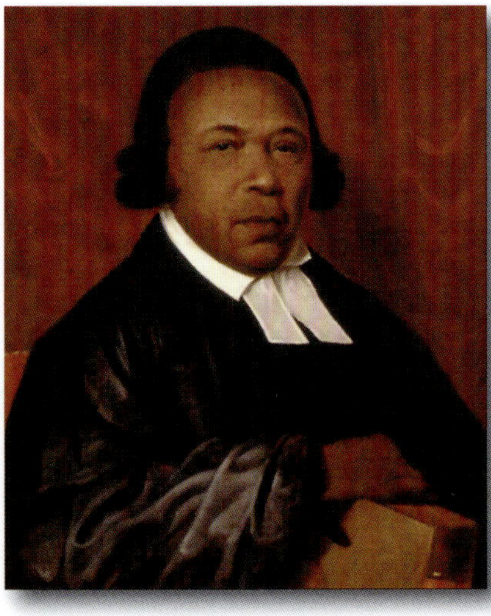

Absalom Jones

Timeline of Events—Caspar Wistar, John Jones, And Benjamin Rush

1729 Birth of John Jones.

1745 Birth of Benjamin Rush.

1751 John Jones obtains MD from University of Rheims and embarks on extended tour of European medical centers.

1756–1763 French and Indian War

- John Morgan serves as surgeon on the Western frontier.
- John Jones treats French commander Baron Dieskau for gunshot wounds of bladder.

1761 Caspar Wistar is born.

1762 William Shippen obtains MD, returns to Philadelphia, and gives America's first medical lectures on anatomy, surgery, and midwifery.

1765 Medical school of the College of Philadelphia is founded. Morgan and Shippen are appointed to professorships in medicine and in anatomy, surgery, and midwifery. A lifelong feud between Morgan and Shippen begins.

1767 John Jones returns to New York and with John Bard founds America's second medical school, King's College (later Columbia) Medical School. Jones is appointed America's first professor of surgery.

1771 New York Hospital is chartered. Jones travels to Europe to raise funds for the hospital.

1775 John Jones publishes America's first medical book, *Practical Remarks on the Treatment of Wounds.*

1776 Declaration of Independence is signed.

1776 New York is captured by the British.

1776 John Jones travels to Albany and enlists in the Continental Army as assistant surgeon.

1776 Battle of Trenton on December 26. Rush helps Washington with his plan to surprise the British by crossing the Delaware River.

1777 At the Battle of Germantown, sixteen-year-old Caspar Wistar, a Quaker, serves as a nurse and is inspired to study medicine.

1777 Battle of Princeton (January). Rush brings the militia to bolster Washington's outnumbered forces.

1777 John Jones's asthma is worsened by the cold climate of Albany, and he decides to leave.

1777–1778	British occupation of Philadelphia. American military commander, Benedict Arnold, meets and begins to conspire with British spymaster, John Andre, to turn over the American fort at West Point to the British. William Shippen's cousin, Peggy, aids them.
1779	Peggy Shippen marries Benedict Arnold, remains in contact with Andre, and aids them in the treasonous plot.
1779	The West Point plot is discovered. Andre is hanged, but Arnold escapes.
1779	The charter of the College of Philadelphia and its medical school is revoked by the state legislature. The school closes and is replaced by the University of the State of Pennsylvania.
1779	Jones relocates to Philadelphia, resigns from the Army, and develops a successful practice.
1780	John Jones is appointed to the staff of Pennsylvania Hospital. There he is a popular teacher of Penn students.
1786	Wistar gets MD from Edinburgh, returns to Philadelphia, and quickly builds large practice.
1788	Wistar appointed chairman of chemistry.
1789	Restoration of charter of College of Philadelphia. Its medical school reopens.
1789–1791	Two Philadelphia medical schools compete.
1792	The two schools are merged to form the University of Pennsylvania.
1790	John Jones is the personal physician of George Washington and Benjamin Franklin. In treating Washington for pneumonia, Jones becomes infected and dies in 1791.
1791	Wistar is appointed adjunct professor of anatomy, surgery, and midwifery. For seventeen years he serves as Shippen's assistant and gives many of his lectures.
1793	The yellow fever epidemic kills 10 percent of Philadelphians. Caspar Wistar and Phillip Syng Physick assist Rush in his treatment of patients by bleeding and purging. Wistar eventually disapproves of Rush's treatment. Washington and Jefferson abandon Philadelphia, and the government collapses.
1800	Wistar publishes finding of megalonyx, a prehistoric giant sloth, one of his multiple paleontological studies. He enlists aid of his assistant, William Horner, in collecting many specimens, eventually forming the museum of the Wistar Institute. Rush lectures to more than 3,000 medical students over forty years. His American theory of disease (only one fever, only one disease, only one treatment) tarnishes the name of United States medicine for half a century.
1808	Shippen dies. Wistar is appointed chairman of anatomy, Physick of surgery, and Thomas Chalkley James of midwifery.

1811, 1814 Wistar publishes first American textbook of anatomy, *A System of Anatomy*.

1813 Rush dies.

1818 Wistar dies.

Notes

[1] Corner, George W. *Two Centuries of Medicine: A History of the School of Medicine, University of Pennsylvania* (Philadelphia: J.B. Lippincott Company, 1965) pp. 34–35.

[2] Ibid., p. 38.

[3] American Philosophical Society Library Staff. Caspar Wistar Memoir in Biographical Memoirs of Members of the American Philosophical Society, *Physicians Vol I, 1787–1935,* edited by Barker and Starzl (Philadelphia: American Philosophical Society, 2013) p. 1.

[4] Ibid., p. 1.

[5] Ibid., p. 1.

[6] *The Art of Philadelphia Medicine,* The Philadelphia Museum of Art, 1965, p. 42.

[7] American Philosophical Society Library Staff. Caspar Wistar Memoir in Biographical Memoirs of Members of the American Philosophical Society, *Physicians Vol I, 1787–1935,* edited by Barker and Starzl (Philadelphia: American Philosophical Society, 2013) p. 1.

[8] Ibid., p. 2.

[9] Ibid., p. 2.

[10] Ibid., p. 3.

[11] Schwartz, Seymour. *Gifted Hands – America's Most Significant Contributions to Surgery* (Amherst, New York: Prometheus Books, 2009) p. 20. According to Sy Schwartz, Jones was "unquestionably the greatest surgeon of the day." He anticipated the credo of modern academic surgery – to be a doctor and something more, not something less.

[12] Rush, Benjamin. *The Autobiography of Benjamin Rush: his Travels through Life Together with His Commonplace Book for 1789–1813* (Westport, Conn: Greenwood Press, 1970) p. 201.

[13] Griesemer AD, Widmann WD, Forde KA, Hardy MA. "John Jones, MD: pioneer, patriot, and founder of American surgery." *World J Surg* (Apr. 2010) 34(4):605–609. p. 606.

[14] Ibid., p. 606.

[15] Schwartz, Seymour. *Gifted Hands – America's Most Significant Contributions to Surgery*, p. 20.

[16] Griesemer AD, Widmann WD, Forde KA, Hardy MA. "John Jones, MD: pioneer, patriot, and founder of American surgery." *World J Surg* (2010) 34(4):605-609. doi:10.1007/s00268-009-0323-9.

[17] Ibid., p. 608.

[18] Ibid., p. 609.

[19] Ibid., p. 609.

[20] Henry, Frederick Porteous. *Standard History of the Medical Profession of Philadelphia* (Chicago: Goodspeed Brothers Publishers, 1897) p. 144.

[21] Kornfeld E. Crisis in the capital: the cultural significance of Philadelphia's great yellow fever epidemic. *Pa Hist* (1984) 51(3):189–205. pp. 193–194.

[22] Henry, Frederick Porteous. *Standard History of the Medical Profession of Philadelphia* (Chicago: Goodspeed Brothers Publishers, 1897) pp. 110–113.

[23] Brodsky, Alyn. *Benjamin Rush, Patriot and Physician* (New York: Truman Talley Books, 2004) p. 326.

[24] Kornfeld E. Crisis in the capital: the cultural significance of Philadelphia's great yellow fever epidemic. p. 198.

[25] North, Robert A. Benjamin Rush, MD assassin or beloved healer? *Baylor University Proceedings,* Vol 13, No 1 (January 2000) p. 7.

[26] Henry, Frederick Porteous. *Standard History of the Medical Profession of Philadelphia,* p. 114.

[27] North, Robert A. *Benjamin Rush, MD assassin or beloved healer?* p. 8.

[28] Ibid., p. 8

[29] D'Elle, Donald. Dr. Benjamin Rush and the American Medical Revolution. *Proceedings of the American Philosophical Society,* Vol 110, No. 4 (Aug. 1966). pp. 228–229.

CHAPTER 3

The Unloved Father of American Surgery

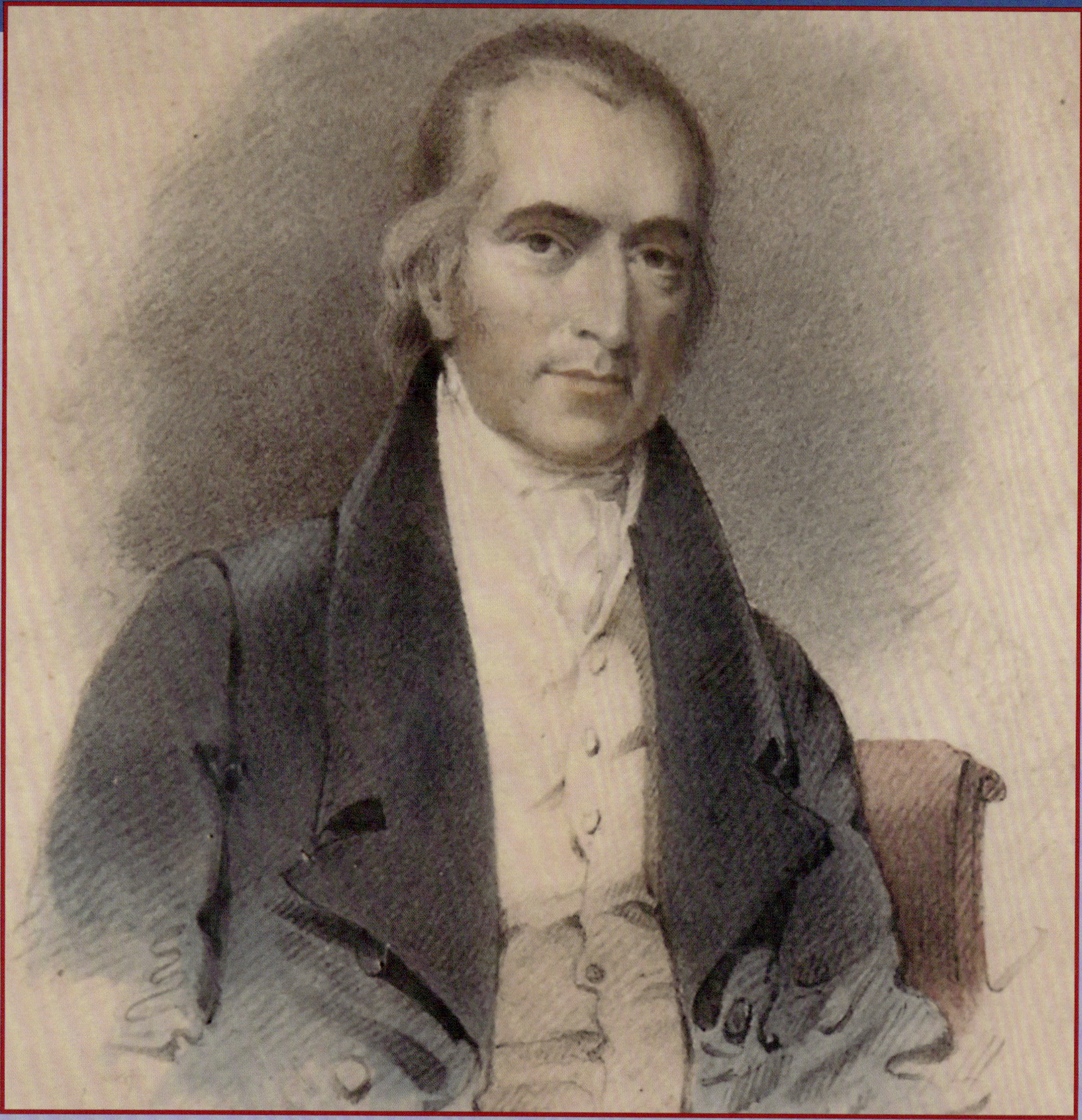

Philip Syng Physick

Philip Syng Physick (1768–1837)

Chairman of Surgery (1805–1819)
Professor of Anatomy (1819–1831)

John Syng Dorsey

His Beloved Nephew, Scribe, and Poet

Professor of Materia Medica (1816–1818)
Professor of Anatomy (1818)

Philip Syng Physick was born in Philadelphia in 1768. He was the grandson of the famous silversmith, Philip Syng, who designed the inkwell used by our founders in signing the Declaration of Independence. As a youth, Philip Physick aspired to being a silversmith like his grandfather. However, his father wanted him to be a doctor. Philip's first experience with surgery was watching an amputation, which created in him a strong aversion to the profession. In spite of this, his father insisted that he study medicine. So after he obtained a BA degree from the University of Pennsylvania in 1785, he studied for three years as an apprentice under Adam Kuhn, the university's professor of materia medica. His father then took him to London in 1788 at age twenty and arranged for him to live with and study under the famous surgeon, John Hunter.[1] Apparently, Physick and Hunter soon bonded. Inspired by Hunter's brilliance and his unique focus on research, Physick applied himself diligently and, before long, became Hunter's favorite pupil.[2] Hunter supported him for the position of house surgeon at St. George's Hospital. He won this prestigious position despite the jealousy of other candidates and the bias against Americans stemming

1768
Birth of Philip Syng Physick

1785
BA University of Pennsylvania

1788–1790
In London, lives with John Hunter, studies under John and William Hunter

1791
House surgeon at St. George's Hospital

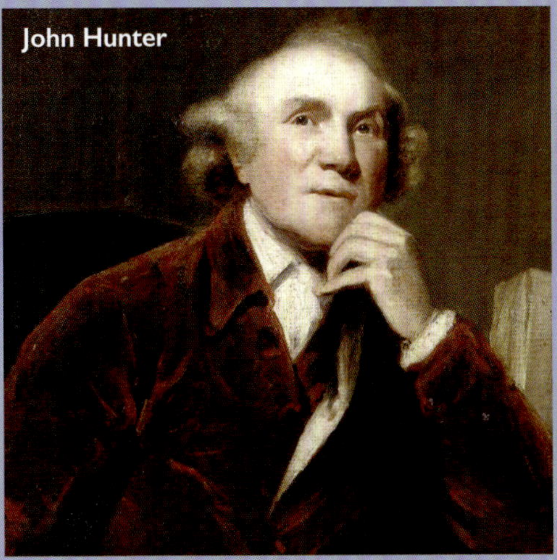

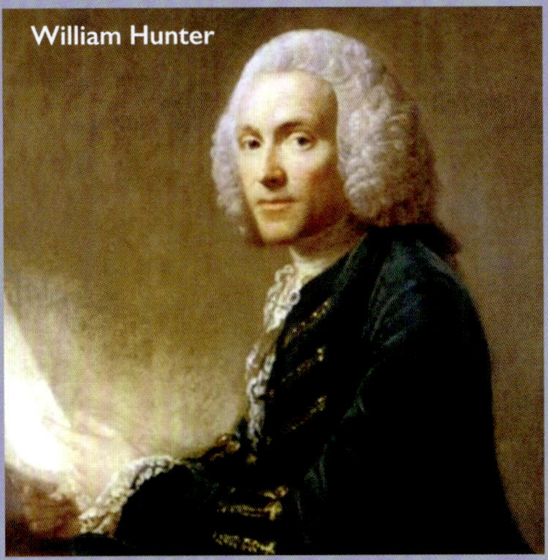

Grandfathers of American surgery

1792
MD University of Edinburgh

1792
Physick returns to Philadelphia. Initially unsuccessful in practice

1793
Physick and Wistar as Rush's apprentices help him treat yellow fever victims by bleeding

1794
With referrals from Rush, Physick's practice thrives

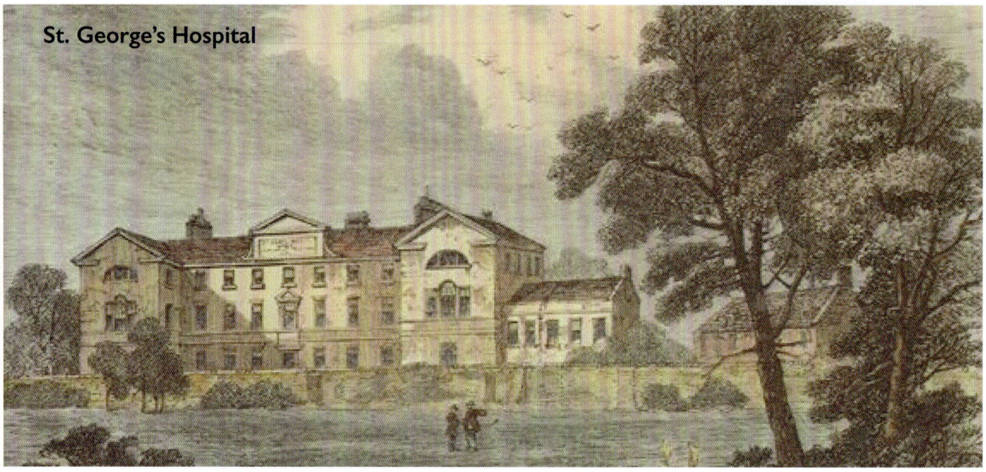

St. George's Hospital

from the recent revolution. On his first day at St. George's, Physick overcame these negative feelings and won the admiration of the surgical staff by skillfully reducing a patient's dislocated shoulder. In 1791, he was awarded membership in the Royal College of Surgeons. Hunter was so impressed with his work that he offered to make Physick his partner in practice if he would remain in London. However, Physick declined this honor and instead, after a year in Edinburgh to obtain his MD degree, came home.

Returning to Philadelphia in 1792, Physick was at first unsuccessful in building a practice but gained prominence and the lifelong support of a powerful mentor by working as Benjamin Rush's understudy during the yellow fever epidemic of 1793. Unfortunately, for the rest of Physick's life, he followed Rush's misguided lead as a strong advocate of bloodletting and powerful laxatives as treatment of yellow fever, as well as for a variety of other diseases. Physick himself contracted yellow fever and attributed his recovery to aggressive bloodletting. Rush subsequently referred his surgical patients to Physick, causing his practice to thrive. Physick's resultant lifelong loyalty to Rush was extreme. He refused ever to join the College of Physicians because of Rush's dispute with and resignation from the College over disagreement with his extreme bloodletting, which most College members recognized as harmful.

The service Physick rendered as a resident at the Bush Hill yellow fever hospital brought him considerable prominence.[3] He was appointed in 1794 as surgeon to the Pennsylvania Hospital and to the Almshouse in 1801. In 1802, he was elected at age thirty-four to membership in the American Philosophical Society. However, he took no notice of the affairs of this prestigious society and never attended a meeting. Perhaps this was an early sign of his tendency to isolate himself.

At the request of the medical students, Physick delivered a course of lectures on surgery at Pennsylvania Hospital. His reputation as a surgeon and teacher grew, and when William Shippen retired in 1805, the university created for Physick its first chair of surgery (without combining it with anatomy and midwifery as it had been during Shippen's professorship).

For the next three decades, Physick was the dominant surgeon of Philadelphia and perhaps the whole United States. His practice was immense, and he was in constant demand as a consultant, but it was his many innovations in surgical treatment that set him apart.[4] These included new methods for removing poisonous substances from the stomach by means of a tube and pump; new methods for treating the ulcers of swollen legs; the successful use of a seton for nonhealing fractures; the use of splints, rest, and sparse diets for treatment of diseased hip joints; success of an operation for an arteriovenous fistula; enucleation as a treatment of cataracts; a snare-like instrument for removing tonsils and hemorrhoids; carbonated beverages for gastrointestinal upsets; improved vascular forceps; a curved needle for suturing arteries; and a bougie-tipped catheter for difficult intubation of the bladder. His most important innovation may have been development of absorbable sutures which he made from kid gloves or catgut.

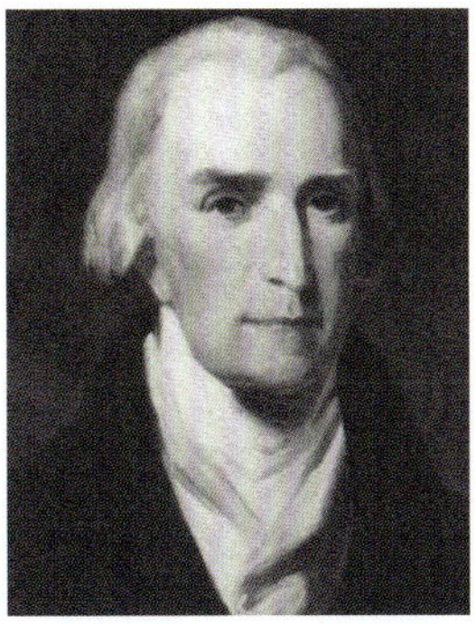
Philip Syng Physick

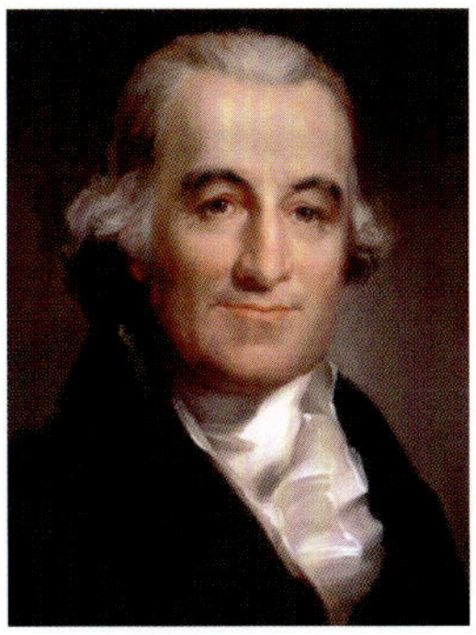
Casper Wistar

Benjamin Rush's apprentices during yellow fever epidemic.

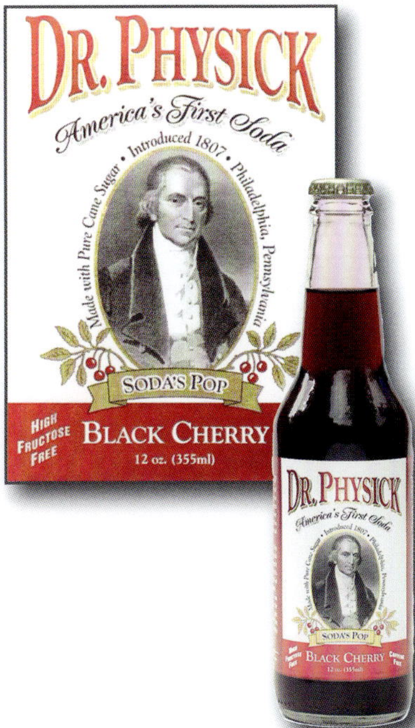

His remarkable inventiveness would have been even more widely appreciated had he not been so unwilling to write. In his whole life, he produced no more than half a dozen brief papers, totaling only thirty or forty pages. To compensate for this deficiency, he deputized his nephew, John Syng Dorsey, to write for him. Dorsey gathered Physick's lecture notes together and produced the first comprehensive surgery text written in America, *The Elements of Surgery*.[5]

As an operating surgeon, Physick was praised as conservative, deft, and unflappable. One operation for which he became particularly well known was cutting for

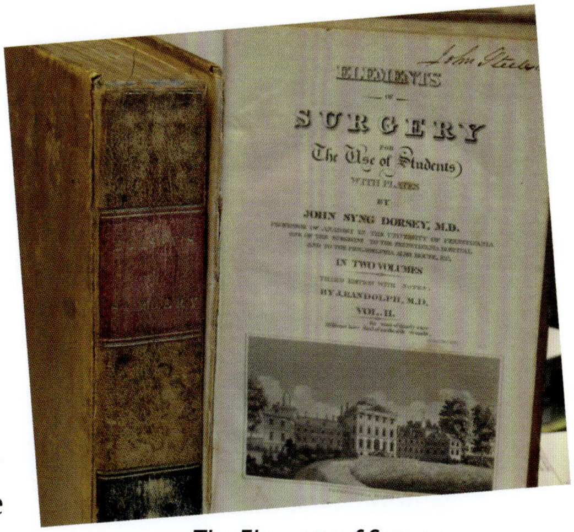

The Elements of Surgery

1805
Physick appointed professor and chair of surgery at Penn

1802–1831
Physick's years of productivity

- 1802—Uses seton to induce inflammation and treat nonhealing fractures
- 1805—Surgical repair of arteriovenous fistula
- 1813—Invents stomach tube to evacuate poisonous substances
- 1816—Uses kid gloves and animal intestines to make the first absorbable sutures
- 1826—Creates colocutaneous fistulas to treat strangulated hernias
- 1828—Devises tonsilatome to excise tonsils and hemorrhoids

Physick writes almost nothing about his accomplishments. His nephew and assistant becomes his scribe

1813
Physick's nephew, John Dorsey, publishes *The Elements of Surgery* based on his uncle's work

bladder stones. In a famous operation, he successfully removed over a thousand small stones from the bladder of seventy-three-year-old US Supreme Court Chief Justice John Marshall. This procedure, carried out in 1831 in the year of Physick's retirement, may have been his last operation. There is a wonderful description of the scene in which these two old men got fortified on brandy in preparation for the operation which was expected to be quite painful before the availability of anesthesia. It is hard to know which old man was more apprehensive.

That Physick's university appointment was professor of surgery rather than of anatomy, surgery, and midwifery (as Shippen's had been) helped identify surgery as a fully developed discipline of its own. Partly because of this, Physick soon became known as the Father of American Surgery.

Although his contributions led to an international reputation, S. D. Gross afforded him only faint praise, saying that there were many other surgeons with "superior mental caliber."[6] Gross contended that although Physick stood for a long time at the head of US surgery, this was mainly because he had the field to himself.[7] Although Gross acknowledged that Physick was well grounded in the principles of surgery, his fame was primarily due to the fact that at the time the field was his exclusive domain. In addition, Gross claimed that if an unusual case or need of an important operation turned up in Philadelphia, it was likely to be sent to John Jones in New York.

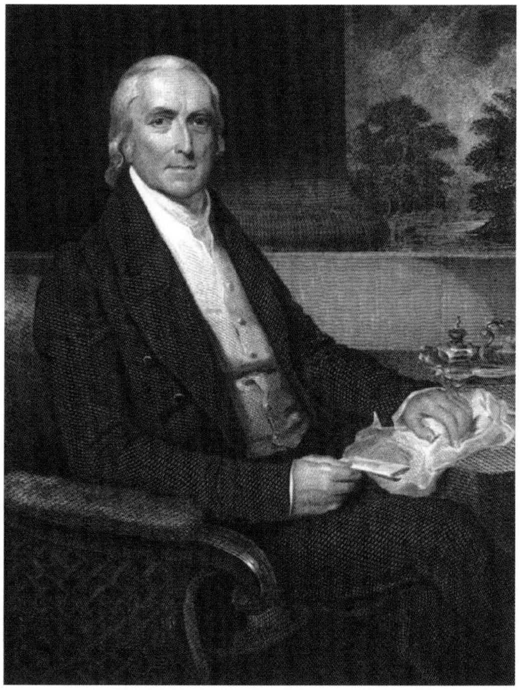

Philip Syng Physick

Gross also attacked Physick on a personal basis as "something of a prig, not popular with his mates, a cold, dyspeptic, unsociable man." Gross never knew Physick until he was a broken old man, but the seeds of these personality traits could be recognized earlier and appear to have made him unpopular with the medical students and to have cost him his job.

Physick's lectures, though careful and authoritative, were usually read verbatim from his script and were dry and boring. At the time, student tuition was the school's major revenue source. The trustees therefore became worried when they noticed that some Penn students were defecting to Baltimore's new school of the University of Maryland, where a charismatic young surgeon was giving lectures in surgery that were much more stimulating than Physick's. Thus, thirty-one-year-old William Gibson was brought in to replace Physick as Penn's surgery chief. The older and much more famous Physick was relegated to a position as professor of anatomy, a discipline in which he had no particular interest or special expertise.[8]

William Horner, Physick's assistant during his early professional career, and later for many years his faculty colleague, probably knew him best. Even when Horner as the school's dean became his boss, he continued for much of his time to serve as Physick's assistant. Horner's assessment of his persona was quite different from that of Gross. He remembered the young Physick as strikingly handsome with features that seemed to be chiseled from marble, a neat and careful dresser, tall, always erect and confident, somewhat vain, reserved and aloof, but good-natured, not outgoing, but willing to participate in polite conversation with humor. Horner had utmost respect for him as "a thoughtful, conservative surgeon, in the operating room deft and unflappable…one of Nature's master-pieces." [9]

In addition to serving as Physick's most qualified, though somewhat effusive, iconographer, Horner's forty-one-page memoir of Physick in the *Proceedings of the American Philosophical Society* provides rare insight into the evolution of a complex personality that darkened with age. Horner relates circumstances that he believes would have made anyone's life unhappy. At age thirty-two, Physick married Elizabeth Emelin, a Quaker. His wife had seven children, three of whom did not survive into adulthood. It was an unhappy marriage, ending in separation. After this and especially after the death in 1818 of his beloved nephew, John Syng Dorsey, on whom he had become so dependent, his life was one of solitude. His personal habits became fixed. He ate the same meal every day and wore the same old-fashioned clothes and powdered his hair as he had when he was young and it was fashionable. Every day was like the last one and the next. It was like the movie *Groundhog Day*. He had no friends or companions. He never traveled, entertained, or allowed himself to be entertained. He became impatient of attempts made to entertain or amuse him. Outside of surgery, he had no interest except in money.[10] His large practice and frugal lifestyle allowed him to accumulate a fortune that, at the time of his death, amounted to about half a million dollars. None of it did he ever share, contribute to charity, or donate to the educational and professional institutions that had sustained him.

In his later years, he was plagued with symptoms Horner cataloged as sequalae of maladies, including chronic sinusitis, pyelonephritis with stone formation, peptic ulcer, and

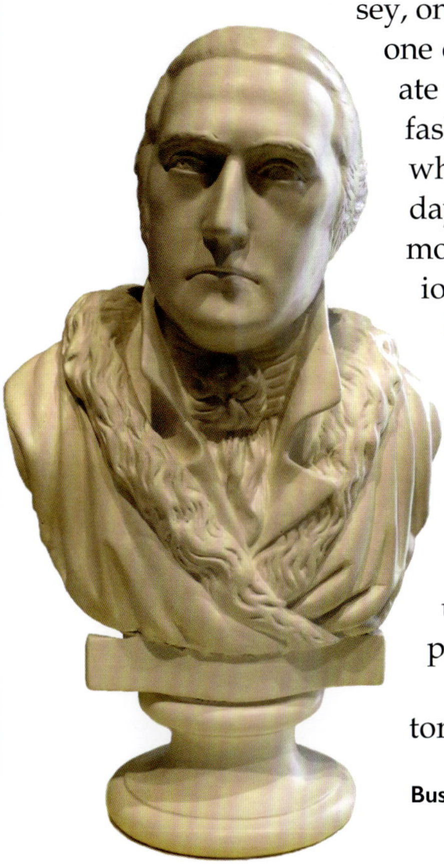

Bust of Philip Syng Physick by William Rush

1800
Unhappy marriage

1818
Death of his beloved nephew John Syng Dorsey

1818
With reluctance, Physick agrees to give up surgical chair and become chair of anatomy. He is succeeded by Gibson as chief of surgery

1818–1837
Decades of declining health, boredom, and misery

1831
Physick retires. His last operation may have been to remove bladder stones from seventy-three-year-old Chief Justice John Marshall

1837
Death of Physick

cardiac valvular disease from rheumatic fever. A near-fatal bout of typhus in 1813 left his face wasted and haggard. For several years he struggled with heart failure and pulmonary edema, unable to sleep except in a sitting position and legs so full of fluid that they broke open and wept.[11]

Physick apparently was always a somewhat odd character. As his health deteriorated with age, this got worse. He became increasingly focused on and troubled by theological matters. He was particularly worried that his body might be dissected or that he might be buried alive. He left instructions that his body not be buried until it had begun to decompose. He arranged for his grave to be guarded for several weeks by armed men after his death in 1837.[12]

Near the end, he confided to Horner that he had never stopped regretting that his father had forced him into medicine. Whatever acclaim medicine had brought him, he said he would have preferred to be a silversmith like his grandfather.

John Syng Dorsey

Professor of Materia Medica (1916–1918)
Professor of Anatomy (1918)

1783
Birth of Dorsey

1802
MD from Penn

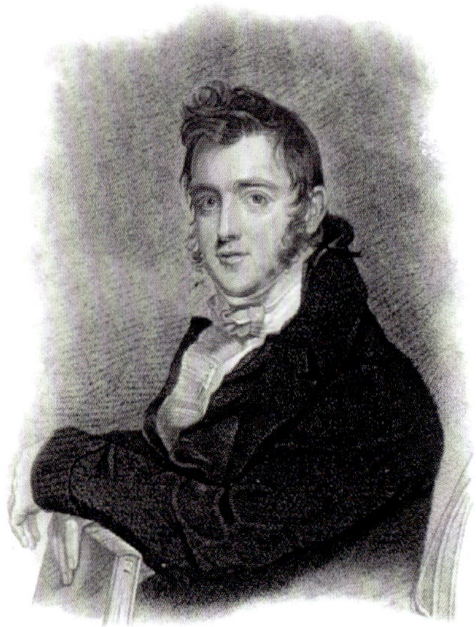

John Syng Dorsey

The story of this unsung hero is one of the department's most unforgettable and saddest.[13] Born in 1783, he was Philip Syng Physick's nephew. Fortunately, he was precocious because he wasn't going to have many years to make his mark. After graduating from Quaker schools in Philadelphia at age fifteen, then two years as an apprentice to his uncle, he enrolled in medical school at Penn. He finished his course work at age nineteen, but needed to petition the faculty for an early diploma since students were not allowed to graduate before age twenty-one.

After another year assisting his uncle, he polished his education by a year spent in the medical institutions of England and France. In Paris, he said he learned nothing and that the French surgeons were less advanced than his uncle. In London, he was befriended and taught by Everard Home, John Hunter's successor and son-in-law. Home also introduced him to his club and to a group of literary friends. It was perhaps during this time that Dorsey developed his interests outside of medicine. He learned to play two musical instruments and learned to draw so well that he illustrated not only his own publications but also those of others. And he began to write poetry.

On his return to Philadelphia, the association with his famous uncle and his engaging personality allowed him to build a successful practice. Because the idiosyncratic Physick was reluctant to write anything, he assigned Dorsey to chronicle his many remarkable accomplishments. In 1807, Physick induced the university to appoint his twenty-four-year-old protégé as adjunct professor of surgery. This was a great help to Physick, and for Dorsey, a unique opportunity to understudy America's foremost surgeon who increasingly relied on his nephew to substitute for him in his practice and for demonstrations and lectures to the medical students. It also forced Dorsey to hone his skills as a writer. Helping him to develop a uniquely concise style was his hobby of composing poetry. Actually, he was pretty good at it.

1807
Dorsey appointed adjunct professor of surgery

1811
To treat aneurysm, Dorsey ligates external iliac artery

1813
Publishes *The Elements of Surgery*

Over the next decade, the leading literary periodical of the time, the *Port Folio,* published forty pages of Dorsey's poems. Their subjects ranged from college drinking songs to the history of science, the incomprehensibility of God, and a variety of romantic topics. Early on, the intent of the verses was probably to help him in courting his future wife, Elizabeth Ralston, whom he married in 1807. Several serious professional critics favorably reviewed his work. A number of his friends and colleagues were also intrigued and complimentary, including even S. D. Gross, the Jefferson surgeon who usually had nothing good to say about Penn doctors such as his uncle.

Also in 1807, Dorsey made plans to write his major opus, a book to be based largely on his uncle's extensive practice, innovations, and lecture notes.

Over the next six years, Dorsey produced a 750-page masterpiece, *The Elements of Surgery*. It was the first comprehensive surgical textbook to be written by an American. It was widely used, not only in this country, but also in Europe over ten years and three editions.

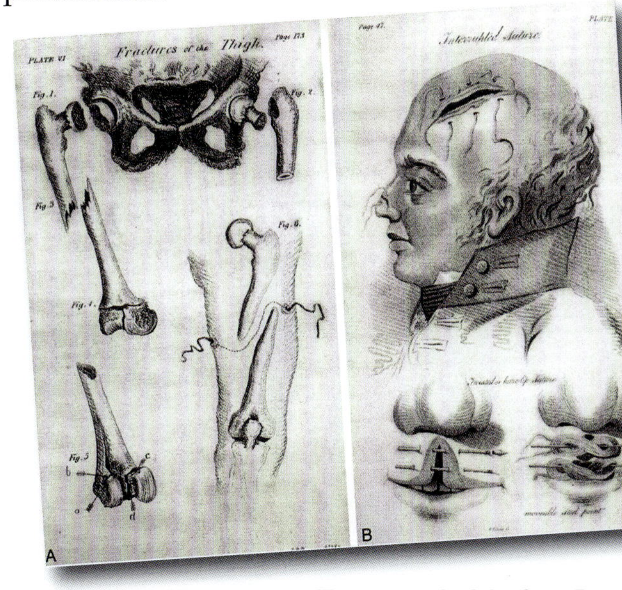

Illustrations by John Syng Dorsey

During this time, in addition to working on his book, he was also helping his uncle in his huge practice and developing his own. He was also an excellent clinical surgeon. In 1811, to treat a patient with a gigantic aneurism in the groin, he ligated the external iliac artery, the first such procedure and perhaps the earliest major vascular operation by an American.

In 1816 at age thirty-three, Dorsey became a university professor in his own right, being appointed chair of the department of materia

1816
Dorsey appointed chair of Department of Materia Medica

1818
Succeeds Caspar Wistar as chair of anatomy. On November 2, Dorsey delivers his first lecture

On November 12, Dorsey dies at age thirty-five from typhus

1818
With reluctance, Physick shifts from chair of surgery to chair of anatomy. Gibson is appointed to succeed Physick as chair of surgery

medica. Two years later, he succeeded Casper Wistar in the important senior chair of anatomy. But by now his time had almost run out. On November 2, he gave his first lecture to the students as the professor of anatomy. A few hours later, the same night, he fell ill with a high fever. It was from typhus. In ten days, he was dead.

Emotionally devastated by the death of his nephew, Physick was also professionally damaged by this unhappy circumstance. For months, the trustees had wondered how to replace Physick with a more interesting lecturer. They speculated that Penn students were defecting to the University of Maryland where the surgical professor was known as a charismatic teacher. With Dorsey's death, the chair of anatomy became available and seemed a suitable site for Physick if he could be persuaded to give up the chair of surgery. Although he was reluctant, Physick, persuaded that it was in the interest of the school, agreed to resign his surgery chair and succeed his deceased nephew as professor of anatomy. Thus, the world-renowned surgeon was shifted to a discipline in which he was neither interested nor very good. William Gibson was brought from Maryland as surgery chairman. Fortunately he was a pretty good choice. But unfortunately Physick, the Father of American Surgery, was never the same.

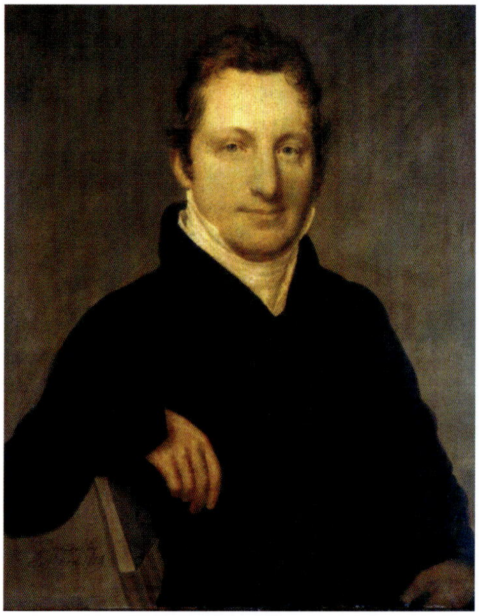

William Gibson
Physick's successor as chairman of surgery

Stories of what might have been are always sad, this one especially so. Dorsey was universally admired and liked for his personal qualities as well as for his promise, which most contemporaries thought would eventually lead to his becoming a major figure in US surgery. Unlike his uncle, he had a generous, happy, attractive manner. Even the crotchety S. D. Gross praised him.

Timeline of Events During the Career of Philip Syng Physick (1805–1831)

1788–1818 Casper Wistar's thirty years on the medical school faculty.

1789–1791 Physick studies anatomy and surgery with John Hunter in London.

1792 Physick obtains MD from Edinburgh University, returns to Philadelphia.

1793 Physick is assistant to Benjamin Rush during yellow fever epidemic.

1792–1808 Wistar is adjunct professor of anatomy, surgery, and midwifery as Shippen's assistant. This is the longest of any of his university appointments.

1802–1829 Medical school is in President's House at 9th and Market Street.

1805–1818 Physick is chairman of surgery.

1805–1831 Some of Physick's research contributions

- 1802—Uses seton to induce inflammation and treat nonhealing fractures
- 1805—Surgical repair of arteriovenous fistula
- 1813—Invents stomach tube to evacuate poisonous substances
- 1816—Uses kid gloves and animal intestines to make the first absorbable sutures
- 1826—Creates colocutaneous fistula to treat strangulated hernia
- 1828—Devises tonsilatome to excise tonsils and hemorrhoids
- 1831—Performs lithotomy on US Chief Justice John Marshall. Removes over a thousand stones.

1809 In Kentucky, Ephraim McDowell performs the world's first laparotomy, removing a huge ovarian tumor; in 1816, he sends report of three successful cases to Physick who refuses to believe or publish it.

1811 Wistar publishes *A System of Anatomy*, the first American textbook of anatomy.

1811 John Syng Dorsey ligates the external iliac artery to treat an aneurysm, America's first major vascular surgery procedure.

1812 War of 1812.

1812 William Gibson in Maryland ligates common iliac artery to treat a gunshot wound, showing that collateral circulation will allow the leg to survive.

1813	Dorsey publishes *Elements of Surgery*, the first American surgery (comprehensive and systematic) textbook. It is based largely on Physick's lectures.
1816	Dorsey is appointed chairman of materia medica in the medical school.
1818	Casper Wistar dies. John Syng Dorsey succeeds him as chairman of anatomy but dies of typhus within days.
1818	Physick resigns chair of surgery and is appointed to succeed Dorsey as chairman of anatomy.
1819	Gibson is recruited from Maryland to succeed Physick as chairman of surgery.
1819	Thomas Chalkley James publishes McDowell's paper on the first successful laparotomy.
1822–1852	William Horner is the first bona fide dean of the medical school, serves for thirty years.
1829–1874	Medical school moves to Medical Hall on 9th Street.
1831	Physick retires.
1837	After years of declining health, Philip Syng Physick dies.

Notes

[1] Horner, William E. Philip Syng Physick Memoir in Biographical Memoirs of Members of the American Philosophical Society, *Physicians Vol I, 1787–1935,* edited by Barker and Starzl (Philadelphia: American Philosophical Society, 2013) p. 11.

[2] Kobler, John. *The Reluctant Surgeon: A Biography of John Hunter* (Garden City, NY: Doubleday & Company, 1960) pp.101–105, 183.

[3] Horner, William E. Philip Syng Physick Memoir in Biographical Memoirs of Members of the American Philosophical Society, *Physicians Vol I, 1787–1935,* edited by Barker and Starzl (Philadelphia: American Philosophical Society, 2013) p. 12.

[4] Rutkow, Ira. Philip Syng Physick (1768–1837). *Arch Surg,* Vol 136 (Aug. 2001), 968.

[5] Ibid.

[6] Gross, Samuel D. *Autobiography of Samuel D. Gross MD with Reminiscences of His Times and Contemporaries Volume II* (Philadelphia: WB Saunders, 1893) p. 241.

[7] Rutkow, Ira. *Philip Syng Physick (1768–1837).*

[8] Harte, Richard. Philip Syng Physick: A Sketch. *U of PA Medical Bulletin,* 18:344 (Feb. 1906).

[9] Horner, William E. Philip Syng Physick Memoir in Biographical Memoirs of Members of the American Philosophical Society. *Physicians Vol I, 1787–1935,* p. 9.

[10] Rutkow, Ira. *Philip Syng Physick (1768–1837).*

[11] Horner, William E. Philip Syng Physick Memoir in Biographical Memoirs of Members of the American Philosophical Society. *Physicians Vol I, 1787–1935* p. 15.

[12] Ibid., p. 17.

[13] Smythe, Roy. The First American Textbook of Surgery. *Annals of Surgery,* Vol 237, No 4, 580–590.

CHAPTER 4

Ill-Tempered Student of Warfare

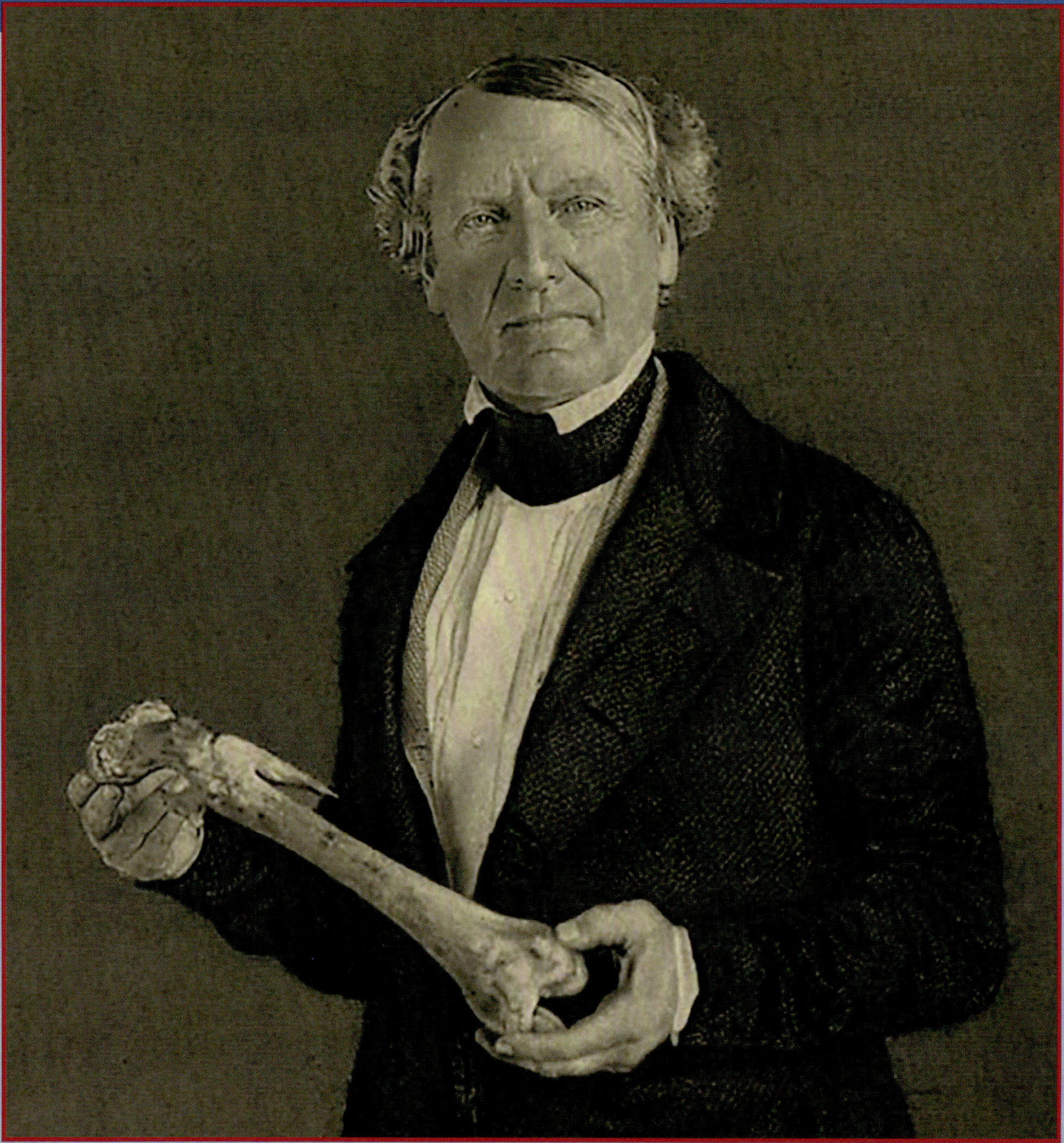

William Gibson (1788–1868)

Chairman of Surgery (1819–1855)

For some reason, William Gibson is not as well remembered as some of the department's other chairmen, perhaps because he is sandwiched in time between Physick, the "Father of American Surgery," and cross-town Jefferson University's "Emperor of Surgery," Samuel Gross. Forgetting Gibson is too bad because his exploits have made him one of my favorites. He must have been an interesting character or, in present-day vernacular, a cool guy.

He was a native of Baltimore and studied at St. John's College in Annapolis and at Princeton in 1803–1804 without getting a degree. In 1806–1807, he attended some of Physick's lectures at the University of Pennsylvania Medical School. He then spent three years wandering around Europe. There, in addition to acquiring his MD in Edinburgh in 1809, he studied with and became the favorite of London's most prominent surgeons, Charles Bell and Astley Cooper.[1] Charles Bell was not only a master surgeon but also a renowned portrait artist. Under Bell's influence and the tutelage of another famous painter, Robert Haydon, Gibson became a good-enough artist to illustrate his own publications. He also studied quite seriously the violin, botany, ornithology, and boxing, the last probably with his friend, the poet Lord Byron. Gibson was also a student of warfare. To cultivate this interest, he attended several battles including the Battle of Carunna during the Peninsular War and later the Battle of Waterloo where, in addition to treating wounded soldiers, he sustained a slight wound of his own.

On his return to his native Baltimore in 1810, he set up practice and began to help organize the first medical department at the University of Maryland. A year later at age twenty-three, Gibson became the founding chairman of surgery at the University of Maryland. His colorful style made him a popular lecturer. That he was also a confident and bold surgeon was demonstrated in 1812 when he ligated the common iliac artery to treat a patient bleeding from a gunshot wound of the groin. Gibson put his finger in the wound and stopped the hemorrhage, but when he

1788
Gibson born in Baltimore

1803
Studies at St. John's College and Princeton

1806–1807
Attends Physick's lectures

1809
MD University of Edinburgh

1811
Becomes University of Maryland's first chairman of surgery at age twenty-three

1812
Treats gunshot wound in American hero General Winfield Scott

1815
Gibson attends Battle of Waterloo, sustains a slight wound

1819
Succeeds Physick as chairman of surgery at Penn

removed his finger, the bleeding restarted. So he kept his finger in the wound and with his free hand, enlarged the wound and with a flexible probe passed a ligature around the bleeding point and tied the ligature. After clearing away the clotted blood, he saw that he had ligated the common iliac artery just below the bifurcation of the aorta. While closing the wound, he noted further bleeding coming from the distal common iliac artery, which he then tied. Since the leg appeared well vascularized, he realized that he had demonstrated for the first time that collateral circulation could maintain viability of the leg after ligation of the common iliac artery. He speculated that this artery could be sacrificed in an operation for aneurysm. Although the patient survived only eighteen days before dying of peritonitis, this operation, the first of its kind, demonstrated that collateral circulation was adequate to maintain viability of the leg.[2] It also contributed to Gibson's fame, which led to his being called to treat a gunshot wound in General Winfield Scott, American hero of the War of 1812, sustained during the Battle of Lundy's Lane.

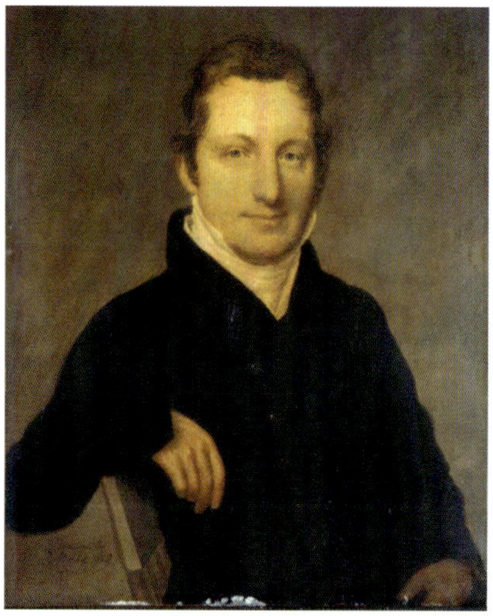

William Gibson

After eight years as professor at Maryland, he was recruited to succeed Philip Syng Physick as professor of surgery at the University of Pennsylvania. Despite Physick's international fame as an innovative surgeon, he was considered by the students to be a dry, uninteresting lecturer. The trustees were concerned that some Penn students were transferring to Maryland for a more interesting course in surgery, thus decreasing the tuition fees on which the University depended. Therefore, Physick, the highly respected "Father of American Surgery,"

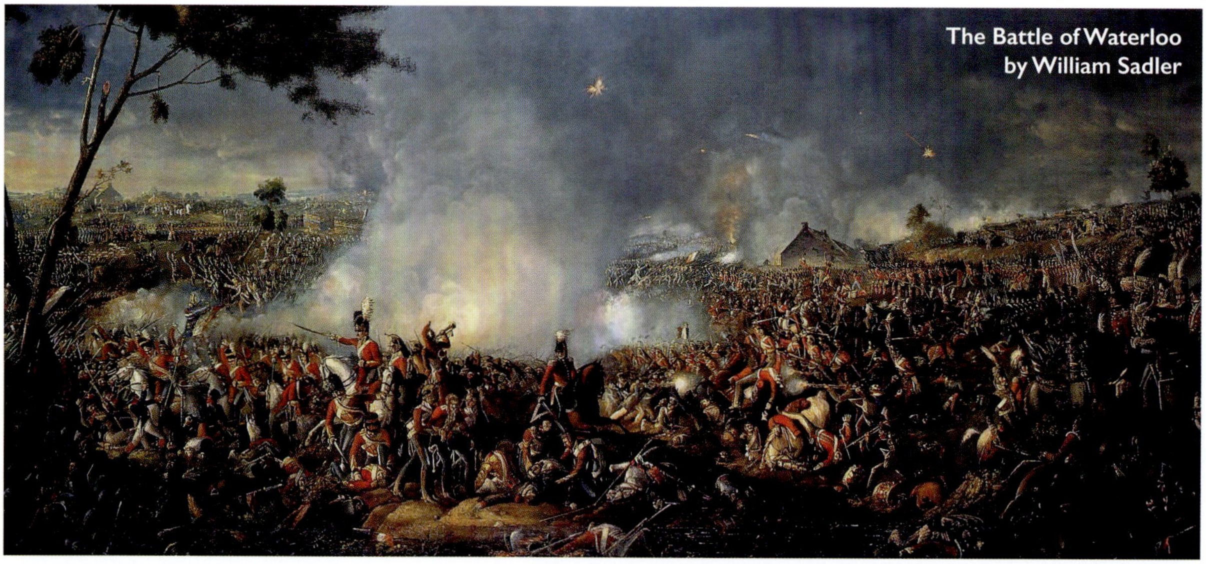

The Battle of Waterloo by William Sadler

was "kicked upstairs" to a position he did not fancy as professor of anatomy. As predicted, Gibson's flair as a lecturer made him a huge success with the students, contributing to an increase in the size of the student body. A favorite with them was Gibson's lecture on gunshot wounds, which he illustrated by shooting live animals in front of the class.[3] In 1818, he became the first to cut the extraocular muscles to treat strabismus,[4] though he did not get around to reporting this until 1840. In another first, he successfully performed two cesarean sections in the same woman.

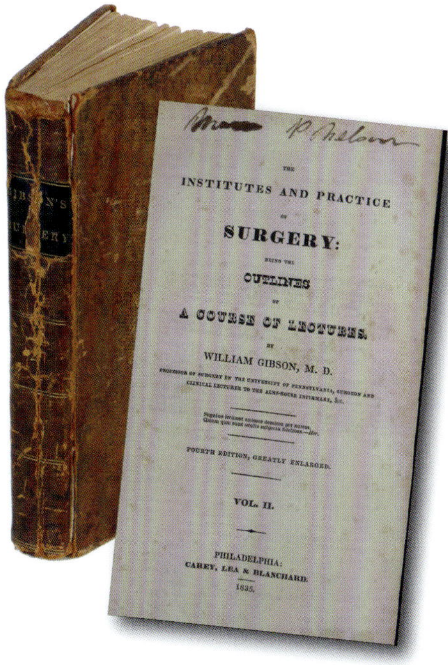

A prolific author in the medical periodicals of the day, Gibson also published an important book in 1824, *The Institutes and Practice of Surgery*. It was the second systematic textbook of the field. Its popularity allowed it to go through eight editions. Another of his widely read books was *Rambles in Europe* that characterized the many famous surgeons of the day whom Gibson had visited in Europe.

Broadly educated, particularly in literature including the classics, Gibson could recite from memory long passages of Latin verse. But not everything about Gibson was admirable. He had a dark side. S. D. Gross described the feisty little Gibson (5'7" tall) as "not an amiable man but one whose ill temper often betrayed him."[5] An example was his driving a fork through his young son's foot during a family argument at the dinner table.[6] Whether in spite of his temper or because of it, Gibson thrived as Penn's chairman of surgery for thirty-six years. After his retirement at age sixty-seven, he enjoyed most of his last thirteen years living in Newport, Rhode Island, where he played two musical instruments and stuffed a huge collection of rare birds, some of which are still preserved in the local museum. He is also known

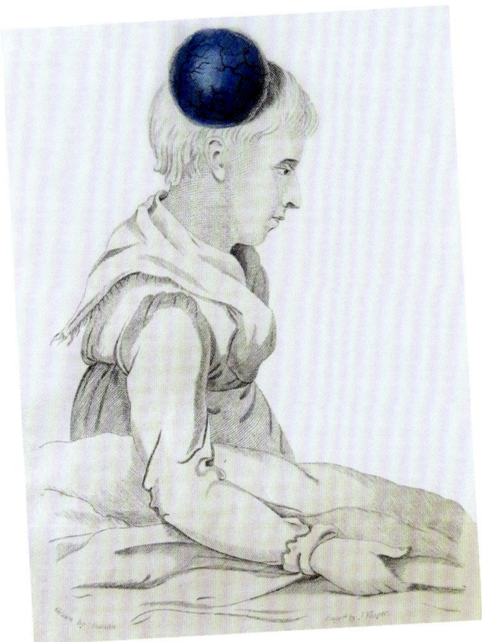

Illustration by Gibson in his surgery textbook.

1824
Publishes second systematic surgery textbook

1842
Crawford Long, Penn Medical School graduate, is first to operate on patient under anesthesia

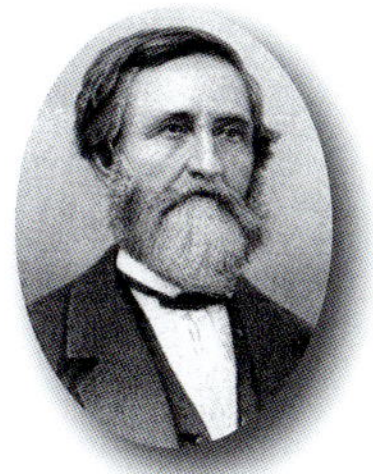

Crawford Long

1846
Anesthesia demonstrated in Boston by William Morton, dentist, and John Collins Warren, surgeon

1847
American Medical Association is founded in Philadelphia

1855
Gibson retires as chairman of surgery

1868
Death of Gibson

to have written a 150-volume diary. One wishes that this lost document could be found to tell us about his amazing career, whether he actually fought in the Battle of Waterloo, and how he came to be wounded there.

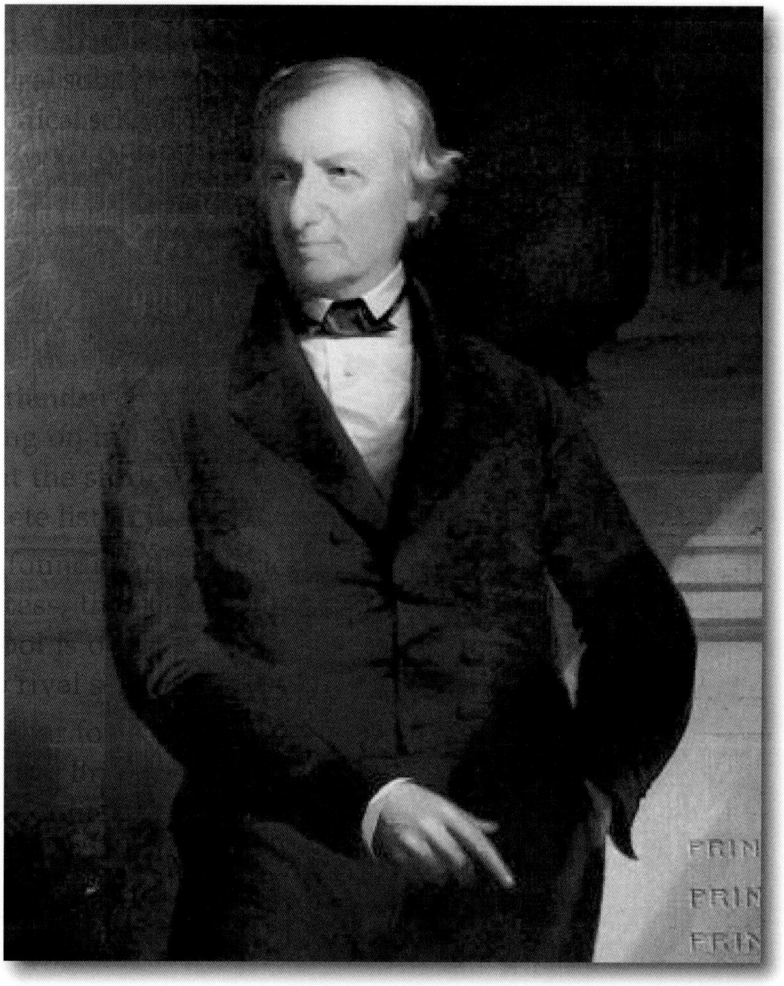

Gibson's portrait as surgery chairman at University of Pennsylvania by John B. Neagle

Timeline of Events During the Career of William Gibson

1809 Gibson obtains MD at University of Edinburgh.

1811 Gibson becomes chairman of surgery at the University of Maryland.

1811 Gibson devises an operation for the extraction of cataracts.

1812 Gibson is the first to ligate the common iliac artery, demonstrating adequacy of collateral circulation.

1815 Penn medical students petition for a course in clinical medicine at Pennsylvania Hospital and the Almshouse.

1818 John Syng Dorsey becomes chairman of anatomy, dies within days.

1818 Philip Syng Physick moves from chair of surgery to succeed Dorsey as chair of anatomy.

1818 Gibson is appointed chairman of surgery at Penn.

1818 Gibson performs operation for strabismus.

1819–1855 During the thirty-seven years that William Gibson is surgery chairman, there are other important events in medicine, although for the most part they are not attributable to Penn surgeons. During thirty of these years, William Horner, a Penn surgeon, is dean of the school (1822–1852) and for twenty of the same years, chairman of anatomy.

1824 Gibson publishes the *Institutes and Practice of Surgery*, the second American surgery text. It goes through eight editions. According to S. D. Gross, the first edition was terrible, but each subsequent edition got better.

1824 Jefferson Medical College is founded. For several years before that, there had been attempts to start this second of Philadelphia's medical schools, but each time, the University of Pennsylvania, not desiring competition, blocked the issue of a charter. This was either the origin or the result of hard feelings between the two schools that persisted for generations. Instead, the bad blood may have been only a reflection of the rivalry between Gibson, Penn's surgeon, and George McClellan, the founder of Jefferson.

1825 By now, there are about a dozen US medical schools. Twenty percent of the students are at Penn.

1835, 1837 Gibson performs two cesarean sections successfully on the same woman.

1842 Anesthesia, one of the great discoveries in all of medicine, is introduced. This accomplishment is credited to a graduate of Penn's medical school, Crawford Long. He deserves a place in anyone's medical pantheon.

1846 Many historians attribute the birth of anesthesia to this date when William Morton famously demonstrated the use of ether in an operation at the "ether dome" of Massachusetts General Hospital. However, it is well-established that Crawford Long, a country surgeon in rural Georgia, successfully used ether as an anesthetic for operations on numerous occasions, beginning four years earlier. Although he neglected to publish this experience until 1848, it is now widely accepted that he was the first. Several other individuals including Horace Wells, Charles Thomas Jackson, and Morton laid claim to this important advance and even tried to patent it, but their claims have been disproven. Crawford Long was born in Georgia, and during college at the University of Georgia, he roomed with Alexander Stephens, who later became Vice President of the Confederacy. Also interesting is that in 1842, Long operated on his two-month-old cousin for cleft lip and palate. This young patient grew up to graduate from Penn's dental school. After a few years of practice in Georgia, he was advised to move west because he had contracted tuberculosis. There he acquired a reputation as a gambler and gunfighter. This was John Henry "Doc" Holliday.

1845 H. H. Smith publishes his book, *Anatomical Atlas Illustrative of the Structure of the Human Body*.

1847 Even after Morton's and Crawford's reports, the administration of ether could be tricky, leading to several failures. In 1847, a group of surgeons including William Horner, Gibson, and Joseph Pancoast were the first to use ether successfully for an operation in Philadelphia.

1847 The American Medical Association is founded at a meeting in Philadelphia. This was the first effort to improve and standardize American medical education. Proposed were elevated standards for medical school admission and graduation and for licensing of physicians. Enactment of the recommendations would take about another hundred years. Even at university schools, faculty members opposed them, anticipating loss of autonomy and reduction of student enrollment and tuition fees. The University of Pennsylvania had delayed several previous attempts to form a national medical society since members of the university felt that this would detract from the individual eminence of their school. The new society was primarily a medical group, although later there was a surgical division. Penn Medicine chairman Nathaniel Chapman was elected as the first president.

1850 In Philadelphia, Women's Medical College is founded. This was the first women's medical school in America and the second in the world, founded two years later than a women's medical college in England.

1850 By this time, Penn medical school has 466 students, the undergraduate college only ninety-five.

1855 Gibson retires.

1868 Gibson dies from mortification of the toe (probably senile gangrene).

Notes

[1] Abrahams, Harold and Mills, David Wyndham H. William Gibson MD Anatomist as seen by a student in 1823. *Transactions and Studies of the College of Physicians of Philadelphia,* Vol 36, No 3, 4th series (Jan 1971) p. 184.

[2] Ashhurst, Astley PC. Presentation of a Portrait of Professor William Gibson, On Behalf of His Granddaughter, Miss Anne H. Gibson. *Transactions of the College of Physicians of Philadelphia*, Vol xiv (1923), p. 117.

[3] Abrahams, Harold and Mills, David Wyndham H. William Gibson MD Anatomist as seen by a student in 1823. *Transactions and Studies of the College of Physicians of Philadelphia,* Vol 36, No 3, 4th series (Jan 1971) p. 187.

[4] Packard, Francis. *History of Medicine in the United States, Vol 1* (New York: Hofner Publishing Company, 1963) p. 1166.

[5] Gross, Samuel D. *Autobiography of Samuel D. Gross MD with Reminiscences of His Times and Contemporaries Volume II* (Philadelphia: WB Saunders, 1893) p. 324–329. This book contains most of the stories in this chapter plus the account of Gross's requested visit to Gibson for consultation for his rheumatism and debility.

[6] Ashhurst, Astley PC. Presentation of a Portrait of Professor William Gibson, On Behalf of His Granddaughter, Miss Anne H. Gibson. *Transactions of the College of Physicians of Philadelphia,* Vol xiv (1923), p. 8. Gibson's granddaughter told this story. While sitting at the dining room table, one of his sons annoyed him. He was told to be quiet but did not. Gibson then drove a carving fork through the boy's foot into the floor and said, "Now will you be quiet?"

CHAPTER 5

A Constitutional Cripple Is the School's Foremost Anatomist, Surgeon, Anthropologist, and Dean

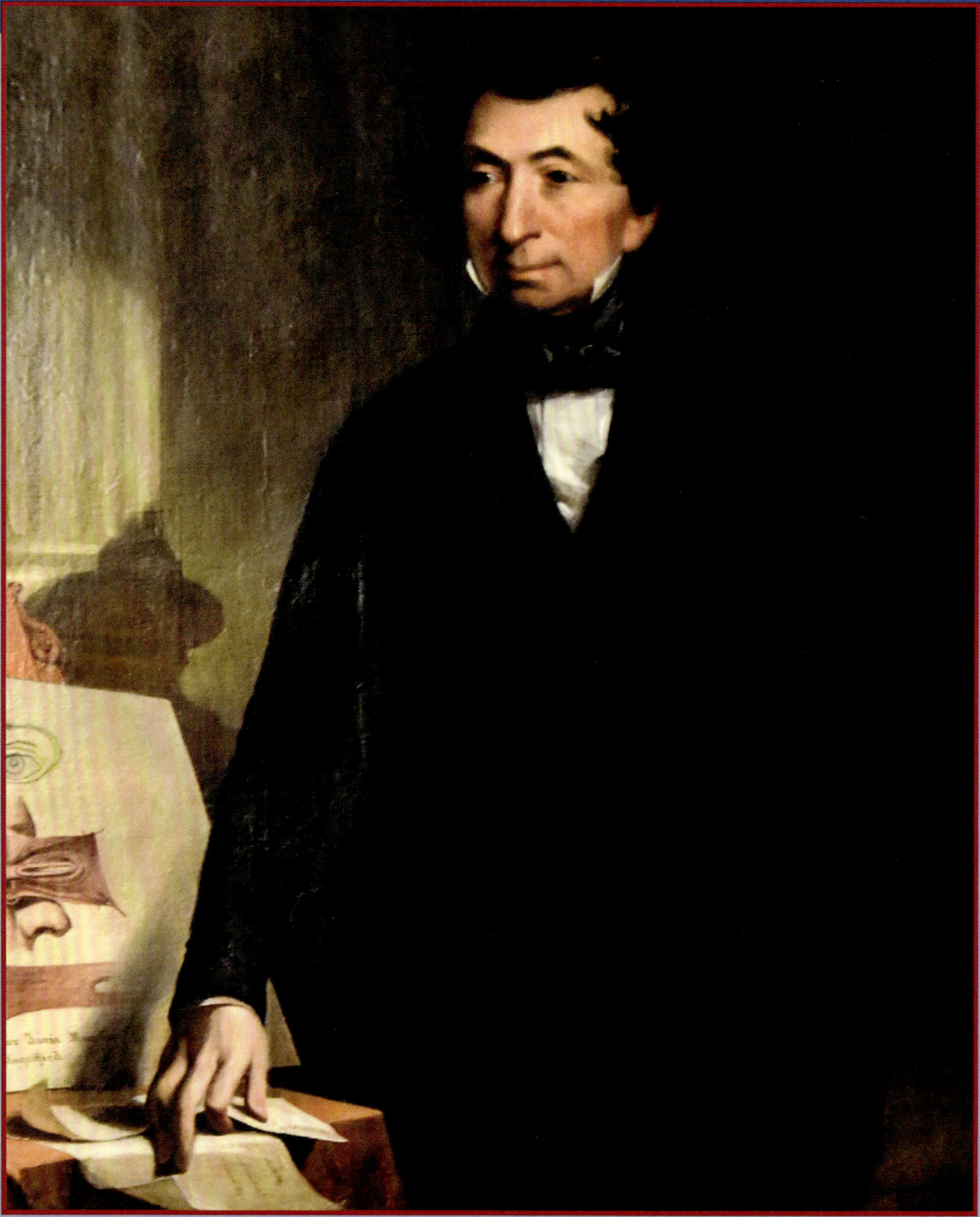

William Edmonds Horner (1793–1853)

Adjunct Professor of Surgery (1822–1831)
Chairman of Anatomy (1831–1853)
Dean (1822–1852)

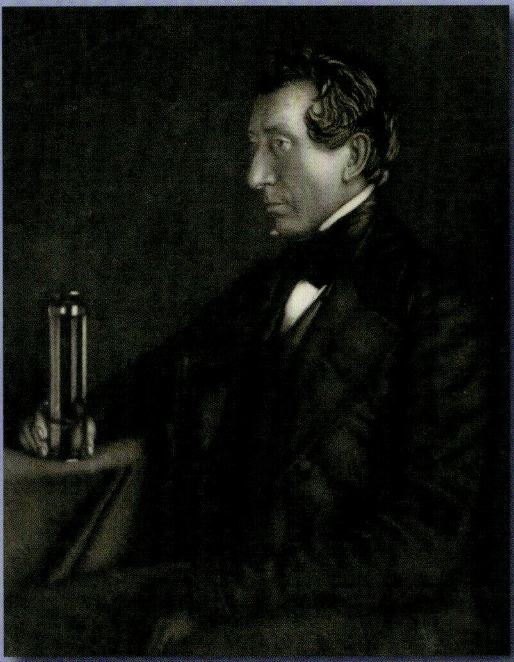

William Horner

It is hard to see why the surgeon William Horner is given little or no notice in the department's archives. He had only an adjunct appointment in the department of surgery but was a key figure in the department of anatomy at a time when surgery and anatomy were essentially interchangeable disciplines. In fact, until this point in the school's history, the department of anatomy had always been headed by a surgeon. Horner was not only one of Philadelphia's best surgeons but was also important to the medical school in the fields of pathology (having written the first American pathology textbook[1]), ophthalmology, anthropology, and administration (longest serving dean). He was also a patriot/soldier, hospital founder, and prolific author.[2]

How he accomplished all that is amazing. From childhood on, he was characterized by himself and others as constitutionally impaired, the victim of daily severe headaches, constant indigestion, and frequent bouts of severe despondency. He described his life as an incessant struggle and claimed that at least a thousand times he had wished himself dead.[3] In addition, his contemporaries rated his intellect as average or below and considered him uninspired to poor as a teacher/lecturer. Yet measured by his accomplishments, he has to be rated as one of the most productive, accomplished, important, and interesting physicians or surgeons of his

1793
Birth of Horner

1812
Volunteers to serve in US Army

1814
MD at Penn

1818
Penn faculty appointment as demonstrator of anatomy for Philip Syng Physick

1818
Wistar dies. Horner catalogues Wistar's collection of human and animal specimens and donates it to become the museum of the Wistar Institute

1821
Studies pathology in France

1822–1831
Adjunct professor of anatomy under Physick

1829
Horner writes first American pathology textbook

1831–1851
Chairman of Department of Anatomy

time, clearly measuring up to or surpassing the department's chairmen in many respects.

The remarkable William Horner was born in 1793 in Warrington, Virginia, and attended private elementary schools near there. He was brought up as an Episcopalian but later in life became a Catholic. After a year of apprenticeship with John Spence, a Virginia physician, he enrolled in medical school at Penn. During the War of 1812, he interrupted his education to volunteer as a surgeon's mate, serving in the Army at Buffalo, New York. Returning to medical school, he graduated in 1814. From 1816 to 1818, he was a dissector under Caspar Wistar. From 1818 to 1820, he was demonstrator of anatomy for Philip Syng Physick and his nephew and assistant, John Syng Dorsey. Following Dorsey's death, he became Physick's backup for many years. In 1821, he studied pathology in France for a year. In 1822, he returned to Philadelphia and was appointed dean of the medical school, serving in this role for thirty years until 1852. Meanwhile, in addition to his surgical practice, he also served as adjunct professor of anatomy under Physick (1822–1831) and then from 1831 to 1851, as chairman of the Department of Anatomy.

As an anatomist, Horner described the tensor tarsi muscle that coordinates eyelid motion with movements of the pupils, the membrane lining the larynx, and how the epiglottis protects the trachea. S. D. Gross, never given to hyperbole, rated him as the best anatomist the country had produced.[4]

As a practicing surgeon, he was the first to successfully repair a severed Achilles tendon (using a seton to stimulate inflammation and healing).[5] In 1837, he described the Z plasty, a procedure still in use by modern surgeons to revise wound scars. In 1843, he collaborated with Physick, Gibson, and Pancoast as the first in Philadelphia to successfully use ether anesthesia. He also collaborated with Physick in describing the extraperitoneal approach for Cesarean sections.

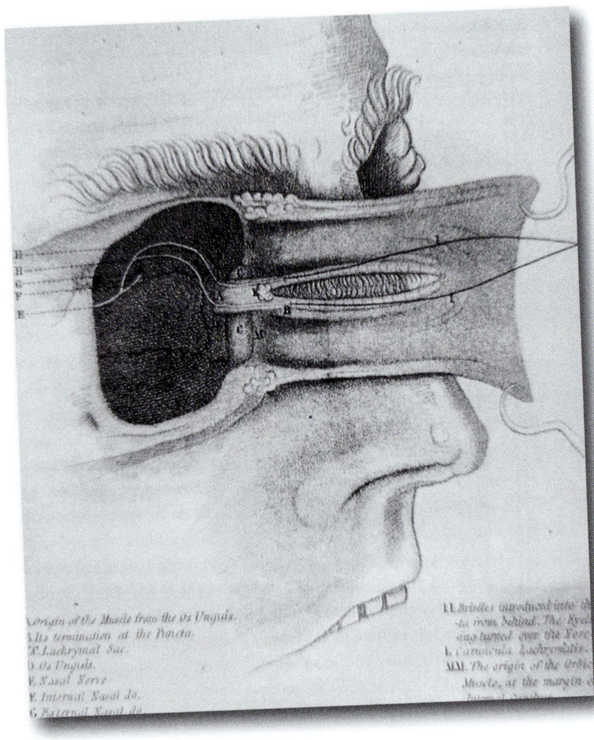

Tensor tarsi muscle

As dean, he was responsible for increasing to 704 the number of required hours of instruction in the medical school curriculum.

In 1849, he founded St. Joseph's Hospital.

As a pathologist in 1832, he studied microscopic

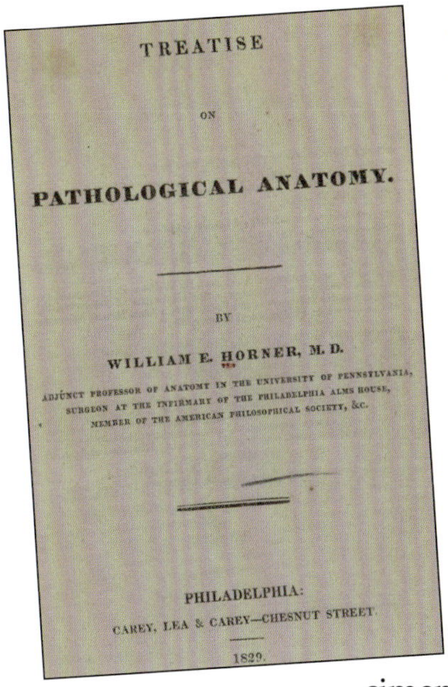

TREATISE

ON

PATHOLOGICAL ANATOMY.

BY

WILLIAM E. HORNER, M. D.

ADJUNCT PROFESSOR OF ANATOMY IN THE UNIVERSITY OF PENNSYLVANIA, SURGEON AT THE INFIRMARY OF THE PHILADELPHIA ALMS HOUSE, MEMBER OF THE AMERICAN PHILOSOPHICAL SOCIETY, &C.

PHILADELPHIA:

CAREY, LEA & CAREY—CHESNUT STREET.

1829.

changes in the intestine occurring during cholera, leading to rice water stools. His 1829 book, *A Treatise on Pathological Anatomy,* was the first pathology text to be published by an American. It was influential as one of the first steps in the United States to use scientific studies to understand disease and its treatment.

As a paleontologist, young Horner joined Caspar Wistar in collecting human and animal specimens for use in their lectures. As Wistar aged, he turned his collection over to Horner who enlarged it and presented over a thousand specimens to the university, whose museum was termed the Wistar-Horner Museum.[6] Eventually, it became the basis of the famous Wistar Institute's collection and museum.

With age, Horner's chronic infirmities became ever harder to bear, and his health continued to decline. He died at age sixty in 1853, probably from a heart attack.

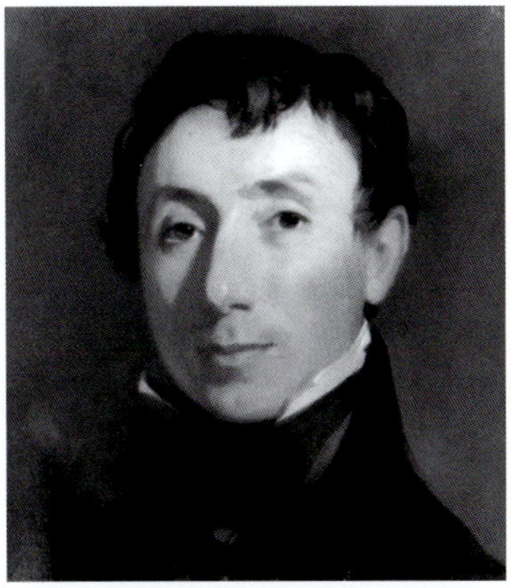

William Horner

1832
Classic microscopic study of intestine during cholera

1853
Death of Horner

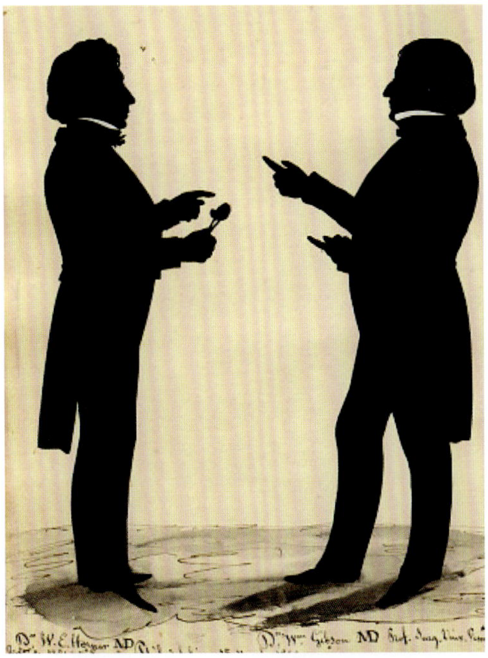

William Horner and William Gibson
March 7, 1843

Notes

[1] Cooper III, David Y, and Ledger, Marshall A. *Innovation and Tradition at the University of Pennsylvania School of Medicine, An Anecdotal Journey* (Philadelphia: University of Pennsylvania Press, 1990) pp. 49–51.

[2] Henry, Frederick P (ed). *Standard History of the Medical Professors of Philadelphia* (Chicago: Goodspeed Brothers Publishers, 1897) pp. 189–190.

[3] Gross, Samuel D. *Autobiography of Samuel D. Gross MD with Reminiscences of His Times and Contemporaries Volume II* (Philadelphia: WB Saunders, 1893) p. 276.

[4] Ibid, p. 274.

[5] Cooper III, David Y, and Ledger, Marshall A. *Innovation and Tradition at the University of Pennsylvania School of Medicine, An Anecdotal Journey* (Philadelphia: University of Pennsylvania Press, 1990) p. 49.

[6] Carson, Joseph: *A History of the Medical Department of the University of Pennsylvania with Sketches of the Lives of Deceased Professors* (Philadelphia: Lindsay and Blakiston, 1869) p. 185.

CHAPTER 6

Unrecognized Administrative Genius of the Union Army

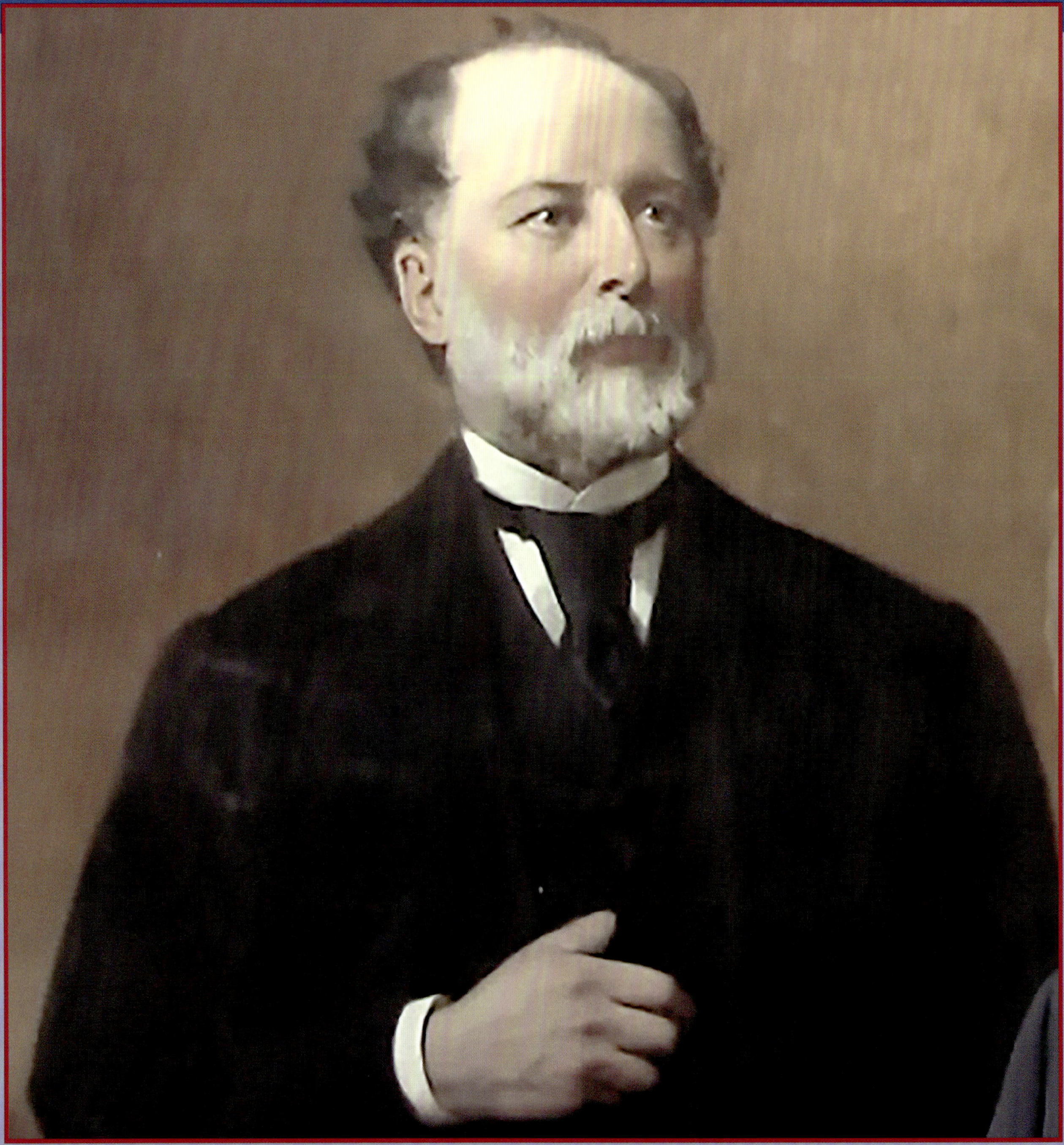

Henry Hollingsworth Smith (1815–1890)

Chairman of Surgery (1855–1871)

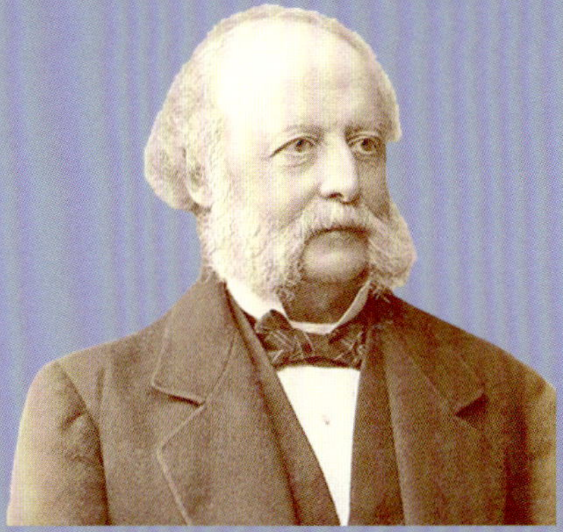

Henry Hollingsworth Smith

Henry Hollingsworth Smith has been pretty much forgotten, even by the surgery department he chaired from 1855 to 1871. Most biographers characterize him as "inconspicuous." Perhaps this is because of his somewhat homely likeness in faded photographs or because we know so little about his personality. This is unfair because a search of the school's archives reveals that Smith had a useful, even distinguished career. This enigmatic chairman was born in Philadelphia and was a graduate of the University of Pennsylvania for college (1834) and medical school (1837). After two years of residency at Pennsylvania Hospital, he polished his education for eighteen months with study in London, Vienna, and Paris. On his return to Philadelphia, he developed a large private practice. He wrote several papers and a book with the medical school's dean, William Horner, whose daughter he married in 1843. In 1849, he joined the faculty at Penn and served mainly as an assistant to Horner.

In 1852, Smith wrote an important book—*A System of Operative Surgery, Based Upon the Practice of Surgeons in the United States: With a Bibliographical Index and Historical Record of Many of Their Operations During a Period of 234 Years.* This book also included an inventory of texts and articles. The medical historian, Ira Rutkow, identifies it as the first systematic and chronological history of American surgery.[1] An additional unique feature is its illustration of operations by photographs (daguerreotypes), many hand colored. The book's multiple reviewers described it as brilliant, including the one from the American Medical Association (AMA). It was praised for its social and political impact and for its important role in establishing surgery as an independent discipline distinct from anatomy, midwifery, and

1815
Smith is born in Philadelphia

1837
MD University of Pennsylvania

1839
After two years training at Pennsylvania Hospital, studies in Europe

1841–1849
Private practice of surgery in Philadelphia

1843
Smith marries Dean Horner's daughter

1849
Appointed to Penn faculty, serves as assistant to Dean Horner

1852
Publishes surgery textbook, the first systematic history of US surgery and the first to illustrate operations in color. It earns favorable reviews, making him famous

1855
Smith is appointed Penn's Surgery chairman. As early as this, D. Hayes Agnew substitutes as lecturer for Smith

1856
Smith publishes another surgery textbook. This one is panned, badly damaging his reputation as a historian and author

1861
Appointed surgeon general of Pennsylvania, requiring him to take leave of absence as chairman. He performs valuable service for Union Army

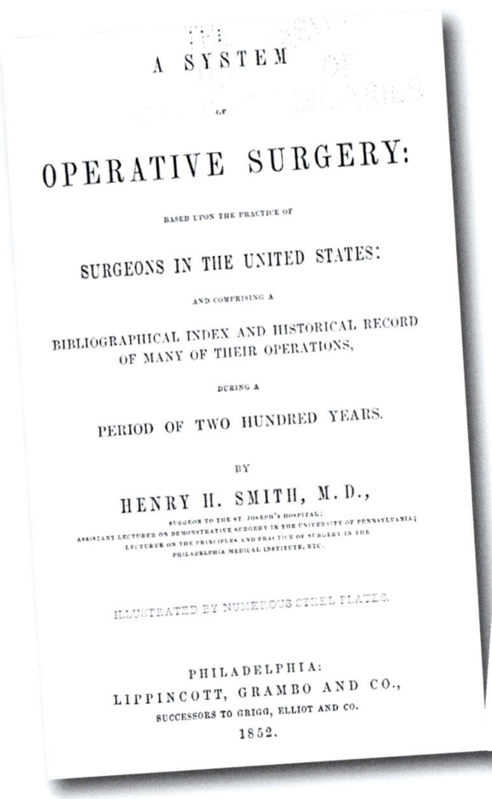
A SYSTEM

OF

OPERATIVE SURGERY:

BASED UPON THE PRACTICE OF

SURGEONS IN THE UNITED STATES:

AND COMPRISING A

BIBLIOGRAPHICAL INDEX AND HISTORICAL RECORD OF MANY OF THEIR OPERATIONS,

DURING A

PERIOD OF TWO HUNDRED YEARS.

BY

HENRY H. SMITH, M.D.,

SURGEON TO THE ST. JOSEPH'S HOSPITAL; ASSISTANT LECTURER ON DEMONSTRATIVE SURGERY IN THE UNIVERSITY OF PENNSYLVANIA; LECTURER ON THE PRINCIPLES AND PRACTICE OF SURGERY IN THE PHILADELPHIA MEDICAL INSTITUTE, ETC.

ILLUSTRATED BY NUMEROUS STEEL PLATES.

PHILADELPHIA:
LIPPINCOTT, GRAMBO AND CO.,
SUCCESSORS TO GRIGG, ELLIOT AND CO.
1852.

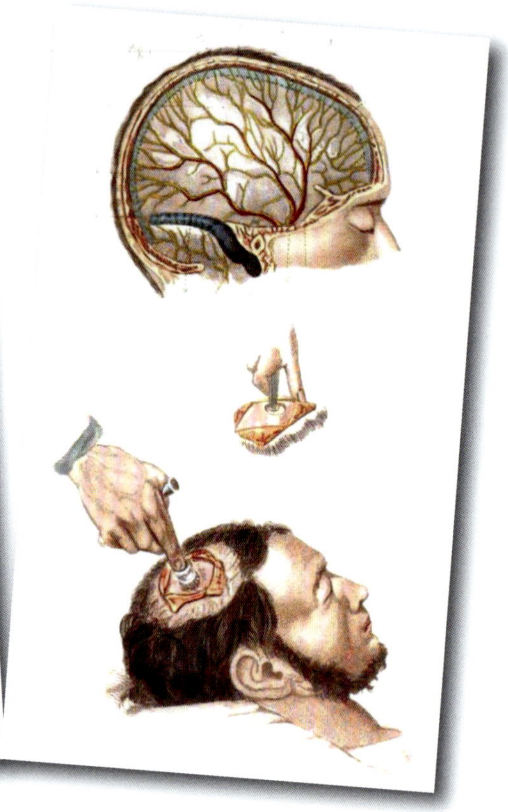

medicine. It may have stimulated the AMA, a few years later, to found a surgical section. Largely on the basis of this well-received book and its establishment of Smith as an authoritative historian, he was, in 1855, promoted at age forty to professor and chairman of Penn's surgery department. It probably didn't hurt that he had married the dean's daughter.

In 1856, Smith published another book, *A Treatise on the Practice of Surgery*. Something had changed. It's hard to understand whether it was style, inadequate research due to demands of the chairmanship, or quite possibly the absence of his career-long supporter and father-in-law, Dean Horner, who by then had died. Whatever the reason, the reviews were scathing and abruptly ruined Smith's reputation as a major historian and scholar.

In 1861, Smith was appointed Pennsylvania's surgeon general and temporarily left his position as chair of surgery. His outstanding military service during this early period of the Civil War deserved to salvage his image and career. Before that, no one had recognized that he was an administrative and organizational genius. He performed very valuable service for the Union Army, virtually transforming care of the wounded soldiers. Amid the chaos of the battles of Williamsburg, West Point, and Cold Harbor, he organized the efficient and safe removal of wounded soldiers from the field for treatment in hospitals of nearby large cities.[2] He arranged to have the dead embalmed on the field, allowing prompt delivery to their families. At the siege of Yorktown, he commandeered a fleet of steamships for use as floating hospitals, effectively evacuating hundreds of casualties.

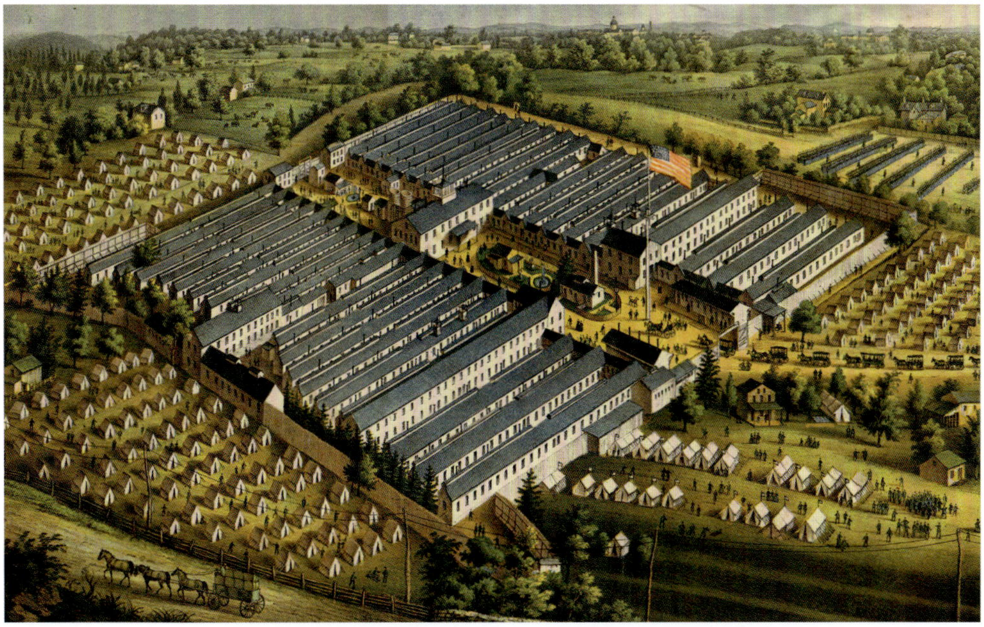

Largest Army hospital, Satterlee (4,500 beds) was located in West Philadelphia, near the present VA Hospital.

1862
Smith returns to civilian life as Penn's chairman of surgery

1862-1865
Isaac Israel Hayes, famous Arctic explorer and Penn graduate, directs Satterlee Army Hospital. It treats 50,000 patients over the course of the war

1870
Agnew resents that Smith had not promoted him for seven years. Agnew threatens to resign

In 1862, after a year in the Army, he resumed his career as Penn's surgery chairman. As a surgeon, Smith was damned with faint praise as thoughtful and conservative, rather than bold and technically aggressive. Still, his colleague, Dean Robert Rogers, chose him as his surgeon when an accident mangled Rogers's right hand, necessitating amputation. A poignant scene is described in which Rogers showed up during one of Smith's lectures to exhibit his nicely healing wound and thank Smith as his surgeon in front of the entire student body.[3] We know little of his relationship with his faculty, but Ira Rutkow describes his style as dictatorial.[4]

Early in their careers, Smith and D. Hayes Agnew appear to have been close companions.[5] As early as 1854, Smith invited Agnew to substitute for him in lectures and clinics, even before Agnew had any association with the university. With Smith's help, Agnew then obtained an entry-level university appointment as a demonstrator in 1863. That, however, proved to be as far as Smith wanted to go in advancing Agnew's career. Over the next seven years, he continued to prevail on Agnew to give many of his lectures and clinics. However, it is notable that he never bothered to secure a promotion for Agnew beyond his low rank as demonstrator of anatomy and surgery. Meanwhile, during these years, Agnew was gradually becoming

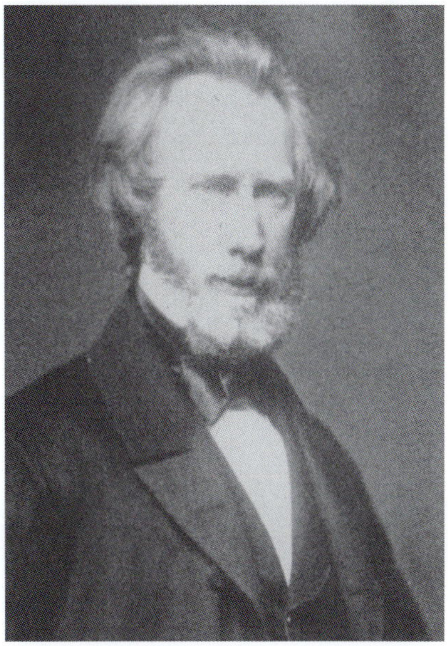

D. Hayes Agnew threatens to resign

1871
Smith is unhappy over the Agnew dispute, resigns as chairman

the most highly experienced and respected surgeon in Philadelphia and was also developing a national reputation. He became recognized as the best teacher of anatomy and surgery that the university had. Eventually, it was clear that his status far surpassed that of Chairman Smith's. The discrepancy between Agnew's faculty rank and his reputation led to resentment of Smith by the students, faculty, alumni, and Agnew himself. Eventually, in 1870, Agnew became so unhappy with the situation that he threatened to resign.[6] It was generally assumed that if he left Penn, he would go to Jefferson, thus strengthening that institution and allowing it to surpass Penn in prestige.

The university could ill afford to lose Agnew, its best teacher and most productive surgeon. His resignation was not accepted. Instead, a special meeting of the faculty was called to elevate Agnew directly from his entry-level position to professor of clinical surgery, a rank essentially equal to that of Chairman H. H. Smith. Not surprisingly, Smith was displeased with this, so much so that within a year (likely under duress), he resigned as chairman. He was only fifty-five years old and would live for another fifteen years.

Despite his significant contributions, Smith never was very much appreciated, perhaps because of conflict with the popular Agnew. He did become president of several medical societies in Philadelphia and Pennsylvania but was never a member of the American Philosophical Society. The school's historian, George W. Corner, called attention to this, emphasizing that Smith was the first professor of any Penn department not elected to this important professional society.[7] Of more significance, he was never elected to membership in the Philadelphia Academy of Surgery or the American Surgical Association.

As a historian, Smith's important contributions have been largely forgotten. Two decades after Smith's acclaimed history of American surgery was published, Samuel David Gross wrote his version of the history of American surgery. In it, he didn't even bother to mention Smith.

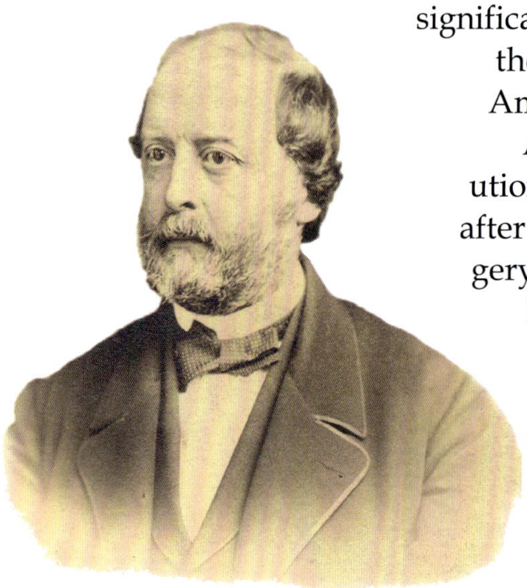

Henry Hollingsworth Smith

Timeline of Events During the Career of Henry Hollingsworth Smith

1810 Thomas Chalkley James becomes Penn's first chairman of midwifery.

1837 Henry Hollingsworth Smith earns MD from University of Pennsylvania.

1837–1839 Two years as resident at Pennsylvania Hospital.

1839–1841 Eighteen months studying in Paris, London, and Venice.

1841–1846 Smith writes book on human dissection, anatomical atlas with Horner, and text on minor surgery.

1843 Smith marries the daughter of Dean William Edmonds Horner.

1849 Smith is appointed junior faculty member at Penn and assists his father-in-law, William Edmonds Horner, the medical school's dean.

1852 Smith publishes *A System of Operative Surgery, Based upon the Practice of Surgeons in the United States: With a Bibliographical Index and Historical Record of Many of Their Operations During a Period of 234 Years*. Positive reviews of the book make him famous.

1853 Dean Horner dies.

1855 Smith is appointed chairman of surgery.

1856 Smith's book, *Treatise on Practice of Surgery*, is unfavorably reviewed, spoiling his reputation as a historian.

1859 John Brown's raid at Harpers Ferry, Virginia. Southern medical students defect from Penn. Led by Hunter McGuire, 119 Jefferson students and 15 from Penn leave for Richmond to continue their medical education. Later, McGuire was Stonewall Jackson's surgeon and years after the war, president of the AMA.

1861–1865 Civil War.

Medical school classes continue during war since more doctors are needed.

Agnew, Smith, John Shaw Billings, and over 1,000 Penn alumni, faculty and students serve—633 in the Union Army; 553 in the Confederate Army. Philadelphia has 10,000 military hospital beds, the most of any city.

Six percent of Union surgeons are Penn graduates; 25 percent of Confederate surgeons are Penn graduates.

Hestonville Army Hospital (Center City) has 200 beds, directed by D. Hayes Agnew.

Two Penn graduates become surgeons general of Union Army—Clement Findley and Joseph Barnes.

A Penn graduate becomes surgeon general of the Confederate army—David Camden de Leon.

Satterlee General Hospital in West Philadelphia at 42nd and Baltimore St. occupies fifteen acres with thirty-four wards, hundreds of tents, and 4,500 beds. It cares for 50,000 patients with only 260 deaths. It is directed by Penn graduate, Isaac Israel Hayes, who had been a famous polar explorer in the Grinnell expedition led by Elisha Kent Kane, another Penn MD.

Mower Hospital in Chestnut Hill occupies twenty-seven acres, with forty-three radiating wards and a 3,600 bed capacity. It cares for 20,000 patients with only 257 deaths. While serving there, D. Hayes Agnew is in charge of half of the surgical patients.

1861–1862	Smith is appointed surgeon general of Pennsylvania and serves with distinction in the Union Army.
	Smith organizes treatment and evacuation of wounded from Battles of Yorktown, Cold Harbor, and Antietam.
1862	Smith returns to Philadelphia and resumes his chairmanship of Penn's department of surgery.
1863	Agnew, after serving as a battlefield and hospital surgeon, returns to his practice in Philadelphia.
1863–1870	Agnew's Penn appointment remains at entry-level as a demonstrator. Smith relies on him as a substitute lecturer, making no attempt to get him promoted.
1865, 1881	Joseph Barnes attends two assassinated presidents—Lincoln and Garfield.
1867	Lister's first paper is published in Lancet on eleven patients with compound fractures successfully treated with antisepsis. His treatment is widely accepted in Europe but not in the United States and England.
1870	Men are admitted to Women's Medical College. In 1993, Women's merges with Hahnemann, and in 2003, it is absorbed by Drexel University.
1870	Agnew threatens to resign unless he is promoted. University calls special faculty meeting to appoint Agnew as professor of clinical surgery.
1871	Smith retires, probably under duress. His rivalry with Agnew has made him unpopular.
1876	US Centennial celebrated. Smith is not asked to participate.
1880	Samuel D. Gross founds Philadelphia Academy of Surgery and American Surgical Association. Smith is never elected to either.
1882	Antisepsis continues to be debated, even at meeting of the American Surgical Association.
1890	Smith dies.

Notes

[1] Rutkow, Ira. Henry Hollingsworth Smith and His Bibliographical Index and Historical Record: The Beginning of American Surgical Historiography. *Annals of Surgery* , 263(4):827–833 (Apr. 2016).

[2] Corner, George W. *Two Centuries of Medicine: A History of the School of Medicine, University of Pennsylvania* (Philadelphia: J.B. Lippincott Company, 1965) p. 117.

[3] Ruschenberger, WSW. *Robert E. Rogers Memoir in Biographical Memoirs of Members of the American Philosophical Society, Physicians Vol I, 1787–1935,* edited by Barker and Starzl (Philadelphia: American Philosophical Society, 2013) p. 92.

[4] Rutkow, Ira. Henry Hollingsworth Smith and His Bibliographical Index and Historical Record: The Beginning of American Surgical Historiography, p. 831.

[5] Adams, J Howe. *Life of D. Hayes Agnew MD LLD* (Philadelphia: FA Davis Company Philadelphia, 1892) p. 141.

[6] Cooper III, David Y and Ledger, Marshall A. *Innovation and Tradition at the University of Pennsylvania School of Medicine, An Anecdotal Journey* (Philadelphia: University of Pennsylvania Press, 1990) p. 117. Adams, J Howe. *Life of D. Hayes Agnew MD LLD,* p. 138.

[7] Corner, George W. *Two Centuries of Medicine: A History of the School of Medicine, University of Pennsylvania,* p. 117.

CHAPTER 7

The Department's Icon: Painting or Man?

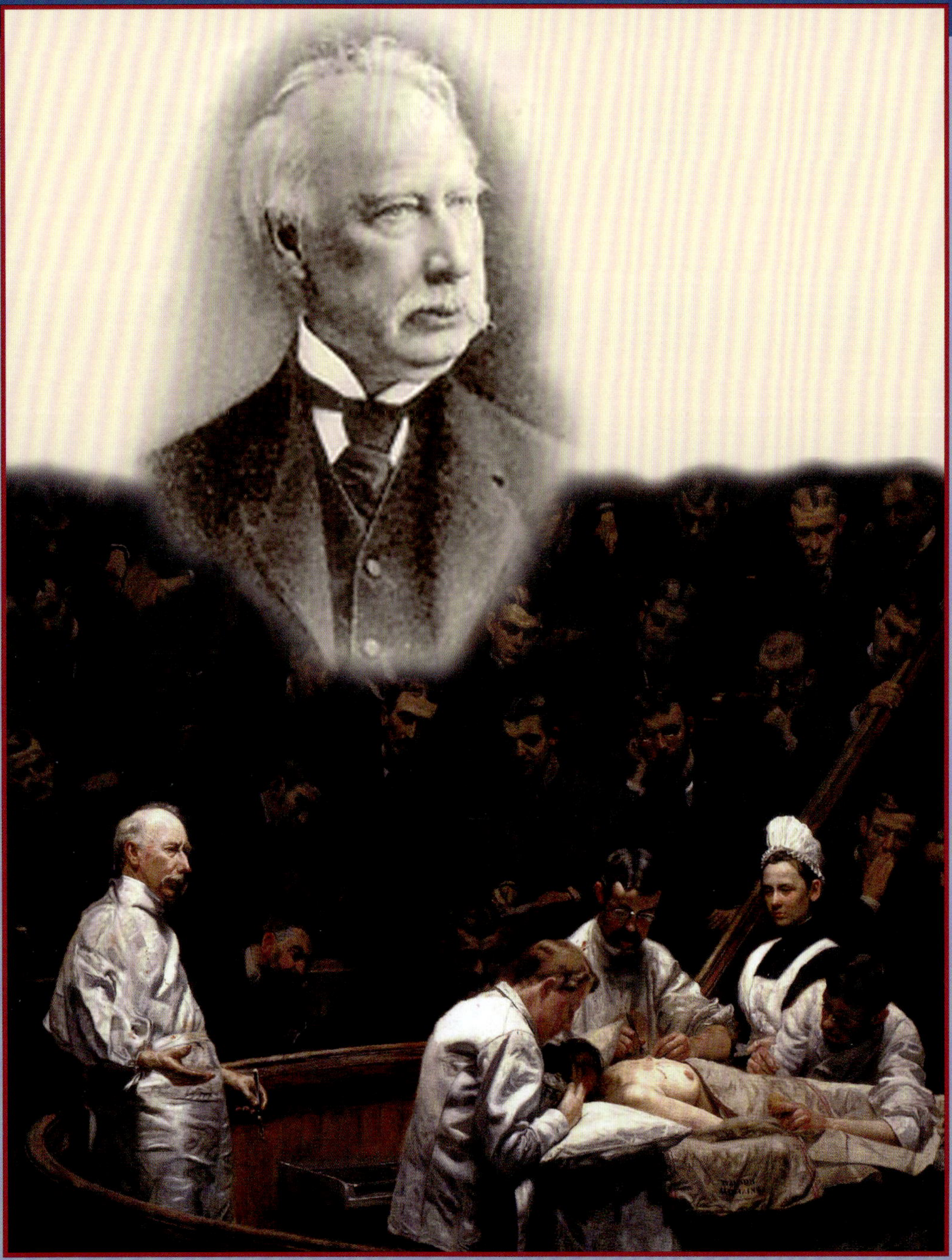

D. Hayes Agnew (1818–1892)

Chairman of Surgery (1871–1889)
John Rhea Barton (JRB) Professor of Surgery (1877–1889)

D. Hayes Agnew is often referred to as our department's iconic figure. When Agnew retired in 1889, Penn's medical students commissioned a portrait of their beloved professor. They couldn't have realized that this would immortalize him. Chosen as the painter was a local artist, now famous but then failing. The $750 fee he got for the painting, *The Agnew Clinic,* helped salvage the career of Thomas Eakins, who at the time was in disrepute, having shortly before lost his job for exposing a nude male model to a class of female students. Ironically, it is now the painting rather than Agnew himself that has become the icon of our department, of the School of Medicine, and even to some extent, of modern surgery itself.

1846–1889

For surgery, the Agnew era is transformative. His years of active practice span the introduction of anesthesia (1846), antisepsis (1867), electric lighting of the operative field (1880s), the Index Medicus of John Shaw Billings to allow a search of surgical literature (1879), the first university teaching hospital for bedside instruction (HUP, 1874), and the first national surgical conference (American Surgical Association, 1880)

Who knows what the iconic painting would be worth today? Its companion piece, *The Gross Clinic,* painted by Eakins thirteen years earlier, recently brought $68 million.[1] This is a story for another day, but it called renewed attention to *The Agnew Clinic.* Before the hype over the value of these two paintings, they were most often discussed by medical historians as representing the transition to modern medicine through the acceptance of antisepsis. The subject of the later painting, D. Hayes Agnew, was our department chairman from 1871 to 1889. A surgical giant in his time, he is now a shadowy figure, mostly forgotten even at our medical school. Few if any students, residents, or faculty know anything about him, except as the subject of Eakins's portrait.

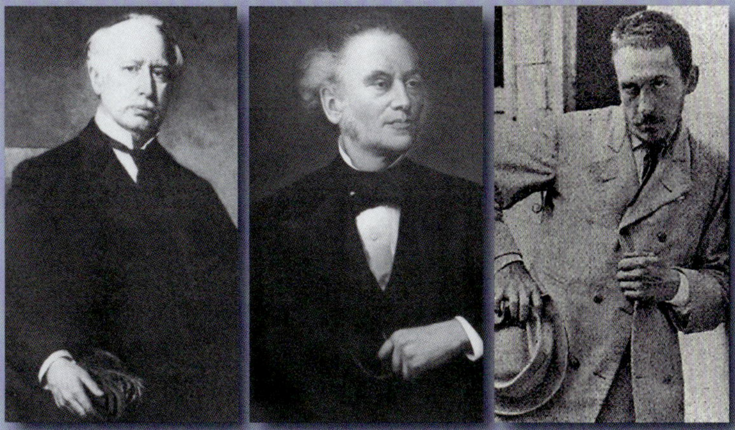

D. Hayes Agnew, S.D. Gross, and Thomas Eakins

1818
Agnew's birth

1838
MD from Penn

1843
Agnew abandons medical career for business venture

1846
Bankruptcy of his iron foundry business, return to medical practice and decision to become a surgeon

1852
Agnew buys School of Anatomy for $600. Begins to dissect and teach anatomy

Even in his day, Agnew modestly avoided notoriety. As a result, he lacked the international fame of the crosstown professor of surgery at Jefferson, the flamboyant Samuel Gross, who was called the "Emperor of Surgery." Agnew deserves better than this.

Nowadays, most of what one hears about Agnew is from the dozens of volumes that art historians have written about him as the subject of the famous Eakins painting. Unfortunately, this considerably obscures the reputation Agnew deserves as a master surgeon, prolific author, and academic leader. The Agnew in the painting is an old man, ready to retire, worn down by a lifetime of long days, sleepless nights, and illness. The other major source of information on him is hyperbole in the rather bland but loving biography written by his nephew, who was one of his students.[2] Agnew's wife carefully supervised and edited this account, probably censoring some of the more interesting parts. Reading between the lines to reconstruct a younger, fully empowered Agnew brings into focus the image of a vigorous man easily capable of competing with the painting as our icon.

Agnew was born and raised near Lancaster, Pennsylvania. His physician father's wealth allowed him to enjoy a carefree youth. His successor, Edward Martin, described him in his eulogy as powerful and athletic, over six feet tall, hard riding, hard reading, and hardworking. "He played the violin, followed the hounds, owned and rode a famous horse, was a lover and trainer of dogs, and was known throughout the countryside as a judge of horses and a dead shot."[3] The family's exalted status was typified by their exhibiting a coat of arms. This was probably responsible for the somewhat aloof, patrician image that Agnew maintained of himself throughout his life. After two years of college, he obtained his MD from Penn in 1838. He then spent several unsatisfying years in general practice with his physician father. This experience was one reason he gave up medicine entirely to manage an iron foundry business that he inherited from his father-in-law.[4]

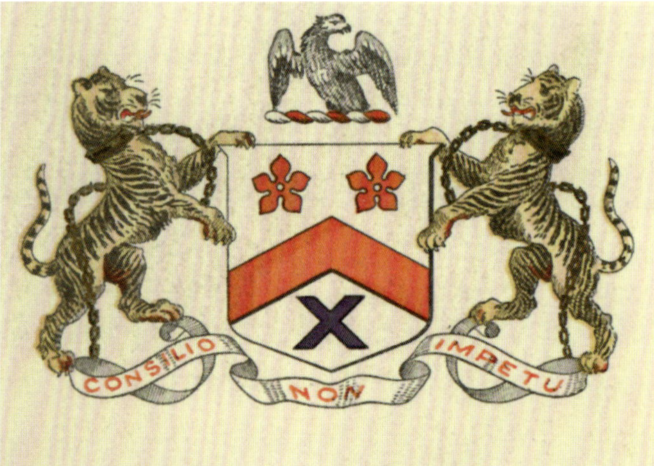

THE AGNEW COAT OF ARMS.

Three years later, when this venture ended in bankruptcy, Agnew decided to pursue a career in surgery. At that time, before there were residencies or formal training programs anywhere, the path to surgery was simply to acquire expertise in anatomy. To accomplish this, in 1852,

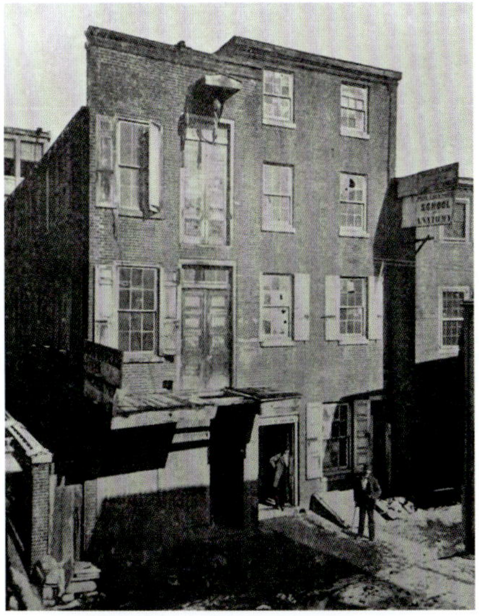

Philadelphia School of Anatomy,
Agnew purchased it for $600.

Agnew purchased the once-famous but now defunct Philadelphia School of Anatomy. He began to dissect, study, and then teach the subject. After hours, since there was no legal way to obtain the cadavers needed for dissection by his students, Agnew became a "resurrectionist"[5] (body snatcher). As a result of hard work and this ghoulish, unlawful activity, Agnew became an expert anatomist. Before long, it was evident that he was also an exceptionally gifted teacher.

During this time, Agnew became a murder suspect when he was found to have in his possession a skull that was perforated by a small round hole.[6] Fortunately, Agnew was able to show that the hole had not been made by a bullet but by a trephine used to treat its owner in life. Later, it became known that to prepare skeletons for student study, Agnew sank cadaver parts in a neighborhood pond where eels did a thorough job of cleaning off the soft tissue from the bones. The owner of the pond sold these eels to a local fish market. They were especially large and were said to have a special "snap" that made them particularly tasty. However, learning this about their diet made the neighbors queasy, and Agnew was forced to abandon this method of preparing bones.

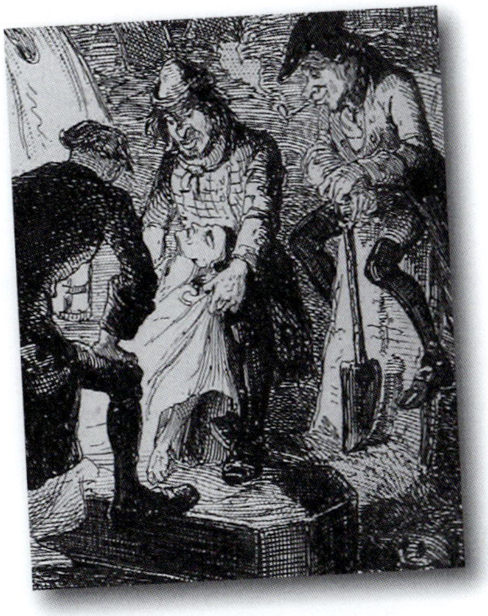

Resurrectionists

As a teacher, Agnew had found at last his true bent. His style was absolutely plain, clear, and very effective. He had none of the eloquence or stagecraft of S. D. Gross. Although ten years older than Agnew, Gross was still at the peak of his fame as a teacher a few blocks away at Jefferson. Nevertheless, because of his effectiveness as a teacher, Agnew began to take students away from Jefferson. Students from Jefferson and other schools enrolled in Agnew's classes, which soon grew from 9 to 267 students. In fact, he eventually had students from all of the nation's states, thirty-four at that time. When he began to practice surgery, it was said that his extraordinary knowledge of anatomy had made him an absolutely confident and precise operator.

His practice interrupted by the Civil War, Agnew acquired a wide reputation as a trauma surgeon. He served on the battlefield during the Battle of Gettysburg. Later, he was assigned to manage 50 percent of the casualties admitted to one of the war's largest Army hospitals, Mower

1852–1863
By dissecting day and night, Agnew teaches himself anatomy and becomes the city's acclaimed instructor in this field

Agnew adds to his anatomy school a school of operative surgery. Aided by his expertise in anatomy, he teaches himself surgery and builds successful practices at Blockley, Pennsylvania Hospital, Wills Eye and Orthopedic Hospitals

1861–1865
Civil War

1871
Appointment as clinical professor and chairman of surgery

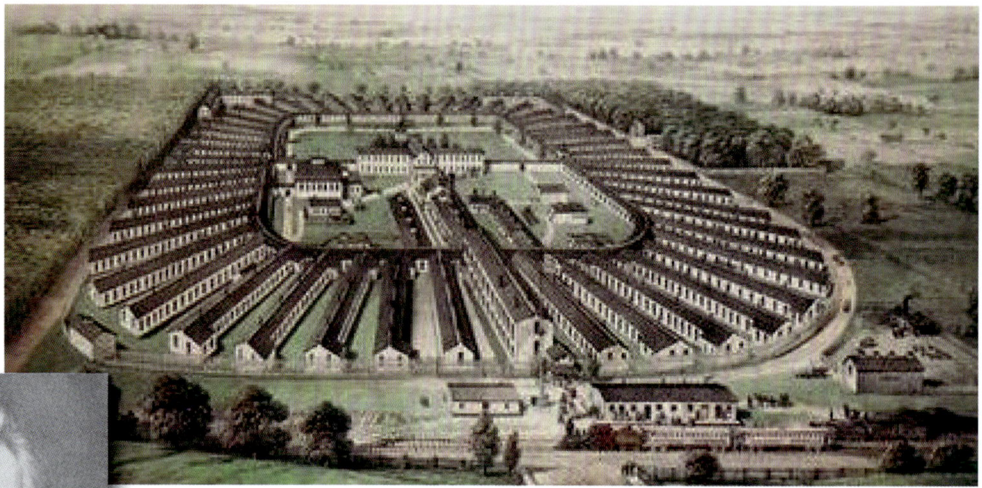

3,600-bed Mower Army Hospital, located in Chestnut Hill

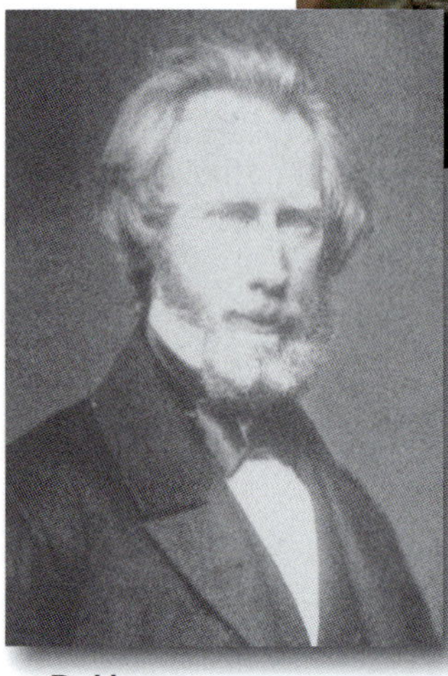

D. Hayes Agnew in 1858.

(3,600 beds), which was in Chestnut Hill.[7] He acquired a reputation as the country's foremost expert on gunshot wounds.

After his Civil War service, Agnew was invited to join the faculty of the University of Pennsylvania. His appointment in 1863 was as a dissector and demonstrator for the chairman, Henry Hollingsworth Smith. Although this appointment was at the lowest level, Agnew was frequently asked to substitute for Smith as a lecturer. Before long, student demand resulted in his being assigned regularly scheduled lectures of his own twice a week. His practice of surgery soon became the largest in the city. It seems likely that Smith took advantage of Agnew's help while keeping him at minimal rank. After seven years with no promotions, Agnew apparently became disappointed and resentful. He submitted his resignation.

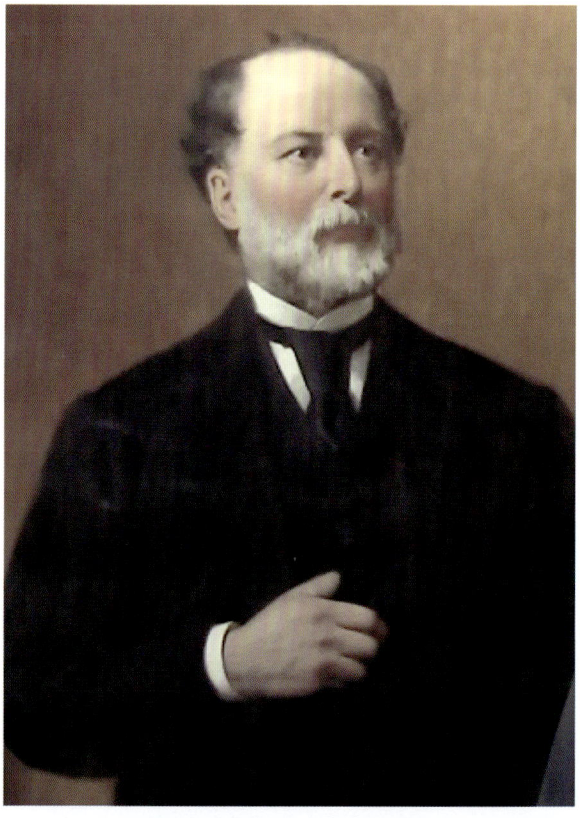

Henry Hollingsworth Smith

The school could hardly afford to lose the faculty member who was its most popular teacher and its most active clinical surgeon. A special meeting of the faculty was called to elect Agnew directly from his entry level rank to full professor.[8] This apparently did not sit well with Smith, who resigned a year later. Agnew was then appointed to succeed him as chairman in 1871. During his tenure, the university built HUP, the country's first teaching hospital, in 1874; and in 1877, appointed Agnew as John Rhea Barton Professor, the country's first endowed chair of surgery.[9] Since then, the John Rhea Barton Professorship has been synonymous with the department chair.

1874
HUP opens. Bedside teaching begins

1876
At the US Centennial, Lister lectures on antisepsis. Some enlightened US surgeons follow his teaching. Others are not convinced, and the argument over antisepsis goes on for more than another decade

As an operating surgeon, Agnew was ambidextrous, deft, and swift in his manipulations without seeming to be. Students crowded to watch his demonstrations, especially if he was cutting for bladder stone. His colleague, Edward Martin, described the scene: "When a patient was prepared with the grooved staff passed into the bladder, Agnew would make one ample peroneal cut into the posterior urethra, drop his sharp pointed knife, *take from his teeth his blunt pointed one,* make with it one further ample cut through a lateral lobe of the prostate, insert his forceps, and remove the stone in less than six seconds, with a deceptive appearance of deliberation." [10]

1877
John Rhea Barton's widow endows professorship in her late husband's name. Agnew is appointed John Rhea Barton Professor

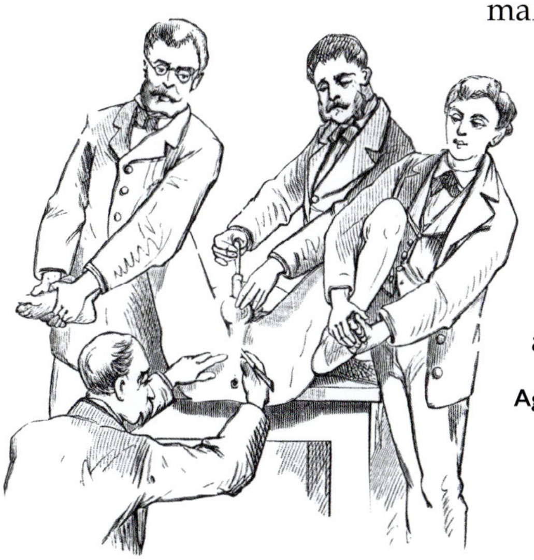

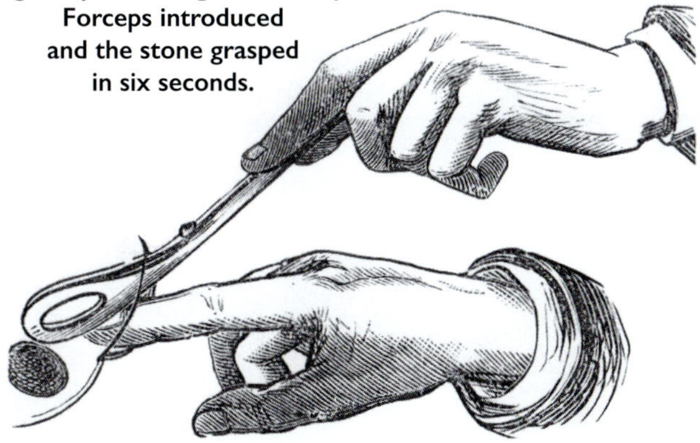

Agnew performing a lithotomy. Forceps introduced and the stone grasped in six seconds.

Agnew was not an experimentalist. His surgical innovations were limited to a few instruments, splints, and an operation for webbed fingers. His local reputation was based on his skill and judgment as a highly experienced clinical surgeon. His national and international reputation was secured by his very successful 3,000 page, three-volume, single-authored textbook of surgery. It replaced Gross's earlier text as the standard for the United States and was translated into several languages, including Japanese. Agnew was a superb teacher with a style that was the opposite of Gross's. As a lecturer, his delivery was simple and straightforward, well-organized, calm, and very effective. Unlike Gross, he was not a dramatist. His unassuming and, by comparison to Gross, somewhat colorless personality and his distaste for political ambition kept him in Gross's shadow. Despite this, many honors came to him, including the presidencies of the College of Physicians of Philadelphia, the Philadelphia Academy of Surgery, and the American Surgical Association.

1878
1881
1883
Agnew's three-volume, 3,000-page, single-author textbook is published. It becomes the most popular surgical text.

1881
President Garfield is shot.

Thirty-six hours later, Agnew is summoned from Philadelphia.

Agnew gives up much of his practice and devotes himself largely to care of the president

Congress eventually awards Agnew $5,000 for his service

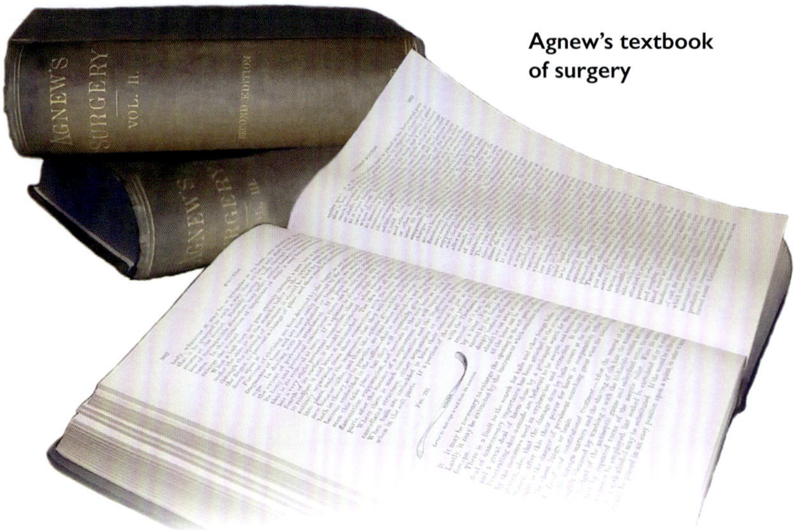

Agnew's textbook of surgery

In 1881, a tragic event would propel Agnew into international fame. On July 2, two hundred days after he was inaugurated, President James Garfield, while walking through a Washington train station, was shot in the back by a "deranged political hack."[11] The president fell to the floor in shock and within minutes was surrounded by local doctors. To evaluate his wound, they at once probed it with unwashed fingers. One inserted a long, unsterile probe which he envisioned to follow the course of the bullet through the liver.

These doctors should have known better. By this time, European surgeons and a great many enlightened US surgeons were practicing anti-

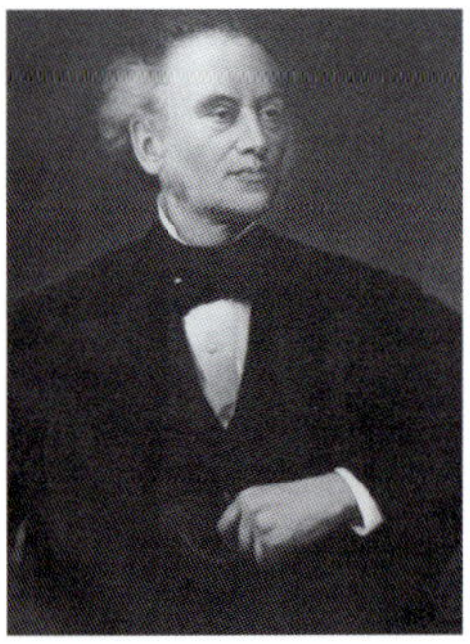

Samuel D. Gross Jefferson's chief of surgery, the most famous and influential surgeon of the time. He was called the Emperor of Surgery.

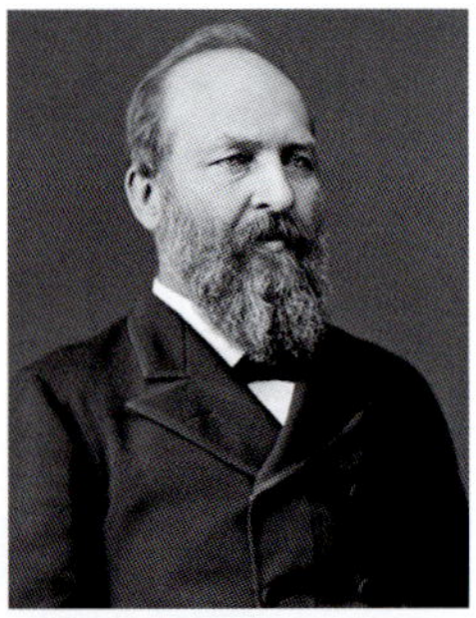

President James Abram Garfield

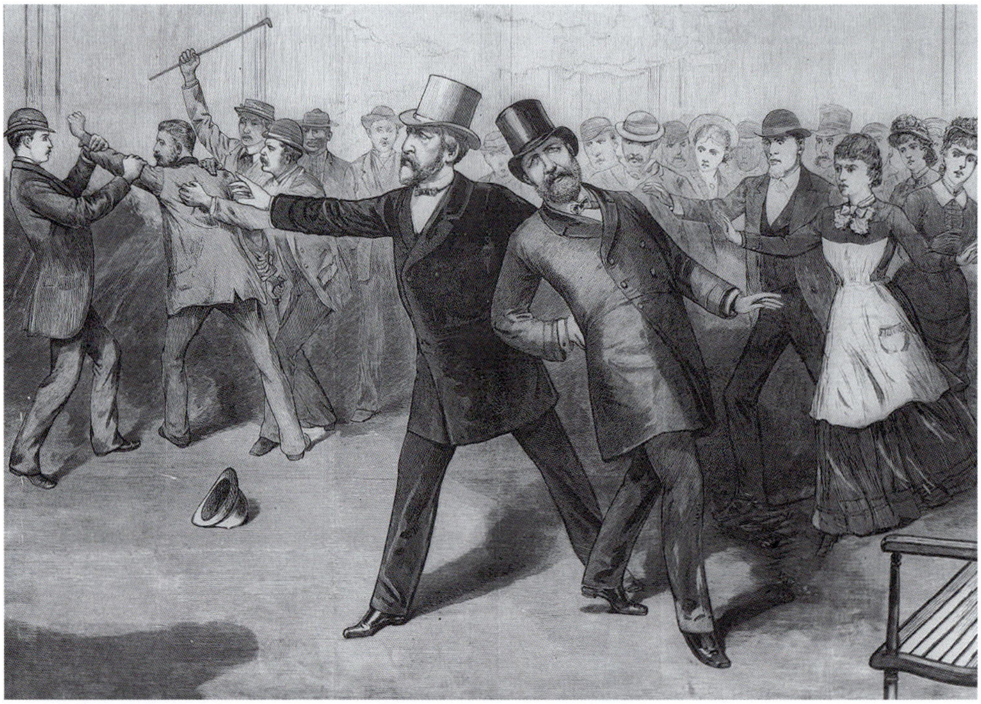

President Garfield is shot by Charles J. Guiteau.

septic methods, despite the opposition of Samuel D. Gross who disputed the usefulness of Lister's antiseptic methods. When the president's wound was not promptly fatal, as his doctors had initially assumed it would be, he was moved to the White House, where the wound was further probed by many of the sixteen doctors who would eventually attend him. The bullet was not located by probing, but the obsession with finding it never ceased. The president's doctors even called in Alexander Graham Bell for what proved to be an unsuccessful attempt to locate the bullet with Bell's metal detector.[12]

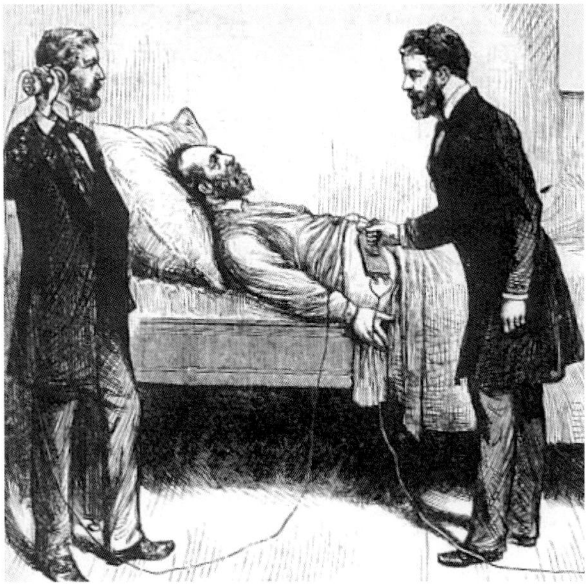

Alexander Graham Bell searching for the bullet with his metal detector.

Obsession for finding the bullet

Operation to remove the bullet is considered too dangerous

Agnew operates on the president but only to drain abscesses

Thirty-six hours after he was shot, Garfield's doctors finally decided they needed to consult a gunshot wound expert. They sent to Philadelphia for Agnew who came at midnight. His train broke a record for high speed, but by then it was too late for his expertise to make any difference. The early, unsterile probing of the wound had already set in motion a lethal infection. Over the next eighty days, Agnew operated on the

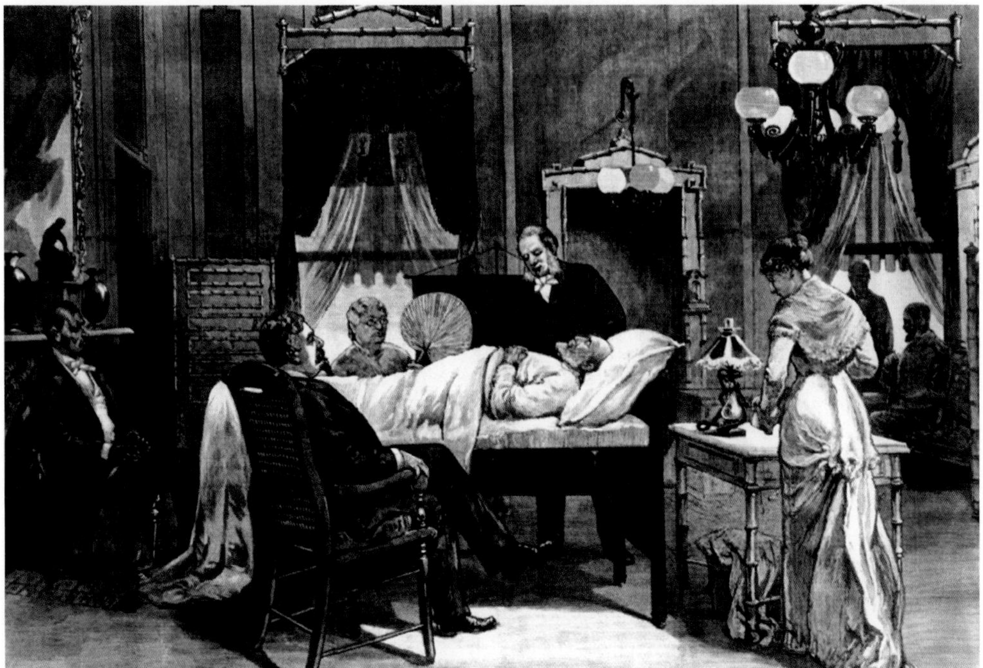

President Garfield on his deathbed. Agnew is seen on the left in the window.

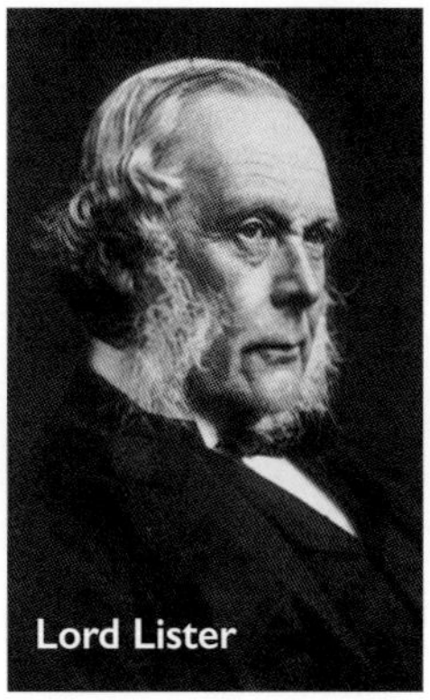

Lord Lister

1875
Thomas Eakins paints *The Gross Clinic*

president several times but only to drain superficial abscesses. Racked with fever and unable to eat, the president lost nearly 100 pounds. Despite attempts to provide nutrition, attempted even by the rectal route, he continued to deteriorate, and he died.[13]

President Garfield's medical case was the first one to be extensively reported in newspapers around the world. Many of them severely criticized the management and his doctors (including Agnew), arguing perhaps correctly that the president would have lived if someone had had the sense to place a small dressing over the bullet hole instead of probing and contaminating it. Of course, the outcome had been determined by unsterile probing of the wound long before Agnew was consulted.

Although Gross was not consulted in the Garfield case, by his influential opposition to the germ theory and antisepsis, he probably had more to do with the president's death than Agnew. In 1876, at the Centennial Exposition of the United States, the widely influential Gross had denied the usefulness of antiseptic technique in a famous debate with Lister. Gross, in fact to the end of his life (1884), never accepted antisepsis or the germ theory. On the other hand, Agnew may have been one of the first to accept Lister's principles[14] and to accept antisepsis. But other indications suggest that during most of his career he was not an "antiseptic surgeon."

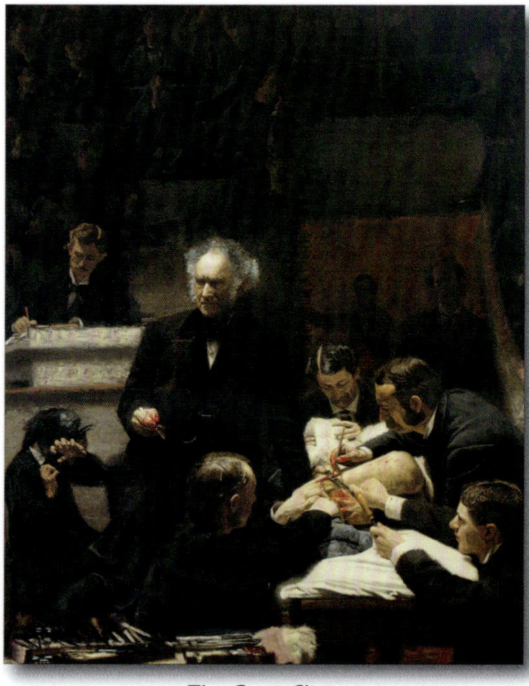

The Gross Clinic
The painting is rejected by Philadelphians as too graphic.

Privately, Agnew would have agreed with the Garfield assassin's unsuccessful defense at his trial that although he shot the president, it was the doctors who killed him. But characteristic of Agnew's personality and aloof image of himself and his profession, he refused to dignify the critics with any response or explanation of this opinion. To newspaper reporters, he simply said, "No comment." To others, he said, "I prefer to stand with my professional brethren."[15]

In his textbook, the section on gunshot wounds makes it clear that Agnew would not have approved of the president's early treatment. It reads:

> All probes should be subjected to the antiseptic bath of carbolized water. A great deal of unnecessary importance has been attached to the extraction of balls and a great deal of harm done by a search

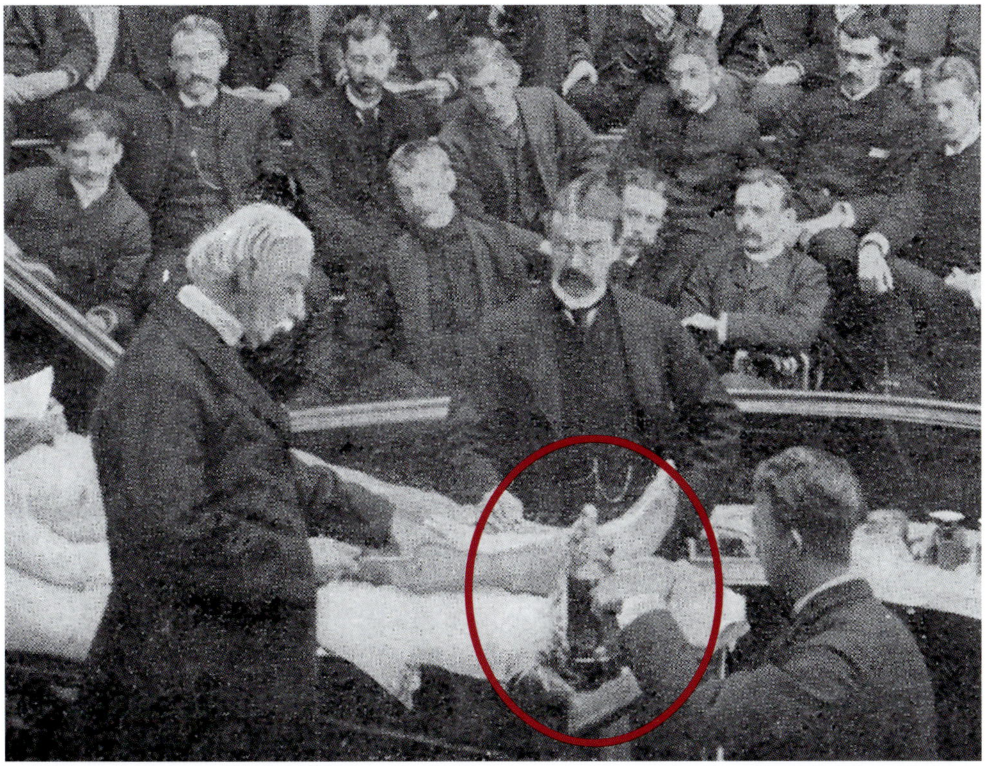

In this undated photograph, Agnew is employing Lister's device to spray antiseptic solution on the wound and into the air. However, Agnew and his assistants are garbed in unsterile street clothes.

1862
J. William White writes detailed review of the case for the newspapers, defending Agnew's decisions and actions

> for missiles. Penetrating shot wounds are aseptic and become septic only by measures used in exploration and extraction. The damage done by balls occurs at the time of their entrance; after this their power for harm is comparatively trifling.[16]

In J. William White's extensive review of the case,[17] he denies claims of others that Agnew explored the wound with his fingers or probes or believed that such maneuvers would be of any use in locating the bullet. White's account goes on to describe the autopsy findings in which the splenic artery aneurysm and fractured vertebra were discovered. The terminal event was rupture of a splenic artery aneurysm that was probably due to injury of the artery by the bullet (although some suggested it could have been caused by a probe). Any small chance that this injury in the artery was minor enough to heal was precluded by the extensive infection in nearby tissues that was the result of early unsterile probing of the wound. In any event, the president was already rapidly dying from his systemic infection before the aneurysm ruptured.

Eight years after the assassination, while Eakins was painting his portrait, criticism of Agnew over management of the Garfield case had been forgotten or assigned to others. Gross had been dead for five years. William Halsted, who would soon be considered America's greatest surgeon, had only just arrived in Baltimore at the new Johns Hopkins Hospital and was not yet famous. During this in-between period, Agnew

1889
The Agnew Clinic painted by Thomas Eakins at the time of Agnew's retirement

was now Philadelphia's, and perhaps the nation's, preeminent surgeon. Thus in 1889, similar to the situation with *The Gross Clinic* fourteen years earlier, Eakins had an opportunity to paint a "big picture" of a famous surgeon.

Analogous in subject and size (6 1/2 × 11 feet) to the earlier *The Gross Clinic,* the painting of *The Agnew Clinic* is strikingly different in every other way.[18] The obvious differences noted by art historians relate to the progress in science and medicine that had taken place during the fourteen-year interval. The entire *Agnew Clinic* scene is brightly and diffusely illuminated by newly invented electric lights. This was advantageous for surgery, but for a painting it was less dramatic than the natural sunlight that Eakins so effectively focused on Gross's face and bloody hand while leaving much of the rest of the scene dimly lit. A second obvious difference is that Agnew and his assistants are garbed in clean, white gowns, rather than Gross's dirty, blood-stained street clothes, and that they are observing sterile technique.

Other less obvious contrasts are perhaps even more interesting but cannot be recognized without understanding the background personalities and careers of the two surgeons. Eakins's genius was the diagnosis and depiction of a subject's character. With Agnew, he is on target, show-

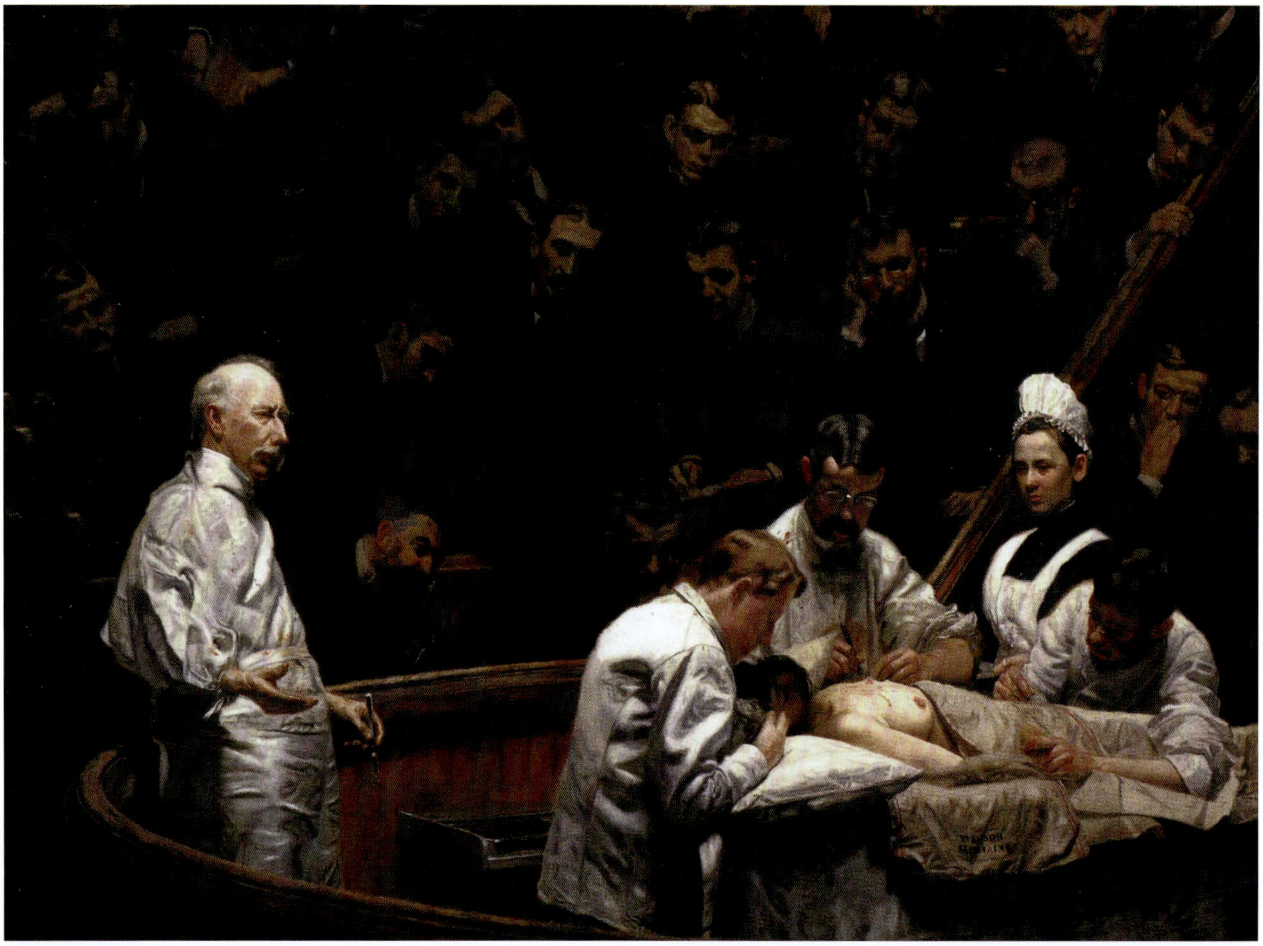

The Agnew Clinic

ing that, unlike Gross, this surgeon is not a showman. Agnew abhorred the theatrical. His teaching style is plain and clear. As an operator, he is not flashy but instead deliberate, precise, and safe. In his operating room, unlike Gross's, there is no excitement, no melodrama. Instead, everything appears to be calm, routine, and under control. This is certainly as we would want it to be if we were the patient being operated upon. But because the scene lacks the excitement and drama of the Gross operating theater, it is not as interesting nor considered as great a painting.

In his spotless white gown, Agnew is patrician. He purposely avoids dramatic effect. To Agnew—the prototypic Victorian gentleman—decorum, quiet dignity and propriety are everything. Bloody hands don't fit the image. He insisted over Eakins's strong objection that the artist paint out the blood that had originally been shown on his hands.[19] The ambidextrous Agnew holds a clean scalpel in his left hand. He appears to have finished his part in the operation. He has stepped away from the operating table, distancing himself from any unpleasantness or discomfort that the operation itself might suggest. Rather than focusing attention on himself, he modestly acknowledges the importance of his team, including a nurse. As compared to *The Gross Clinic,* the painting suffers from its lack of melodrama, theatricality, and yes, even from the lack of blood.

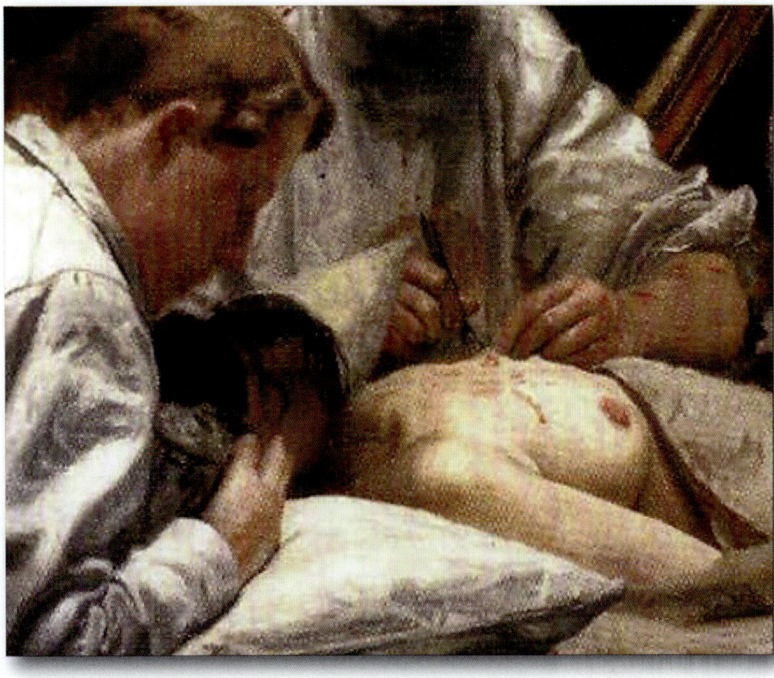

Eakins's commitment to realism dictated that, rather than flattering Agnew, he portray him as he was, aging and perhaps even a bit dull. At the time of his retirement, the voltage had gone down in the seventy-one-year-old Agnew.[20] One wishes that Eakins could have painted him as a younger man, perhaps as a Civil War battlefield surgeon, while robbing graves to provide cadavers for his students, or while cutting for bladder stone, holding in his teeth his second knife.

Except for one important detail, Philadelphia Victorians might have applauded *The Agnew Clinic* as evidence that Eakins had learned his lesson from the previous criticism of *The Gross Clinic.* Instead, *The Agnew Clinic* was rejected. The important detail was the choice of operation shown, a mastectomy. The art critics labeled it "repulsive to the public and not cheerful for ladies to look at."[21] Although some art historians have assumed that this was his signature operation, in fact this procedure was one Agnew hated, an operation he believed was never curative.

He would only resort to a mastectomy to get rid of an ugly lesion of far-advanced cancer. It was an operation that, for him, carried a 10 percent operative mortality, a 60 percent chance of local recurrence, and only a 9 percent chance of long-term survival.[22]

Despite Eakins's reputation for realism, his obsession for nude women prevailed, with the result that he did not portray the operation realistically. We know from the diary of Nurse Mary Clymer, who is depicted as an assistant in the operation, that when Agnew did perform a mastectomy, he always carefully covered the woman's other breast.[23] Who then was likely to choose this operation: the professor who hated the operation or the artist who loved to paint the naked female?

Agnew's idea of a good time was to spend Sundays after church quietly at home in study of the scriptures and a few hymns. Although he loved and could recite passages from Shakespeare, Agnew would never attend the theater, which he considered "a symptom of moral deterioration of the community." He resigned from the staff of Pennsylvania Hospital rather than teach a class attended by female students—not wishing to embarrass them by discussion of sexually transmitted diseases.[24] Epitomized and constrained by Victorian values, Agnew was universally admired and loved by his contemporaries. A review of his life reveals virtually nothing to criticize. By today's standards, he might be considered slightly boring, especially as the old man of Eakins's *The Agnew Clinic.* But in his day, the younger Agnew was anything but dull. He, rather than the painting, deserves to be our department's icon.

Timeline of Events During the Career of D. Hayes Agnew

1818–1833	Carefree youth as member of wealthy family.
1833–1835	Agnew attends Jefferson College in western Pennsylvania (1833–34) and Newark College in Delaware (1834–35).
1838	MD from Penn, followed by two years in general practice with physician father.
1843–1846	Agnew abandons medicine for business. He goes bankrupt and decides to become a surgeon.
1852–1862	Agnew buys a defunct, private anatomy school and teaches anatomy and surgery there. This is the extent of his training in surgery. He becomes such a good teacher that he attracts students from every state.
1858	Agnew frequently substitutes for Penn's chairman Smith as a lecturer.
1861–1863	Agnew is a Civil War battlefield surgeon and director of one of the war's largest hospitals in Philadelphia.
1863	Agnew is appointed "demonstrator" at Penn. After he is kept at this lowest level of faculty rank for seven years, he threatens to resign.
1867	Lister's first paper on the success of antisepsis. The two decades of American refusal to accept Listerism overlap the time period that Agnew serves as chairman of Penn Surgery. Antisepsis is still hotly debated at the 1882 meeting of the American Surgical Association and is not fully accepted until Agnew is ready to retire in 1889. It is a shameful story.
1871	D. Hayes Agnew is appointed clinical professor of surgery in 1870 after threatening to resign because for seven years he had received no promotions, despite being the most respected teacher of surgery and having the largest practice of surgery in the city. Concern that he might move to the rival medical school, Jefferson, encourages trustees to appoint him first as clinical professor and, a year later, as a university professor and chairman of the department of surgery.
1871	John Rhea Barton dies. Shortly thereafter, his wife makes a gift of $50,000 to the university for a professorship in surgery. His is a famous name because this chair is always held by the University of Pennsylvania's chairman of surgery. This obscures the fact that Barton was an outstanding surgeon in his own right.
1874	Largely through the fundraising and efforts of William Pepper Jr., the nation's first university-owned teaching hospital (HUP) is opened. A group of clinical professors are appointed to do bedside teaching. Agnew becomes one of them, and then a university professor as well as the chairman of the department.

1874–1904	Penn's Medical School moves to Medical Hall at 36th and Spruce St.
1875	Thomas Eakins paints *The Gross Clinic*. Most critics condemn it.
1876	The United States centennial celebration features a world's fair in Philadelphia directed by William Pepper Jr. and is attended by many thousands of visitors. Eakins's painting, *The Gross Clinic*, is exhibited at the fair, but because it is too graphic for Philadelphians, it is hidden in an out-of-the-way military building. At the Centennial, Lord Lister gives a lecture promoting antisepsis, but S. D. Gross and most American surgeons are not convinced.
1877	Agnew is appointed John Rhea Barton Professor.
1877	Dissection becomes part of the medical school curriculum (fourteen hours per week). Before this, anatomy was taught only by lecture.
1880	S. D. Gross founds American Surgical Association and Philadelphia Academy of Surgery.
1881	William Pepper Jr. becomes provost. Optional fourth year is added to medical school curriculum.
1881	President Garfield is assassinated. D. Hayes Agnew is called to take care of him, but earlier contamination of his wound by his doctors has already made his death from sepsis inevitable.
1882	Nathan Francis Mossell is the first Black graduate of the medical school.
1884	In New York, Halsted begins study of local anesthesia with cocaine; becomes addicted.
1884	William Osler is recruited to the Penn faculty by William Pepper Jr. He works at Blockley, mainly in pathology. Emphasizes bedside teaching.
1885	Edward Muybridge comes to Penn, collaborates with neurology chairman, Francis Dercum, in motion studies, the forerunner of movies.
1887	Philadelphia surgeon Thomas Morton performs the first appendectomy in which the diagnosis of appendicitis is made preoperatively. Earlier, other Americans, Fitz, Bull, Sands, and McBurny made contributions. Their operations were mainly on perforated appendices.
1889	Eakins paints *The Agnew Clinic*. Agnew retires. Osler moves to the new Johns Hopkins Hospital in Baltimore that is designed by John Shaw Billings, who will become a University of Pennsylvania faculty member in 1891. Both Osler and William Halsted start residencies, which are the prototype of the modern specialty training programs in medicine and surgery.
1889	Department of orthopaedics founded, splitting it from surgery. DeForest Willard is chairman.
1892	Agnew dies.

Notes

[1] S. Salisbury. City Art Icon About to be Sold, *Philadelphia Inquirer*, 11 November 2006 A01, A11.

[2] Adams, J. Howe. *History of the Life of D. Hayes Agnew MD LLD* (Philadelphia: FA Davis Company Philadelphia, 1892).

[3] Martin, Edward. D. Hayes Agnew. *Surgery, Gynecology and Obstetrics* (Feb 1928) p. 2.

[4] Adams, J. Howe. *History of the Life of D. Hayes Agnew MD LLD* (Philadelphia: FA Davis Company Philadelphia, 1892) pp. 71–72.

[5] University of Pennsylvania Archives.

[6] Adams, J. Howe. *History of the Life of D. Hayes Agnew MD LLD* (Philadelphia: FA Davis Company Philadelphia, 1892) pp. 71–72.

[7] Adams, J. Howe. *History of the Life of D. Hayes Agnew MD LLD* pp. 131–135.

[8] Cooper III, David Y and Ledger, Marshall A. *Innovation and Tradition at the University of Pennsylvania School of Medicine, An Anecdotal Journey* (Philadelphia: University of Pennsylvania Press, 1990) p. 117.

[9] Morton, Thomas G. *History of the Pennsylvania Hospital 1751–1895* (Philadelphia: Times Printing House, 1897) p. 504.

John Rhea Barton was a nephew of Benjamin Smith Barton (prof. of materia medica at Penn). He never had a University of Pennsylvania faculty appointment, but he was a prominent member of the staff of Pennsylvania Hospital where he practiced actively from 1823 to 1836. He had obtained his MD from Penn in 1818 and then was an apprentice at Pennsylvania Hospital from 1813 to 1818. He was said to be a fine clinical surgeon with an emphasis on mechanical innovations. His name is associated with a figure-of-eight bandage of the head for treatment of fractures of the mandible and to a fracture of the distal radius. He is credited with creating a pseudoarthrosis to act as an artificial hip joint for disabling ankylosis. He also developed a bran dressing to absorb drainage from the wound of compound fractures.

Barton retired in 1840, having accumulated enough money from his practice to fund a thirty-year retirement. Shortly after his death, his wife's gift to the university funded what became the country's first endowed chair in surgery.

[10] Martin, Edward. *D. Hayes Agnew,* p. 5.

[11] Stanley-Brown, EG. The Location of the President's Bullet. *Proceedings of the Charaka Club* (1985) 12:45–104.

[12] Frank Leslie's *Illustrated Newspaper*, Vol 52, No. 1351 (20 Aug, 1881) 412–13.

[13] Reyburn, R. Clinical History of the Case of President James Abram Garfield. *JAMA* (1894) XXII(17): 621–624. The autopsy revealed that the bullet, after entering to the right of the spine, fractured the eleventh and twelfth ribs. It then traversed the body of the first lumbar vertebra, before traveling to the left, where it lodged retroperitoneally, inferior to the pancreas. It was firmly encased in the scar tissue and could have caused no further trouble. Nearby were extensive intraperitoneal and retroperitoneal abscesses. The immediate cause of death appeared to be a ruptured splenic artery aneurysm.

[14] DaCosta, JC. Biographical Sketch of Professor Samuel D Gross. *Proceedings of the American Philosophical Society* (Jan. 1885) pp. 78–85.

Samuel D. Gross was as great a surgeon as the United States produced in the nineteenth century. His colleagues referred to him as the "Emperor of American Surgery." Not surprisingly, the memoir written by his disciple Dr. DeCosta omits an important blemish on Gross's otherwise stellar care—his stubborn and highly influential opposition to antisepsis. Also not mentioned in the memoir is the reason Dr. Gross's fame has endured or even increased in the twenty-first century—his depiction as the surgeon in Thomas Eakins's *The Gross Clinic,* considered by some art critics to be America's best painting. Ten years before the time of the painting, Joseph Lister had introduced antiseptic technique, and it had already been widely accepted in Europe, preventing many deaths from postoperative infection.

In Eakins's painting of *The Gross Clinic,* Dr. Gross's disregard of antisepsis is obvious from his unsterile garb, instruments, and hands. W. W. Keen recalled that Gross sometimes paused during operations to sharpen his knife on the sole of his boot. A few young American surgeons, including Keen, were stimulated to practice antisepsis by their attendance of Lister's demonstration of his techniques during his visit to Philadelphia in 1876. But for another ten years, many surgical patients in the United States lost their lives from infection because American surgeons followed Samuel Gross's advice and refused to adopt antiseptic techniques.

[15] White, JW. Memoir of D. Hayes Agnew. 24. Although Agnew believed a direct response to the press regarding criticism over the Garfield case was beneath his dignity, he did allow his junior assistant, J. William White, to prepare a response. White wrote, "Had he [Agnew] divorced his interests from those of some of the gentlemen who saw the case earlier, he could easily have avoided all responsibility for those portions of the treatment most open to hostile criticism."

[16] Agnew, David Hayes. *The Principles and Practice of Surgery,* 3 vols, 2nd ed (Philadelphia: J.B. Lippincott Company, 1889) 1:302.

[17] White, JW. A Review of the More Important Surgical Problems of President Garfield's Case. *Medical News* 40 (24 June 1882): 680.

[18] Barker, Clyde F. The Jayne Lecture, Thomas Eakins and his Medical Clinics. *Proceedings of the American Philosophical Society*, Vol 153, No 1 (March 2009). pp. 38–42.

[19] Ibid., p. 40.

[20] Adams, J Howe. *History of the Life of D. Hayes Agnew MD LLD*, p. 332.

The Agnew Clinic was presented to the school on the 1889 graduation held at the Academy of Music. Also being celebrated were Agnew's retirement, Osler's departure for Hopkins, and Osler's famous address, "Aequinimitas." The aging Agnew, unsteady on his feet, almost fell while acknowledging the applause.

[21] Smith, MS. The Agnew Clinic: Not Cheerful to Look At. *Prospects* 11 (1987): 161–83.

[22] Agnew, David Hayes. *The Principles and Practice of Surgery,* 3 vols, 2nd ed (Philadelphia: J.B. Lippincott Company, 1889) 3:71.

[23] Mary V. Clymer Lecture Notes ca. 1887–89. Archives of the History of Nursing, University of Pennsylvania. No pagination.

[24] Adams, J. Howe. *History of the Life of D. Hayes Agnew MD LLD*, p. 145.

CHAPTER 8

A Forgotten Scholar

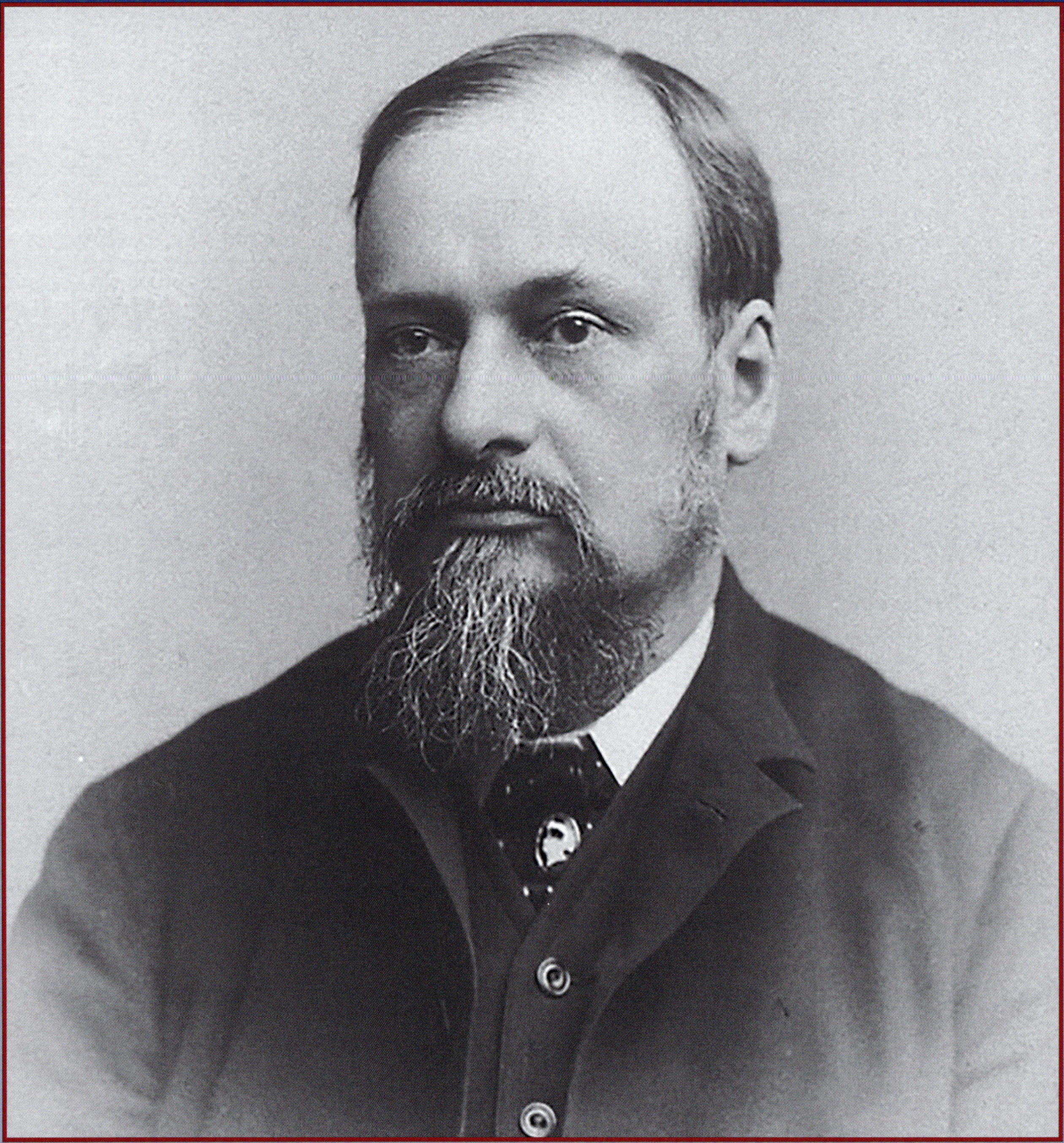

John Ashhurst Jr. (1839–1900)

JRB Professor and Chairman of Surgery (1889–1900)

John Ashhurst Jr. is frequently overlooked in histories of the department, perhaps because the school has no portrait to remind us of him. This is curious because he was one of the most distinguished and probably the smartest chairman. He succeeded Agnew in 1889 and served as John Rhea Barton Professor until 1900.

Even as a child, John Ashhurst was recognized as having a remarkable intellect.[1] He was unusually attracted to books. He was reading before he was four and by sixteen had acquired a library of 3,000 volumes. Throughout life, his favorite forms of relaxation were reading Greek and Latin literature, solving mathematical problems, and playing the piano at which he was an expert. Homeschooled as a child, he entered college at Penn at age fourteen and compiled the highest average ever attained by a student at the university. He graduated from medical school at Penn in 1860 and was awarded a master's degree the same year. After internship at Pennsylvania Hospital, he served during the Civil War at military hospitals in Chester and Germantown.

Early in his surgical practice, he worked mainly at Episcopal Hospital where he became internationally known as an expert in bone and joint surgery. Later, he developed special skills in plastic surgery and surgery of blood vessels. His colleagues considered him the most learned American surgeon. He was perhaps the world's foremost authority on medical and surgical bibliographies.[2] He was the chief reviewer of the *American Journal of Medical Sciences* and the editor of the *Transactions of the College of Physicians,* the *Transactions of the International Medical Congress,* and the six volumes of the *International Encyclopedia of Surgery.* In 1871, he published the first edition of his own textbook, *Principals and Practice of Surgery.* Even though textbooks by Samuel D. Gross and D. Hayes Agnew were still available, Ashhurst's eminence and skill as a writer made his book the one most widely studied and quoted through its six editions. Interestingly, John Ashhurst's son, Astley Paston Cooper Ashhurst, was, like his father, a Penn surgical professor and also authored a respected textbook of surgery.

1839
Birth of Ashhurst

1860
Ashhurst is a brilliant student. Graduates from Penn at age nineteen with master's degree

1861–1865
After internship at Pennsylvania Hospital, serves in Army during Civil War

1888
Ashhurst admits he did not accept Lister's antiseptic method until the year before

1889
Succeeds Agnew as chairman of surgery

1898
Ashhurst suffers disabling stroke

1900
Ashhurst retires and dies

Ashhurst's first two decades of surgical practice preceded the acceptance of antisepsis in America, and he never espoused Lister's methods with enthusiasm. In fact, Ashhurst was said to be the last surgeon to operate in a frock coat. In 1888, he presented at a meeting of the American Surgical Association his experience with 120 joint excisions performed for tuberculosis, destructive arthritis, compound dislocations, and fractures. In this paper, he admitted that he had "switched over to Lister's antiseptic methods" only the year before.[3] He said the greatest benefit had been lessening the necessity for frequent changes of dressings. Yet his results were exceptionally good, and in his extensive practice, serious postoperative infections were rare. This was perhaps due to his obsession with cleanliness. On his wards, he often cleansed and dressed every patient's wounds with his own hands. This process was not perfunctory. It began with turpentine, hot water, and soap, followed by permanganate of potassium, and finally washed off with alcohol.[4]

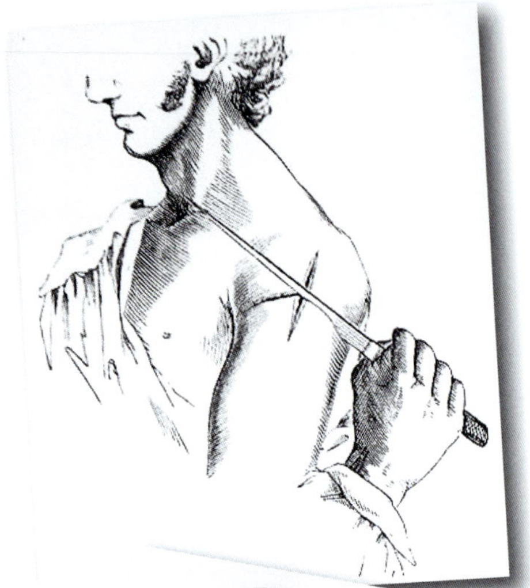

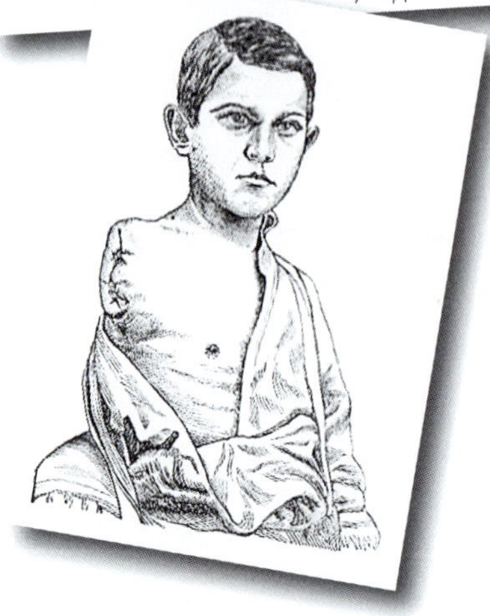

In 1889, John Ashhurst became chairman of the University's department of surgery. As chairman, he was an indefatigable worker who never took a vacation. Nationally prominent, he was a member of all the important surgical societies and vice president of the American Surgical Association.

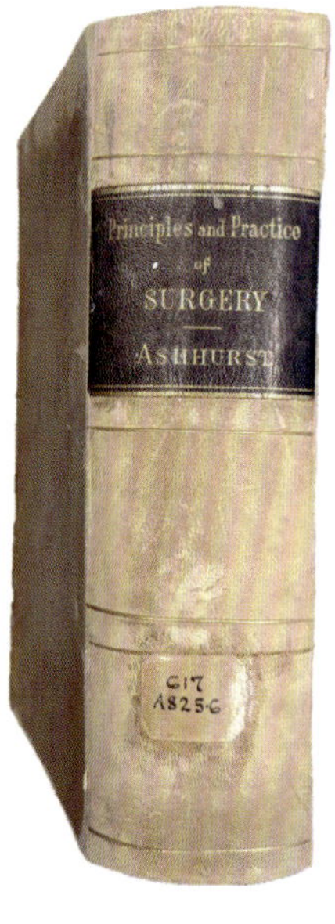

Ashhurst's textbook and illustrations

In August of 1898, Ashhurst suffered a cerebral hemorrhage that completely paralyzed his left side. Although his intellect was unimpaired, he was inactive for the next two years until his death at age sixty-one. He had a special feeling for the Philadelphia College of Physicians, the presidency of which, in 1898 to 1899, he considered his highest honor. His huge library which he left to the college constitutes much of its collection of rare medieval and classical works. The college named its main reading room after him, and the only known portraits of Ashhurst hang there.[5]

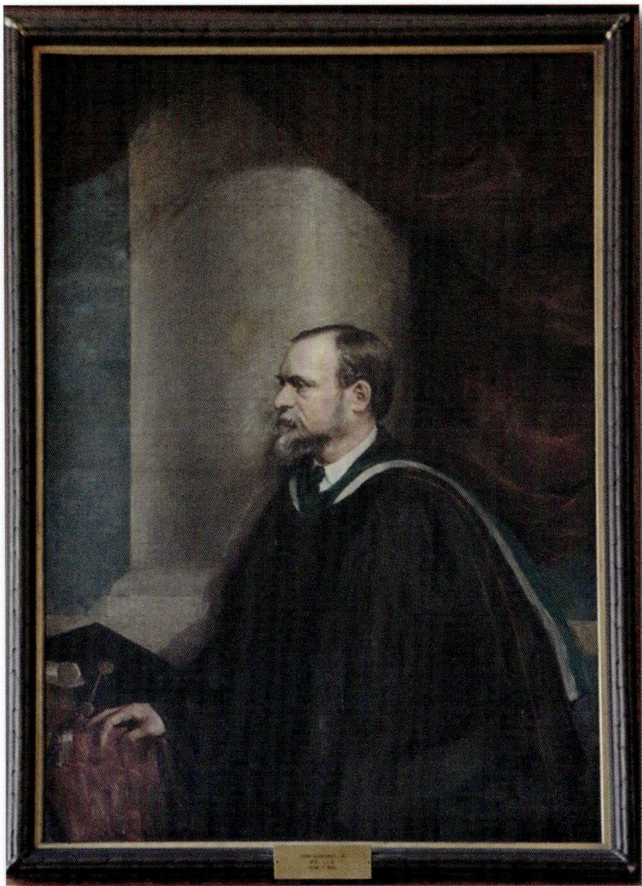

Ashhurst Room, The College of Physicians of Philadelphia

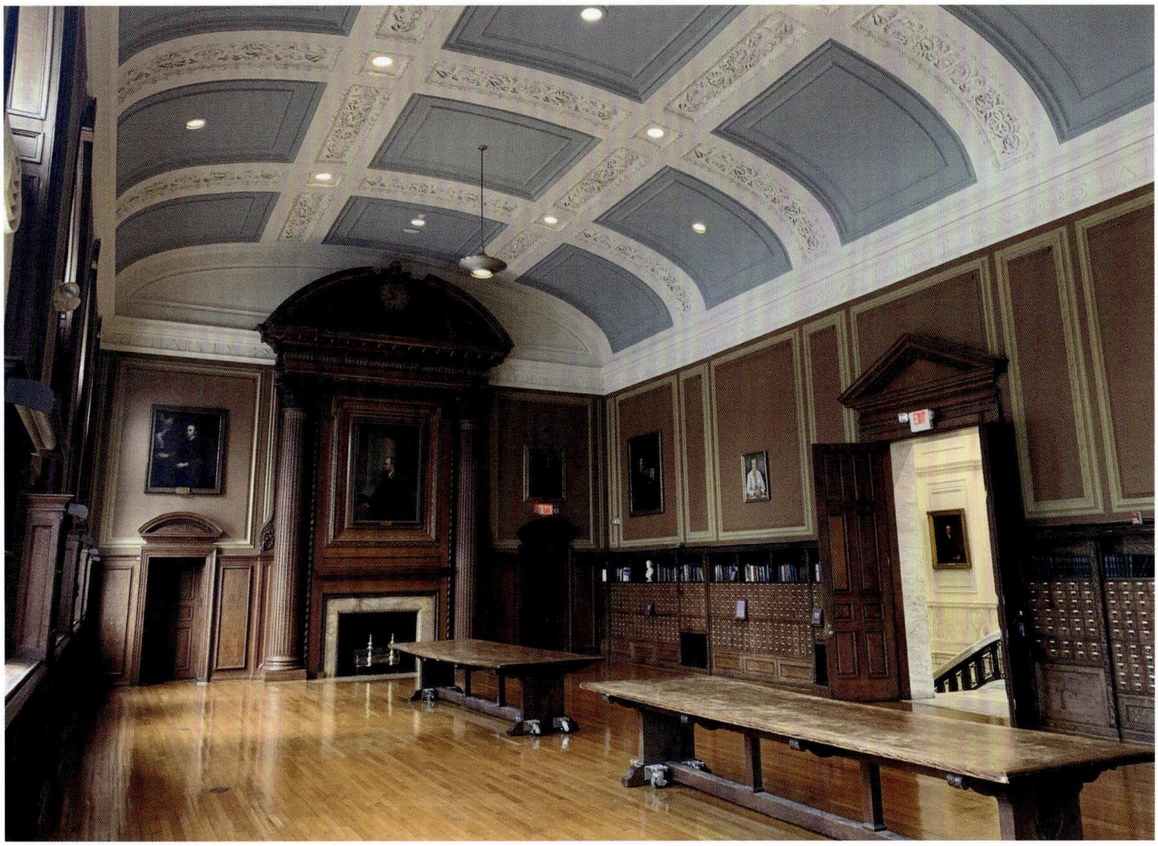

Timeline of Events During the Career of John Ashhurst Jr.

1889 Ashhurst is appointed chairman of the department of surgery. During his ten years as chairman, many important medical events occur. Our incomplete archives fail to address Ashhurst's role in them.

1889 Johns Hopkins Hospital opens.

1889 Osler establishes a modern residency, and shortly thereafter, Halsted establishes his surgical residency. Later, in a classic publication from a speech at his twenty-fifth Yale reunion, Halsted reveals the four aspects he considers crucial for an optimal residency: a single professor (chief) fully in charge; graded responsibility of residents to independence over a period of many years; mandatory research by the residents; and the specific intent to train professors/teachers. Halsted's residency proved to be very successful in training highly respected surgeons, many of whom become department chairmen at other medical schools. Other universities take note of the success of Halsted's residency program and begin to copy it. Penn sends a delegation to Baltimore to evaluate the Hopkins residency, rejects the Halsted model, and decides to continue the Penn system. There is no emphasis at Penn to train future leaders, and virtually none are trained.

1889 William Pepper offers John Shaw Billings an appointment at Penn as director of the department of hygiene and director of HUP. Billings designs buildings for the Department of Hygiene and for a clinical laboratory named for Pepper's father. The Pepper clinical laboratory is the first of its kind.

1890 Arthur W. Goodspeed and William N. Jennings Leonard (a surgical fellow under J. William White) perform the world's first X-ray at Penn without realizing what they have done. In 1895, five years after Goodspeed and Leonard's first X-ray at Penn, Roentgen at Wurzburgh University publishes his paper on X-rays. Following this, many investigators begin to experiment and employ X-rays—Penn being perhaps the first—utilizing J. William White's patients. The first major presentation of X-rays used for fractures and other clinical purposes is given in 1897 by J. William White at the annual meeting of the American Surgical Association. Leonard becomes the first head of radiology as a section of the department of surgery. He burns his hands with X-rays and eventually dies as a result.

1891 John Shaw Billings accepts William Pepper's offer of an appointment as director of HUP and chairman of the department of hygiene. Billings actually arrives in Philadelphia only in 1895 and begins a lecture series on public health. Few students are interested in this field. Compared with Billings's other monumental accomplishments, perhaps this was his only failure. He is physically in Philadelphia for only eight months before moving to New York where he designs the New York Public Library.

1892	The Wistar Institute for Anatomy and Biology is founded. Much of its museum is based on the Wistar/Horner collection of anatomical specimens. It is named for Caspar Wistar.
1893	Johns Hopkins School of Medicine opens.
1893, 1895	J. William White presents to the American Surgical Association his treatment of prostatic enlargement by castration, first in animals and then in patients. He does not realize that many of his patients have prostate cancer rather than benign prostatic hypertrophy, thus missing the influence of endocrine manipulation on tumors, which later is the basis of Charles Huggins's Nobel Prize.
1893	President Cleveland undergoes a "secret" operation on a yacht. W. W. Keen of Jefferson is part of the operating team.
1895	Pepper Laboratories of Clinical Medicine (designed by Billings) opens. It is the first of its kind.
1896	White and W. W. Keen publish the *American Textbook of Surgery*, the first textbook with separate authors for each chapter, chosen for their expertise in a special field. For example, Harvey Cushing wrote the long section on neurosurgery.
1898	Edward Martin, who will become chairman of Penn Surgery in 1910, plays a major role in the Spanish-American War, successfully controlling the epidemic of typhoid fever with public health measures. He sends many of the most severe cases by troop train for care at HUP. The trains are staffed by HUP nurses. Expenses are borne by Penn. Juan Guiteras (a member of the Walter Reed team) and others from Penn serve in this war.
1898	Ashhurst suffers a stroke that disables him for his last two years as chairman.
1900	Ashhurst dies.

Notes

[1] Kelly, Howard A, and Burrage, Walter L. *American Medical Biographies* (Baltimore: The Norman, Remington Company, 1920), pp. 41–43. Essay on John Ashhurst by Astley P. C. Ashhurst.

[2] Harte, Richard H. Memoir of John Ashhurst, Jr. *Transactions of the College of Physicians of Philadelphia*, Third series, Volume the twenty fourth (1902) xliii-lvii.

[3] Ashhurst, John Jr. A Contribution to the Study of Excisions of the Larger Joints. *Transactions of American Surgical Association* (1931) 49: 503–506.

[4] Harte, Richard H. *Memoir of John Ashhurst, Jr.*, p. 9. Like Ashhurst, Agnew attributed his good results to his obsession with neatness and cleanliness, rather than Listerism. Photographs show that he eventually adopted Listerism, but exactly when is uncertain.

[5] Berkowitz, Julie. *College of Physicians of Philadelphia Portrait Catalogue* (College of Physicians of Philadelphia, 1984) pp. 6–7.

CHAPTER 9

Playboy or Surgeon-Scientist?

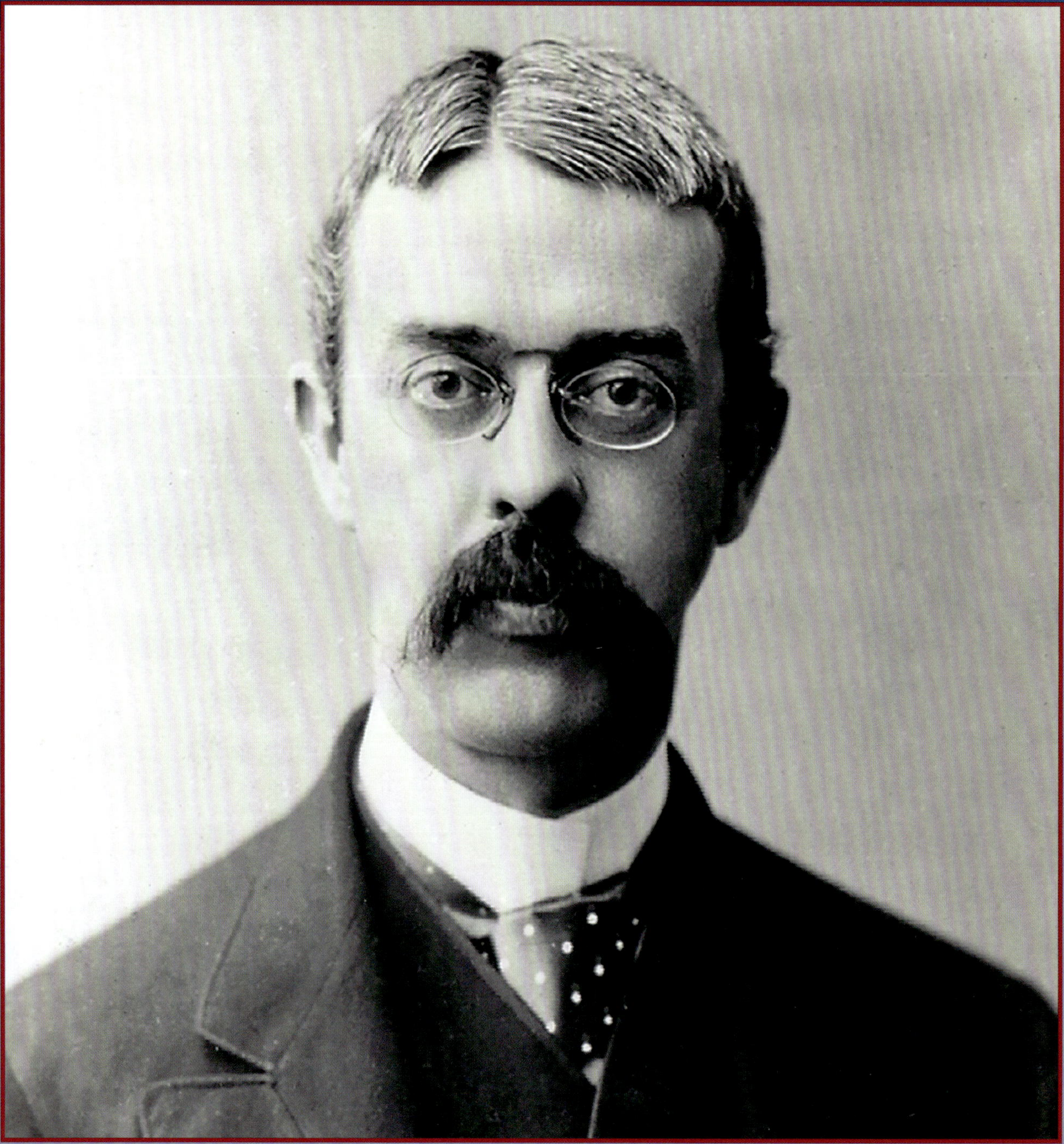

J. William White (1850–1916)

JRB Professor and Chairman of Surgery (1900–1910)

J. William White's long and colorful career was one of the most interesting. In his youth, he was an adventurer, sportsman, and sometimes an irresponsible brawler. The older White was a productive scholar. Born in 1850, White came from a prominent Philadelphia family. He had a fiery, aggressive spirit and became famous for his hair-trigger temper. In his youth, his family's wealth and indulgence allowed him to do pretty much whatever he pleased. His biographers, including me, have had a lot of fun reviewing his colorful early escapades. Unfortunately, this has somewhat obscured that as he matured, he became an accomplished academic surgeon of international stature.

He attended public and Quaker elementary schools and then, since at the time there were no entrance requirements, he directly entered medical school at Penn when it had only a two-year curriculum. These shortcuts allowed him to graduate at age twenty-one at the head of his class with both an MD and a PhD in chemistry.[1]

To occupy himself for the next year, he searched for and signed up for an adventure. As a member of Louis Agassiz's famous Hassler scientific expedition (1871–72), he helped survey marine biology and

1871
MD, PhD at Penn.
It would be another 130 years before Penn would have its only other surgery chairman with a PhD

1871–1872
Member of Agassiz's expedition around South America

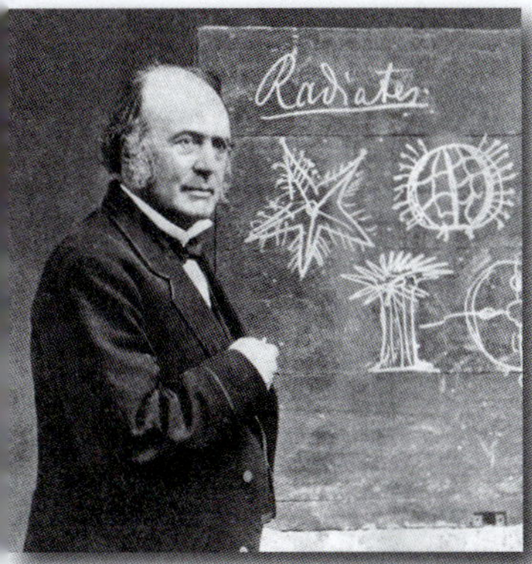

Louis Agassiz
Harvard's famous naturalist

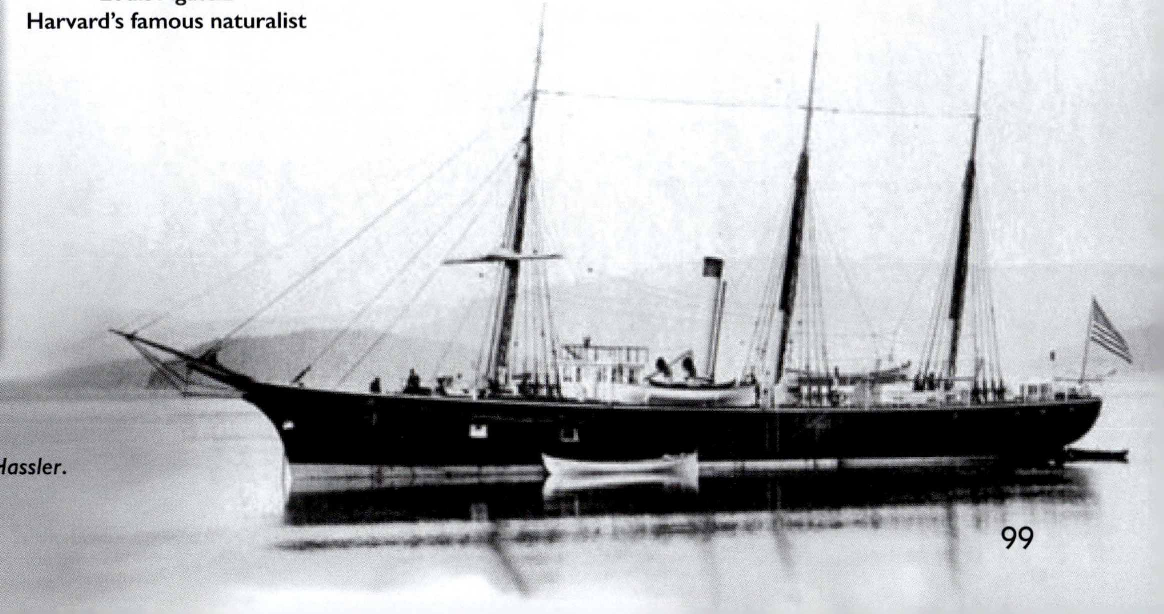

The expedition ship *Hassler*.

1874
After the voyage, White is appointed to Penn faculty. For many years, he serves as Agnew's assistant

1879
White fights Philadelphia's last duel

dredge up specimens from the ocean floor in a tour of the West Indies, Galapagos Islands, and, by rounding Cape Horn, both coasts of South America.[2] White, an amateur photographer, played an important role as the only one taking pictures. He was also hired by the *New York Herald* to write about the trip. The voyage ended up in San Francisco. On the way back to Philadelphia by train, White stopped in Salt Lake City where he heard Brigham Young give a sermon, advising the audience to avoid doctors.

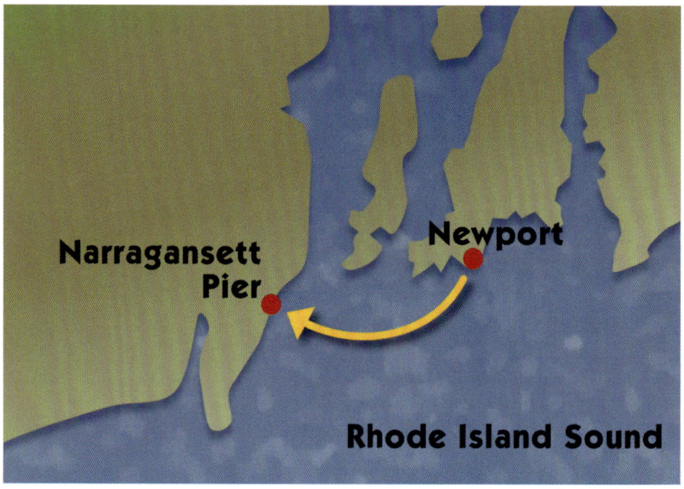

Arriving home at age twenty-two, "Billy" White still had a lot of living to do. Before the heyday of intercollegiate team sports, he was about as athletically active as a young man could be, vigorously engaging in big-game hunting, steeplechasing, boxing, Alpine mountain climbing, and distance swimming.[3] Always a romantic, White fantasized that he, as Lord Byron had done, would swim the Hellespont, the ocean passage from Europe to Asia Minor which, in Greek mythology, Leander traversed in a fatal attempt to reach his mistress, Hero. But for a Philadelphian, the Hellespont was inconveniently located, so White decided to substitute what he envisioned as a similarly difficult swim in Rhode Island. It was, in fact, a much longer one—ten miles from Newport to Narragansett. This swim in a cold, choppy ocean took five hours, but White made it with ease.[4]

An even more famous event of White's early years was widely reported in the newspapers. This was his participation in the last formal duel to be fought in Philadelphia.[5] In 1879, twenty-nine-year-old White became physician to the First City Troop, which in peace time was really nothing more than an exclusive social club. White showed up at a Troop party in the club's fancy dress uniform. A trooper challenged the doctor's right to wear this official garb. An argument ensued, and the hot-tempered White punched the trooper, knocking him to the floor. Satisfaction was demanded, and a formal duel was scheduled.

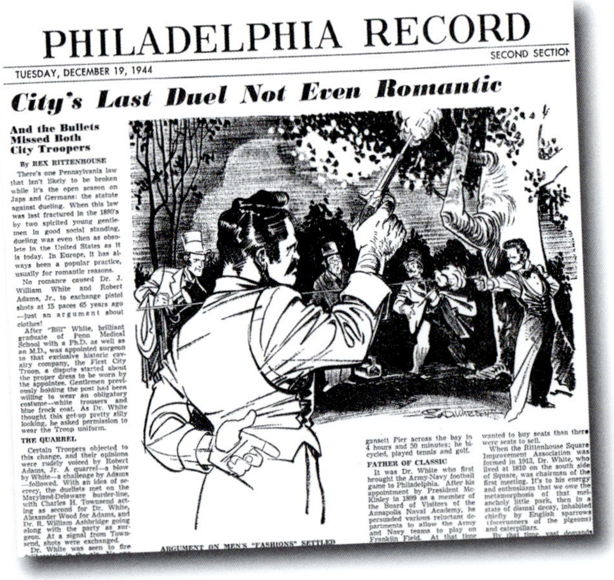

PHILADELPHIA RECORD

TUESDAY, DECEMBER 19, 1944 — SECOND SECTION

City's Last Duel Not Even Romantic

And the Bullets Missed Both City Troopers

By REX RITTENHOUSE

There's one Pennsylvania law that isn't likely to be broken while it's the open season on Japs and Germans: the statute against dueling. When this law was last fractured in the 1880's by two spirited young gentlemen in good social standing, dueling was even then as obsolete in the United States as it is today. In Europe, it has always been a popular practice, usually for romantic reasons.

No romance caused Dr. J. William White and Robert Adams, Jr., to exchange pistol shots at 15 paces 65 years ago—just an argument about clothes!

After "Bill" White, brilliant graduate of Penn Medical School with a Ph.D. as well as an M.D., was appointed surgeon to that exclusive historic cavalry company, the First City Troop, a dispute started about the proper dress to be worn by the appointee. Gentlemen previously holding the post had been willing to wear an obligatory costume—white trousers and blue frock coat. As Dr. White thought this get-up pretty silly looking, he asked permission to wear the Troop uniform.

THE QUARREL

Certain Troopers objected to this change, and their opinions were rudely voiced by Robert Adams, Jr. A quarrel—a blow by White—a challenge by Adams—followed. With an idea of secrecy, the duelists met on the Maryland-Delaware border-line, with Charles H. Townsend acting as second for Dr. White, Alexander Wood for Adams, and Dr. R. William Ashbridge going along with the party as surgeon. At a signal from Townsend, shots were exchanged.

Dr. White was seen to fire ...

ARGUMENT ON MEN'S "FASHIONS" SETTLED

... gansett Pier across the bay in 4 hours and 50 minutes; he bicycled, played tennis and golf.

FATHER OF CLASSIC

It was Dr. White who first brought the Army-Navy football game to Philadelphia. After his appointment by President McKinley in 1899 as a member of the Board of Visitors of the Annapolis Naval Academy, he persuaded various reluctant departments to allow the Army and Navy teams to play on Franklin Field. At that time ... wanted to buy seats than there were seats to sell.

When the Rittenhouse Square Improvement Association was formed in 1913, Dr. White, who lived at 1810 on the south side of Square, was chairman of the first meeting. It's to his energy and enthusiasm that we owe the metamorphosis of that melancholy little park, then in a state of dismal decay, inhabited chiefly by English sparrows (forerunners of the pigeons) and caterpillars.

By that time, vast demand ...

Since duels were against the law in Philadelphia, White and the trooper, along with their seconds and a surgeon, met in a secret place south of the Mason-Dixon line where duels were apparently okay. The duel was fought with pistols. The trooper aimed at White and shot first. Fortunately, he missed. White, by then having cooled off, discharged his pistol in the air.

In 1874, White was appointed to the Penn faculty where his first years were spent as assistant to D. Hayes Agnew. In 1882, he wrote a long defense of Agnew's treatment of assassinated President Garfield for the newspapers, countering assertions that Agnew was among the doctors who, ignoring antisepsis, looked for the bullet by probing the wound with unwashed fingers or dirty instruments, thus fatally infecting the president.[6] In 1886, White was promoted to clinical professor of genitourinary surgery. But even three years later, Eakins's painting, *The Agnew Clinic,* shows him still as Agnew's assistant. Later, when White became department chairman, he did not choose Eakins for his own portraitist but instead his friend, John Singer Sargent, who was at the time a much better-known painter than Eakins.[7] The socially well-connected White also listed as his close friends the author Henry James, President Theodore Roosevelt, and Sir Joseph Lister.

1881
President Garfield is assassinated. Agnew is summoned to care for him

1882
White writes account of Garfield's wounds, defending Agnew's role and denying that he probed the wounds with unwashed fingers

1883
Unable to control his temper, White often uses his fists to settle arguments. This even makes the newspapers

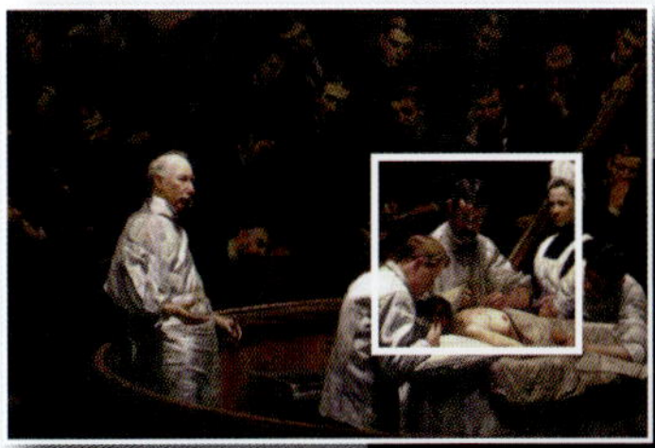

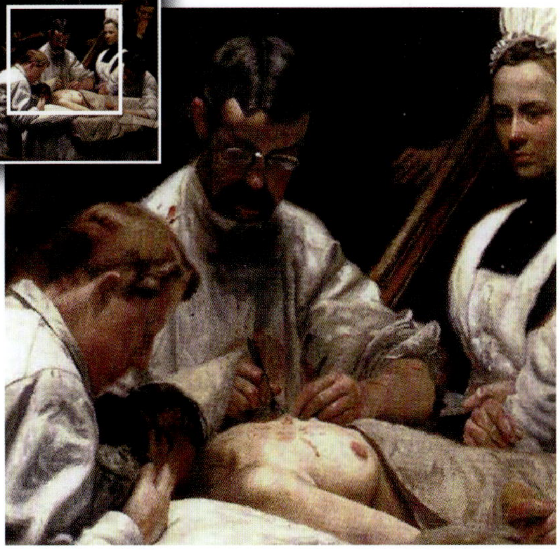

As Agnew's assistant, J. William White finishes the operation.

He was in his day an internationally known surgical leader. He was the first to use X-rays in diagnosis and management of fractures. His report of this experience to the American Surgical Association was made in 1895, only months after Roentgen's first paper.[8] This report was the first at the American Surgical Association and one of the first anywhere of their clinical use. Also included in this paper was the first use of X-rays for identifying gall stones and kidney stones. It also speculated on their possible use in treatment of cancer.

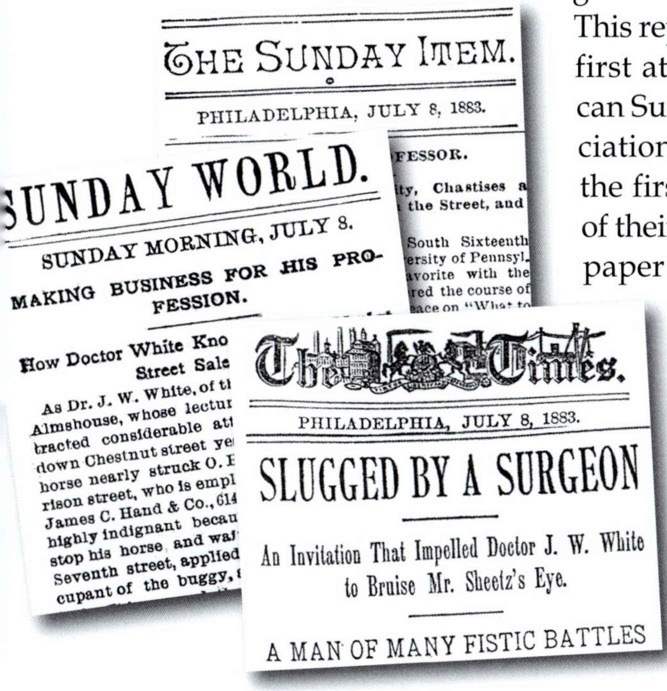

THE SUNDAY ITEM.
PHILADELPHIA, JULY 8, 1883.

SUNDAY WORLD.
SUNDAY MORNING, JULY 8.
MAKING BUSINESS FOR HIS PROFESSION.
How Doctor White Kno... Street Sale...
As Dr. J. W. White, of th... Almshouse, whose lectur... tracted considerable att... down Chestnut street ye... horse nearly struck O. F... rison street, who is empl... James C. Hand & Co., 614... highly indignant becau... stop his horse, and wa... Seventh street, applied... cupant of the buggy, ...

The Times.
PHILADELPHIA, JULY 8, 1883.
SLUGGED BY A SURGEON
An Invitation That Impelled Doctor J. W. White to Bruise Mr. Sheetz's Eye.
A MAN OF MANY FISTIC BATTLES

White wrote several books on anatomy, genitourinary surgery, and in 1892, with W. W. Keen, edited the *American Textbook of Surgery,* the first

1893
Report to American Surgical Association of castration as a treatment for enlarged prostate

1895
White first to use X-rays in diagnosis and treatment of fractures

1899
White hosts Theodore Roosevelt at Franklin Field as the stadium (built by White) opens

1900
White succeeds John Ashhurst as John Rhea Barton Professor and Chairman of Surgery. This precipitates a bitter feud with his colleague, John B. Deaver, who had also been a candidate for the chair. Their resultant rivalry is described in detail in Chapter 11 on Deaver

multi-author surgical text, an important innovation since different authorities were invited to write the sections in their fields of expertise.

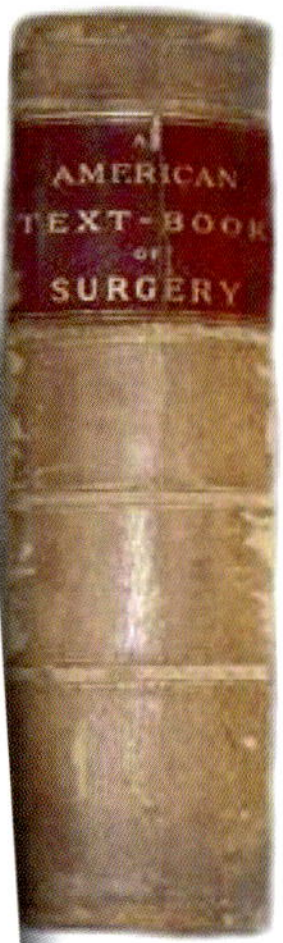

White barely missed doing what could have been some landmark clinical research. In his gynecology practice, he noticed that after removal of the ovaries, women's uterine fibroids shrank. This suggested to him the project for which he is best known. In 1893, his experiments showed that castration shrank the prostate of dogs. It had been forgotten that John Hunter had noticed this phenomenon 100 years earlier. White then found that the same procedure could alleviate the symptoms of patients with enlarged prostates. In 1895, he presented 111 such cases to the American Surgical Association.[9] He was not aware that one-third of the patients he treated by this method had prostate cancer instead of or in addition to benign prostatic hypertrophy. If he had noticed this, he might have been credited as the first to recognize that hormonal manipulation could be used as successful treatment of some human cancers, a finding that decades later led to Charles Huggins's Nobel Prize. Since White did not make this connection, he is now mostly remembered for his youthful escapades and his persistent interest in sports rather than for science.

EDITORIAL ARTICLES.

THE USE OF SKIAGRAPHY FOR THE DETECTION AND LOCATION OF FOREIGN BODIES IMPACTED IN THE ŒSOPHAGUS.

[In connection with the case of Dr. Le Conte's, published in this number of the Annals of Surgery, in which was shown the value of skiagraphy to determine the location of a bullet embedded in the soft tissues at the root of the neck, it may be of interest to give the following editorial abstract of a report of a case in which, by means of Röntgen rays, the presence and location of a foreign body impacted in the œsophagus were determined, and great help in carrying out successful treatment of the case was secured.]

Even late in his career, White's interest in athletics continued. He founded the university's department of physical education and was its first chairman.[10] From 1882 to 1900, he was vice president and then president of the university's Athletic Association. He used his own funds to recruit and subsidize many of the university's star athletes. He funded the university's first gymnasium. He was responsible for building Franklin Field and, through his friend Theodore Roosevelt, having the Army-Navy game played there.

ANNALS OF SURGERY.

THE RESULTS OF DOUBLE CASTRATION IN HYPERTROPHY OF THE PROSTATE.[1]

By J. WILLIAM WHITE, M.D.,

OF PHILADELPHIA,

PROFESSOR OF CLINICAL SURGERY IN THE UNIVERSITY OF PENNSYLVANIA; SURGEON TO THE UNIVERSITY, PHILADELPHIA, AND GERMAN HOSPITALS.

I SHALL ask the indulgence of the Association, if in the paper I am about to read I seem to go a little beyond the exact limitation of the title. I have divided it into,—(1) a Theoretical, (2) a Clinical, and, (3) an Experimental portion.

I shall consider in part first a theory of causation which, though I must admit it to be vague, has seemed to help me to an understanding both of the results of the operation and of some of the clinical features of the growths.

The second part contains a review of some illustrative cases; a summary of a considerable number (111 in all); and a consideration of the objections thus far urged against the operation and of its relative merits and future prospects.

In the third portion I have given the experimental and other evidence in regard to the value of,—(*a*) Unilateral castration; (*b*) Ligation of the vas; (*c*) Ligation of the spermatic and deferential arteries; (*d*) Ligation of the entire cord. Tables of the 111 cases and of the fatal cases are appended.

[1] Read at the meeting of the American Surgical Association, New York, May 28, 1895; and at the meeting of the American Genito-Urinary Association, Niagara Falls, May 29, 1895.

In 1900, White succeeded John Ashhurst as John Rhea Barton Professor and Chairman of Surgery. This precipitated a bitter feud with his colleague John B. Deaver, who had also been a candidate for the chair. Their resultant rivalry is described in detail in chapter 11 on Deaver.

In 1906, White was responsible for recruiting J. Edward Sweet to the university as an associate professor in Penn's department of experimental surgery, the first such department in the United States.[11]

In 1906, White discovered a mass in his lower abdomen and, assuming he had cancer, traveled to Minnesota to be operated on by Dr. William Mayo. The mass turned out to be an abscess from perforation of a colonic diverticulum.[12] Although White continued as JRB Professor and chairman, he never returned to clinical practice and operating.

In 1910, a period of turbulence ensued at the medical school over Charles Frazier's proposed reform of the faculty and emphasis on research. At this stage, White was satisfied with his position as the chairman of the department of surgery and was opposed to any disruptive change, as were his conservative senior surgeon colleagues.[13] Bitterness of the fight over these issues further decreased his appetite for hospital and university politics, prompting him to resign as chairman of surgery. The next few years, as detailed in his diary, were spent on world travel with his wife and on his hobbies.

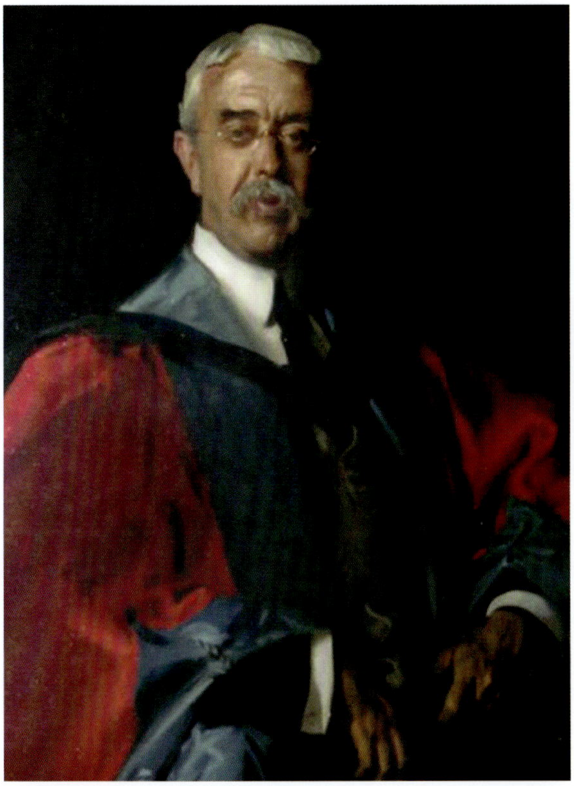

James William White, MD, PhD **by John Singer Sargent**

Beginning in 1914 with the onset of World War I, White was ready for another cause, a patriotic one. He became very active in supporting England and France in their struggle with Germany and actively promoted the United States' entry to the war.[14] In 1914, he organized and established the American Ambulance Hospital, a 180-bed hospital in Paris, staffed by University of Pennsylvania personnel. He also wrote a widely circulated book titled, *Primer of the War for Americans.*

In 1916, he died of metastatic cancer.

At the end of his life, in disposing of his estate of $800,000, which was real money in 1916, White did his best to make sure he would be

1906
White is appointed John Rhea Barton Professor of Surgery and recruits J. Edward Sweet to head at Penn the first department of surgical research

1906
White undergoes an operation at Mayo Clinic

1906 (Dec. 1)
White arranges for Army-Navy game to be played at Franklin Field in Philadelphia

1910–1911
After leading conservatives in opposition to proposed faculty reform, White retires as surgery chairman, becomes University trustee

1914–1918
World War I. White strongly supports England and France

1914
Organizes and funds American Ambulance Hospital in Paris

1916
White's death

remembered. He left $150,000 to endow the J. William White Professorship in surgical research, first held by Ravdin and recently held by Ali Naji. Smaller amounts were left to his many clubs, including the Franklin Inn Club for an annual dinner to be held in his honor. The money has not held up sufficiently for dinner or even for the cocktails, but the club still toasts White at its annual dinner. He left $5,000 to the university with the instructions that it be invested and held in a separate fund for 100 years. White specified that the accumulated money was then to be used for publication of a biography based on his extensive diary that has been preserved in the university archives.[15] One wonders what the university has done with this money, which should have become available in 2016 and whether the book will ever be written.

Timeline of Events During the Career of J. William White

1871	White receives both MD and PhD in chemistry from University of Pennsylvania.
1871–1872	White travels with Louis Agassiz on the Hassler Expedition around the coast of South America to San Francisco.
1879	White fights in Philadelphia's last pistol duel.
1893	White reports that castration shrinks the prostate.
1895	White reports to American Surgical Association some of the earliest experience with X-rays.
1900	White appointed John Rhea Barton Professor and Chairman of Surgery.
1901–1909	Charles Frazier is dean of School of Medicine.
1901	Seminal publication by Charles Frazier and William Spiller on division of the sensory root of the fifth cranial nerve for relief of trigeminal neuralgia (tic doulouroux).
1901	Walter Reed and his team demonstrate that yellow fever is transmitted by mosquitoes. Juan Guiteras, a member of Reed's team, taught pathology at Penn from 1889–1895.
1903	Society of Clinical Surgery founded by Harvey Cushing—Frazier is founding member.
1904	Medical Laboratories Building (now John Morgan Building) is constructed.
1906	The Rockefeller Institute opens in New York. Simon Flexner, Penn's pathology chairman, is recruited to direct it.
1906	J. Edwin Sweet is recruited from the Rockefeller Institute by White to head a department of experimental surgery, the first such department in the United States. Sweet is accused of cruelty to animals by the antivivisection movement and is brought to trial in 1914. After serving in the Army during World War I, Sweet resumes his research at Penn. In 1926, Sweet moves to Cornell.
1906	White is operated on at the Mayo Clinic. His abdominal mass is benign. He remains chairman of surgery but never returns to clinical activity.
1909	Anticipating criticism by the upcoming Flexner report, Dean Charles Frazier and Provost Charles Harrison attempt to emphasize research by replacing old faculty and appointing young national leaders. J. William White leads the opposition, and the attempt fails. New faculty are ousted, and Frazier and Harrison both resign.

1909	A. N. Richards is appointed chairman of pharmacology. He is the only survivor of the young faculty recruited by Frazier and Harrison in their attempted reform.
1909	Penn establishes the nation's first department of research medicine.
1910	The first EKG is taken in the Pepper laboratories.
1910	The Flexner report is published. Its findings of deficiencies lead to closure of many American medical schools. Penn is ranked in a top group but is less than highly praised for academic or research activities.
1910	White retires as chairman of surgery, becomes university trustee.
1911 (Jan 1)	Edward Martin becomes chairman of surgery.
1911	The Clinical Congress of North American Surgeons meets in Philadelphia. Edward Martin is president of the Clinical Congress. He and his friends of the Society of Clinical Surgery are important in forming this precursor to the American College of Surgeons.
1911	The first human kidney transplant is performed by former Penn faculty member, Levi J. Hammond, at the Clinical Congress.
1912–1913	The American College of Surgeons is founded. Edward Martin is one of the founders and a member of the Board of Regents.
1914	White establishes American Ambulance Hospital in Paris.
1916	White dies.

Notes

[1] Repplier, Agnes. *J. William White, M.D., a biography* (Boston: Houghton Mifflin company, 1919) p. 7.

[2] Ibid., p. 9–28.

[3] Master Surgeons of America. *Surgery, Gynecology and Obstetrics*, 35:665 (1922) p. 666.

[4] Repplier, Agnes. *J. William White, M.D., a biography*, p. 74.

[5] City's Last Duel, Rittenhouse, Rex. *Philadelphia Record* (Tues., Dec. 19, 1944) with drawing.

[6] White, JW. A Review of the More Important Surgical Problems of President Garfield's Case. *Medical News* (24 June 1882) 40:680.

[7] Repplier, Agnes. *J. William White, M.D., a biography*, p. 178.

[8] White, JW. The Use of Skiagraphy on the Detection and Localization of Foreign Bodies Impacted in the Esophagus. *Ann Surg* (1896 Aug.) 24(2): 238–242.

[9] Ravitch, Mark. *A Century of Surgery Vol I, 1880–1980* (Philadelphia: J.B. Lippincott Company, 1981) p. 166.

[10] Master Surgeons of America. *Surgery, Gynecology and Obstetrics*, 35:665 (1922) p. 666.

[11] Cooper III, David Y, and Ledger, Marshall A. *Innovation and Tradition at the University of Pennsylvania School of Medicine, An Anecdotal Journey* (Philadelphia: University of Pennsylvania Press, 1990) p. 146.

[12] Repplier, Agnes. *J. William White, M.D., a biography*. p. 139.

[13] Corner, George W. *Two Centuries of Medicine: A History of the School of Medicine, University of Pennsylvania* (Philadelphia: J.B. Lippincott Company, 1965) p. 234.

[14] Master Surgeons of America. *Surgery, Gynecology and Obstetrics*, 35:667 (1922).

[15] Martin, Edward. James William White, PhD., M.D., LL.D. *Transactions of the American Surgical Association*, 34:43 (1916) xlv.

CHAPTER 10

How a Little Club Inspired Surgery's Largest Professional Society

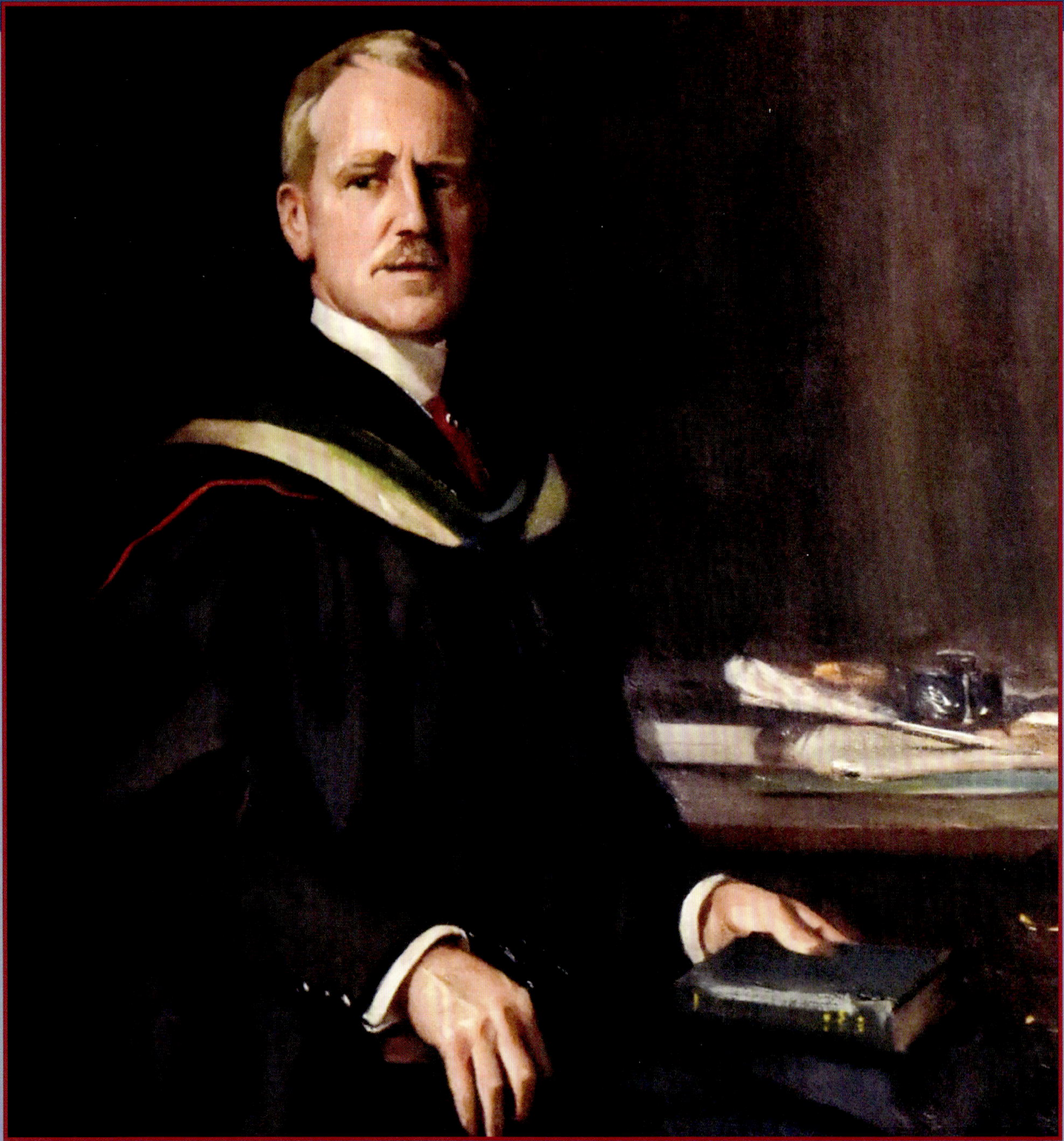

Edward Martin (1859–1938)

JRB Professor and Chairman of Surgery (1910–1918)

Edward Martin's distinguished career is especially interesting for the broad variety of his accomplishments. He left important marks not only in surgery but also in the diverse fields of military service, public health, civic politics, education, and philanthropy. At age fourteen, he enrolled in college at Swarthmore, graduating magna cum laude and Phi Beta Kappa in 1878. He was also a member of the crew and football teams. Four years later, he obtained a master's degree from Swarthmore. In 1883, he graduated from medical school at Penn, where he was AOA and a member of the university's championship crew.

1878
AB Swarthmore College

1882
Master's degree Swarthmore

1883
MD University of Pennsylvania

1885–1900
Assistant to Agnew and White

Early in his faculty years at Penn, he served as an assistant to both D. Hayes Agnew and J. William White. Like his closest mentor White, he was particularly interested in urology. He became widely known as an expert on male infertility. Some refer to him as the father of this field.[1] His research led to a treatment for obstructive azoospermia. Of eleven operations he performed to correct blocked passages of the vas deferens, seven remained patent, allowing three pregnancies.[2] In 1909, he coauthored with J. William White the standard textbook of the day on genitourinary diseases.

Martin was also a broadly experienced and innovative general surgeon.

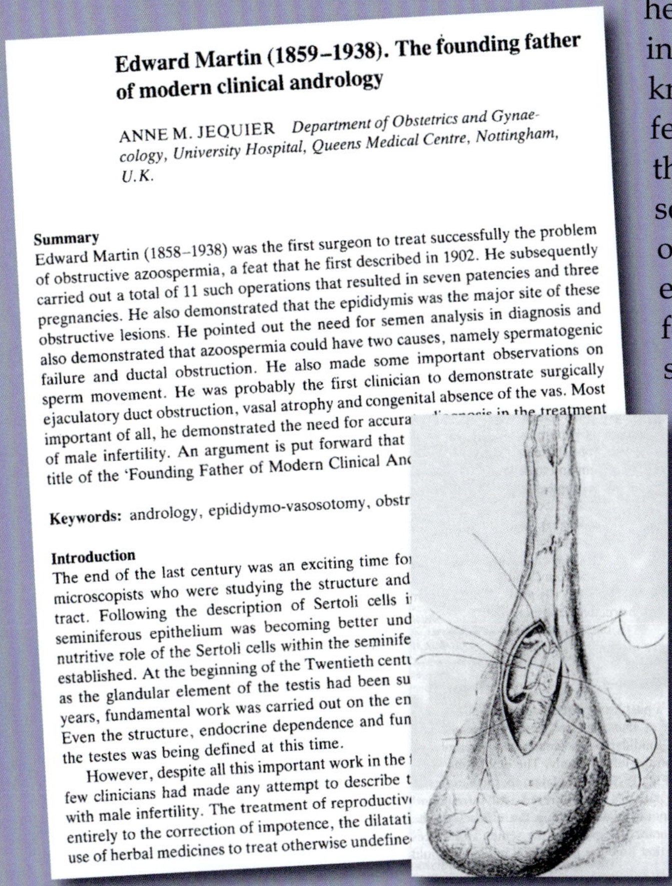

Edward Martin (1859–1938). The founding father of modern clinical andrology

ANNE M. JEQUIER *Department of Obstetrics and Gynaecology, University Hospital, Queens Medical Centre, Nottingham, U.K.*

Summary
Edward Martin (1858–1938) was the first surgeon to treat successfully the problem of obstructive azoospermia, a feat that he first described in 1902. He subsequently carried out a total of 11 such operations that resulted in seven patencies and three pregnancies. He also demonstrated that the epididymis was the major site of these obstructive lesions. He pointed out the need for semen analysis in diagnosis and also demonstrated that azoospermia could have two causes, namely spermatogenic failure and ductal obstruction. He also made some important observations on sperm movement. He was probably the first clinician to demonstrate surgically ejaculatory duct obstruction, vasal atrophy and congenital absence of the vas. Most important of all, he demonstrated the need for accura[...] in the treatment
of male infertility. An argument is put forward that
title of the 'Founding Father of Modern Clinical An[...]

Keywords: andrology, epididymo-vasosotomy, obstr[...]

Introduction
The end of the last century was an exciting time fo[...]
microscopists who were studying the structure and
tract. Following the description of Sertoli cells i[...]
seminiferous epithelium was becoming better und[...]
nutritive role of the Sertoli cells within the seminife[...]
established. At the beginning of the Twentieth centu[...]
as the glandular element of the testis had been su[...]
years, fundamental work was carried out on the en[...]
Even the structure, endocrine dependence and fun[...]
the testes was being defined at this time.

However, despite all this important work in the [...]
few clinicians had made any attempt to describe t[...]
with male infertility. The treatment of reproductiv[...]
entirely to the correction of impotence, the dilatati[...]
use of herbal medicines to treat otherwise undefine[...]

1898
Spanish-American War

A variety of his work was presented or discussed at meetings of the American Surgical Association. Topics included were outpatient treatment of fractures of the lower extremity, some of the earliest attempts to treat shock with adrenalin,[3] study of gum acacia as a blood substitute, the use of morphine for postoperative pain, and the benefit of preoperative breathing exercises.[4] As an experimentalist, he was interested in the Eck fistula and investigated anastomosis of a mesenteric vein to the iliac vein for portal hypertension.[5]

When neurosurgeon Charles Frazier refused to try William Spiller's suggestion that section of the anterolateral columns of the spinal cord would relieve unrelenting lower body pain, Spiller went to Martin. Martin then successfully performed the first cordotomy of this type.[6]

In teaching, Martin was one of the first to use lantern slides. Working with the Eastman Kodak company, he also made a movie illustrating the treatment of appendicitis.[7]

Martin's nonmedical interests and activities included experiments in heavier-than-air aviation prior to the success of the Wright brothers.

Martin also had an extensive military record. During the war with Spain in 1898, he served in Cuba as battalion leader of the Third Regiment of the Pennsylvania National Guard. In that war, only 385 of Leonard Wood and Teddy Roosevelt's Rough Riders and other American soldiers died in battle. At the same time, a typhoid epidemic killed more than 2,000 of the soldiers. Martin was credited with developing and enforcing policies and sanitary precautions that stamped out the disease in the US camps in Cuba.[8] Martin also directed that many of the most severe cases be sent by special trains for treatment at HUP.[9]

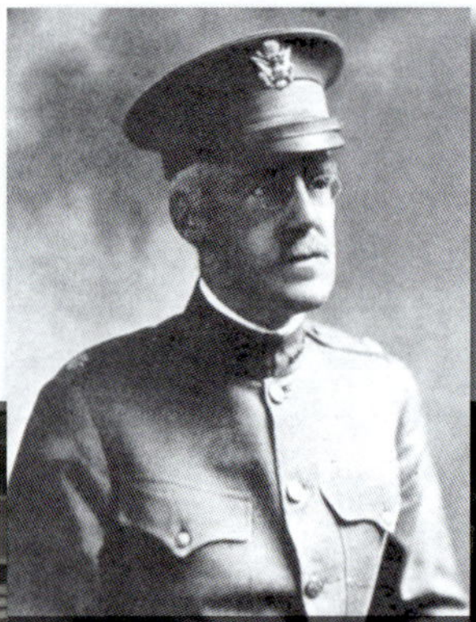

Colonel Edward Martin

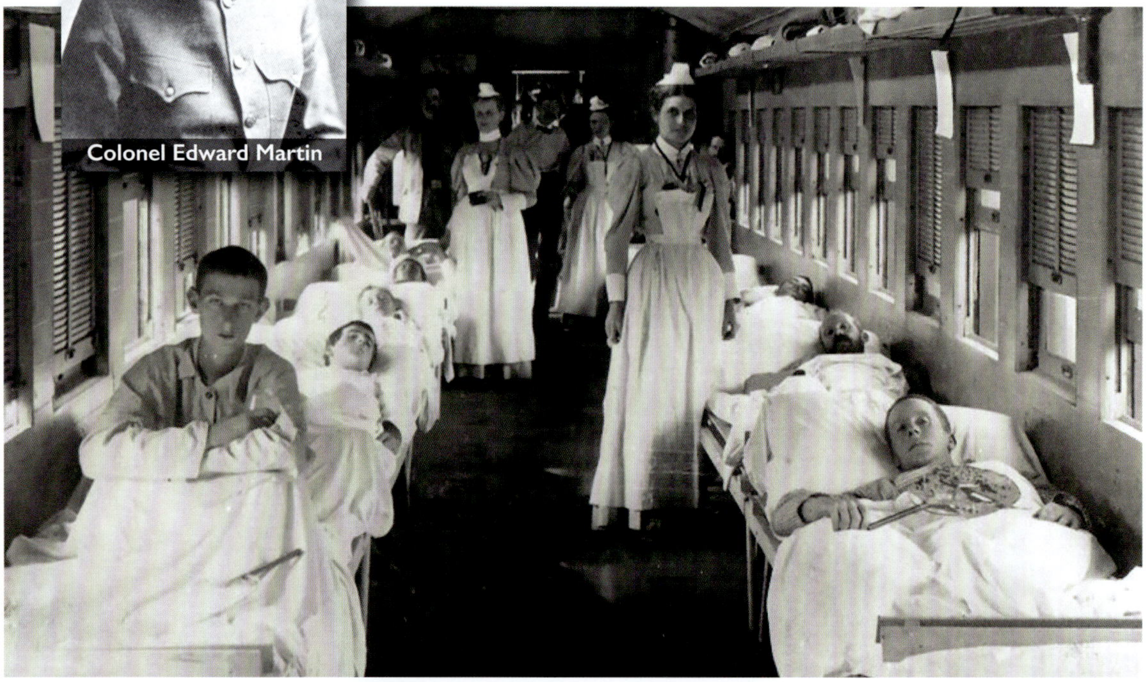

Martin's train transports typhoid victims for care at HUP.

The part played by Edward Martin and his friends in the Society of Clinical Surgery in the founding of the American College of Surgeons is an interesting story.[10] Founded in 1903 by Harvey Cushing, membership in the Society of Clinical Surgery is one of surgery's most coveted. Election to its limited membership can only occur before age fifty-five (until recently, this age limit was forty-five). Another unique aspect is that during the annual meeting, always held at a university hospital, the members are invited into the host's operating rooms where they stand elbow-to-elbow with the surgeon and discuss the procedure while it is going on. Most probably think the value of belonging is limited to the prestige of being elected and the opportunity to make friends with other leaders of academic surgery. But study of the society's history reveals that at one time, it served another important purpose. It was a parent of the American College of Surgeons. How this small travel club inspired the world's largest surgical organization has been largely forgotten.

1903
Society of Clinical Surgery founded

1908
Franklin Martin attends and is inspired by a meeting of Society of Clinical Surgery

In 1900, Harvey Cushing, Alton Ochsner, and William Mayo attended a meeting of the International Surgical Congress in Paris. To them, this Congress seemed an endless series of dull papers. During a break, they sat on a bridge overlooking the Seine complaining to one another that since they were too young for election to major surgical societies, they were undervalued. They decided to start a society of their own. Its members would be academic surgeons interested in teaching and research, but the purpose of their new society would be more practical. The members would get together at various university centers and learn from watching each other operate. Importantly, no one over the age of forty-five could be elected to membership. They called it the Society of Clinical Surgery.

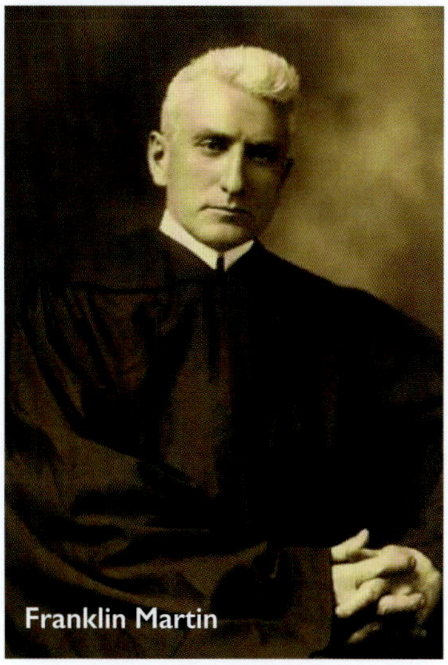
Franklin Martin

A few years later, Franklin Martin (not a member) was invited to a meeting of the new society. He was intrigued by the openness of its format. He wondered if he could capture its essence and provide for many the educational experience then being enjoyed by only the few members of the Society of Clinical Surgery.

As he later told the story, Franklin Martin, the founding editor of *Surgery, Gynecology and Obstetrics* (later named *Journal of the American College of Surgeons),* decided to invite the 3,000 subscribers of his journal to a meeting in Chicago where they would be invited to watch operations by the city's best surgeons.[11] Because of the large number of guests, it would have to occur in small groups at multiple hospitals. The guest surgeons (1,600 of them) applied to attend the meeting which he called the Clinical Congress of the Surgeons of North America. It lasted two weeks and was a huge success.

1910
Clinical Congress of Surgeons of North America in Chicago. Sixteen hundred attendees watch surgical operations

1910
Flexner Report

1910
Edward Martin succeeds White as chairman of surgery

1911
Martin performs first cordotomy

1911
Second Congress of Surgeons of North America meets in Philadelphia. Edward Martin is president of Congress

1913
Clinical Congress of Surgeons of North American meets in Washington, DC, changes name to Clinical Congress of American College of Surgeons

He then persuaded another Dr. Martin (not a relative) to organize further meetings of this clinical Congress. This one was Edward Martin, HUP's John Rhea Barton Professor and Chairman. To plan the next Congress in Philadelphia, Edward Martin met with a group of his friends from the Society of Clinical Surgery, including Rudolph Matas, Alton Ochsner, the Mayo brothers, and J. M. T. Finney. Among the multiple clinics held in various Philadelphia hospitals during the 1911 Congress was a demonstration by Alexis Carrel of his vascular suturing technique. Also at Episcopal Hospital, the world's first human kidney transplant was performed by Philadelphia surgeon, Levi. J. Hammond (see 1911 timeline at end of chapter). The Congress was attended by more than a thousand surgeons and was a resounding success.

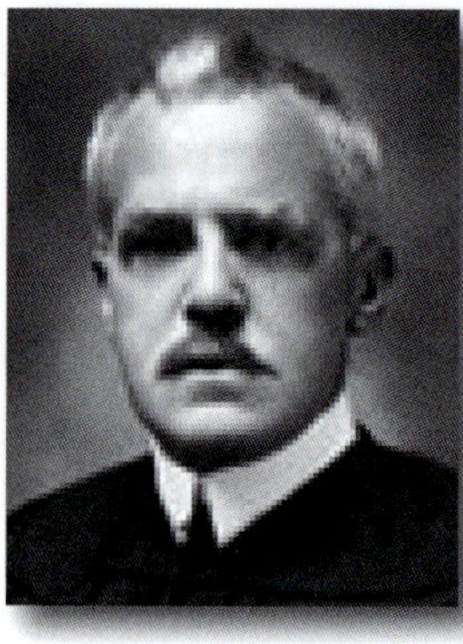

Edward Martin

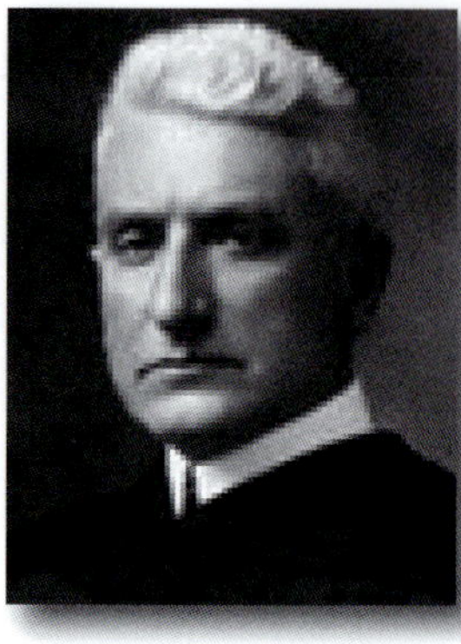

Franklin H. Martin

After another successful meeting of the Congress in New York, the 1913 meeting was planned for Washington, DC. Again, Edward Martin was the president, and the planners of the meeting were the leaders of the Society of Clinical Surgery. They decided to change the name of the Clinical Congress to the American College of Surgeons. The first Board of Regents was comprised of Edward Martin and the other members of the Society of Clinical Surgery.

Over the years, attempts have been made by the American College of Surgeons to emulate the meetings of the Society of Clinical Surgery, especially the opportunity for watching and discussing ongoing operations. Movies of operations were among the first methods. Edward Martin was a pioneer of this. When television became available in the 1940s, live operations were shown to an audience by closed-circuit TV. Attendees could discuss the case as it progressed. This was an entertaining and very popular segment of the College's program. It was eventually discontinued because it encouraged the surgeon to hurry a complex operation in order to finish it on schedule. As a resident, I had an opportunity to scrub on a few of these live TV operations and to observe the consequences of the pressure.

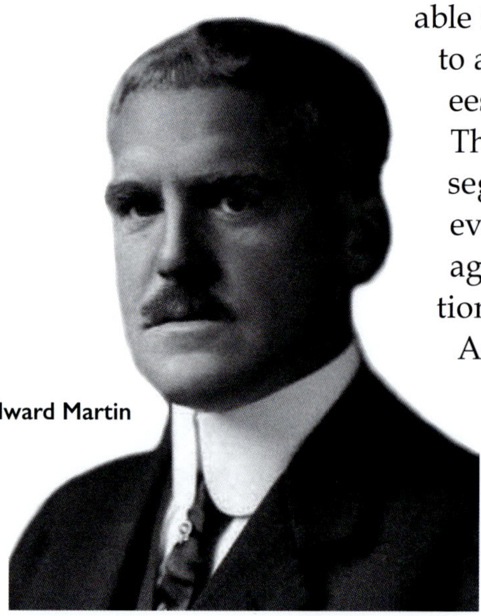

Edward Martin

So what is the present status of the Society of Clinical Surgery now that its relationship with the American

College of Surgeons is long forgotten? Its members still enjoy the intimacy and informality of watching each other operate. HUP's Edward Martin and the Society's role in this history may not be remembered, but his legacy is continued through the large number of HUP members—including Todd Bauer and Rachel Kelz, the current officers. Edward Martin would no doubt be pleased with the present leadership.

In 1902, Martin became clinical professor of surgery at Women's Medical College and from 1903 to 1910, clinical professor of surgery at Penn. In 1910, he was appointed John Rhea Barton Professor and Chairman of Surgery in our department.

During World War I, Martin was promoted to colonel and was the first director of Base Hospital 20, the HUP-staffed unit in France.[12] He also headed the Army Medical Reserve Officer Training camp and was a member of the powerful Medical Section of the Council of National Defense, which determined who should be drafted into the armed services.

Nationally respected, he was a member of the American Surgical Association, the Society of Clinical Surgery, the American Philosophical Society, and the American Association of Genitourinary Surgeons.

Locally, Martin was best known for his civic activities. Because of his interest and experience in public health and sanitation, he was appointed Philadelphia's director of public health and charities.[13] Later he became commissioner of health for Pennsylvania. He also served three terms—twenty-seven years—on the Philadelphia Board of Education, including three years as chairman. Honorary doctorates were awarded to Martin by Swarthmore, Penn, and Temple.

Rather unexpectedly, in 1918 at age fifty-nine, Martin retired after only eight years as chairman of Penn's surgery department to serve as chief of surgery at Walter Reed Hospital. When questioned about his motive for this, he answered that he felt he should give up surgery or give up golf and that he preferred to give up surgery.

Martin was always loyal and particularly generous to his alma maters. Through his friendship with Fred B. Kirby, a wealthy college classmate, he obtained a million-dollar gift to fund the Edward Martin Biological Laboratory Building at Swarthmore.[14] Another million dollars was left in his name for medical student scholarships at Penn. He once tried to use his golfing skills for the benefit of the Penn department of surgery. He made a bet with Charles Geist, the wealthy owner of the Seaview Golf Club near Atlantic City.[15] If Martin won, $100,000 would fund a chair in his name in our Department of Surgery. If he lost, $1,000 would go to Geist. This wager was reported in the local newspapers, illustrated by cartoons. Martin was a serious golfer, but apparently, he lost since there is no Martin Chair at Penn.

Before and during his subsequent twenty years in retirement, the debonair Martin was reported to be something of a ladies' man. Although assumed to be happily married, he sometimes admitted female admirers to the hospital for extended stays that were never explained. Hidden

1918
Martin directs HUP's Base Hospital 20 in France

1918–1923
Edward Martin is director of Public Health and Charities. Serves twenty-seven years on Philadelphia Board of Education

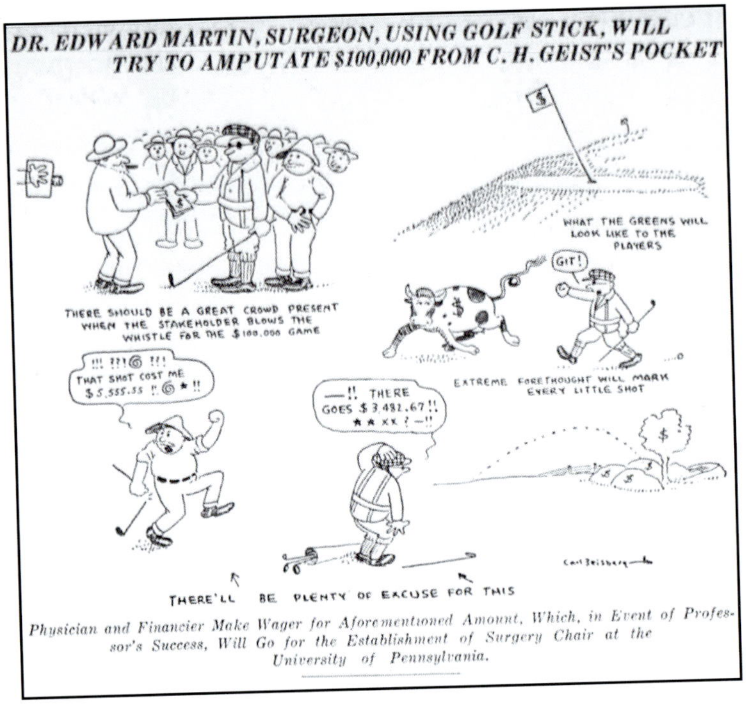

Cartoon from the *Evening Ledger*—May 27, 1915

away somewhere is an inkwell that used to be exhibited in a display case of the John Morgan building. The most interesting feature of this artifact is a round hole in the right upper corner.[16] The hole was made by a bullet that caused a superficial wound in Martin's chest on its way to the inkwell. Although the details of the episode are obscure, we know that the bullet was fired from the gun of a jealous husband and that the shooter was the director of HUP.

Martin's portrait in the John Morgan Building shows him to be a handsome man. Ironically, it was necessary for the artist to obscure the fact that Martin had lost most of his nose to squamous cell cancer. For years he was forced to wear a prosthetic nose.[17]

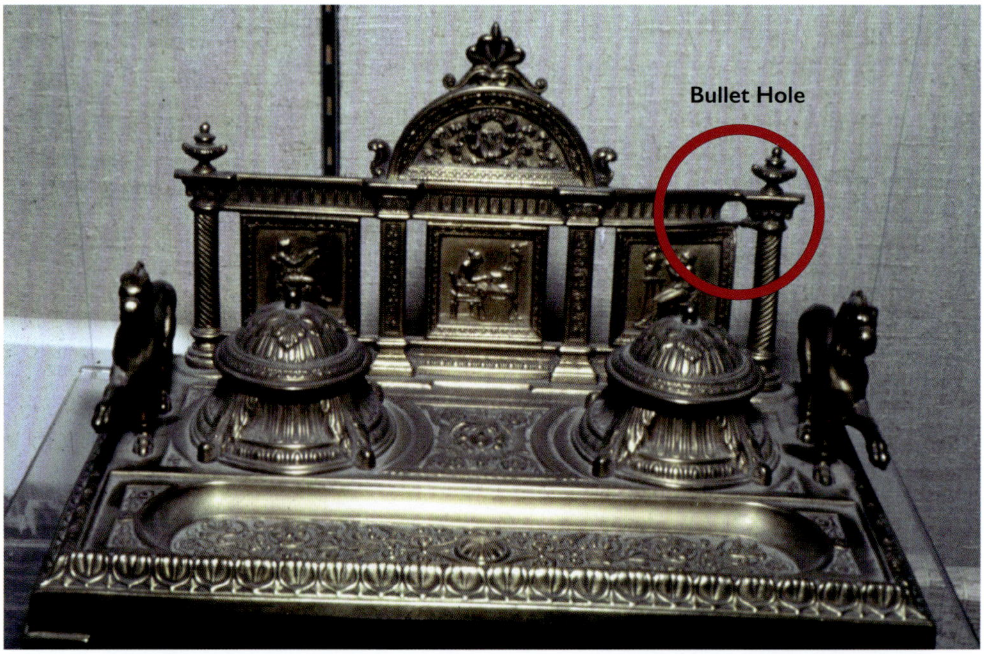

Timeline of Events During the Career of Edwin Martin

1878 Martin graduates from Swarthmore Phi Beta Kappa and member of crew and football teams.

1882 Nathan Francis Mossell is the first Black graduate of Penn medical school.

1883 Martin obtains MD from University of Pennsylvania.

1885–1900 Martin is assistant to D. Hayes Agnew and J. William White.

1898 Spanish-American War. Martin's hygiene policies stamp out the typhoid epidemic that is killing more soldiers than battle wounds.

1910 The Flexner Report is published. Its findings of deficiencies lead to closure of many American medical schools. Penn is placed in a top group but is not praised for academic and research activities. Penn dean Edgar Fahs Smith, in response to criticisms of the Flexner Report, conceives the idea of a graduate school to further educate medical school graduates. Graduate School is formed.

1910-1918 Martin is chairman of Penn's department of surgery.

1911 The second Clinical Congress of North American Surgeons meets in Philadelphia. Edward Martin is president of the Clinical Congress. It is inspired by meetings of the Society of Clinical Surgery, which allow members to watch operations. Over several years, the Congress morphs into the American College of Surgeons.

1911 The first human kidney transplant is performed at the Clinical Congress by former Penn faculty member, Levi J. Hammond. As a donor, he uses the kidney of a man killed in an accident twenty-four hours earlier. Prolonged warm ischemia would have made success impossible despite the *New York Times'* favorable report. On the same day, Hammond performs a testicle transplant, attempting to avoid ischemic damage by cooling the donor organ.[18] Alexis Carrel also presents a paper at the same meeting.

1911 Alfred Stengel is appointed chairman of medicine. He reorganizes the department into divisions and, in response to the Flexner Report, attempts to emphasize research.

1912 Henry K. Pancoast is the first US professor of roentgenology. He is the first to note the influence of radiation on development of leukemia and to recognize its promise for treatment of cancer.

1913 The American College of Surgeons is founded. Edward Martin is a founder and member of the first Board of Regents.

1914 Women are admitted to the University of Pennsylvania Medical School.

1915 Charles Wolferth is HUP's first medical resident.

1916 The Graduate School of Medicine of the University of Pennsylvania is founded. The Graduate Hospital opens in 1919. George Muller, a senior surgeon at Penn and future president of the American College of Surgeons and the College of Physicians of Philadelphia, becomes the chairman of the graduate division and chief of surgery at Graduate Hospital. Muller leaves Penn in 1936 to become chairman of surgery at Jefferson. Chevalier Jackson opens the first broncoscopic clinic in the United States. He is the first chairman of bronchoscopy and esophagoscopy at Graduate Hospital.

April 1917–Nov. 1918 The United States participates in World War I. HUP personnel staff Base Hospital 20 at Chatel Guyon, a resort in France. Edward Martin is the first director. John B. Carnett is the organizer of the unit and serves the longest as director. Eldridge Eliason is the chief of surgery.

1918 Martin resigns as Penn chairman of surgery and becomes chief of surgery at Walter Reed.

1918 The influenza epidemic hits Philadelphia, and the death rate exceeds that of any other US city; 1,200 die in one month. In 120 days, twenty-two million die worldwide. HUP is quarantined with no visitors allowed. Penn medical students are pressed into service. Isaac Star, a future dean, writes a classic paper about his experience.

1918 After the war, Carnett, director of Base Hospital 20, is among faculty members not reappointed to HUP by chairman John B. Deaver. Instead, Carnett becomes chief of surgery at Graduate Hospital.

1918 The first two women graduate from medical school at the University of Pennsylvania, Gladys Girardeau and Alberta Peltz.

1918 I. S. Ravdin graduates from medical school.

1918 Elizabeth Glenn becomes the first woman intern at HUP. She later marries I. S. Ravdin and becomes associate dean. During World War II, she will pretty much run the medical school in the absence of Dean Pepper.

1935 Martin receives honorary doctorate of science from Temple.

1936 Martin is president of Philadelphia Board of Education.

1938 Martin dies.

Notes

[1] Jequier AM. Edward Martin (1859–1938): The founding father of modern clinical andrology. *Int J Androl* (1991) 14(1):1–10. doi:10.1111/j.1365-2605.1991.tb01057.x.

[2] Ibid.

[3] Ravitch, Mark. *A Century of Surgery Vol I, 1880–1980* (Philadelphia: J.B. Lippincott Company, 1981) p. 204.

[4] Eliason, Eldridge. Memoir of Edward Martin 1859–1938. *Annals of Surgery*, 108(3):476 (Sept. 1938).

[5] Ravitch, Mark. *A Century of Surgery Vol I, 1880–1980,* p. 451.

[6] Cooper III, David Y and Ledger, Marshall A. *Innovation and Tradition at the University of Pennsylvania School of Medicine, An Anecdotal Journey* (Philadelphia: University of Pennsylvania Press, 1990). p. 108.

[7] Eliason, Eldridge. *Memoir of Edward Martin 1859–1938.*

[8] Ibid.

[9] *To Spread the Light of Knowledge, 250 Years of the Nation's First Medical School* (Philadelphia: Trustees of the University of Pennsylvania) p.103. Edward Martin arranged for six trains with 267 patients to be sent to HUP. Only one patient died.

[10] Martin, Franklin. *Presidential Address American College of Surgeons: The Past, the Present, the Future: Story of Soc Clin Surg – ACS.* Delivered at ACS Congress (1928) p. 19.

[11] Martin, Franklin. *Presidential Address American College of Surgeons: The Past, the Present, the Future: Story of Soc Clin Surg – ACS.* Delivered at ACS Congress (1928).

[12] Eliason, Eldridge. *Memoir of Edward Martin 1859–1938.*

[13] Cooper III, David Y and Ledger, Marshall A. *Innovation and Tradition at the University of Pennsylvania School of Medicine, An Anecdotal Journey*, p. 478.

[14] Eliason, Eldridge. *Memoir of Edward Martin 1859–1938.*

[15] *Morning Ledger Philadelphia* (Thurs., Mar. 27, 1915).

[16] Cooper III, David Y and Ledger, Marshall A. *Innovation and Tradition at the University of Pennsylvania School of Medicine, An Anecdotal Journey*, p. 119.

[17] Ibid., p. 119.

[18] Baron, Pamela, Schulsinger, David, Sheynkin, Yefim. The Curious Case of Dr. Levi Hammond: Transplantation Galore of 1911. *Journal of Urology* (Apr. 2015) Vol 193, No 4S, p e584–585. doi: 10.1016/j.juro.2015.02.487.

CHAPTER 11

Slashing His Way to World Fame

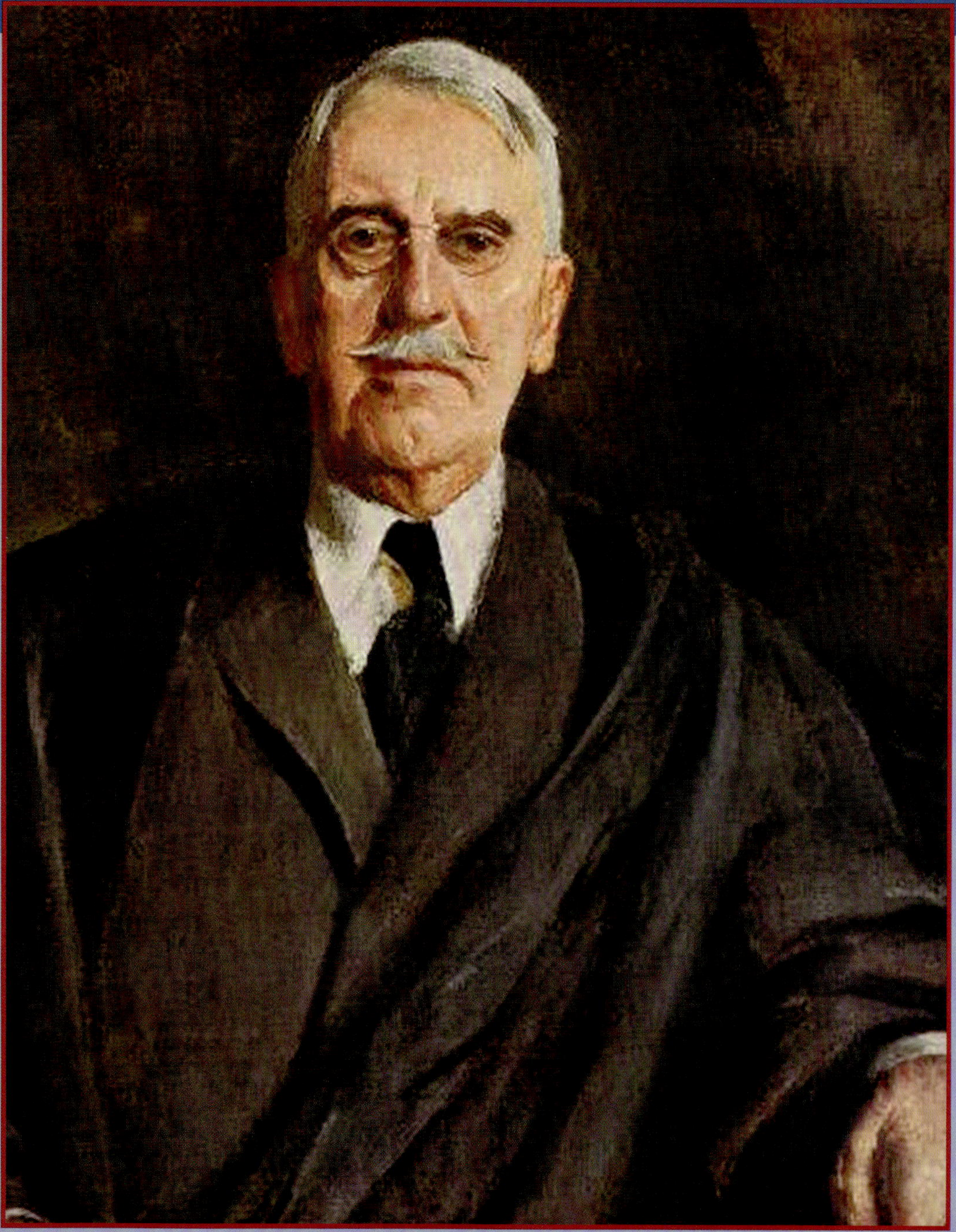

John B. Deaver (1855–1931)

JRB Professor and Chairman of Surgery (1918–1922)

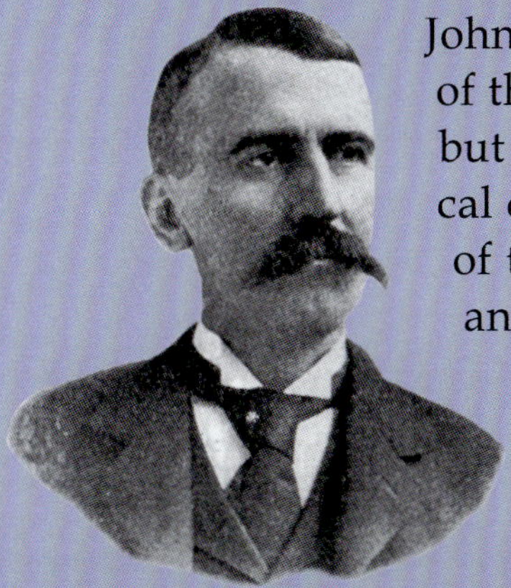

John Blair Deaver

John B. Deaver's four-year term (1918–1922) was one of the shortest of any surgery department chairman, but over his extensive career, this flamboyant surgical colossus was probably the most famous and one of the most colorful of the bunch.[1] With better luck and fewer years lost to exile from the university, he would surely have had greater impact on the development of the department.

John B. Deaver was born near Lancaster, Pennsylvania, in 1855. His father was a doctor, a country general practitioner. Three of his father's sons became doctors. As a child, Deaver attended West Nottingham School in Maryland, but instead of going to college, he taught in Lancaster public schools to earn money for medical school, graduating from Penn in 1878.[2] Then for a few years, he and his two doctor brothers practiced surgery together in rural Pennsylvania, operating as a team on patients stretched out on their kitchen tables, one brother as surgeon, one as first assistant, and the other as anesthetist.[3]

In 1881, the twenty-six-year-old Deaver joined the faculty at the University of Pennsylvania. At first, he devoted himself mainly to the study of anatomy in which he became an authority, a popular teacher, and the author of four widely read textbooks.[4] Building on his extensive knowledge of anatomy, he also became a confidant surgeon. Intent on

1855
John Blair Deaver is born near Lancaster, Pennsylvania

1878
MD from Penn

1878–1881
Community practice of surgery by Deaver

1881
Deaver appointed to Penn faculty, in first years concentrates on study of anatomy

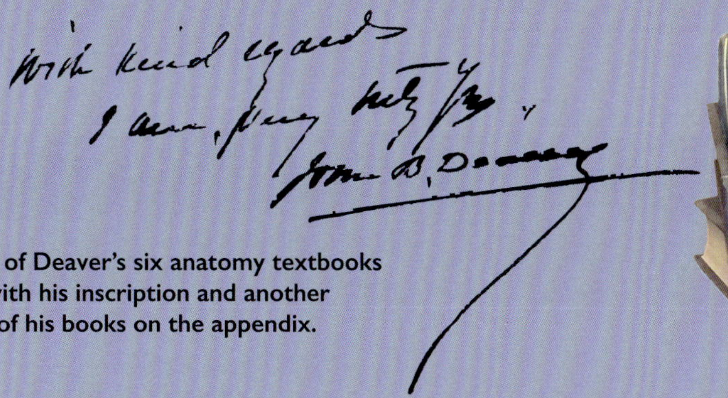

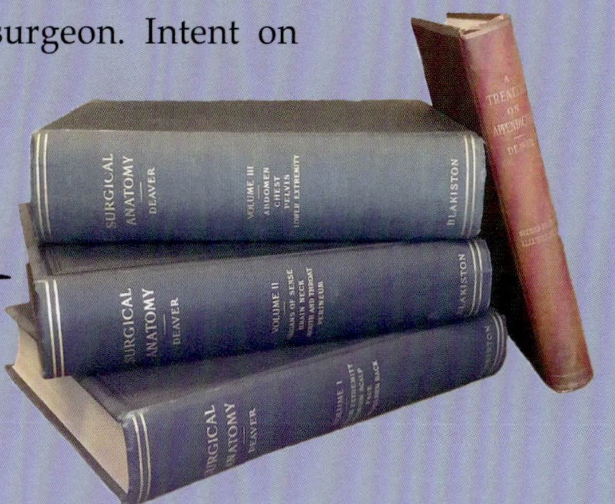

Three of Deaver's six anatomy textbooks with his inscription and another of his books on the appendix.

1885
Deaver begins to build his surgical practice

1889
Deaver becomes chief of surgery at German Hospital

1890
Despite lack of college education, Deaver becomes prominent medical author

1900
Deaver and White compete to succeed John Ashhurst as Penn surgery chairman. They become and remain lifelong enemies

White wins out and becomes Penn chairman

In spite, Deaver removes White's privileges at the German Hospital

developing a large practice, he operated not only at HUP but also at the German Hospital (renamed Lankenau Hospital during World War I). Largely responsible for his success was a fantastic work ethic. Deaver arose each morning before 5:00 a.m. and met his residents for rounds at 5:30.[5] He had no interest in pre- and post-operative care. On rounds, he saw only the patients selected by his residents as needing special attention.[6] This gave him more time to operate, which was his overriding passion. Fortunately, his judgment and physical diagnostic skills were exceptionally good, for he had a distrust of laboratory findings and a distaste for research.[7] As his practice grew to one of the city's largest, so did his national and international reputation.

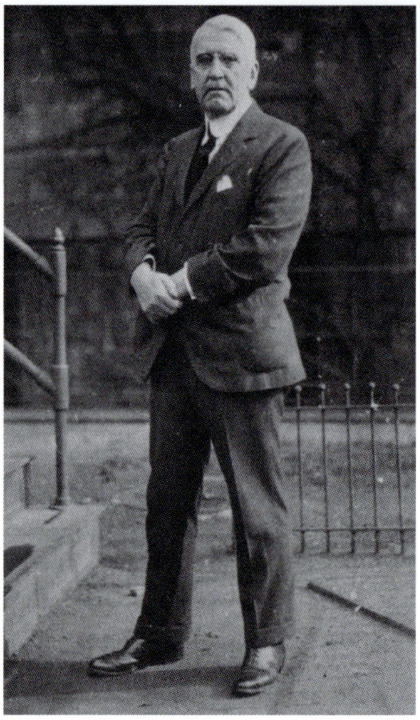

John B. Deaver
Always a country boy

Yet Deaver always remained a country boy from Lancaster. He was crusty, totally uninhibited, and lacking in social graces.[8] All of his life, he was embarrassed that he had not attended college.[9] He blamed this and his rural background for an inability to write proper English. However, his energy and editorial help (ghostwriting) by his young associates allowed Deaver to author 256 papers and six books.[10] At first, he paid his colleague George Muller one dollar for each paper he wrote. As proceeds from Deaver's growing practice allowed, he later paid I. S. Ravdin twenty-five dollars a paper and eventually paid Ravdin's wife, Dr. Elizabeth, 250 dollars a paper.[11] As a result, despite his lack of polish and his earthy language, he was heralded as a scholar and as a respected teacher, especially in anatomy.

A Famous Feud: Deaver versus White

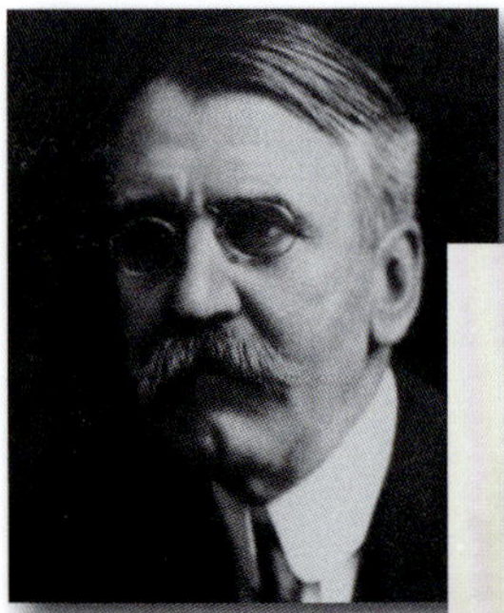

John B. Deaver

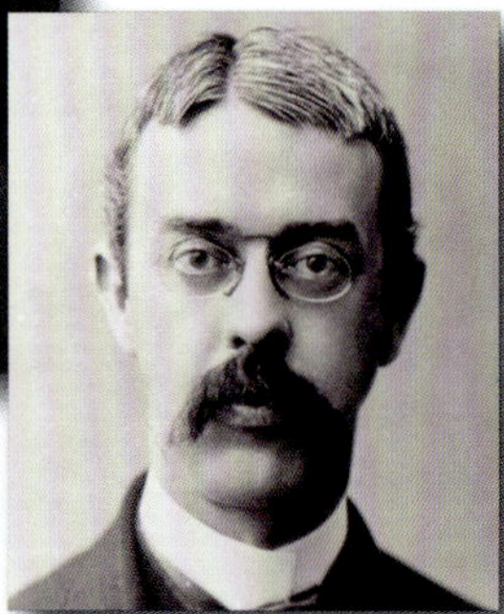

J. William White

Deaver and J. William White, his polished and socially prominent faculty colleague, developed an antipathy toward each other bordering on enmity.[12] This got worse in 1900 when Deaver and White became the obvious candidates to succeed John Ashhurst as chairman of the department of surgery. White was chosen. This may have been because of White's more acceptable social graces and family prestige or his considerable record in research. But Deaver thought himself better qualified, which in some respects, he was. Anyway, they became frank enemies. The angry Deaver then arranged to have White's practice privileges terminated at the German Hospital where Deaver had become the chief.[13] White retaliated by getting Deaver dismissed from the Penn faculty, thus forcing him to leave HUP.[14] For the next ten years, Deaver conducted his practice entirely at the German Hospital, now Lankenau. While he was in exile there, the proliferation of his surgical practice made him a legend.[15] His speed and confidence as an operator and his flamboyant showmanship depended on his incredible knowledge of anatomy rather than care or skill in dissection. His roughness and impatience in the operating room, although allowing acceptable outcomes, caused him to be described as a "slasher."[16] He performed as many as twenty-five operations a day. His Saturday afternoon operating schedule, using three to four tables at a time, became a mecca for spectators who came from all over the United States and abroad to watch this circus.[17]

1900–1910
In retaliation, White has Deaver fired from HUP faculty. He takes his practice entirely to German Hospital

1900–1910
Deaver's huge practice at German Hospital makes him famous. He also writes and lectures widely

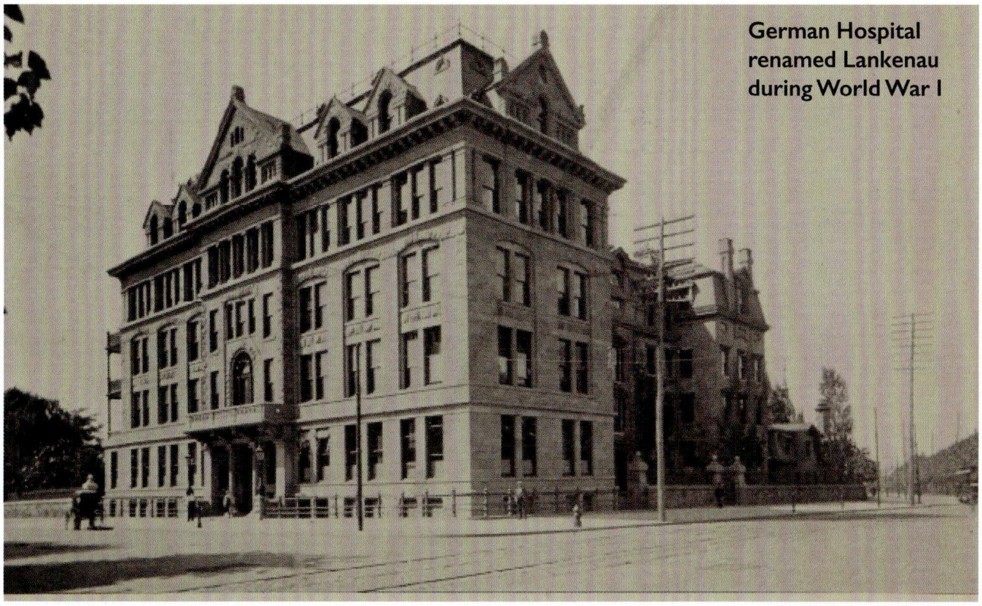

German Hospital renamed Lankenau during World War I

An internationally recognized authority on abdominal surgery, Deaver was one of the first to advocate early operations for appendicitis. In one year, he counted up 650 appendectomies.[18] One hundred and sixty of his appendicitis patients once held a celebratory dinner for him. He was also especially proficient in surgery of the biliary tree and for cancers of the pancreas, colon, stomach, uterus, and breast. He referred to the Cesarean section as his operation. His prolific bibliography on these topics bolstered the growth of his reputation.[19] In fact, he became so well-known that people from all over the country and even beyond came to him for advice or operations. Among those consulting him were actress Lillian Russell and US presidents Wilson and Coolidge. The railroad magnet Henry Huntington traveled from California for Deaver to operate on him. Unfortunately, he died during the operation.[20]

1900–1910
Deaver's world famous Saturday clinic at German Hospital

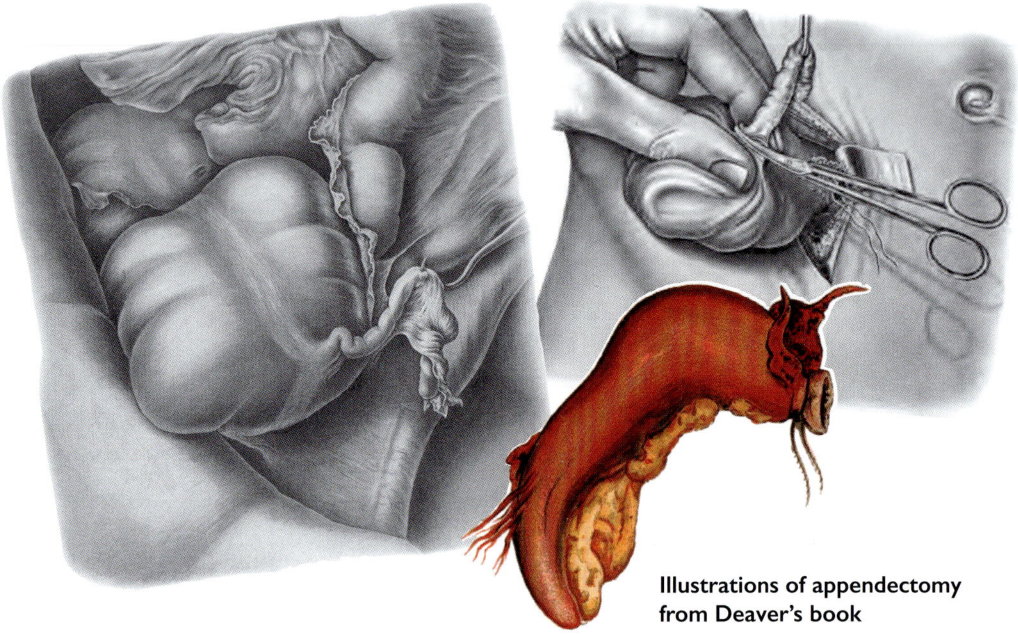

Illustrations of appendectomy from Deaver's book

It is generally conceded that Deaver did more operations than any other surgeon before or since.[21] He was known for aphorisms such as "cut well, sew well, get well" and "an inch and a half, a minute and a half and a week and a half," referring to the length of the incision, the time of the appendectomy, and the duration of the hospitalization.[22] He also said that no surgeon could be proficient until he had filled his own graveyard. His critics altered this to "Death by Deaver."

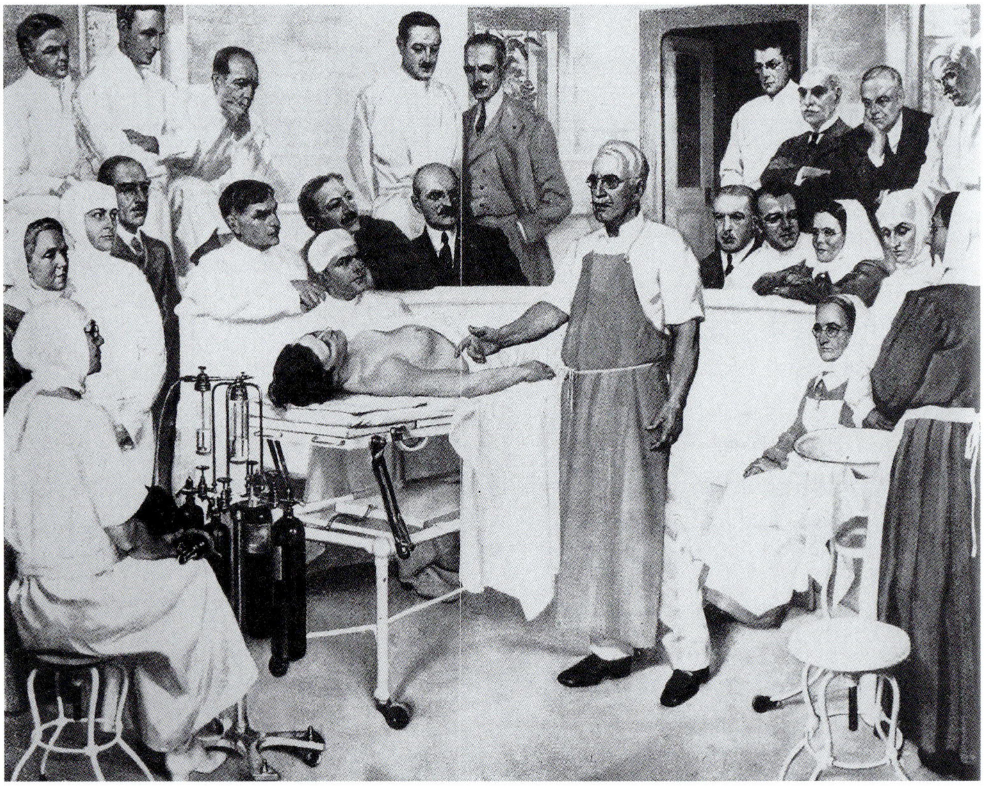

John B. Deaver's Saturday afternoon surgical clinic. Using three to four tables, he performs as many as twenty-five operations. An international audience watch.

In 1910, Deaver's enemy, J. William White, retired as department chairman. Once White was out of the way, his successor as chairman, Edward Martin, allowed Deaver to return to the university.[23] Eight years later, Martin retired, and Deaver was finally recognized by his appointment as John Rhea Barton Professor and Department chairman. [24] He was sixty-three years old. This happened in 1918 during World War I. Because many of the department's surgeons were away on military assignments, there were only three senior surgeons left at HUP, two of whom were not very active. At first, this suited Deaver very well because he always liked to do as many operations as possible.[25] But as the caseload became oppressive, he began to allow the residents to do a few of the easy operations, something he had never before permitted, preferring to do all aspects of every operation himself. As the residents became more experienced, they were allowed to do more and eventually even the most difficult cases, very much to the benefit of their education.[26]

As a teacher of operative surgery, Deaver was generous with his time, especially with his favorite resident, I. S. Ravdin. If the young Ravdin called for help or advice during an operation, Deaver would show up in the operating room, never scrubbing, but always remaining to provide support or give advice until the crisis was resolved.[27]

In 1918, as the war ended and former HUP faculty surgeons completed their military assignments, they assumed that their previous faculty positions would be waiting for them. Deaver had other ideas. He was determined to maintain his wartime monopoly of HUP's surgical cases. Now as the department chairman, he controlled appointments. He decided not to reappoint any of the former faculty.[28] As Dr. Ravdin tells the story, he convinced Deaver that some of the returning surgeons could be valuable faculty members who deserved to be reappointed. Deaver relented in some cases, but he saw a way that he would at least be able to retain all of the abdominal surgery for himself. He decided to divide up the body and assign each of the returning surgeons to a specific portion.[29] The youngest surgeons would be limited to the treatment of bones—fractures and amputations. Others would have surgery of the chest or hernias or the anus (proctology). Some would not be reappointed at all, such as a particularly deserving young surgeon, John Carnett, who had been the director of World War I's Base Hospital 20. But he was also a protégé of Deaver's old enemy, J. William White. Banished from HUP,

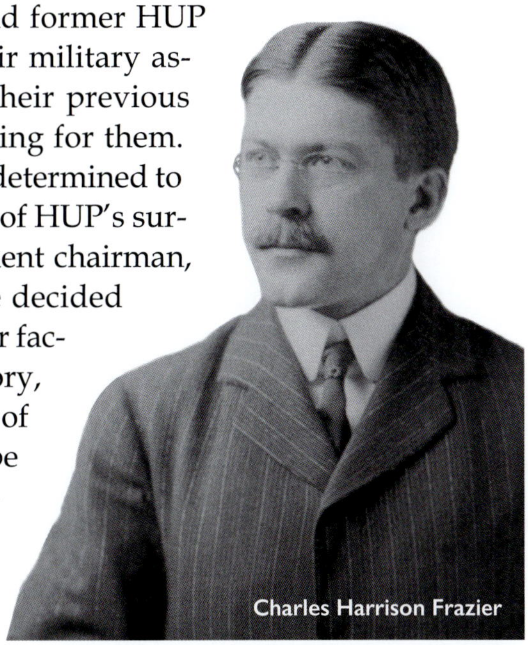

Charles Harrison Frazier

1910
Deaver's enemy White retires as chairman. Deaver's privileges are restored at HUP

1918
Deaver appointed chairman of surgery

1918
World War I ends. Deaver is reluctant to reappoint returning Army surgeons to the HUP faculty

1918
Deaver's reappointment of returning Army surgeons to HUP faculty is selective. Each surgeon is assigned to a particular body part, for example, Charles Frazier to the brain and thyroid

1918–1922
While he is HUP's chief of surgery, Deaver is important mentor of I. S. Ravdin

1921
Deaver elected president of American College of Surgeons

1922
Reluctantly, Deaver gives up Penn's surgery chairmanship. His time has already been extended beyond the usual age limit of sixty-five

1931
Deaver dies

Carnett was allowed to become a faculty member at the Graduate Hospital. He became chief there but soon suffered an untimely death. Charles Frazier, who had already shown interest in neurosurgery, was told he was limited to operations above the clavicle (in addition to the brain, this included only the thyroid).[30]

In retrospect, Deaver's apportionment of the body parts was a concept ahead of its time. It was the department's first move toward specialization, an idea that in coming decades would contribute to the progress of American surgery. However, it is worth remembering that this innovation had nothing to do with Deaver's foresight or desire to advance and modernize his department. Instead, his motivation was entirely selfish, to feed his obsession by protecting his enormous practice of abdominal surgery.[31]

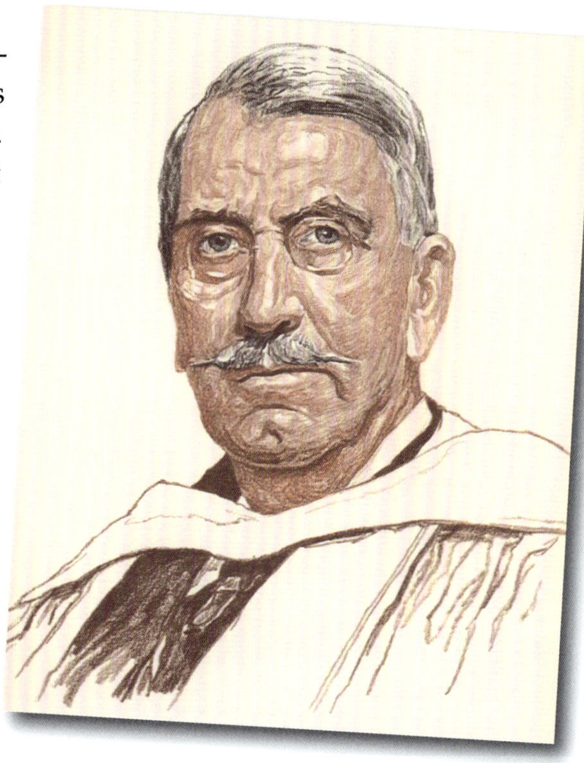

President of the American College of Surgeons
John B. Deaver

The eccentric and colorful style of this larger-than-life surgeon no doubt had a lot to do with his fame and his professional reputation. He was widely sought as a lecturer by professional groups and never turned down an invitation to speak.[32] He became a member of all the important surgical societies. He was a founder of the American College of Surgeons and, in 1921, became its fifth president.

Deaver's most important contribution to the department's future was through his relationship with I. S. Ravdin. Although Ravdin was tagged as a Frazier man, he was also Deaver's favorite. While Ravdin was still an intern, Deaver assigned him to the administrative position of chief resident, although there were other house officers more senior.[33] When Ravdin finished his residency, he had planned to return to his native Indiana to set up a community practice of surgery. Instead, Deaver persuaded him to remain in Philadelphia, first as clinical assistant to another master surgeon, George Muller, and then as administrative director of the new Graduate Hospital.[34]

Deaver never really retired, but after his time as department chair, he had time for golf. Even then, his restless and aggressive style prevailed. On Saturdays, he played by himself for thirty-six holes, wearing out two caddies and running from one hole to the next.[35] At age seventy-three, after surviving two years of a mysterious anemia, he died in 1931.[36]

Timeline of Events During the Career of John B. Deaver

1878	Deaver graduates from medical school, practices rural surgery with his two doctor brothers.
1880–1898	Deaver is appointed in the university's department of anatomy, writes and teaches anatomy.
1886	Deaver is appointed surgeon at German Hospital.
1889	Deaver becomes chief of surgery at German Hospital.
1900	White is appointed chairman of surgery at HUP. Deaver removes White's privileges at the German Hospital. White retaliates by removing Deaver's credentials at HUP.
1900–1910	Deaver's Saturday Operations Clinic at German Hospital makes him world famous.
1906	White is operated on by William Mayo for benign lesion. He retires from surgical practice and devotes himself to international travel, civic affairs, and becomes University trustee.
1910	Flexner Report is published.
1910	Dean Charles Frazier and Provost Harrison attempt to promote research by replacing old faculty with young academic stars. This reform fails.
1910	Edward Martin becomes JRB Professor and chairman of surgery.
1911	Deaver is allowed to return to HUP.
1916	J. William White dies.
1918	Deaver succeeds Edward Martin to become John Rhea Barton Professor and Chairman of the Department.
1918	I. S. Ravdin graduates from Penn medical school and becomes a HUP intern. During wartime shortage of house staff, Ravdin's training is accelerated. After only a few months, Deaver promotes him to the position of chief resident at HUP. HUP's senior surgeons (Deaver, Muller, and Frazier) are all enemies, each with an autonomous clinical service. Ravdin becomes the favorite of all three.
1918	The influenza epidemic kills 50 to 100 million victims worldwide. Sixteen thousand Philadelphians die from it. Philadelphia is the hardest-hit US city, in part, because of a super-spreader event in Philadelphia for selling war bonds. The third- and fourth-year classes of Penn medical school are closed. Twenty-five percent of HUP doctors and nurses are in France in the Army.

1918	As the war ends, HUP doctors assume they can return to their peacetime appointments, but Chairman Deaver is reluctant to reappoint former faculty to the HUP staff. Those turned away include John B. Carnett, a former junior faculty member who was the fundraiser, organizer, and leader of Base Hospital 20 in France. Carnett goes to Graduate Hospital where he becomes chief of surgery.
1919	Graduate School of Medicine and its hospital become international training facilities and centers of research. The graduate program is especially useful for refresher courses for returning military doctors after both World War I and II. Some of Penn's most distinguished investigators are based there (see Chapter 21). Chevalier Jackson establishes the country's first bronchoscopic and esopholoscopic clinics at Graduate Hospital.
1919	Ravdin is sent by Deaver to Graduate Hospital as George Muller's assistant. There he develops a successful practice and relationships with many Philadelphia practitioners who, in the future, will help him build his huge practice at HUP.
1921–1922	Deaver serves as president of the American College of Surgeons.
1921	A. N. Richards begins doing his classic experiments to show how the kidney makes urine.
1922	Charles Harrison Frazier succeeds Deaver as John Rhea Barton Professor and Chairman of Surgery at Penn.
1922	Frazier brings Ravdin back to HUP from Graduate Hospital as his assistant and the department's "executive director."
1931	Deaver dies.

Notes

[1] *Our Medical Heritage,* Lancaster City & County Medical Society, pp. 177–178.

[2] Ivy, Robert H. Personal Recollections of Holders of the John Rhea Barton Professorship at the University of Pennsylvania School of Medicine *Transactions and Studies of the College of Physicians of Philadelphia* 4th Ser, Vol 42, No 3 (1975) p. 249.

[3] Ibid., p. 249

[4] Ibid., p .249

[5] *The Reminiscence of Isidor Ravdin,* Columbia University Oral History Collection Part II No 156. Isidor Ravdin, Saul Benison, Barbara Land, Columbia University Oral Research Office, New York Times Oral History Program (1971) p. 54.

[6] Ibid., p. 54

[7] Ibid., p. 54

[8] Ivy, Robert H. *Personal Recollections of Holders of the John Rhea Barton Professorship at the University of Pennsylvania School of Medicine,* p. 249.

[9] Ashhurst, APC. Memoir of John Blair Deaver. *Annals of Surgery,* 95 (1932) p. 637.

[10] Ibid., p. 639

[11] *The Reminiscence of Isidor Ravdin,* pp. 56–57.

[12] Ivy, Robert H. *Personal Recollections of Holders of the John Rhea Barton Professorship at the University of Pennsylvania School of Medicine,* p. 249.

[13] Ashhurst, APC. Memoir of John Blair Deaver, p. 638.

[14] *The Reminiscence of Isidor Ravdin,* p. 40.

[15] Ashhurst, APC. Memoir of John Blair Deaver, p. 638.

[16] Ibid., p. 639

[17] Ashhurst, APC. Memoir of John Blair Deaver, p. 640.

[18] Dr. John B. Deaver, Noted Surgeon, Dies. *New York Times* (Sept. 26, 1931).

[19] Ashhurst, APC. Memoir of John Blair Deaver, p. 639.

[20] Henry E. Huntington Dies After Operation in East. *The Los Angeles Times* (May 24, 1927) p. 1.

[21] Ashhurst, APC. Memoir of John Blair Deaver, p. 639.

[22] Cooper III, David Y and Ledger, Marshall A. *Innovation and Tradition at the University of Pennsylvania School of Medicine, An Anecdotal Journey* (Philadelphia: University of Pennsylvania Press, 1990) p. 121.

[23] Ivy, Robert H. *Personal Recollections of Holders of the John Rhea Barton Professorship at the University of Pennsylvania School of Medicine,* pp. 250–251.

[24] Ashhurst, APC. Memoir of John Blair Deaver, p. 638

[25] *The Reminiscence of Isidor Ravdin,* p. 54.

[26] Ibid., p. 54.

[27] Ibid., p. 53.

[28] Ibid., p. 60.

[29] Ibid., p. 61.

[30] Cooper III, David Y and Ledger, Marshall A. *Innovation and Tradition at the University of Pennsylvania School of Medicine, An Anecdotal Journey,* pp. 108–109.

[31] *The Reminiscence of Isidor Ravdin,* p. 64.

[32] John B. Deaver speeches, MSS 2/036-01. Historical Medical Library of the College of Physicians of Philadelphia. http://localhost:8081/repositories/2/resources/1352.

[33] *The Reminiscence of Isidor Ravdin,* p. 51.

[34] Ibid., p. 69.

[35] Ivy, Robert H. *Personal Recollections of Holders of the John Rhea Barton Professorship at the University of Pennsylvania School of Medicine,* p. 250.

[36] Ibid., p. 251.

CHAPTER 12

Comeback of a Failed Reformer

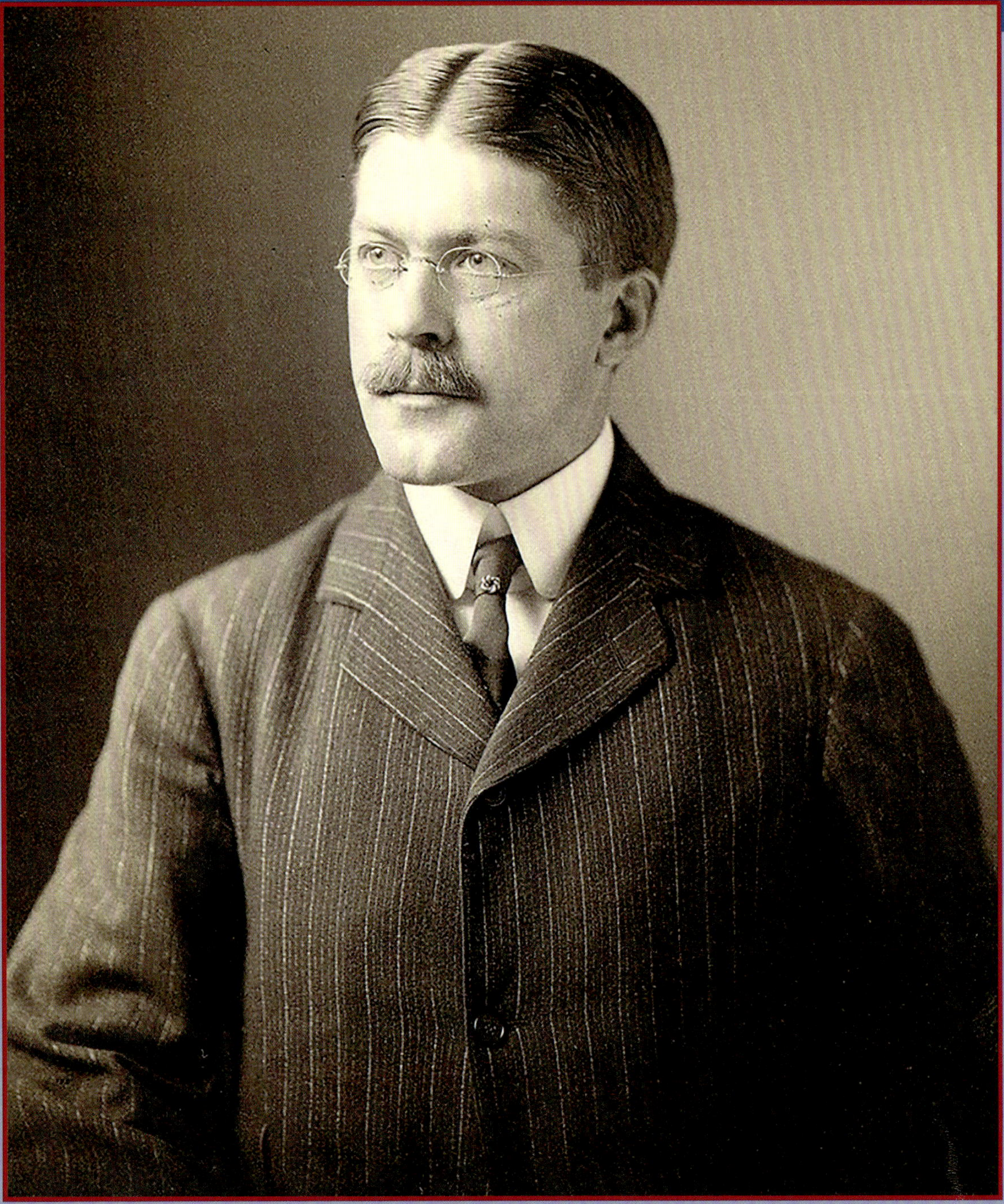

Charles Harrison Frazier (1870–1936)

JRB Professor and Chairman of Surgery (1922–1936)

Largely unrecorded for decades in the bland archives of the department are the peaks and valleys of this chairman's turbulent history. During the peaks, he may have been the leader most responsible for Penn Surgery as an academic department. He had neither the international acclaim of his predecessor in the chair—the flamboyant John B. Deaver—nor the technical gifts of his successor, the elegant Eldridge Eliason. But for lasting impact, he surpassed both of them and perhaps all the others. The story of Charles Frazier's rise, fall, and eventual vindication reads almost like an adventure novel.

1870
Charles Frazier is born into a prominent Philadelphia family

1892
Frazier's MD from Penn

1896
Frazier's first Penn faculty appointment

1900
Frazier appointed clinical professor of surgery

He was a short but powerfully built man with piercing blue eyes, a fiery temper, and a resounding voice.[1] This combination led to a presence that struck terror in the hearts of students, interns, residents, and many faculty colleagues. In a social setting, he could be gracious and charming, but he was viewed by most as autocratic and tyrannical. Tom Langfitt, a recent chief of Penn neurosurgery, said he was the prototypical neurosurgeon.

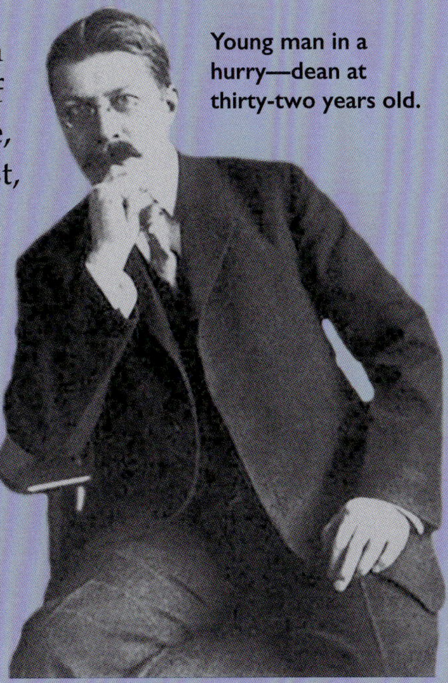

Young man in a hurry—dean at thirty-two years old.

Along with so many of the early Penn faculty, Charles Frazier came from one of Philadelphia's elite families. His uncle, Charles Custis Harrison, was the provost, the university's highest officer during the era before Penn had presidents.[2] George Leib Harrison, his cousin, was the department of surgery's most important philanthropist whose estate would eventually endow the Harrison Department of Surgical Research.[3] Charles Frazier graduated from college in 1889 and medical school in 1892, both at Penn. After interning at HUP and Episcopal Hospital under White and Ashhurst and

1903
Frazier is dean of Penn's medical school. He becomes disappointed with Penn's academic performance

1907
Frazier establishes HUP's social services

1909
Frazier submits to the trustees his plan for faculty reform and emphasis of research

1910
Publication of the Flexner Report

1910
Frazier's plan for reform is endorsed by trustees

a year in Berlin studying pathology, surgery, and neurology under Virchow and von Bergmann, he joined the Penn faculty in 1896.

Family connections probably played a role in his rapid progress to appointment as professor of surgery and then in 1903 as dean when he was only thirty-two years old. As the school's dean, rather than perpetuating the status quo of a faculty populated largely by his relatives and family friends, Frazier unexpectedly worked to change Penn Medicine's tradition of inbreeding and its mediocre performance in research. He also fought successfully for academic reforms, such as tightening entrance requirements from two to four years of college.

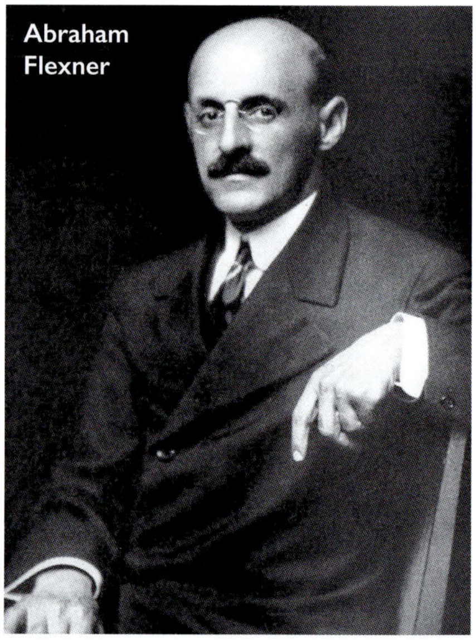
Abraham Flexner

Not satisfied with these accomplishments, he was determined to bring about greater changes, and he thought he knew how. He also believed there was some urgency to this, since Abraham Flexner was about to complete his famous survey of American medical schools and issue an influential report evaluating each school.[4] Frazier anticipated that Penn would be embarrassed by receiving a mediocre grade. In hopes of avoiding this, he drafted a plan to reorganize the faculty and drastically modernize the school's priorities, thus improving its image at this critical time.[5] He thought he was in a position to implement the plan by using the power of the provost, his uncle.

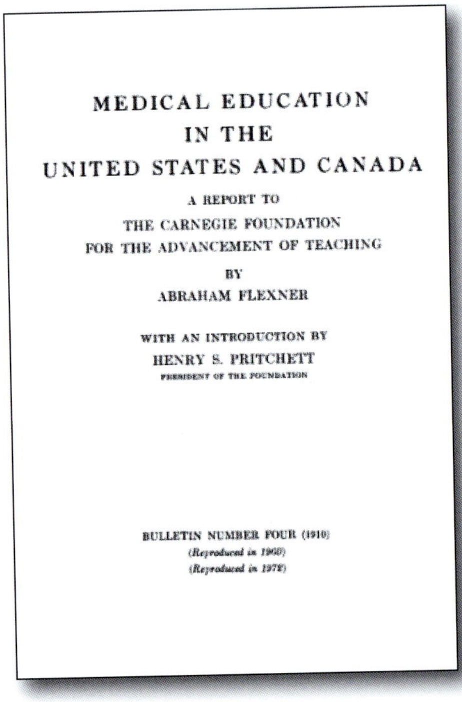
MEDICAL EDUCATION
IN THE
UNITED STATES AND CANADA
A REPORT TO
THE CARNEGIE FOUNDATION
FOR THE ADVANCEMENT OF TEACHING
BY
ABRAHAM FLEXNER
WITH AN INTRODUCTION BY
HENRY S. PRITCHETT
PRESIDENT OF THE FOUNDATION
BULLETIN NUMBER FOUR (1910)
(Reproduced in 1960)
(Reproduced in 1972)

Provost Harrison was also worried about the impending Flexner Report that he feared would damage Penn with faint praise of the school's academic programs.[6] He was persuaded that his nephew's plan was sound and that he could pull it off.

Some young faculty, alumni, and students realized that reform was needed, but most senior faculty opposed it. More than anyone else, Frazier was responsible for orchestrating a dramatic shakeup. His reputation was on the line.

The provost was not a doctor. As a highly successful businessman, he was used to having his own way.[7] He had little regard for the polite, deliberately paced formalities customary in the academic world. He was a man of action. Therefore, the provost,

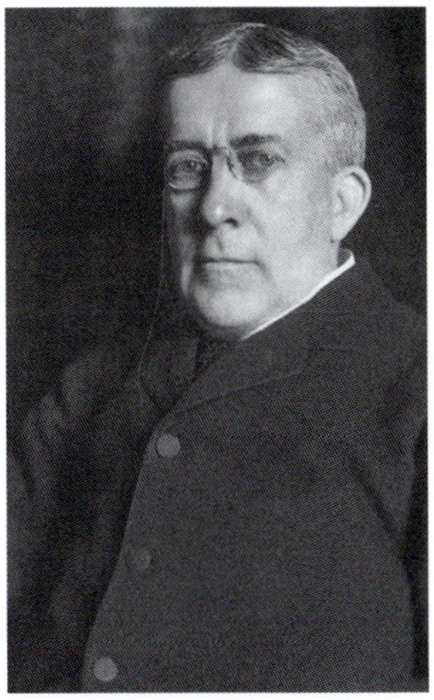

Charles Custis Harrison
Provost

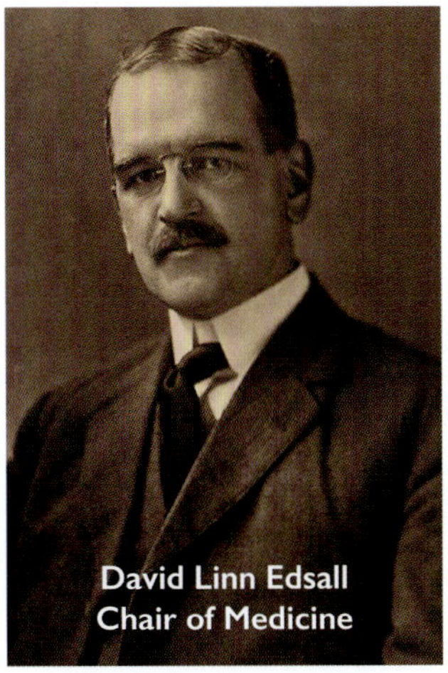

With Frazier the leader
of the young Turks.

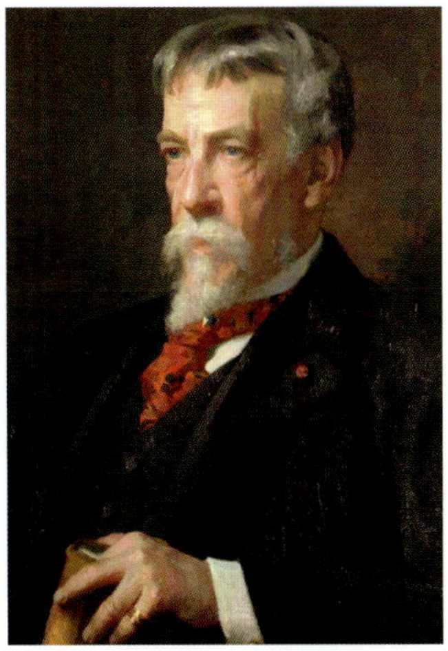

S. Weir Mitchell
Board of Trustees Leader

1909–1910
The Edsall Affair

1910
Opposition to the reform by conservatives is led by surgical chair J. William White

1910
The reform fails. New faculty are ousted

quite independently of the board of managers or any faculty knowledge or support, went directly to the university trustees for approval of Frazier's plan for reorganization.[8] It would abruptly replace most of the senior faculty with young, research-oriented outsiders. The trustees and especially their leader, S. Weir Mitchell, liked the plan and endorsed it.

David Edsall, one of Penn's only young academic stars, was appointed chair of medicine, replacing the beloved but aging James Tyson who was considered part of the "dead wood."[9] Bright young leaders identified by Edsall were recruited from other parts of the country (Chicago, California, Harvard, and Northwestern) and appointed as chairs of most other departments.[10] In addition, all faculty, even the surgeons, would be expected to spend at least half of their time doing research, teaching, or other academic work for the school rather than on their private practice.[11] These and other anticipated changes of the plan, such as limitation of active faculty appointments to age sixty-two for surgeons, were given front-page coverage in the local newspapers. It looked very much as if Frazier and his uncle had succeeded in what they viewed as "dragging the medical school out of self-satisfied complacency and scientific stagnation."[12] It seemed to be a fait accompli.[13]

But wait, not so fast! The conservative old guard fought back, vigorously resisting the changes. The ensuing battle was bitterly fought. The hard-headed surgery chairman, J. William White, was the leader of the opposition.[14] The department's other surgeons, mostly conservatives with lucrative private practices, were the faction most powerful in overcoming the change. When the smoke cleared, the old guard had prevailed. The newcomers would soon be ousted or given so little support that they resigned, including Edsall, who left for Washington University and then soon became Harvard's distinguished dean. Badly embarrassed by the reversal, Provost Harrison resigned, as did Frazier as dean. With the default of these two leaders of the reform, the whole thing collapsed.

1910–1922
Frazier concentrates on clinical practice. He performs more than 700 operations for tic douloureux with a mortality of less than 0.5 percent.

During long operations, the hard driving Frazier often wore a flask of milk on his belt. A tube from the flask was threaded under his shirt and mask to drip milk into his mouth which he swallowed to neutralize the effect of gastric acid on his duodenal ulcer

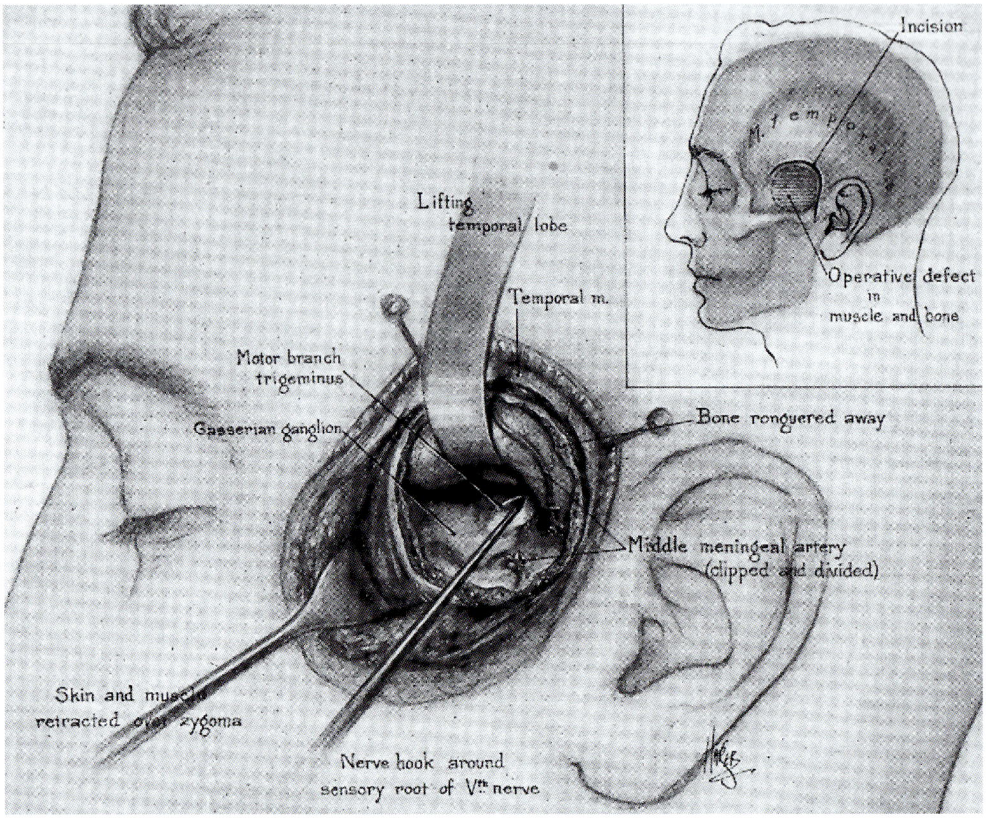

Exposure for section of sensory root of 5th cranial nerve in Frazier's operation for tic doulouroux.

The failure of this reform had profound and lasting results. It allowed Johns Hopkins, the new upstart school, to extend its lead in research and supplant lofty Penn from its traditional position as medicine's academic king. Ten years later, Frazier, the leader of the rebellion, wrote that he was still smarting, still devastated by the debacle.[15]

Despite the setback, the impact of Frazier's failed reform was not entirely negative. At least it called attention to deficiencies in the school, which was relying too heavily on its glorified past. In addition, the one young recruit who chose to remain at Penn instead of bailing out was the new chair of pharmacology. In coming generations, he would become a giant of American medicine and the school's most important leader, A. N. Richards.[16] But it would take thirty-five years before Frazier's protégé, I. S. Ravdin, would, at least in surgery, accomplish much of Frazier's dream to elevate academic activity to a level even with Penn's traditional emphasis on private clinical practice. To some extent, this battle still goes on as it probably always will.

Frazier had always been interested in neurosurgery, and for the rest of his life, he turned his attention to research and the development of this new field. He is now remembered best for his pioneering role and eminence in the emerging field of neurosurgery. Except for his contemporary, Harvey Cushing, he became recognized as perhaps the nation's leader in this new specialty.[17] Of his many innovations, his best known work is on tic douloureux. As early as 1901, working with neurologist William Spiller, Frazier had shown that preganglionic section of the sensory root of the fifth cranial nerve was as effective and lasting for relief of the pain of trigeminal neuralgia as avulsion of the Gasserian ganglion, and a much safer operation.[18] Cordotomy, or section of the anterolateral columns of the spinal cord for relief of pain, was another product of the collaboration of Spiller and Frazier.[19] Less well-known was Frazier's improved treatment of pituitary lesions and his management of head trauma and peripheral nerve injuries.[20] His trainees in neurosurgery headed their own programs at many institutions, including the University of Michigan, the Crile Clinic, and the Mayo Clinic.[21]

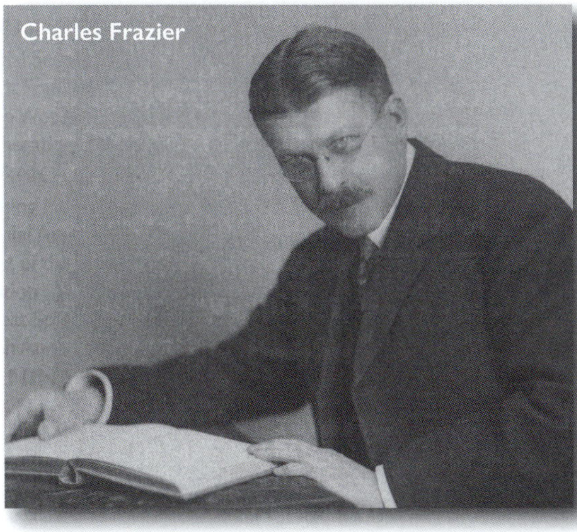
Charles Frazier

During World War I, Frazier was disappointed not to be given an overseas Army assignment. Instead he was placed in charge of Base Hospital II, a military hospital at Cape May, New Jersey, taking care of wounded soldiers. There he treated 500 patients with peripheral nerve injuries and 200 patients with gunshot wounds to the head.

Frazier's relationship with his surgical colleagues had been cooled by his attempt to reorganize the faculty and emphasize research over private clinical practice. The powerful John B. Deaver also opposed these changes and was particularly hostile to Frazier. In 1918, Deaver became chairman of the department of surgery. One of his first actions was to forbid Frazier to operate on any part of the body below the clavicle.[22] This ended Frazier's activity as a versatile general surgeon, although it allowed him to become the department's specialist in thyroid surgery. It was claimed that he performed as many as 300 thyroidectomies per year, mostly for toxic goiter. For the rest of his career, in addition to neurosurgery, he maintained a large thyroid practice, a thyroid clinic, and fellowship. Deaver's dictum was an additional reason for Frazier to focus on surgery of the brain and cranial nerves, which he had already begun to emphasize. Being forced to confine himself largely to neurosurgery helped Frazier become a world leader in the field.

When Deaver retired in 1922, Frazier was appointed John Rhea Barton Professor and Chairman of Surgery, serving in this position until 1936. As chairman, he continued to improve the research and academic aspects of the department. Another important innovation was his appointment at HUP of a group of postinternship fellows. This was the first step toward modern residency training.[23] One of his fellows became an

1911
Cordotomy for unrelenting lower body pain is suggested by Spiller, first performed by Edward Martin, and later improved by Frazier

1914–1918
World War I. Frazier directs an Army hospital in New Jersey

1918
Influenza epidemic

1918
John B. Deaver is appointed surgery chairman, limits Frazier to brain and thyroid surgery

1922–1936
Charles Frazier succeeds Deaver as surgery chairman

1925
Frazier starts a fellowship program for postinternship training in surgery

important leader in the department, L. Kraeer Ferguson.

While he was a junior in college at Wilmington, Pennsylvania, L. Kraeer Ferguson volunteered to serve in the Army, was sent to France, and was awarded his degree in absentia in 1918.[24] After the war, he attended the Université d'Aix-Marseille before returning to the US in 1919. He finished medical school at the University of Pennsylvania in 1923, served his internship at HUP in 1925, and completed surgical training there in 1928 as the first resident in Charles Frazier's formal training program. After a year of study in Germany at Frankfurt am Main, he returned to Philadelphia and was appointed to the surgical faculty of the University of Pennsylvania. With Detlev Bronk in the Johnson Foundation, he published research papers on the nervous control of intercostal respiration. In 1929, he was appointed chief of the surgical outpatient clinic at HUP. Based on this experience, he wrote *Surgery of the Ambulatory Patient,* a book that became a standard text on the subject through multiple editions. He served for many years on the staff of Philadelphia General Hospital (PGH) and was chief of surgery there from 1937 to 1955.

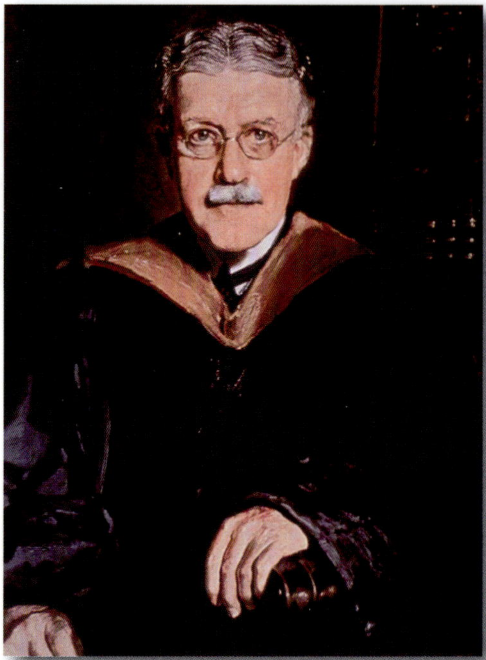

Charles Frazier as John Rhea Barton Professor and Chairman of Surgery. Portrait by Frederick Roscher, 1930.

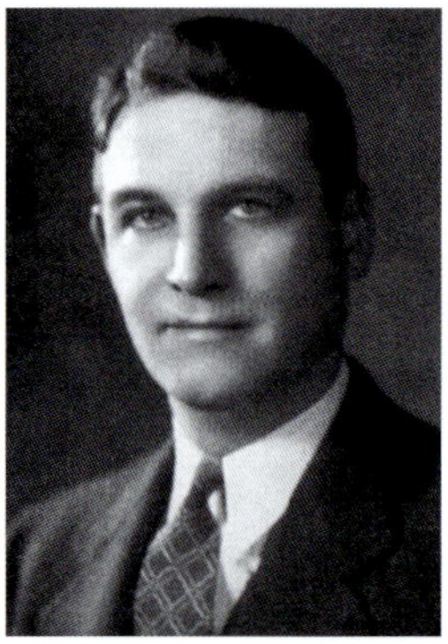

L. Kraeer Ferguson

During World War II, Ferguson served as a member of the University of Pennsylvania naval unit. He was chief of surgery on the hospital ship *Solace* in the Pacific theater of war. His group compiled a record low mortality rate. Of 4,039 battle casualties, only seven patients died. In 1946, Ferguson was appointed clinical professor of surgery at the University of Pennsylvania, and in the following year, professor and chairman of the department of surgery of Women's Medical College and professor of surgery at the Graduate School of Medicine of the University of Pennsylvania. He held both of these positions until 1960 when he retired from Women's Medical College and became chairman of the department of surgery of the Graduate School. In 1962, he suffered a partial paralysis of his left hand and retired from surgical activity. However, he remained active as a teacher and consultant at Graduate Hospital. Ferguson's clinical focus was gastrointestinal surgery, which was the topic of his more than 150 publications, including the book, *Current Perspectives in Gastroenterology,* published with William Blakemore in 1967. He was a member of all the important surgical organizations including the American Surgical Association and served as an officer in many of them.

Maybe the most important aspect of Frazier's chairmanship was his relationship to his assistant, I. S. Ravdin, who always identified Frazier as his most important mentor. In 1918 when Ravdin finished his residency, the only job opportunity offered him by Deaver, then department chairman, was a position at Graduate Hospital.[25] Thus, Ravdin's future seemed to be that of just one more surgical practitioner at a local hospital. But in 1922, Frazier took over as department chairman and needed an assistant. He promptly sent for Ravdin, rescuing him from his exile at Graduate Hospital. Frazier made Ravdin the department's executive director, a new position which was effectively the chairman's second in command.[26] Then in 1927, he sent Ravdin to Scotland and England for training in basic research.[27] This was the making of Ravdin as an academic surgeon and the key to the future of our modern department.

Unfortunately, Frazier's eventual demise was an ugly one. In 1935, I. S. Ravdin accompanied his chief to Johns Hopkins where Frazier underwent a botched prostatectomy by the famous urologist, Hugh Young. Ravdin, a pioneer in blood transfusions, helped resuscitate Frazier from shock caused by the extensive intraoperative bleeding, but his convalescence was prolonged and metastases were soon discovered.[28] Incontinence caused by the operation made the rest of Frazier's brief survival miserable. Refusing to give up, Frazier continued to operate even when he had to be strapped to the table to prevent falling.[29]

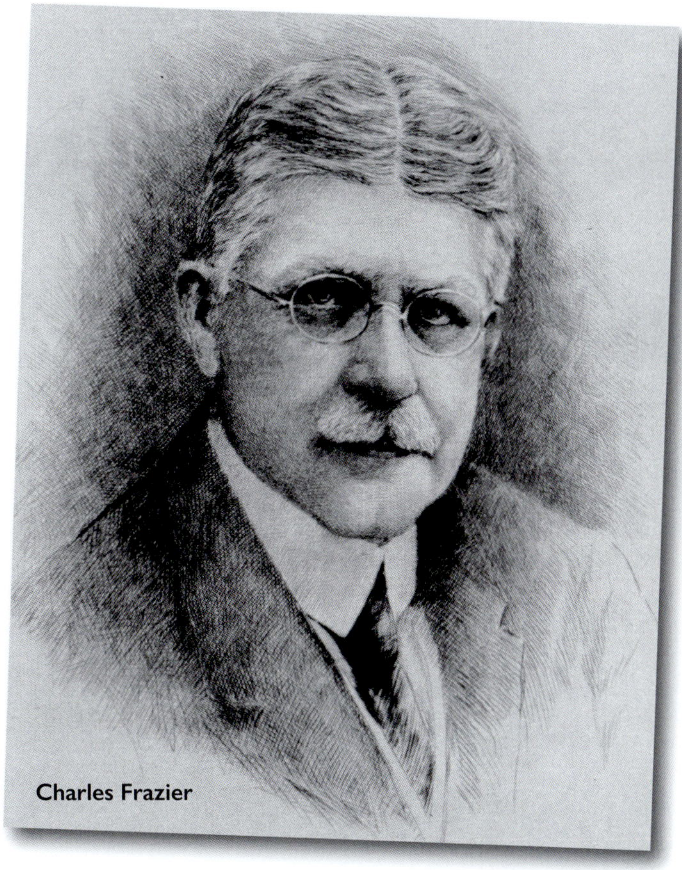

Charles Frazier

Frazier's most lasting impact on the department's progress was his role in obtaining its large endowment. In 1936, his family connection led to a $2.7 million bequest for the department's research.[30] Thus, thirty years after his failed academic reform, Frazier was able, through his family's generosity and the efforts of his protégé, I. S. Ravdin, to accomplish reform in surgery, creating at last a truly academic department.

1925–1927
Frazier is president of Society of Clinical Surgery

1927
Frazier sends I.S. Ravdin to England for a year of research

1935
Charles Frazier is operated on for prostate cancer

1936
Frazier's cousin George Leib Harrison leaves $2.7 million for the Department of Surgery's research. Ravdin uses the endowment to begin building a research faculty

1936
Frazier dies and is succeeded by Eldridge Eliason

But before Ravdin came into the kind of power needed to achieve this vision, another decade and a world war would go by. After Frazier's retirement and death in 1936, two candidates contended for the chairmanship. One was Eldridge Eliason, a conservative favoring Penn's traditional emphasis of clinical practice (the status quo). The other was I. S. Ravdin, a fiery young advocate of surgical science. Ravdin was much more widely known and respected nationally but Dean William Pepper saw Eliason as a safer bet and chose to appoint him as chairman.

Ravdin and the modern department would have to wait.

Timeline of Events During the Career of Charles Frazier

1892	Frazier receives MD from Penn.
1893–1894	Frazier interns at HUP and Episcopal Hospital.
1895	Frazier studies surgery, neurology, and pathology in Europe under Virchow and von Bergmann.
1896	Frazier is appointed to Penn faculty.
1901	Frazier and Spiller report that section of the preganglionic fifth nerve is a better and safer operation for tic douloureux than excision of the Gasserian ganglion.
1903	Thirty-two-year-old Frazier becomes the school's dean. With his uncle the provost, he attempts to promote research by replacing senior faculty with young, outside investigators.
1910	Opposed by the established conservatives, the reform fails. Frazier and Harrison are embarrassed and resign.
1914–1918	World War I.
1918	Spanish Flu epidemic.
1918	As chairman, John B. Deaver restricts Frazier to operations above the clavicle, limiting him to operations on the brain and thyroid.
1922	Former Dean Charles Frazier (1903–1909) succeeds John B. Deaver to become chairman of the department of surgery. Frazier brings Ravdin back to HUP from his exile in private practice at Graduate Hospital and appoints him as the department's executive director. In this new position, Ravdin serves as Frazier's assistant.
1924	Pharmacologist Carl Schmidt finds ephedrine in China and introduces it to the United States. He begins to train a series of surgeons and anesthesiologists.
1925–1927	Frazier is president of the Society of Clinical Surgery.
1927	Frazier sends Ravdin to Scotland and England where Ravdin spends a year in basic research instead of simply observing famous European surgeons operate, as other American doctors have done.
1928	On Ravdin's return, Frazier appoints him as director of the department's research and as the first J. William White Professor of Surgical Research.
1929	The Eldridge Reeves Johnson Foundation for Medical Physics is founded with Detlov Bronk as director. Bronk is awarded National Medal of Science. He later becomes director of Rockefeller Institute.
1930	The university's formal affiliation with Children's Hospital of Philadelphia is established.

1931 Francis Wood and Charles C. Wolferth prove that ischemia of the heart causes angina.

1931 John B. Deaver dies. Muller succeeds him as Chief of Surgery at Lankenau Hospital; Muller is also chief at Graduate. Muller is a major figure in Penn's department of surgery. He is a graduate of the University of Pennsylvania medical school class of 1899. He interned for three years under Deaver at the German Hospital before spending his early career at HUP as Frazier's assistant.

1932 George Cox Institute is established for study of diabetes.

1933 George Muller is appointed professor of clinical surgery at the University of Pennsylvania.

1933 Blue Cross is established.

1933 John Gibbon and his wife Mary begin to work at Penn in the department's laboratories on their heart-lung machine.

1934 T. Greer Miller and William Osler Abbot design the Miller-Abbot long double lumen tube for treatment of intestinal obstruction.

1935 Frazier is operated on at Hopkins for prostate cancer. Shock from intra- and postoperative bleeding is alleviated by blood tranfusions by Ravdin, a pioneer in this procedure.

1935 Charles Frazier's cousin, George Leib Harrison, designates his $2.7 million endowment for research to his personal physician, John B. Carnett. Carnett dies before Harrison, and the bequest goes to the department of surgery for its research and academic programs.

1936 The Harrison Department of Surgical Research is established. Ravdin becomes Harrison Professor and controls the endowment.

1936 Failing to become Penn's chairman, Muller goes to Jefferson as chairman of surgery. While at Penn, he was president of the Philadelphia College of Physicians, Academy of Surgery of Philadelphia, County Medical Society, and American Association of Thoracic Surgery. He is one of the earliest thoracic surgeons. In 1939, he becomes president of the American College of Surgeons.

1936 Frazier dies.

1936 Provost William Pepper appoints conservative candidate, Eldridge Eliason, as surgery chairman despite I. S. Ravdin's far greater national reputation. This postpones any chance of reforms that Ravdin would have advocated.

Notes

[1] Cooper III, David Y and Ledger, Marshall A. *Innovation and Tradition at the University of Pennsylvania School of Medicine, An Anecdotal Journey* (Philadelphia: University of Pennsylvania Press, 1990) p. 109.

[2] Meyerson, Martin and Winegrad, Dilys Pegler. *Gladly Learn and Gladly Teach: Franklin and His Heirs at the University of Pennsylvania, 1740–1976* (Philadelphia: University of Pennsylvania Press, 1978) pp. 102, 133.

[3] Cooper III, David Y and Ledger, Marshall A. *Innovation and Tradition at the University of Pennsylvania School of Medicine, An Anecdotal Journey,* pp. 150–151.

[4] Corner, George W. *Two Centuries of Medicine: A History of the School of Medicine, University of Pennsylvania* (Philadelphia: J.B. Lippincott Company, 1965) pp. 229–230.

[5] Cooper III, David Y and Ledger, Marshall A. *Innovation and Tradition at the University of Pennsylvania School of Medicine, An Anecdotal Journey,* p. 139. Langfitt, Thomas W: Charles Harrison Frazier. His Influence on the Development of Early Neurosurgery in America and on the Development of the University of Pennsylvania School of Medicine. *Surg Neurol* (1990) 34, p. 130.

[6] Meyerson, Martin and Winegrad, Dilys Pegler. *Gladly Learn and Gladly Teach: Franklin and His Heirs at the University of Pennsylvania, 1740–1976,* p. 135.

[7] Ibid., p. 102.

[8] Corner, George W. *Two Centuries of Medicine: A History of the School of Medicine, University of Pennsylvania,* p. 123. Aub, Joseph C. and Hapgood, Ruth. *Pioneer in Modern Medicine: David Linn Edsall of Harvard* (Boston: Harvard Medical Alumni Association, 1970), p. 85. Cooper III, David Y and Ledger, Marshall A. *Innovation and Tradition at the University of Pennsylvania School of Medicine, An Anecdotal Journey,* p. 140.

[9] Aub, Joseph C. and Hapgood, Ruth. *Pioneer in Modern Medicine: David Linn Edsall of Harvard,* p. 88.

[10] Ibid., p. 85, 89

[11] Ibid., p. 87. Cooper III, David Y and Ledger, Marshall A. *Innovation and Tradition at the University of Pennsylvania School of Medicine, An Anecdotal Journey,* p. 140.

[12] Cooper III, David Y and Ledger, Marshall A. *Innovation and Tradition at the University of Pennsylvania School of Medicine, An Anecdotal Journey,* p. 139.

[13] Aub, Joseph C. and Hapgood, Ruth. *Pioneer in Modern Medicine: David Linn Edsall of Harvard,* p. 88. Cooper III, David Y and Ledger, Marshall A. *Innovation and Tradition at the University of Pennsylvania School of Medicine, An Anecdotal Journey,* p. 140.

[14] Aub, Joseph C. and Hapgood, Ruth. *Pioneer in Modern Medicine: David Linn Edsall of Harvard,* p. 93. Corner, George W. *Two Centuries of Medicine: A History of the School of Medicine, University of Pennsylvania,* pp. 234–235.

[15] Corner, George W. *Two Centuries of Medicine: A History of the School of Medicine, University of Pennsylvania,* p. 236.

[16] Ibid., p. 236.

[17] Rhoads, Jonathan E. and Langfitt, Thomas W. Charles Harrison Frazier, M.D. 1870–1936. *Surg Neurol* (1977 May 7) (5) p. 253.

[18] Boockvar, John A. *Neurosurgery Department History,* https://www.pennmedicine.org/departments-and-centers/neurosurgery/about-us/history.

[19] Ibid.

[20] World Biographical Encyclopedia, *Charles Harrison Frazier,* https://prabook.com/web/charles_frazier/3759146.

[21] Rhoads, Jonathan E. and Langfitt, Thomas W. Charles Harrison Frazier, M.D. 1870–1936. *Surg Neurol* (1977 May 7) (5) p. 254.

[22] Cooper III, David Y and Ledger, Marshall A. *Innovation and Tradition at the University of Pennsylvania School of Medicine, An Anecdotal Journey,* p. 108.

[23] Rhoads, Jonathan E. and Langfitt, Thomas W. Charles Harrison Frazier, M.D. 1870–1936. *Surg Neurol* (1977 May 7) (5) p. 254.

[24] Blakemore, William S. Memoir of L. Kraeer Ferguson. *Transactions of the Philadelphia Academy of Surgery*, Volume XXXI, pp. 15–18.

[25] *The Reminiscence of Isidor Ravdin,* Columbia University Oral History Collection Part II No 156. Isidor Ravdin, Saul Benison, Barbara Land, Columbia University Oral Research Office, *New York Times Oral History Program 1971*, p. 69.

[26] Ibid., p. 76.

[27] Ibid., p. 88.

[28] Ibid., p. 114.

[29] Cooper III, David Y and Ledger, Marshall A. *Innovation and Tradition at the University of Pennsylvania School of Medicine, An Anecdotal Journey,* p. 110.

[30] Ibid., p. 150.

CHAPTER 13

A Gentleman Athlete Trains a Generation of Master Surgeons

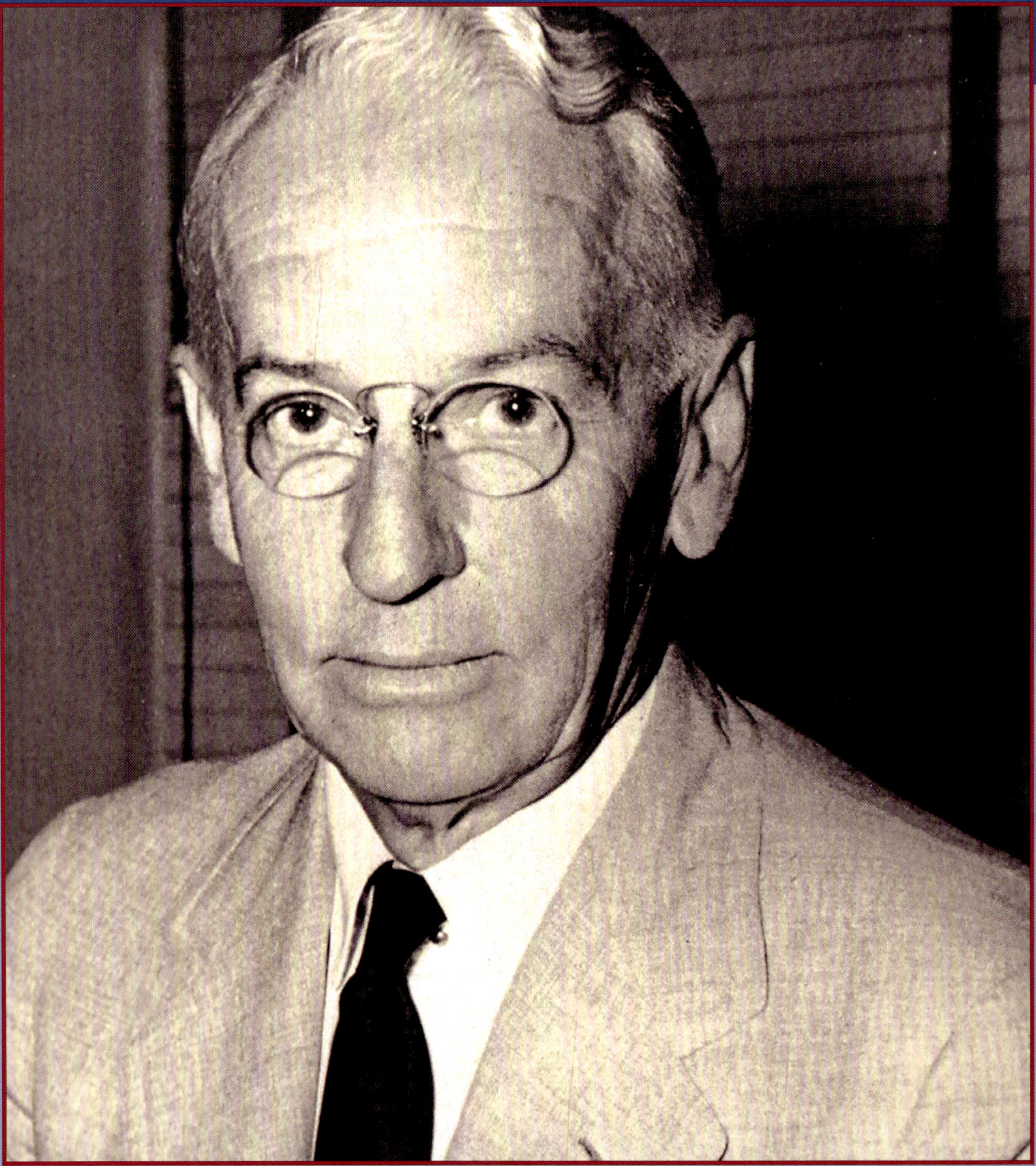

Eldridge L. Eliason (1879–1950)

JRB Professor and Chairman of Surgery (1936–1945)
Eliason Residents: Craftsmen and Something More

Eldridge Eliason's career proves that not every successful surgical chairman needs to be a rock star or a brilliant eccentric. Sometimes a steady conscientious approach is good enough. Eliason's turn as chairman was not about progress or change but about maintaining a good, solid status quo. He had less impact on the department's evolution than movers and shakers like Charles Frazier, I. S. Ravdin, or even the brief leadership of John B. Deaver. But there are some good stories about him.

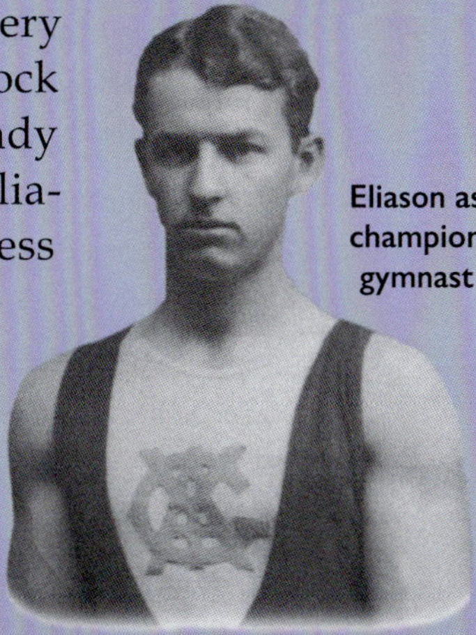

Eliason as champion gymnast

1879
Birth of Eliason

1901
BA Yale, Phi Beta Kappa. Captain of baseball team. National intercollegiate gymnastics champion

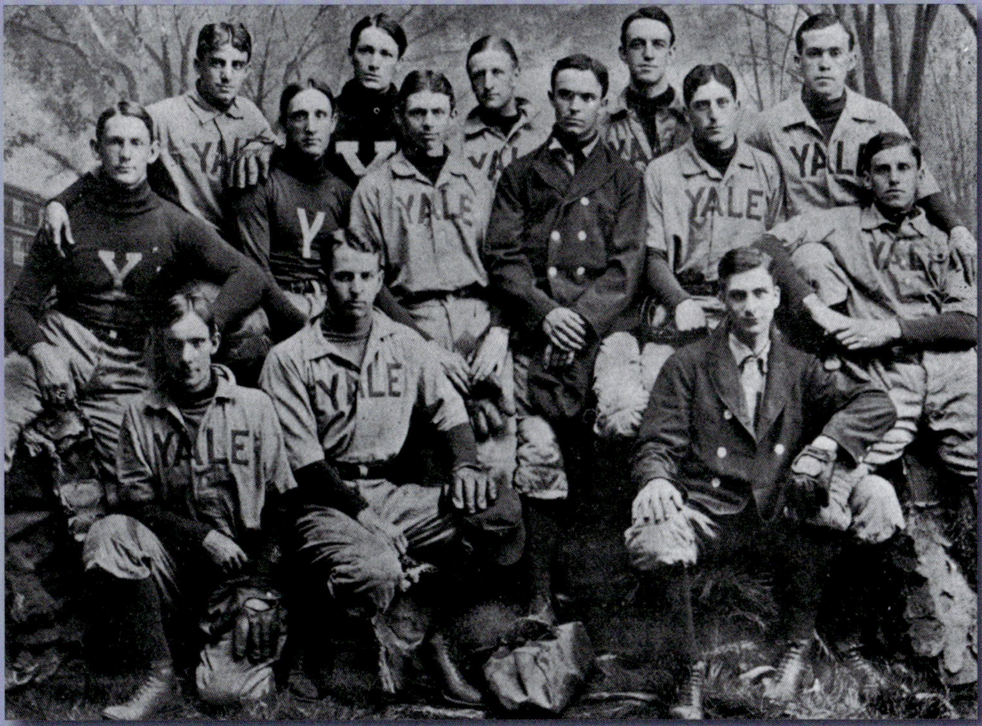

Yale University Baseball Team, 1901 (Eliason in front row, 2nd from left)

1905
MD Penn

1905–1907
Intern under Ashhurst and White

1906–1930
Coach of Penn gymnastics team

1907
Appointed to Penn Surgery faculty

Eldridge Eliason, the John Rhea Barton Professor from 1936 to 1945, was surely the department's best athlete. While at Yale, he captained the baseball team and was the American and Canadian national intercollegiate gymnastics champion. The story goes that he applied for medical school at Jefferson, but on traveling to Philadelphia for an interview, he was given incorrect directions and turned up at Penn.[1] Realizing his mistake, he announced he would leave. However, the dean recognized him from watching him compete against Penn in gymnastics and persuaded him to enroll at Penn. After internship and residency under Ashhurst and White, he remained at Penn for the rest of his professional life, except for a year in France as chief of surgery at Penn's World War I Army Hospital Base 20. Throughout his life, Eliason stayed in shape by doing gymnastics daily. For more than fifteen years, he coached the University of Pennsylvania's gymnastics team.[2]

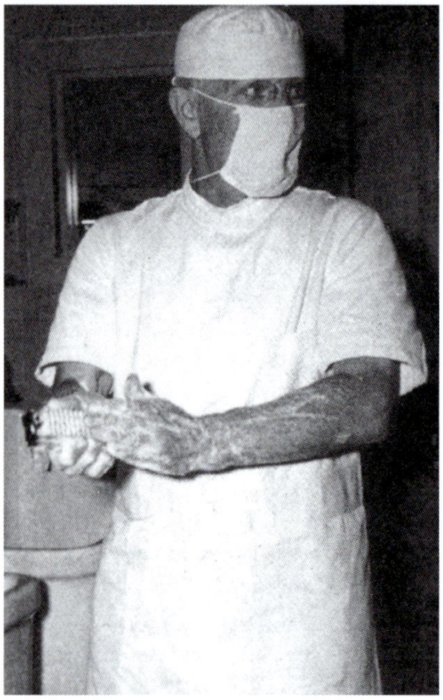

Tailored scrubs, silk mask.

Eliason was a handsome bachelor, much admired by the nurses who made sure that his tailored scrub suits were pressed and that his special silk masks were always available. In return, Eliason was respectful and supportive of nurses. He wrote a textbook on surgical nursing that was widely read through many editions.[3]

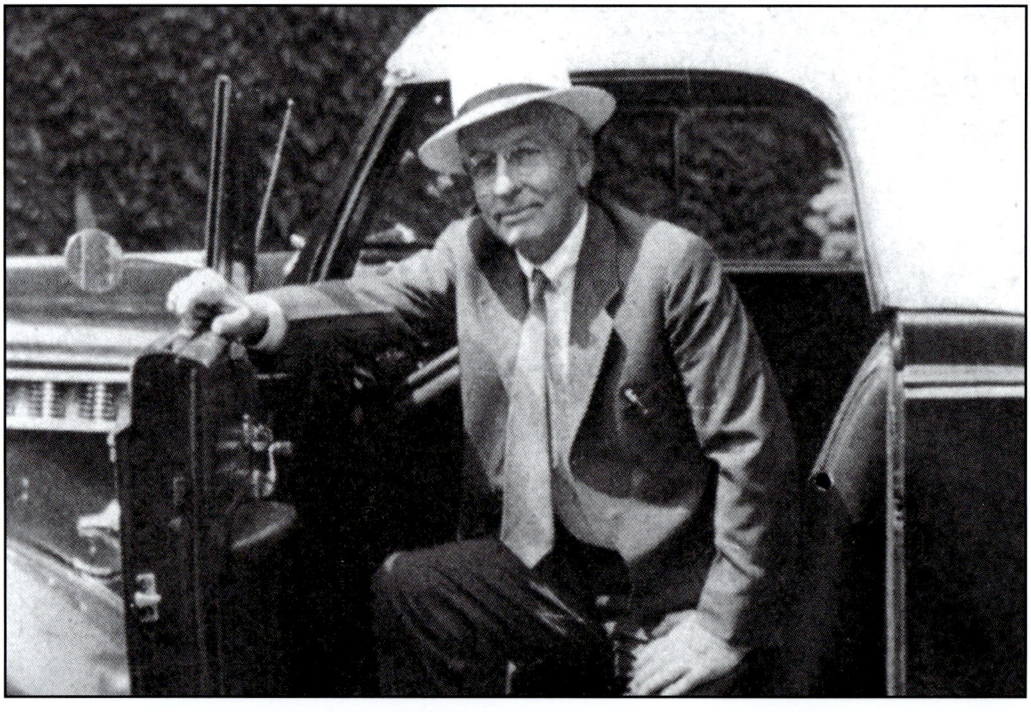

A fast Packard convertible contributed to his glamorous image.

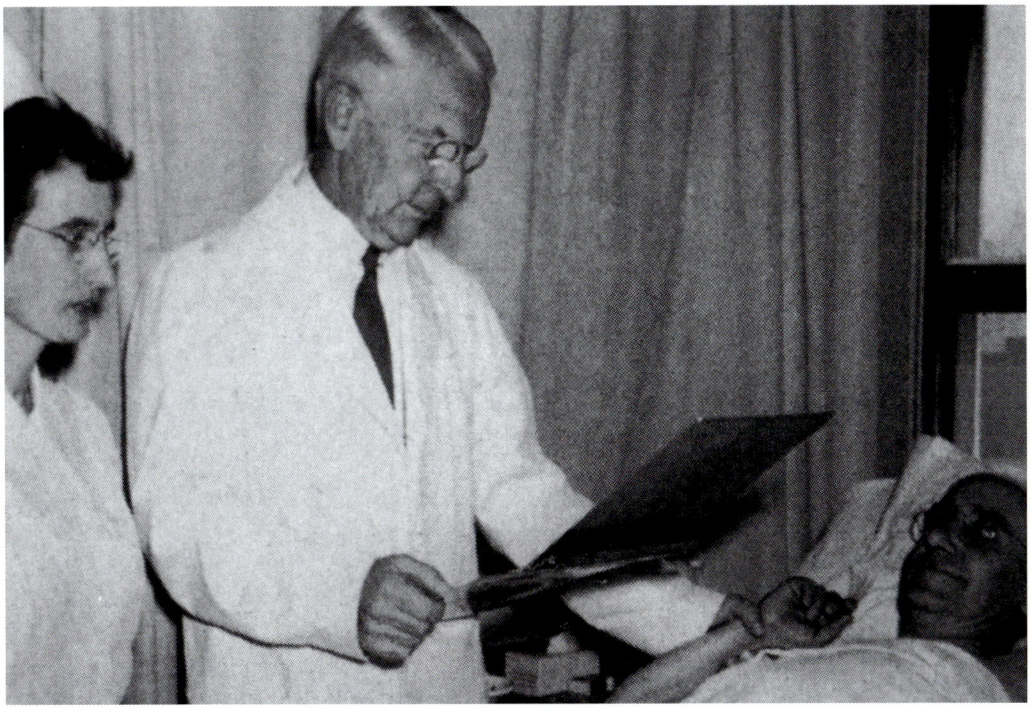

Eliason focuses on clinical practice and teaching.

1918
World War I, chief of surgery at Base Hospital 20 in France

1935
Harrison Endowment of $2.7 million for research is controlled by Ravdin. Eliason is not involved with or interested in research

He was very serious, very smart, even-tempered, conservative, noncontroversial, and universally well-liked. Like other Penn chairmen, he was nationally prominent and a member of all the prestigious surgical societies, including the American Surgical Association. Notably, he was a member of the Society of Clinical Surgery and president of the Philadelphia Academy of Surgery. His emphasis was taking good care of his patients and training good surgeons, not bad ambitions for a surgical professor. He was a good teacher and an exceptionally fine technical surgeon. He had little interest in research and discouraged his residents from being distracted by attempting it. In fact, he did not believe a clinical surgeon should try to be an investigator.[4] He dismissed those who did as "salt-water surgeons." In this attitude, he was not so different than most of our other surgical chairmen, the exceptions being Frazier and, later on, Ravdin. Whether because of selection or training, Eliason residents also became known for their technical expertise. The best example of this was the cardiac surgeon, Julian Johnson, who was certainly the best surgeon I ever saw. Residents trained by Ravdin and Rhoads, in contrast to Eli's residents, were expected to focus their attention on scientific and academic aspects of surgery and, like their chiefs, were not particularly known for their technical skills.

Perhaps because of this difference in emphasis, Eliason and Ravdin were never friends. But their serious enmity began in 1936 when they were the two logical candidates to succeed Charles Frazier as John Rhea Barton Professor and Department Chairman. To advise him in the selection, Dean William Pepper solicited letters of advice from surgical leaders of other schools. Of thirty-two responses, all but one

1935
Ravdin, while accompanying Frazier to Hopkins for prostate surgery, learns from Welch about the William Halsted residency. Ravdin plans to copy it

1936
Charles Frazier retires as chairman of surgery. Ravdin and Eliason are contenders as his successor; Eliason is chosen

1936–1945
Eliason is chairman of surgery, University of Pennsylvania

1936–1945
Relationship of Ravdin and Eliason is cool

1937
American Board of Surgery founded. Five years of post-graduate training for surgeons is mandated

1942
Eliason is president of the Philadelphia Academy of Surgery

recommended the nationally more prominent I. S. Ravdin.[5] We will never know why, but Pepper then chose Eliason as the next chairman, perhaps because he was senior to Ravdin or because he had a bigger practice, but I think most likely because the dean thought that he would be easier to control than the feisty Ravdin.

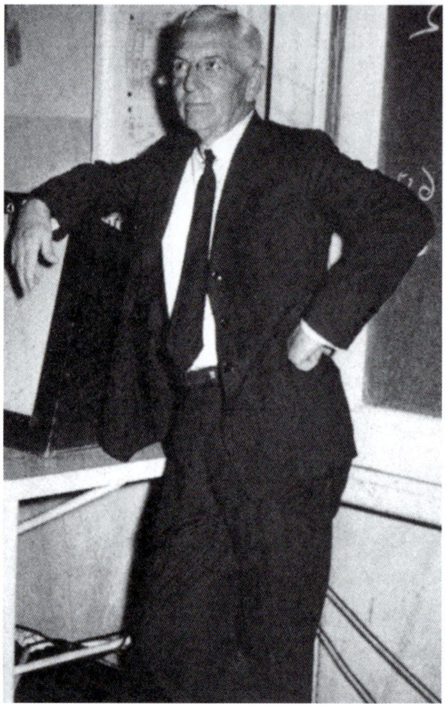

Eliason: John Rhea Barton Professor and Chairman.

As the chairmanship selection process was playing out, Ravdin's energy and persistence in maneuvering were largely responsible for a $2.7 million bequest coming to the department from the estate of George Leib Harrison, Charles Frazier's cousin. This Harrison endowment was to be devoted to support of surgical research, including a research professorship. Since Ravdin was already the department's director of research, he was appointed to the professorship and given control of the endowment funds. As the new Harrison professor, he would have similar, but not quite equal, status to the more senior John Rhea Barton chair.

Eliason and Ravdin met to discuss how the two professors would work together. They eventually agreed that Eliason would be chief of a large clinical service and responsible for student teaching. Ravdin would have a smaller clinical service and continue to direct research. But in addition, Ravdin wanted to select the residents and oversee their training. At their meeting, Eli agreed with this plan, but before long he reneged on their agreement and took over the selection and management of the residency.[6] Ravdin never forgave him for this betrayal. To Ravdin, this completely undermined Eliason's reputation for integrity. Since he was outranked, Ravdin had to accept this arrangement, but in retaliation, he sequestered the Harrison endowment, keeping it entirely for research and for himself. Thus, his budget exceeded by a factor of ten the funds Eliason had available for the entire clinical and student teaching programs.[7] This discrepancy probably didn't help their relationship.

On the clinical side, there was little cooperation between the two professors. Each one had a separate and independent service with its own group of residents. Ravdin was convinced that for a first-rate department, this was an unworkable model. He resolved that if he were ever in charge, there would be only one professor and that he would have complete control.[8] It would be the good fortune of the department that in another nine years, Ravdin would get his chance.

During the years leading up to and during World War II, not much change took place under the leadership of Eliason other than research that was done in the Harrison Department by Ravdin and his associates. In fact, Eliason's greatest contribution to the progress of the department may have been his training and recruitment to the faculty of Julian Johnson, who was to become a major force in the department.

1942–1945
Ravdin is in India as commander of the 20th General Hospital

1950
Death of Eliason

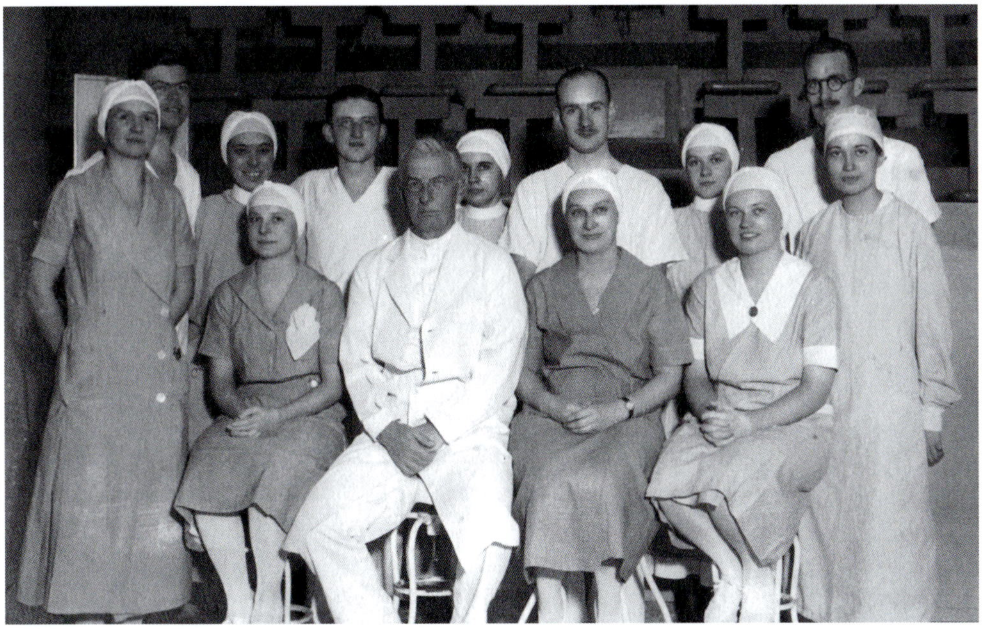

Eliason Service Team

Eldridge Eliason's Residents: Craftsmen and Something More

In 1937, with the founding of the American Board of Surgery, five years of postgraduate surgical training was mandated. It was the beginning of modern residencies. HUP trainees could be identified as either Ravdin or Eliason residents. With each group, the influence of their leader was clearly evident and, in most cases, followed them throughout their professional lives. As one of I. S. Ravdin's residents, I grew up agreeing with his view that it was important for academic surgeons to participate in research. Eliason disputed this, proclaiming openly that a good surgeon's full attention needed to be focused on his clinical activity, especially during his period of training. This attitude may have contributed to the particularly fine technical abilities developed by his residents. But to be fair, examination of the careers of the Eliason residents reveals that they were an outstanding bunch, perhaps mainly as clinical surgeons, but hardly without other accomplishments.

This group all became university professors and chiefs of the surgical departments of their hospitals. They were all members of the American Surgical Association. One was director of the American College of Surgeons, and another was president of the American College of Surgeons. One became surgeon general of the US Navy. Not a bad record for a mentor Ravdin accused of aiming only at clinical expertise in his trainees.

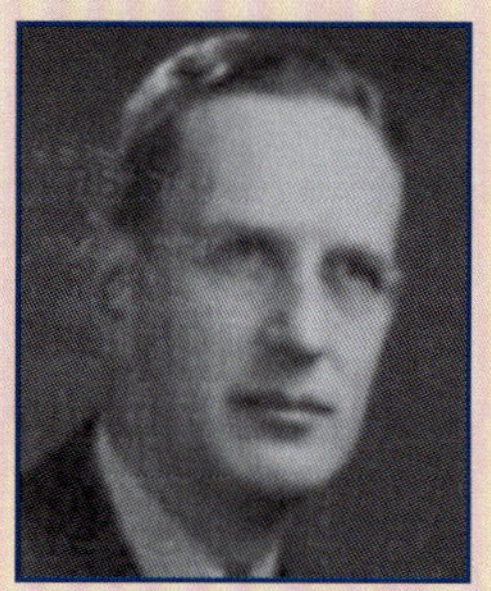

John Paul North (1901–1977) graduated from Princeton in 1922 and from the medical school of the University of Pennsylvania in 1926.[9] He interned at HUP and took his surgical training there under Eldridge Eliason, completing it in 1932.

When the HUP Army Unit 20th General Hospital was formed in 1942, Dr. North was at first chief of general surgery, and then, when the unit got to India, the chief of all the surgical services, while Dr. Ravdin became commanding officer. Two and a half years later, North returned to the United States and became chief of surgery at the Army's Kennedy General Hospital in Memphis, Tennessee. For his outstanding service in the Army, he received the Legion of Merit. After the war, he joined the Veterans Administration and served as chief of surgery in two veterans' hospitals in Texas. He also became professor of clinical surgery at Texas Southwestern Medical College. It is noteworthy that Julian Johnson, in writing his memoir, praised him as a clinical surgeon as well as an administrator, also noting that he was well-liked, admired, and respected for his great charm and sensitivity.

From 1961 to 1969, he was director of the American College of Surgeons, thus one of the most important individuals in surgery. He was universally admired for his leadership skills which were important at this pivotal time for the ACS. In his retirement, he lived in Dallas where he was greatly respected and admired as he had been everywhere. His memberships in professional societies included the American Surgical Association, the Southern Surgical Association, the Western Surgical Association, and a dozen others. Julian Johnson commented on his host of friends who remembered him with affection and admiration for his gracious charm, sensitivity, and steadfast loyalty to his principles and friends. Another signal of high regard was the formation of the John Paul North Society formed by sixty-four of his residents.

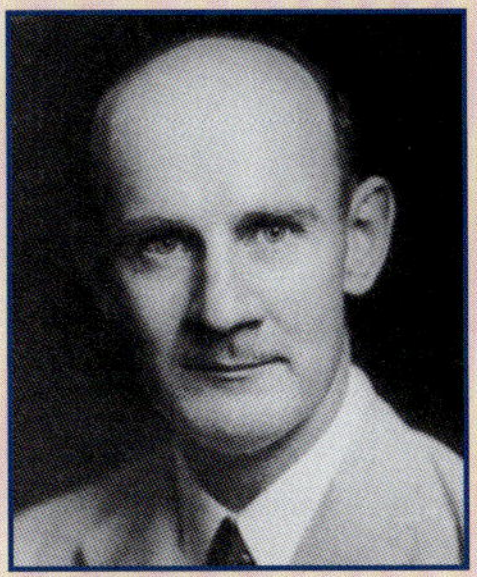

Charles W. McLaughlin Jr. (1906–1990) Charles McLaughlin was born in Iowa and went to the medical school of the University of Iowa for two years, then transferred to Washington University in St. Louis where he got his MD.[10] He was then a resident at Montréal General Hospital, followed by a year in pathology at McGill. He then came for three years to the University of Pennsylvania where he was a fellow under Dr. Eliason.[11] Following that, he joined the faculty of the University of Nebraska, where he remained until retirement. He had a variety of interests within general surgery and also pediatric surgery.

During World War II, he was in the Navy, seeing combat in the Pacific where his ship, the *Essex,* was hit by kamikazes. Later, he became the director of the medical service of the Strategic Air Command located in Omaha. In the last part of his clinical career, he was active in cancer surgery, particularly in breast cancer. In addition to his very active teaching and clinical activity at the University of Nebraska, he had a long history of service to the American College of Surgeons, serving on its Board of Governors, its Board of Regents, and finally as president of the American College of Surgeons in 1974.

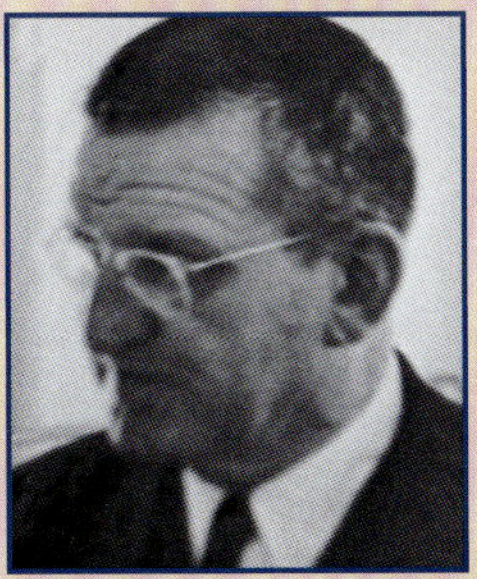

William H. M. Erb Sr. (1907–1987) graduated from medical school at the University of Pennsylvania in 1930.[12] He served his internship at HUP in 1930–1932. After a year on Dr. Frazier's thyroid service at HUP, he was a fellow from 1933 to 1936 with Dr. Eliason. After that, he studied for nine months in Germany, a month in England, and a month in Scotland. Later, he became affiliated in practice with Drs. Ferguson and Stevens at Presbyterian Hospital. He also taught at Women's Medical College and Riddle Memorial Hospital. He served on the staff of the Philadelphia General Hospital from 1937 to 1974, and in 1965, became president of the hospital's medical staff. For many years, he was in charge of the residency program at PGH. His mentorship was considered so valuable that some HUP residents elected to spend their chief year at PGH rather than HUP. He was president of the Philadelphia Academy of Surgery from 1972–74 and gave the annual oration of the Academy in 1975.

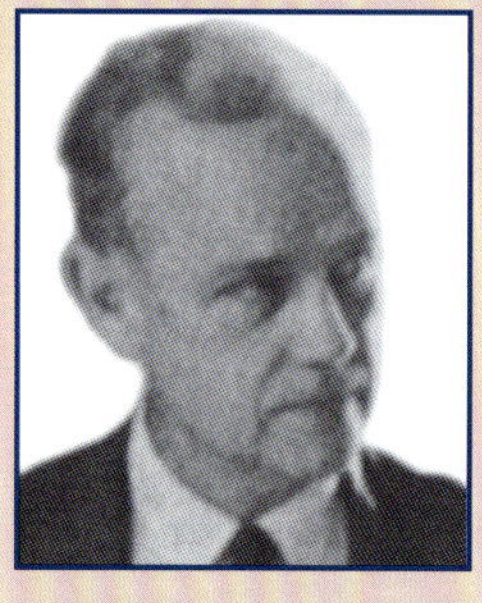

Julian Johnson (1907–1987) Although Johnson trained under Eliason, his career was more tightly linked with Ravdin. See Chapter 18 for his biographical sketch.

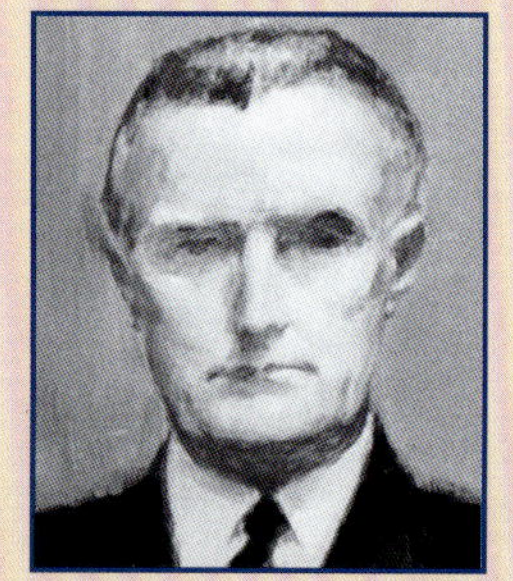

Robert B. Brown (1908–1977) graduated from Allegheny College in 1929 and in 1933 from the medical school of the University of Pennsylvania, where he ranked first in his class.[13] Bill Fitts, in writing his memoir for the American Surgical Association, recalled him from his house staff days as a superb technical surgeon. His colleagues often selected him if their families needed surgical care. Dr. Brown had two fellowships at HUP, the first in thyroid and neurosurgery with Charles Frazier in 1935 to 1936 and the second, a five-year fellowship under Eldridge Eliason, which he completed in 1941. He reported for active duty in the Navy in 1942. In 1943, he served on the *Solace*, the Navy unit organized by Kraeer Ferguson, which served in the South Pacific. In 1945, he served as chief of surgery on board the hospital ship *Tranquility*. At the same time, his enthusiasm for teaching induced him to offer his services to I. S. Ravdin as a volunteer faculty member. Dr. Ravdin, the surgical staff, and the Penn medical students were grateful for his contributions. Dr. Brown next joined the *USS Repose* which operated in the Korean area of hostilities. For his work there, he was awarded the Bronze Star. His clinical and administrative activities were largely responsible for the excellent care given to more than 8,000 patients admitted to the hospital ship during that time. In 1951, he was chief of surgery at the Naval Hospital in Bethesda, Maryland, and also served as clinical professor of surgery at Georgetown University School of Medicine. In 1960, he was commander of the Naval Hospital in Bethesda and was approved by the president for the rank of rear admiral. Throughout this period of great administrative responsibility, he also remained active as a clinical surgeon. In January 1965, he was appointed by the president to be surgeon general of the Navy and chief of the Bureau of Medicine and

Surgery. He was also promoted to the rank of vice admiral and awarded the Distinguished Service Medal. He received many military service medals and concomitantly was elected to membership in many surgical societies, including the American Surgical Association, the Halsted Society, the Society for Vascular Surgery, the Southern Surgical Association, and the American Association for the Surgery of Trauma. For several years, he suffered from generalized rheumatoid arthritis and in 1977, developed a fatal lymphoma.

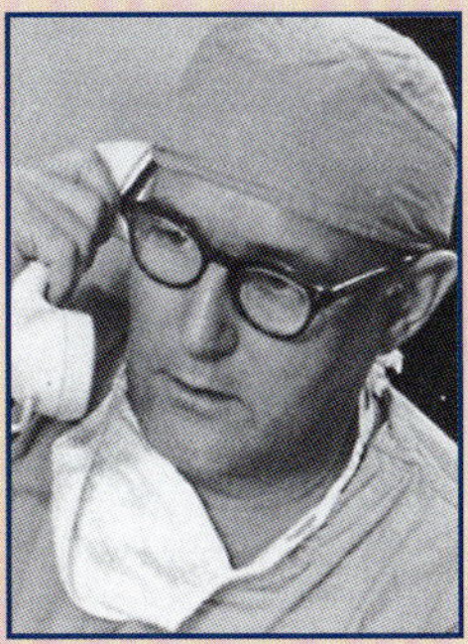

Lloyd Stevens (1914–2021) graduated from Penn medical school in 1937 as first in his class and recipient of the Packard Prize in clinical medicine. His internship and residency in surgery were at the Hospital of the University of Pennsylvania from 1937 to 1944. Eliason was department chairman but much of his training was under Ravdin. From 1944 to 1979, he was on the faculty at the University of Pennsylvania and the surgical staff of HUP, Graduate Hospital, the Medical College of Pennsylvania, and Philadelphia General Hospital where he was visiting chief of surgery from 1950 through 1976. From 1959 to 1979, he was director of surgery at Presbyterian Medical Center. He was also surgeon to the Philadelphia Eagles football team from 1945 to 1949.

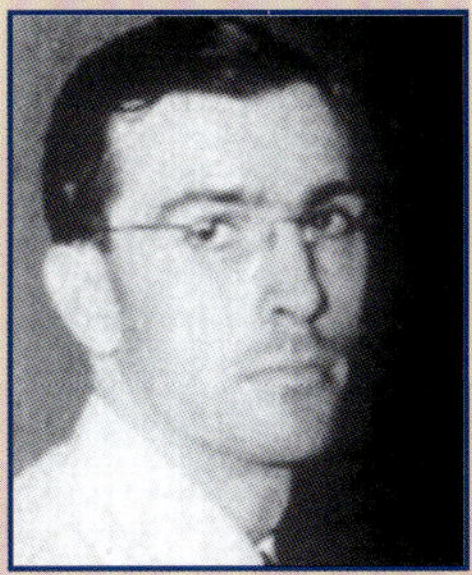

Bob Welty (1914–1989) graduated from medical school at the University of Pennsylvania in 1938. He served most of his training under Eldridge Eliason, finishing it in 1946 with the final eight months under I. S. Ravdin just as he returned from the wartime 20th General Hospital. Thus, Welty was the last Eliason chief and the first Ravdin chief resident. From 1946 to 1948, he was in practice with L. K. Ferguson and Lloyd Stevens. In October 1948, he married Elizabeth May, a graduate of Cornell Medical School and the medical residency of New York Hospital. She was at the time of their marriage an instructor in medicine at HUP. In 1949, they moved to Spokane, Washington, where they practiced for the next thirty-six years, he in surgery and she in medicine. Bob also became clinical associate professor at the University of Washington School of Medicine and president of the North Pacific Surgical Association. In 1987, the Weltys made a pilgrimage back to HUP to attend Jonathan Rhoads's eightieth birthday symposium. While they were here, they told me that they had arranged to give the university $1.5 million for endowment of a professorship in the name of Eldridge Eliason. Sadly, only two years later, Bob Welty died. Elizabeth Welty continued to practice and, after retirement, filled her life with civic activities in Spokane, also becoming a trustee in the local college (Whitman), which awarded her an honorary degree. She served on a number of boards, such as the Spokane Symphony Orchestra, Spokane Public Radio, and the Spokane Opera. She never forgot her affection for Penn and made several additional generous contributions to the School of Medicine, and another, approaching $1 million, to the department of surgery.

Timeline of Events During the Career of Eldridge Eliason

1901 Eliason graduates from Yale where he is captain of the baseball team and the intercollegiate gymnastics champion of the United States and Canada.

1918 During World War I, Eliason is a lieutenant colonel and the first commander of the US Army Hospital Base 20.

1936 Charles Frazier retires. In considering his successor, Dean Pepper solicits advice from many external consultants, all but one of whom identify Ravdin as superior to the other major candidate, Eldridge Eliason. In spite of this, Eliason is selected, perhaps because he is senior to Ravdin or perhaps because he has a larger clinical practice.

1936–1945 Eliason focuses on clinical practice and on training outstanding clinical surgeons like himself (Julian Johnson, William Erb, Lloyd Stevens, Robert Brown, John Paul North, Charles McLaughlin, and Robert Welty).

1936–1943 Ravdin focuses on research. His research is on liver function and physiology, liver disease, and the toxicity of ether. He trains several prominent surgeons (Jonathan Rhoads and Charles Johnston). He recruits to the faculty several prominent surgical investigators (John Lockwood, Norman Freeman, and Harold Zintel).

1936 George Leib Harrison endows the department with $2.7 million for research and academic purposes. The funds are controlled by Ravdin and exceed by a factor of ten the funds the department has for clinical activities. The endowment results in establishing the Harrison Professorship of Surgical Research. Ravdin is appointed Harrison Professor.

1936 One of HUP's three senior surgeons, George Muller, goes to Jefferson as chairman of surgery.

1936 The first sulfa drug (sulfanilamide) becomes available.

1937 Founding of American Board of Surgery; five years of surgical training is mandated.

1938 Jonathan Rhoads studies vitamin K and the coagulation system. Heparin becomes available.

1940 Ravdin develops acute cholecystitis. He chooses to be operated on by the young Jonathan Rhoads with senior surgeons Eliason and Columbia's Chairman Whipple serving as consultants and assistants at the operation. Ravdin makes a complete recovery.

1941 On December 7, the Japanese bomb Pearl Harbor, bringing the United States into World War II. Ravdin is assigned by the secretaries of the Army and the Navy to travel the next day to Pearl Harbor to inspect the facilities and care for US soldiers and sailors. He takes with him sulfanilamide, the blood substitute albumin, and a bottle of whiskey.

1943 The 20th General Hospital is formed and moves to Assam, India, to support the US invasion of Japanese-occupied northern Burma. Colonel Ravdin directs the surgical service and then becomes the overall leader. He is promoted to general.

1945 The war ends and General Ravdin is invited to succeed Eliason as the John Rhea Barton Professor and Chairman of Surgery. He accepts only on condition that there will be only one professor of surgery and he will have complete control of the department. There will no longer be separate professors and services, such as the Eliason service and the Ravdin service before the war.

1946 On January 1, Ravdin becomes chairman of the department.

1946 Jonathan Rhoads is diagnosed with advanced tuberculosis. He is hospitalized for most of the year in Albuquerque, treated successfully with streptomycin, but suffers impaired balance from the drug's eighth nerve toxicity.

1950 Eliason dies.

Notes

[1] Cooper III, David Y and Ledger, Marshall A. *Innovation and Tradition at the University of Pennsylvania School of Medicine, An Anecdotal Journey* (Philadelphia: University of Pennsylvania Press, 1990) p. 253.

[2] Ferguson, L. Kraeer. Eldridge Eliason 1879–1950. *Transactions of the American Surgical Association* (1950) 68, p. 559.

[3] Ibid., p. 559.

[4] Personal conversation with Dr. H. G. Barker, a Ravdin resident.

[5] The Reminiscence of Isidor Ravdin, *Columbia University Oral History Collection Part II* No 156. Isidor Ravdin, Saul Benison, Barbara Land, Columbia University Oral Research Office, *New York Times Oral History Program* (1971), p. 133.

[6] Ibid., p. 134–135.

[7] Ibid., p. 136.

[8] Ibid., p. 136.

[9] Wade, Preston A. Memoir of John Paul North. *Transactions of the American Surgical Association*, Vol. XCV, pp. 77–78.

[10] Oral History Transcript: Charles W. McLaughlin, Jr. (1979) *Washington University School of Medicine Oral History Project.*

[11] For McGlophlin's detailed description of his HUP fellowship, see Barker, Clyde F. and Daly, John M, (eds). *Jonathan E. Rhoads Eightieth Birthday Symposium* (Philadelphia: J. B. Lippincott Co, 1989) pp. 268–270.

[12] Ranieri, TA. Memoir of William Henry Moyer Erb, Sr., M.D. 1907–1987. *Transactions of the Philadelphia Academy of Surgery*, Volume XXXIV, pp. 72–75.

[13] Fitts, William T. Memoir of Robert Bruce Brown 1908–1977. *Transactions of the American Surgical Association*, Vol. XCVI, pp. 61–63.

CHAPTER 14

An Army General Transforms Penn Surgery

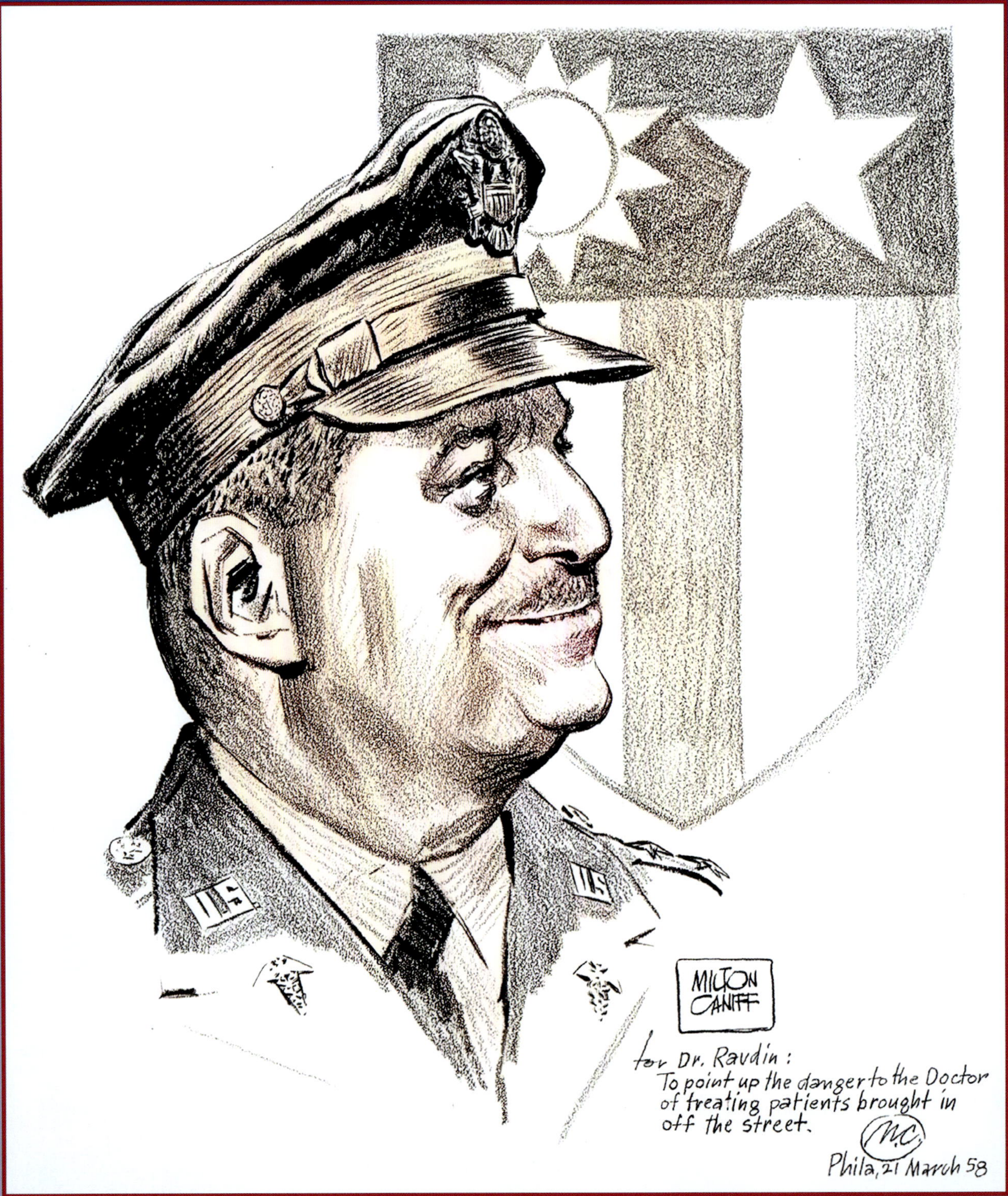
MILTON CANIFF
for Dr. Ravdin:
To point up the danger to the Doctor of treating patients brought in off the street.
M.C.
Phila, 21 March 58

I. S. Ravdin (1894–1972)

JRB Professor and Chairman of Surgery (1946–1960)

Ravdin's Chief Residents: The Finest Generation?

As one of I. S. Ravdin's residents, it is hard for me to conceive that, with passing decades, this fascinating character's fame has largely faded from memory, even in the department he created. Certainly he was the most colorful of Penn surgery leaders. And he was the most powerful! He could accomplish more with one pound on the table than any of his successors could through consensus building and a dozen committee meetings.

His military service in World War II was the making of I. S. Ravdin's career, but he had previous military experience in 1916 when drafted into the Army to accompany General Black Jack Pershing and George Patton

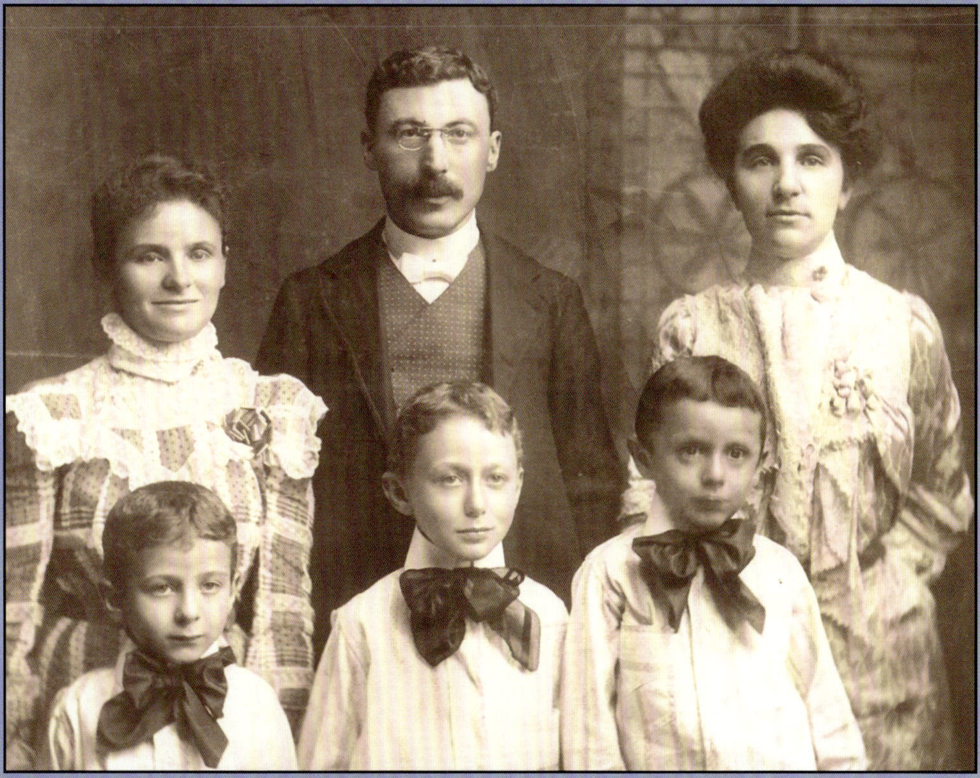

"(back row l to r) Wilhelmina and Marcus Ravdin, cousin Ida Jacobson (front row) I. S. (Isidor Schwaner), Bernard, Hiram

1860s to 1880s

I. S. Ravdin's father is born in Riga, Latvia, his mother in Königsberg, Prussia.

They immigrate to America in the early 1880s.

His father graduates in medicine from Memphis Hospital Medical College.

His grandfather and great-grandfather are also doctors

1894

Ravdin is born in Evansville, Indiana

1912

Ravdin graduates from high school and runs away from home to Memphis where he buys and publishes a magazine (*The Southern Voter*). He publishes religious sermons of ministers from Arkansas and north Texas. After several years, he goes home and enrolls in Indiana University

1916
Army Private Ravdin chases Mexican rebel Pancho Villa with George Patton and General Pershing

on a mission to pursue the Mexican rebel chief Pancho Villa. There, according to Ravdin's son, he learned to chew tobacco because on night patrol, cigarette smokers were likely to get a sniper's bullet between the eyes. Unfortunately, Rav was forever after a heavy smoker.[1]

Born and raised in Indiana, Ravdin also attended college and two years of medical school there before finishing medical school at Penn. He then began his internship at HUP. Because of the war, HUP had only a few other interns or residents. After only four months, Ravdin was appointed chief resident, an administrative position usually going to a senior resident.[2] This also accelerated his clinical training so that he acquired earlier experience with large operations than was likely during normal times. In fact, his training turned out to be more like an apprenticeship than a standard residency. To his advantage, the mentors teaching him, Charles Frazier and especially John B. Deaver and George Muller, were master surgeons. It also helped that although these three surgeons did not get along with each other, they all liked Ravdin and paid special attention to his surgical training.

After finishing his training, Ravdin planned to return to Indiana to start a community practice of surgery. Deaver, then the chairman, and

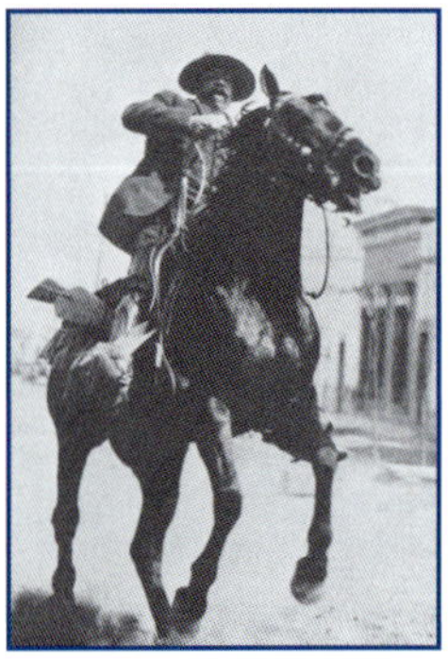

Pancho Villa

General Black Jack Pershing

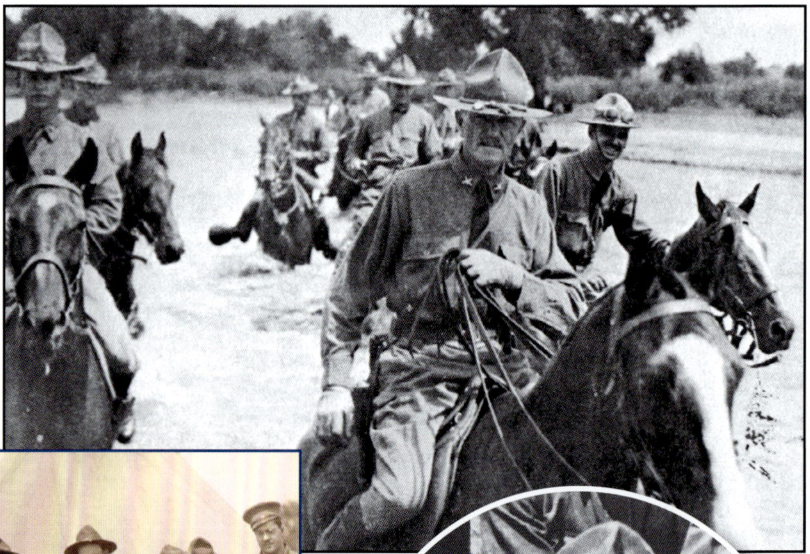

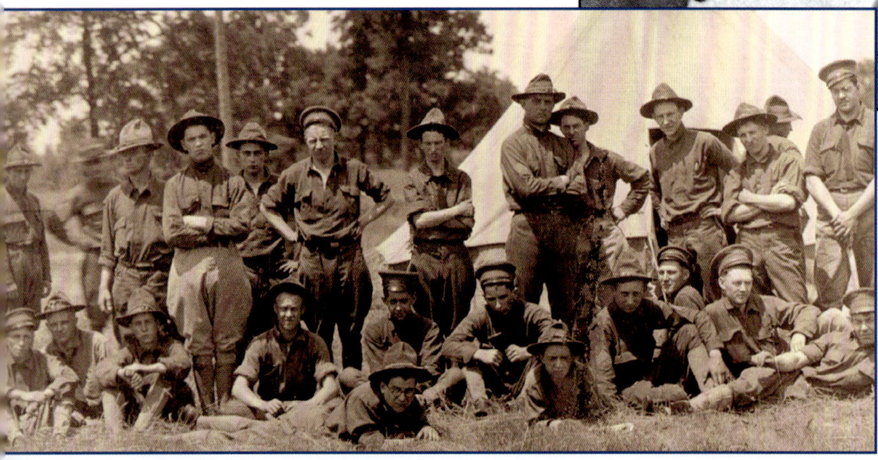

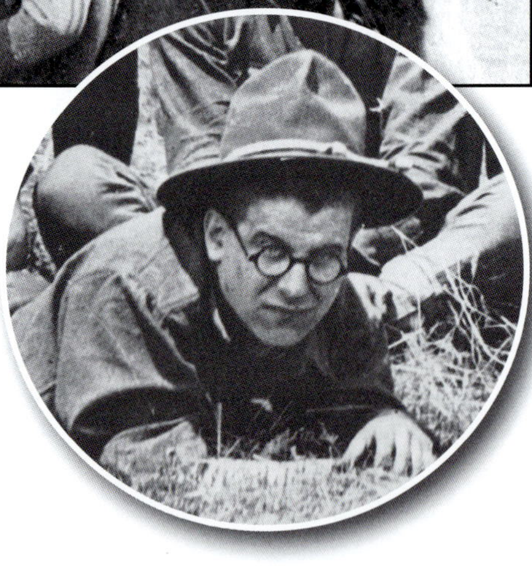

1916 Private I. S. Ravdin as National Guardsman pursues Pancho Villa with Pershing and Patton. The start of a lifetime committment to the Army.

others urged him to stay in Philadelphia. He was offered a job as head of the new Graduate Hospital that shortly before had formed as a merger of Penn with two older schools and hospitals, Polyclinic and Medico Surgical Hospital.[3] Ravdin elected to stay in Philadelphia, began a successful practice at Graduate Hospital, and gained valuable experience as an independent surgeon. But in 1922 when Frazier became chairman, he brought Ravdin back to HUP as his assistant.[4]

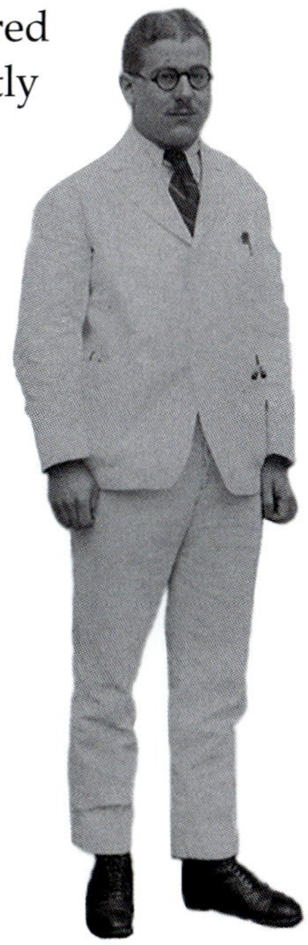
I. S. Ravdin as an intern

In 1927, the thirty-three-year-old Ravdin went abroad for a year of research under Sir Edward Sharpey Schafer, the physiologist who pioneered studies of pituitary and other hormones, and Sir Henry Dale, the Nobel Laureate, who was then England's top scientist.[5] From them, Ravdin learned laboratory techniques and, more importantly, the value of collaborating with basic scientists.

Returning to Penn, he was appointed director of the Department of Surgery's research. Ravdin then focused on laboratory investigation with the energy that characterized his life. Over the next fourteen years, he averaged a publication approximately every thirty days, many of them in basic science journals. He defined the capacity of the gallbladder to concentrate and alter bile.[6] He reproduced syndromes of malnutrition in animals, showing that hypoproteinemia delayed gastric emptying and impaired wound healing. And, he began to study methods of nourishing patients who couldn't eat.

He stimulated the research of his colleagues and trainees in shock, blood substitutes, surgical infection, antibiotics, and wound healing. Two of the department's projects, which began their gestation during this time, would change the care of patients around the world. John Gibbon, working in Penn's Harrison Department of Surgical Research from 1935 to 1942, demonstrated in animals the feasibility of cardiopulmonary bypass.[7] Ravdin's own interest in nutrition, after years of further research

1918
After college and two years of medical school at Indiana University, Ravdin graduates from Penn Medical School, becomes HUP intern; after only four months is promoted to chief resident

1918–1919
US enters World War I

1921
Ravdin marries Dr. Elizabeth Glenn. She was HUP's first female intern

1919–1922
Ravdin has private surgery practice at Graduate Hospital and serves as assistant to George Muller

1922
Ravdin is called back to HUP by Frazier, appointed department's executive director (Frazier's assistant)

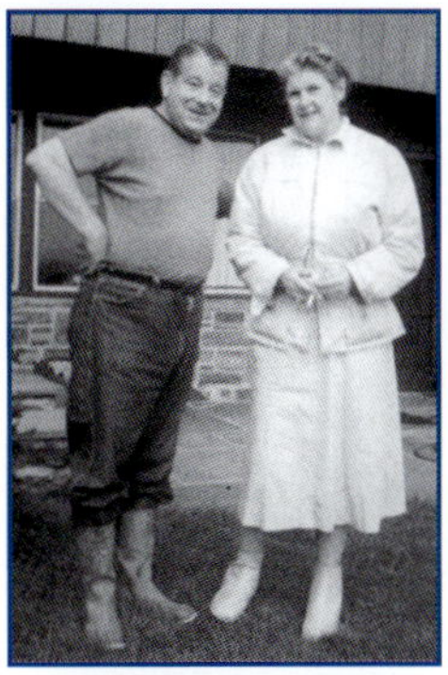
Rav and his wife, Elizabeth

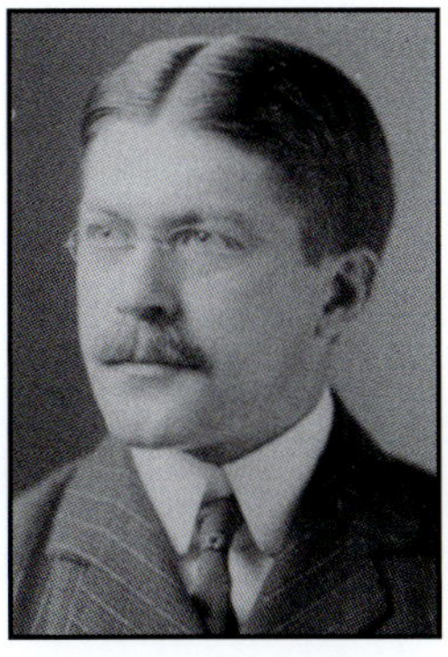
Charles Frazier

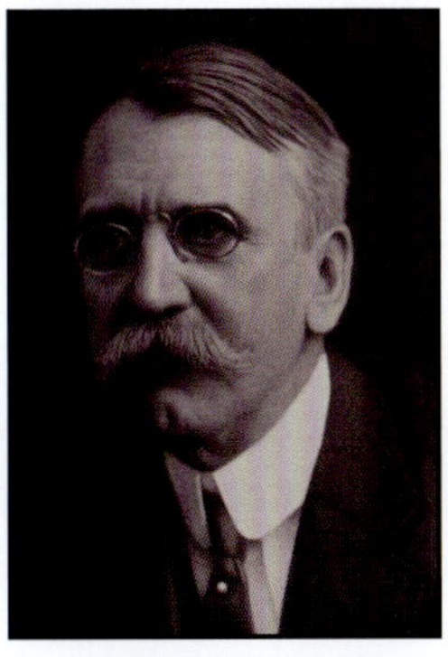
John B. Deaver

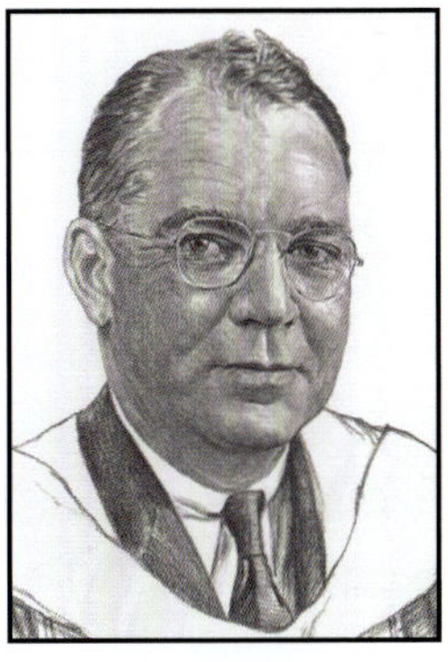
George Muller

Three crusty surgeons dominate HUP surgery. They have independent services and hardly speak to each other. Ravdin is a favorite with all of them.

1927
A year of research for Ravdin in Edinburgh and London

1928–1942
Ravdin combines HUP practice with basic science research; becomes the department's director of research

1935-1942
Working in Penn's Harrison Department of Surgical Research, John and Mary Gibbon make progress with their heart-lung machine

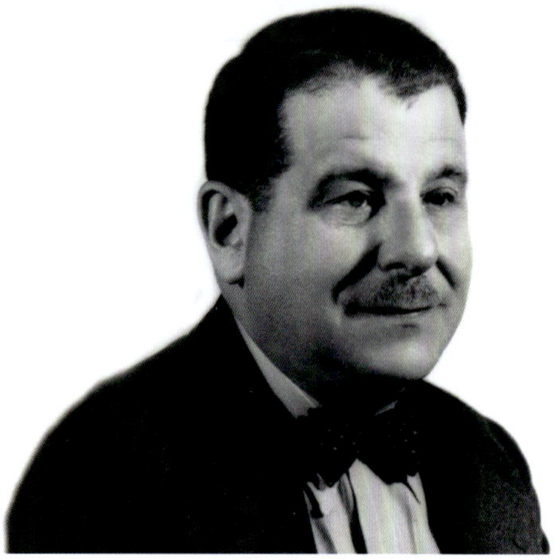

A year of full-time research

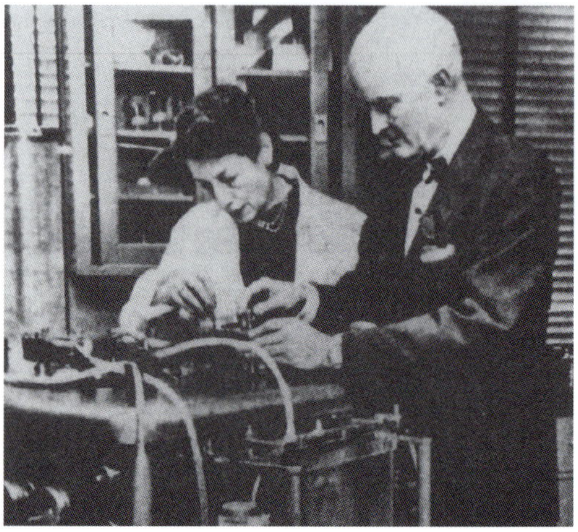

John and Mary Gibbon with heart-lung machine

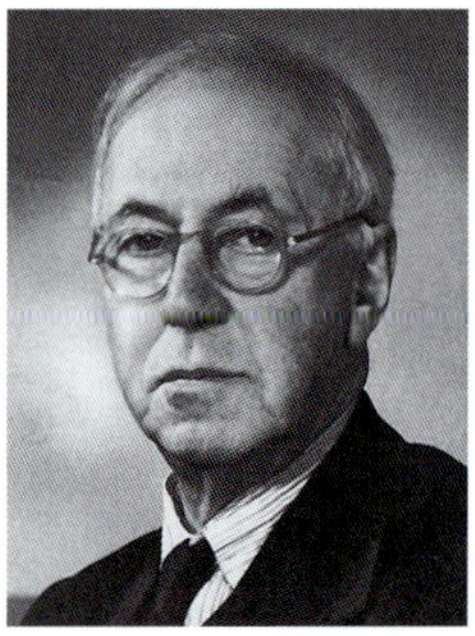

Sir Henry Dale

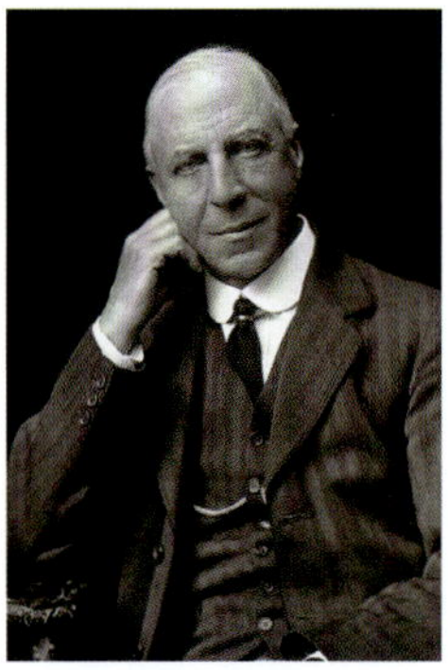

Sir Edward Sharpey Schafer

in Jonathan Rhoads's laboratory, culminated in the landmark report by Dudrick, et al., on parenteral hyperalimentation.[8]

In 1936, Frazier died, and Eldridge Eliason, Penn's senior surgeon, was appointed chairman of the department. By then, Ravdin also held a professorship, so in keeping with the Penn tradition, there were now two separate and quite different surgical services (one headed by Eliason and the other by Ravdin). These services functioned autonomously, selecting and training their own separate group of residents. Eliason, a technical virtuoso, encouraged his residents to focus on operative skills. In contrast, Ravdin's residents were expected to spend time in the laboratory and to consider every operation an exercise in abnormal physiology and biochemistry. Ravdin trainees became leaders in academic surgery. But in technical expertise, they were no match for Eliason's residents.

Underlying the superficial collegiality of the two chiefs was a keen rivalry, which sometimes approached enmity.[9] As the director of research, Ravdin was in complete control of the $2.7 million endowment that came to the department in 1935 for surgical research. The annual income from this endowment far exceeded the amount available to Eliason from all other sources for running the department's clinical and teaching programs. This discrepancy did not improve the alliance of the two professors. Their relationship was also illustrated in an interesting scenario in 1940 when Ravdin needed an operation for acute cholecystitis.

Ravdin's choice as the operating surgeon was one of his own trainees, a man not yet an assistant professor who had finished his residency only the year before, the young Jonathan Rhoads. One imagines that Penn's chairman (Eliason) and Columbia's (Alan Whipple, who Ravdin summoned from New York) were somewhat put off by being assigned as assistants at the operation.[10] Typically, Ravdin really wanted to direct the procedure himself which, since he was awake under spinal anesthesia, he began to do. Whipple is said to have exclaimed, "Rav, scrub up or shut up!"[11] Ravdin recommended a cholecystostomy. This was done. Rav got well and never had any more trouble with his gallbladder that was never removed.

The day that Pearl Harbor was bombed, Ravdin was asked by the secretaries of the Army and Navy to fly to Hawaii to report on the care being given to the wounded.[12] On a small, one-engine plane navigated by the stars, he carried with him a large supply of the blood substitute albumen, a jar of the new drug sulfanilamide, and a bottle of Jack Daniel's whiskey, none of which he feared would be readily available in the islands.[13] He found that the care being given American soldiers by Army doctors, such as Leonard Heaton, was excellent.[14]

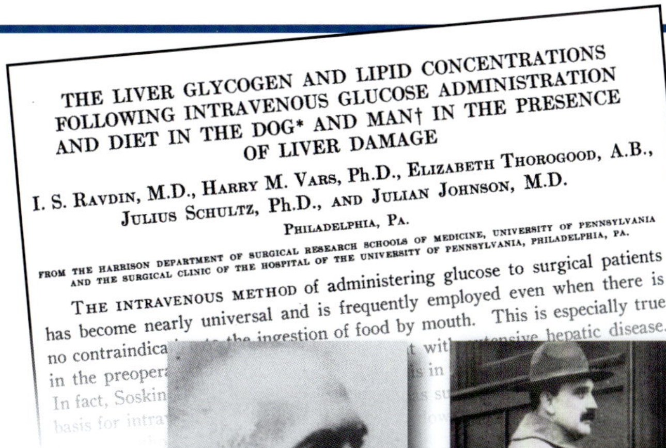

THE LIVER GLYCOGEN AND LIPID CONCENTRATIONS FOLLOWING INTRAVENOUS GLUCOSE ADMINISTRATION AND DIET IN THE DOG* AND MAN† IN THE PRESENCE OF LIVER DAMAGE

I. S. RAVDIN, M.D., HARRY M. VARS, Ph.D., ELIZABETH THOROGOOD, A.B., JULIUS SCHULTZ, Ph.D., AND JULIAN JOHNSON, M.D.

PHILADELPHIA, PA.

FROM THE HARRISON DEPARTMENT OF SURGICAL RESEARCH SCHOOLS OF MEDICINE, UNIVERSITY OF PENNSYLVANIA AND THE SURGICAL CLINIC OF THE HOSPITAL OF THE UNIVERSITY OF PENNSYLVANIA, PHILADELPHIA, PA.

THE INTRAVENOUS METHOD of administering glucose to surgical patients has become nearly universal and is frequently employed even when there is no contraindica... the ingestion of food by mouth. This is especially true in the preoper... with extensive hepatic disease. In fact, Soskin... basis for intra...

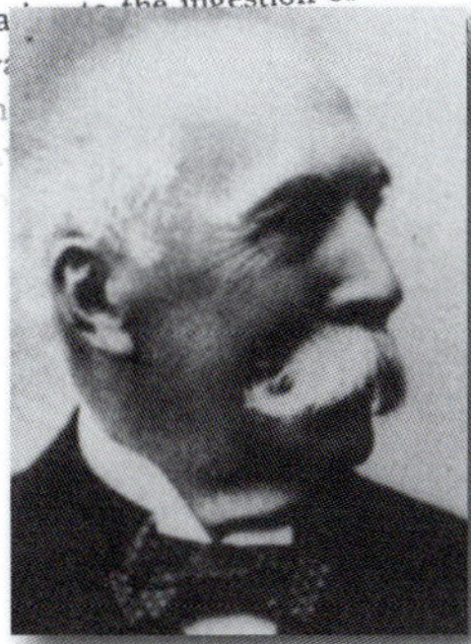

George Leib Harrison

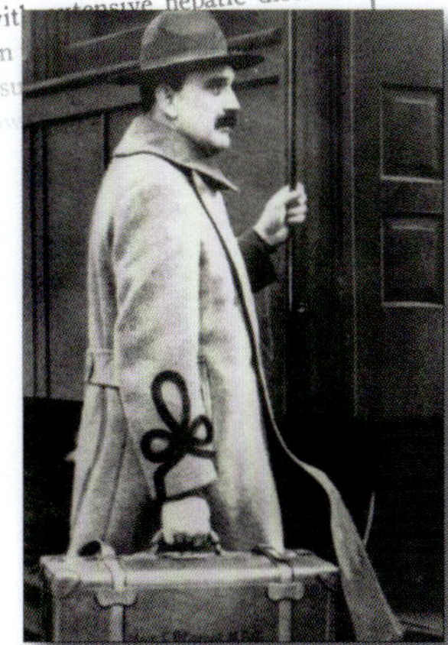

John Berton Carnett

His next assignment was to recruit and staff an Army hospital, largely from Penn personnel. For the first time, he would be fully in charge of his own show. I believe his extraordinary war experience was the defining factor in his distinctive leadership style. Leaving Jonathan Rhoads in Philadelphia to maintain the integrity of the Ravdin service at Penn, Rav took his unit to Ledo, a town near the border of India with enemy-held Burma. His 20th General Hospital was placed there to provide support for the Allies' impending invasion and control of Japanese-held northern Burma, which was deemed indispensable for opening the Burma Road. This road was the

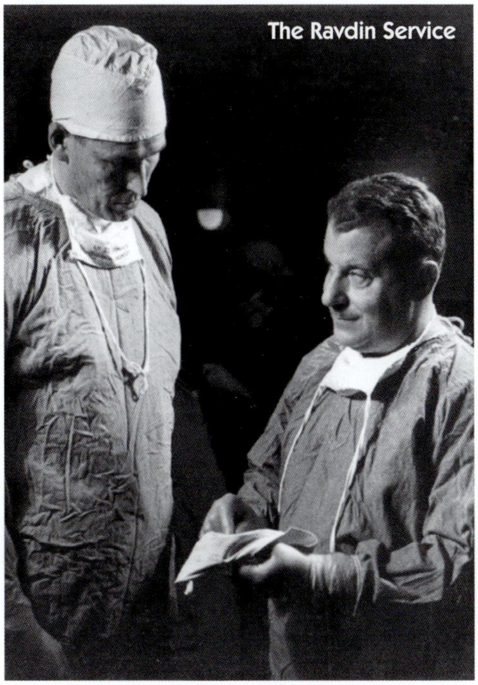

The Ravdin Service

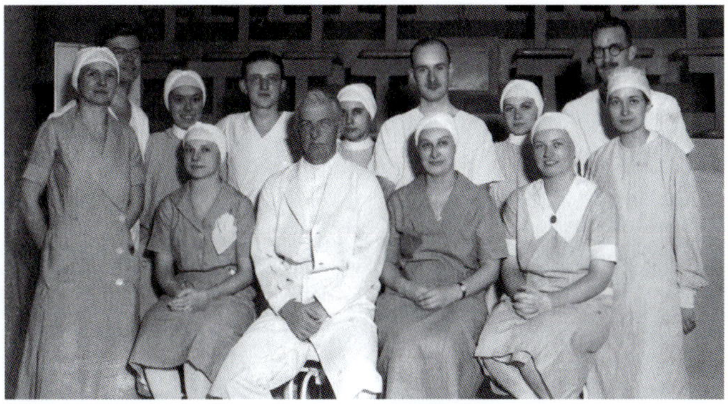

The Eliason Service

1935
George Leib Harrison's endowment of $2.7 million is at first intended for John Carnett's research, but when Carnett dies before Harrison, it goes to support research in the Department of Surgery of the University of Pennsylvania

1936
The endowment allows formation of the Harrison Department of Surgical Research, Ravdin becomes its director and Harrison Professor of Surgery.

There are now two professors at HUP, Eliason and Ravdin

1936
George Muller leaves Penn to become chairman at Jefferson, also becomes president of the American College of Surgeons in 1940

1936
Frazier is operated on at Hopkins for prostate cancer.

While accompanying Frazier, Ravdin makes friends with Hopkins dean William Welch, who tells him about the Halsted residency. Ravdin decides to establish one like it

1936
Frazier dies

1936
Ravdin is passed over as candidate for chairman of surgery. Eliason becomes John Rhea Barton Professor and Chairman of the Department of Surgery.

There are now two separate services, two professors, and two separate residencies at HUP

1937
American Board of Surgery is founded; mandates five-year surgical residencies

1939
Jonathan Rhoads finishes his residency under Ravdin

1940
Ravdin develops acute cholecystitis and is operated on by Rhoads; Eliason and Whipple assist

Young Rhoads operates on his chief

The Assistants

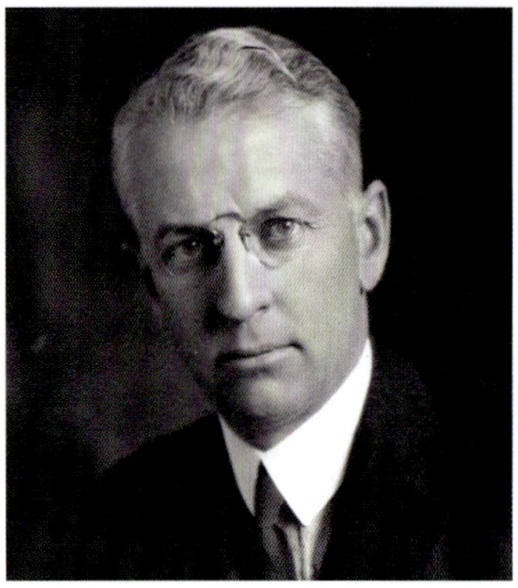

Eldridge Eliason

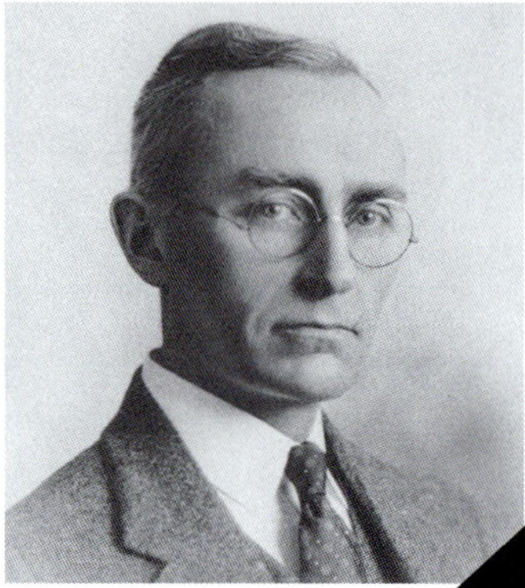

Allen Whipple

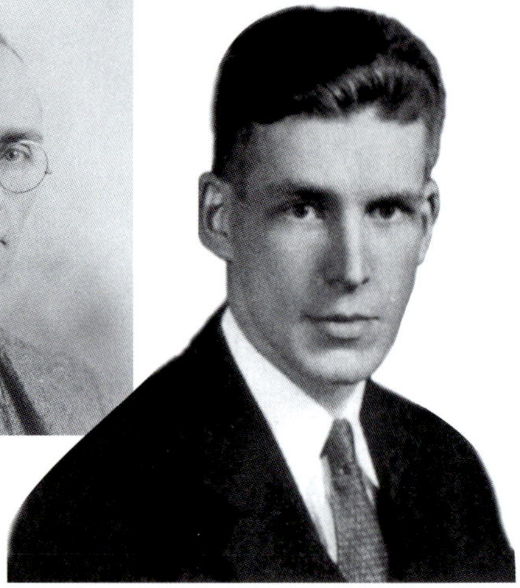

Jonathan Rhoads, the Operative Surgeon

only possible land route for supplying the Chinese army. Otherwise, supplies had to be flown to China with great risk and expense over the "Hump" (Himalayan Mountains).

Ravdin arrived at the assigned hospital site during the monsoon season to find only a clearing in the jungle, which was knee-deep in mud, and a few bamboo huts. Rav's administrative genius and ability to cut through Army red tape were soon evident. Within months, his staff and some native recruits had somehow strung electric lines, dug drainage ditches, and built roads, an airstrip, a power plant, and dozens of buildings that soon accommodated a census of 2,500 patients.[15] The 20th General Hospital became a town occupying forty acres. Ravdin described himself as its mayor. General "Vinegar Joe" Stillwell (Commander of American Forces in the China-Burma-India theater) regularly made rounds with Rav on Sunday mornings and described it as "the best God damn hospital in the army."[16]

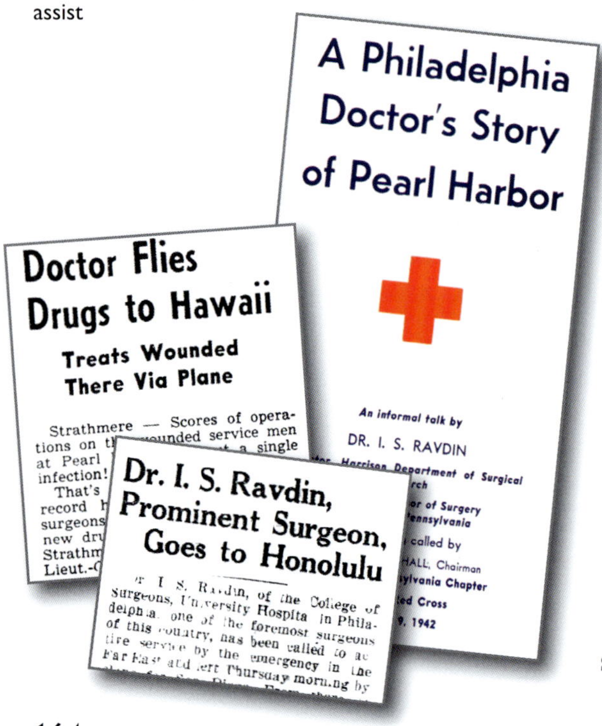

Spearheading the offensive in Burma was an elite group of volunteer jungle fighters, which soon became famous as "Merrill's Marauders." General Merrill led his men in a series of commando raids through jungles, over mountains, and across rivers, often as much as 100 miles behind enemy lines. The famous actor, Jeff Chandler, played Merrill in a major Hollywood movie in 1962. Food and ammunition could reach his men only by airdrop. Crucial to their morale was Merrill's promise that the wounded would be evacuated by small planes to Rav's 20th General Hospital. In three months of action, the Marauders sustained casualties of 80 percent. On a single day,

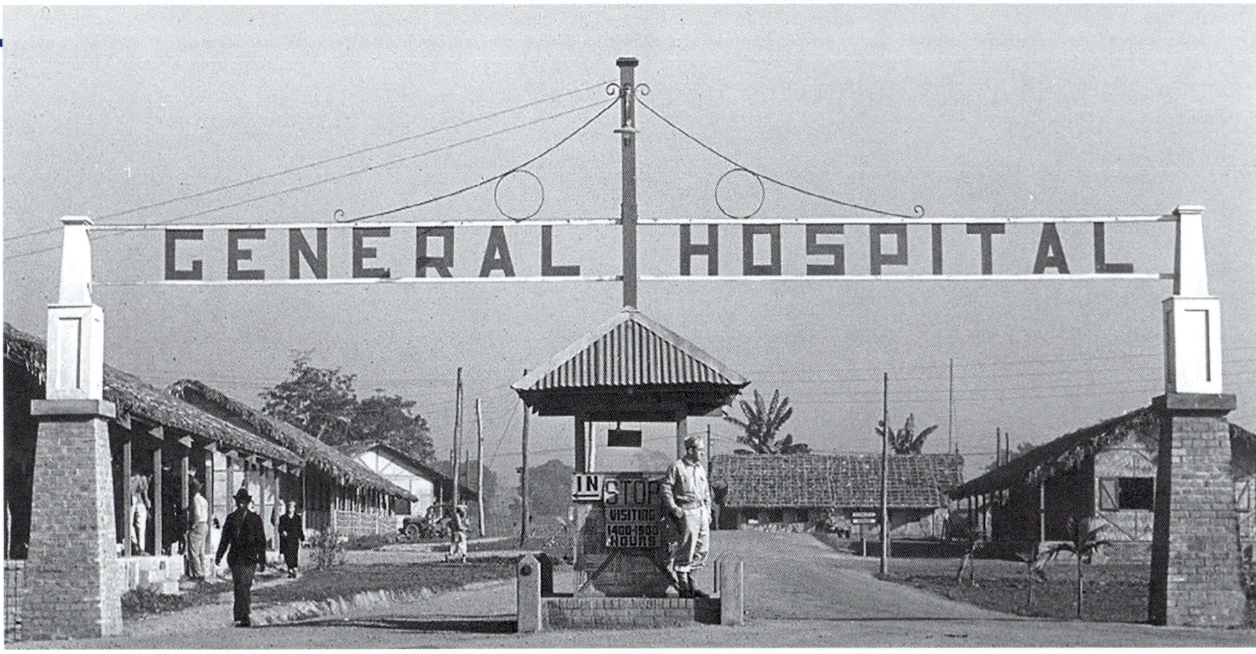

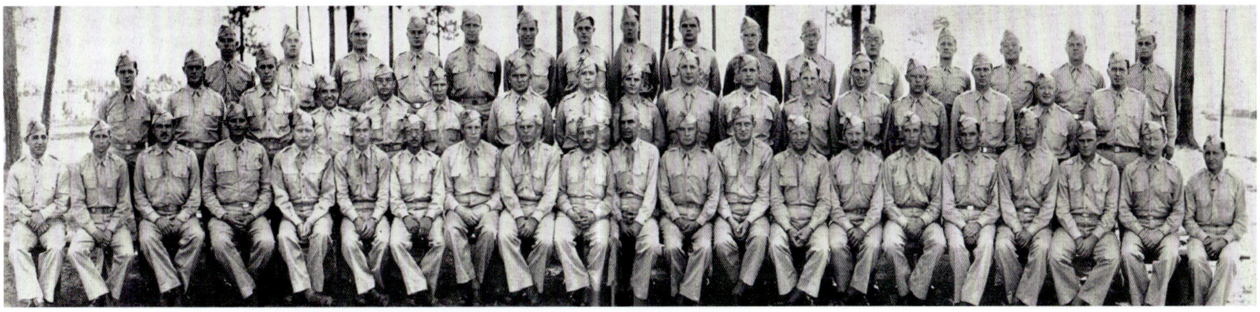

General Ravdin's 20th General Hospital Team

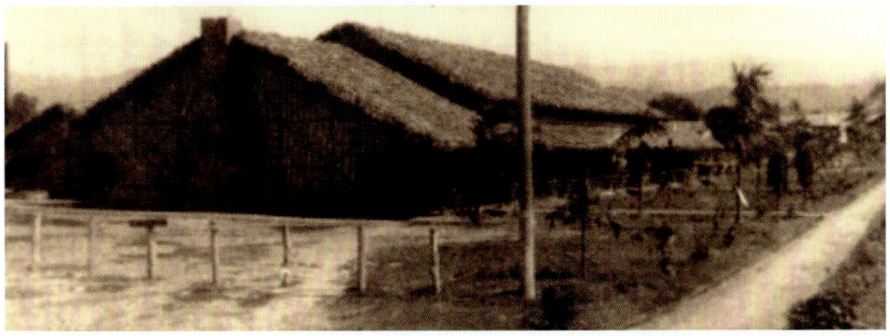

Operating rooms at the 20th General Hospital are in thatched huts.

Planning the Recapture of Northern Burma

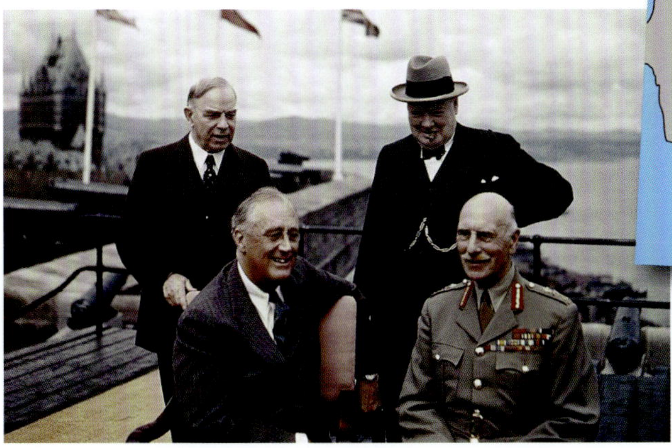

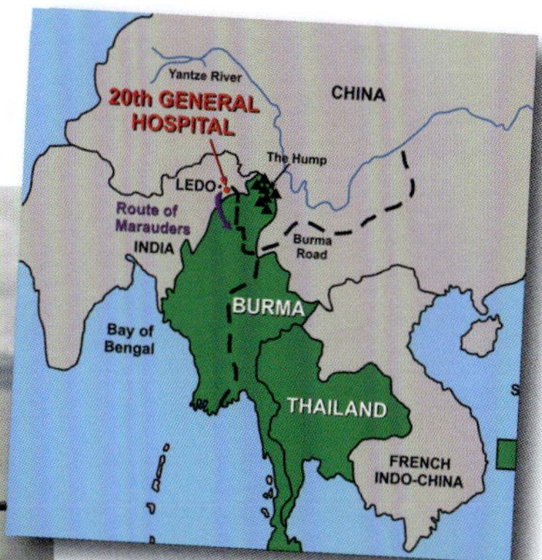

Mackenzie King, Franklin D. Roosevelt, Winston Churchill, and the Earl of Athlone at La Citadelle in Quebec

1941 (December)
After the Japanese bomb Pearl Harbor, Ravdin is sent there to assess the treatment of casualties.

Ravdin makes sure his trip to Pearl Harbor is well publicized

1942
Ravdin organizes the 20th General Hospital from HUP personnel including 73 doctors, 150 nurses and 600 enlisted men

1942–1943
May 15–January 5 training at Camp Claiborne, Louisiana for 20th General Hospital

1943 (August)
Roosevelt and Churchill meet in secret in Quebec to plan how the Ledo and Burma roads can restore land route for supplying Chinese

Part of the plan is for 3,000 volunteer jungle fighters (Merrill's Marauders) to protect engineers building the road.

Traveling by ship through the Panama Canal, the 20th General reaches Bombay by March 3 and then travels by train to reach its destination at the small town of Margherita during the monsoon season

1943–1945
The 20th General Hospital becomes World War II's largest hospital.
Ravdin is commander

1943–1945
For the hospital, Ravdin's staff builds 289 buildings and an air strip. For food, they plant a vegetable garden. And for meat, they breed pigs and geese.

The 20th General is not only WWII's largest hospital but the one that most resembles a peacetime university hospital. It has a staff of expert specialists, a modern laboratory, and a teaching conference schedule that attracts an audience from other military units in the area

1945
Ravdin is presented Legion of Merit by General Louis Pick, chief of Army engineers. Pick directed building of the Ledo and Burma Roads, one of history's great construction projects

sixty-three of them were admitted to the 20th General. Merrill himself was twice hospitalized for heart attacks. He and Rav became lifelong friends. It was Merrill who delivered the star that made Ravdin the only general to command an overseas hospital in wartime.[17] Ten years later, he got a second star, making him the only person on non-active military service to be promoted to major general.

Another important patient of the 20th General was Queen Victoria's grandson, Supreme Allied Commander in Southeast Asia, Lord Louis Mountbatten. One day, as Mountbatten was riding in his jeep through

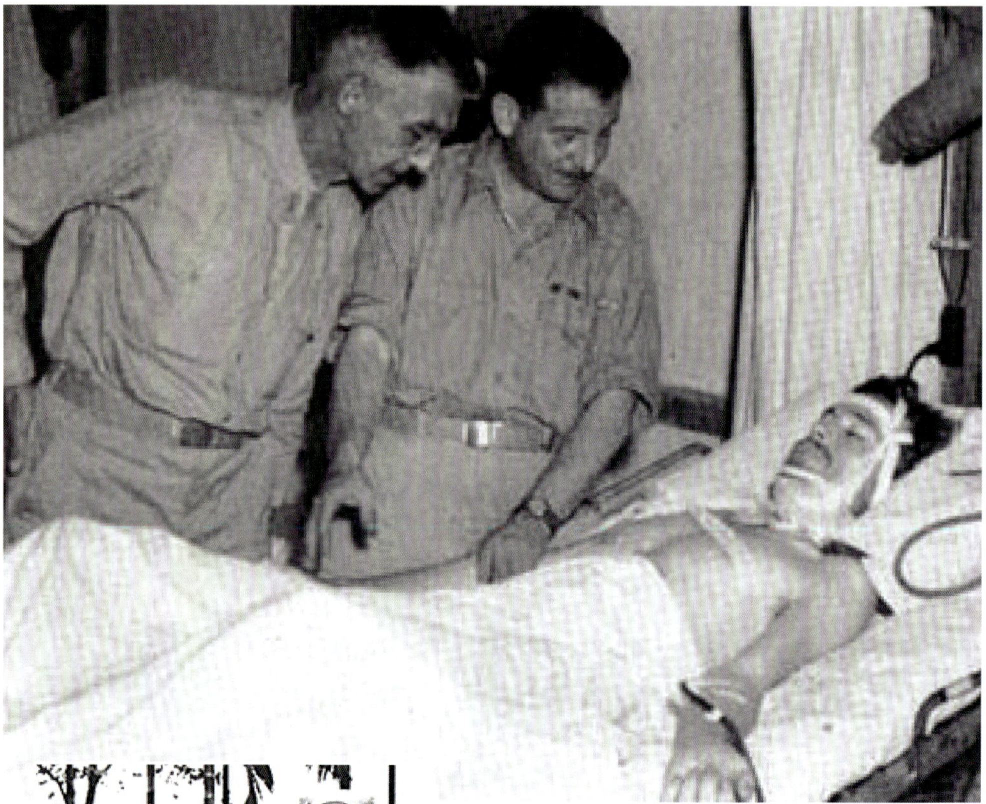

General "Vinegar Joe" Stillwell and "Mayor" Ravdin make rounds together Sunday mornings.

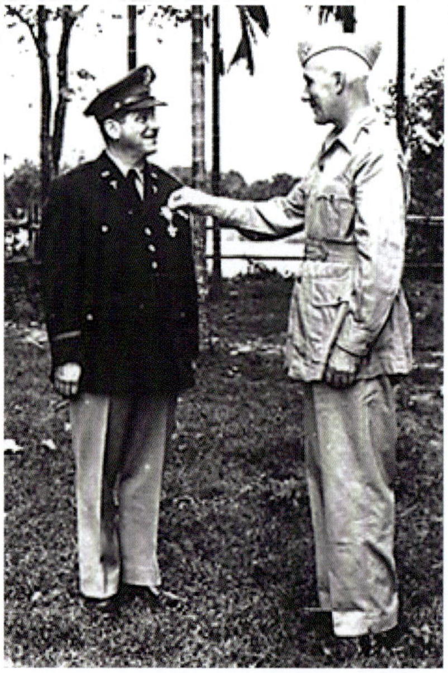

Brigadier General Lewis A. Pick presents Radvin with Legion of Merit.

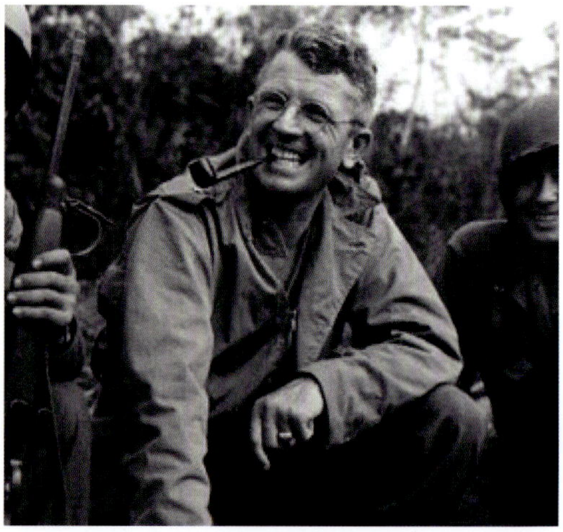

General Frank Merrill

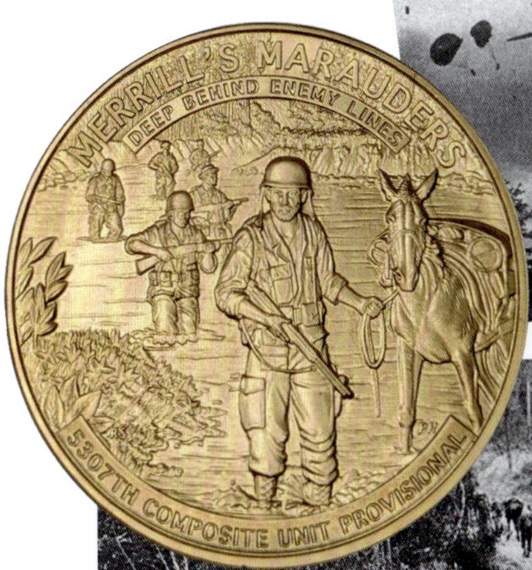

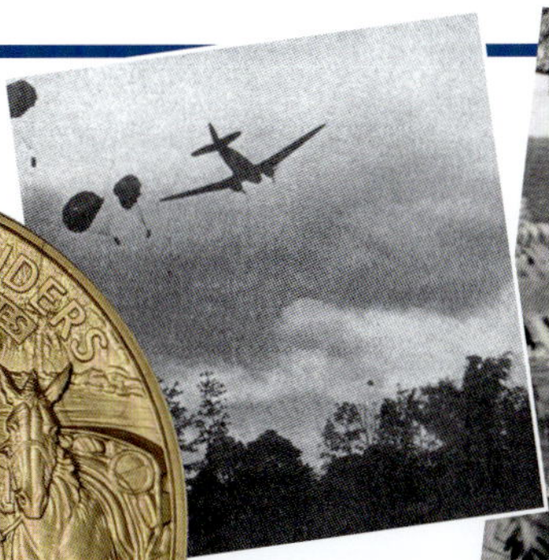

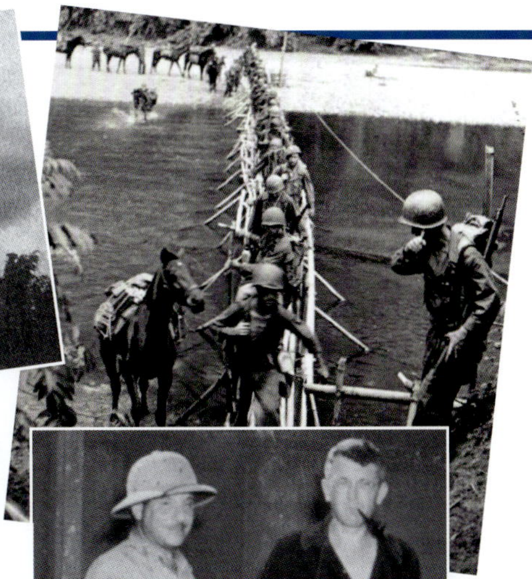

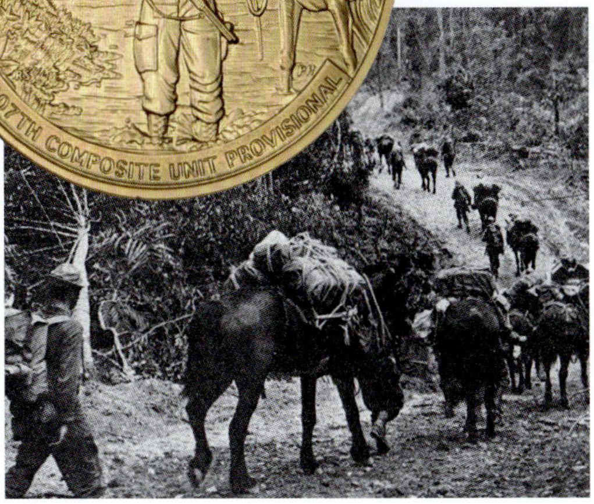

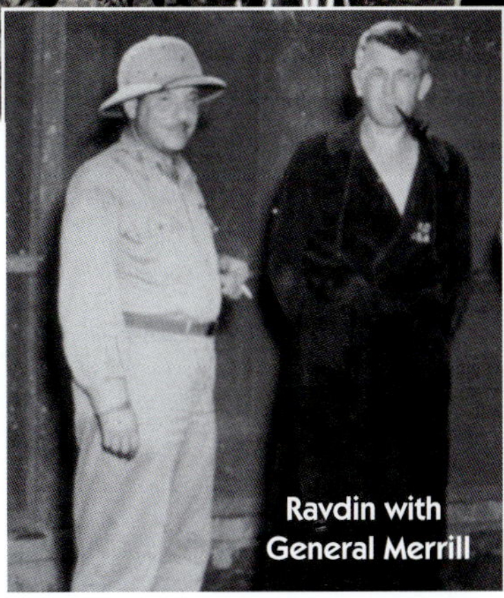

Ravdin with General Merrill

1944

On February 24, 3,000 Marauders begin a 1,000-mile march over the Kumon Bum Mountains. This trip nearly cripples them.

Multiple promises of relief or reinforcements never materialize.

On May 17, the Marauders take Myitkyina airfield. Only 200 are left in condition to fight.

In August, Marauders are disbanded.

In the attempt to apologize for lack of support and in recognition of their courage, every member of the Marauders is decorated

the jungle, his left eye was pierced and blinded by a piece of bamboo. He was flown to the 20th General for treatment. In admitting his famous patient, Ravdin, whose father was an ophthalmologist, found that the anterior chamber of his eye was filled with blood. He quickly called Captain Harold Scheie, the 20th General's ophthalmologist, to take care of him.

1944

Mountbatten's eye injury

SC 4/455/V

SOUTH EAST ASIA COMMAND HEADQUARTERS.

18th March, 1944.

Dear Colonel Ravdin,

I am writing to thank you personally, and through you all members of the 20th U.S. General Hospital staff concerned, for the way I was looked after during my week in the hospital with an injured eye.

If anything could increase my affection and regard for our American allies, my week at Ledo would undoubtedly do so.

This letter is being taken to you by Captain Scheie, who has been kindness itself to me. I am particularly grateful to you for having allowed him to accompany me to Delhi where he made a great hit with all members of my mess.

Yours sincerely,

Louis Mountbatten

P.S. Since dictating the above I have just heard the splendid news of your promotion, and hasten to offer you my most heartfelt congratulations.

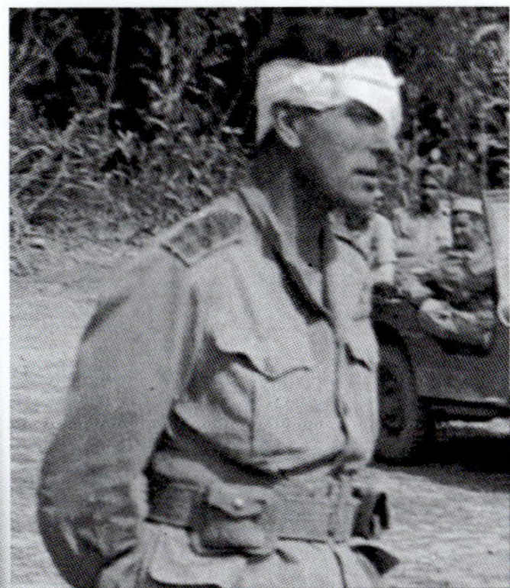

Lord Louis Mountbatten

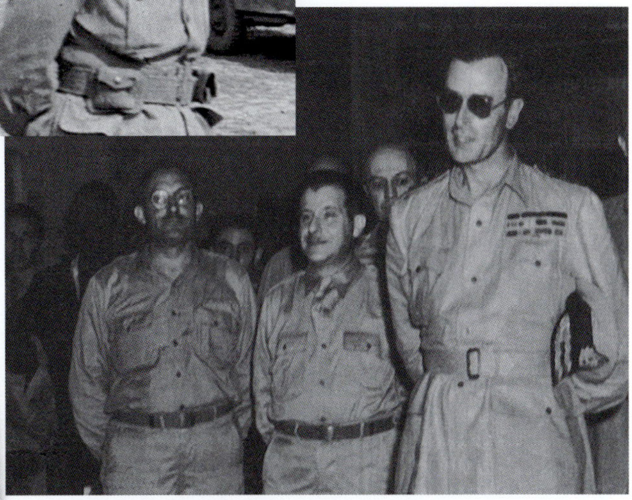

General Ravdin and Lord Mountbatten dedicating the air-conditioned unit, probably one of the first intensive care units anywhere.

1944
20th General staff publishes 100 papers while in India.

One of these by Norman Freeman describes treatment by sympathectomy of 114 patients with causalgia.

Ravdin believes Bill Fitts's experience with onlay bone graft for femoral fractures exceeds the number done in any US hospital

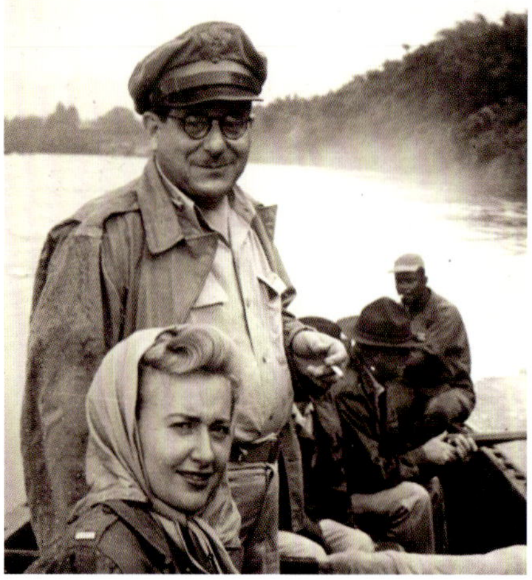

General Ravdin heading home from India.

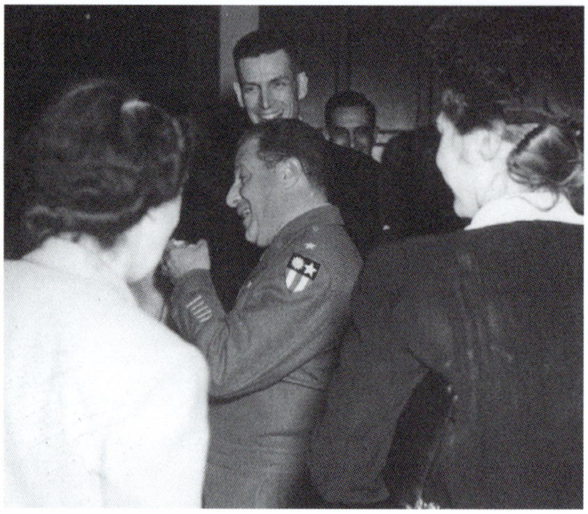

Welcome home celebration

1945
Ravdin promoted to brigadier general

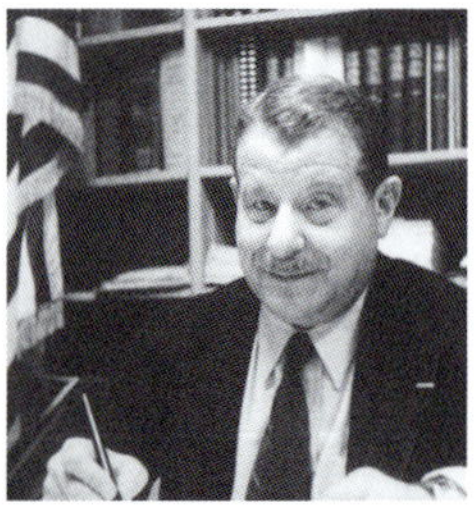

Post-war, his general's flag was always by Ravdin's desk.

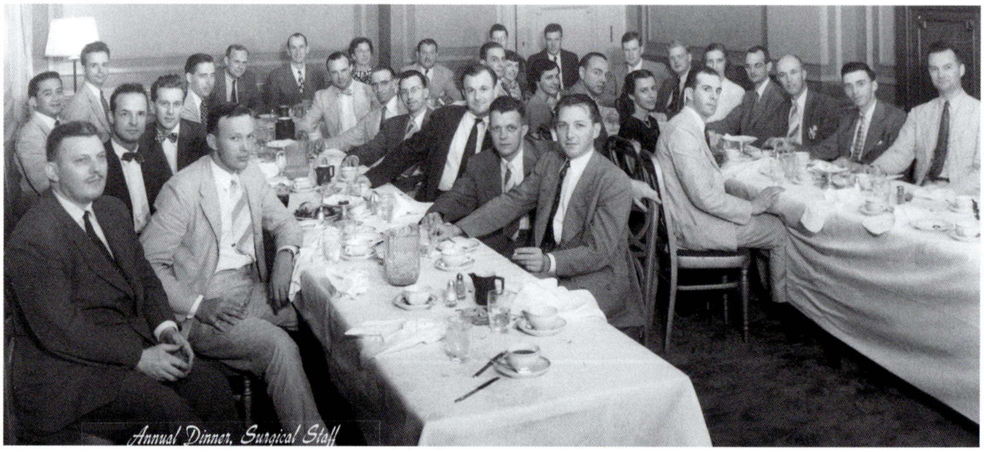

Ravdin's faculty and residents met regularly for dinner, a tradition inspired by wartime relationships of the 20th General Hospital team.

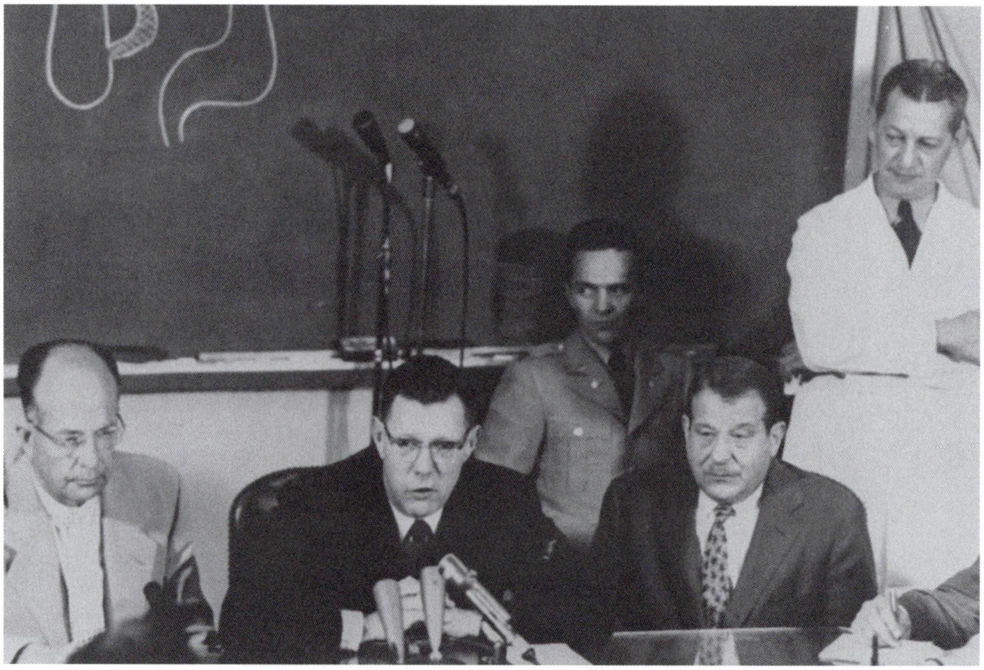

I. S. Ravdin discussing President Eisenhower's operation

A week later with his vision still at risk, Mountbatten insisted on leaving to deal with a Japanese counteroffensive, which was threatening to cut the Allies' supply lines. Ravdin sent Captain Harold Scheie, later Penn's ophthalmology chair, with Mountbatten to complete the treatment, which was ultimately successful.[18]

Always the consummate politician, Ravdin used his influence with these powerful friends to secure resources for his hospital and patients. Scrub typhus was a common ailment, which caused fever to be uncontrollable in the tropical climate and carried mortality as high as 20 percent. Ravdin persuaded General Stillwell to remove the air conditioners from his officers' quarters at the Imperial Hotel in New Delhi and install them in the 20th General Hospital. Lord Mountbatten flew in to dedicate the new air-conditioned intensive care unit [19] where the mortality of scrub typhus soon fell to less than 1 percent.[20]

As the war ended and General Ravdin started for home, he was asked to succeed Eliason as Penn's chairman of surgery, to the delight of Jonathan Rhoads (seen behind Ravdin in the photo at top right of pg. 168). He accepted only on condition that he become the one and only surgical chief.[21] From now on, there would be only one surgical service, and Ravdin would call all the shots. At HUP, he promptly appointed a geographic, full-time, university-based faculty comprised entirely of men who were either his own former residents or who had served under him in India.[22] Eliason-trained surgeons were strangely missing (except for Julian Johnson, who had been on Rav's 20th General Hospital's team). Ravdin ran his department and soon ran the entire University Hospital and School of Medicine pretty much the same way he ran the 20th General Hospital—as its commanding general. In fact, his general's flag was always kept at the side of his desk. Somehow, men who had worked for him in India were appointed dean of the medical school, chairman of medicine, and chiefs of neurosurgery, ENT, ophthalmology, plastic surgery, and thoracic surgery.[23] Small wonder that Rav's power went unchallenged.

During his fifteen years as chairman, the growth in the department's stature was exceeded only by Ravdin's own personal recognition. He was not only a member of all the important surgical organizations but president of them and a dozen others. He received eleven honorary degrees and became an honorary fellow of five foreign surgical colleges.[24]

In 1956, a perceived national crisis brought Ravdin to public attention. While chairing a meeting of the Board of Regents of the American College of Surgeons, Ravdin was interrupted by a message that President Eisenhower was being admitted to Walter Reed with abdominal pain and that the presidential airplane, the *Columbine,* was being sent to fetch him. After examining the president, Ravdin advised immediate surgery for intestinal obstruction. Walter Reed's chief of surgery, General Leon-

1945

August 5
Hiroshima atomic bomb.

August 14
Japan surrenders.

December 1945
20th General Hospital closes

1946
Ravdin returns from India and becomes John Rhea Barton Professor and Chairman of Department

1946
Determined to be fully in charge of his department, Ravdin gets rid of faculty members trained by others, appoints a geographic full-time salaried faculty, and starts a residency program modeled in large part after Halsted's.

C. Everett Koop finishes his residency in 1946. Ravdin appoints him chief of the division of pediatric surgery at CHOP. He serves in this position for thirty-three years, before becoming US Surgeon General

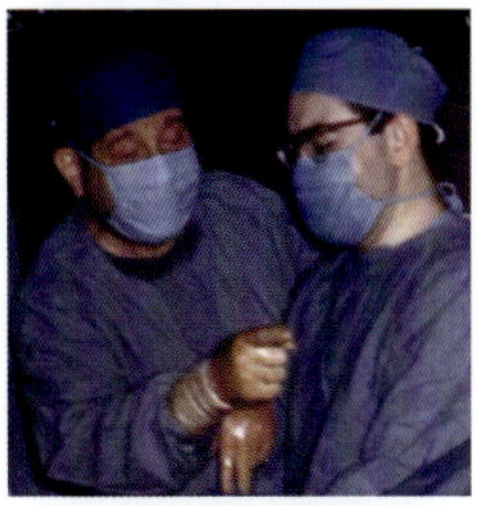

Rav disciplines an assistant.

1951
Norman Freeman, former Ravdin resident, now at UCSF, performs world's first resection of abdominal aortic aneurysm

Ravdin as Cult Figure

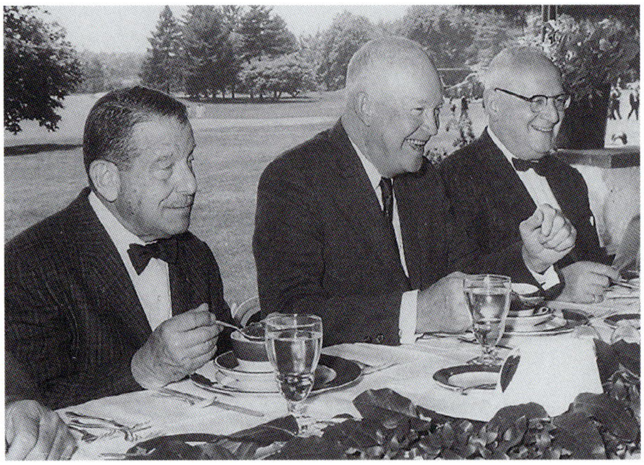

At fundraiser, Rav is honorary caddie for golf match: Eisenhower and Arnold Palmer vs. Jimmy Demaret and Ray Bolger.

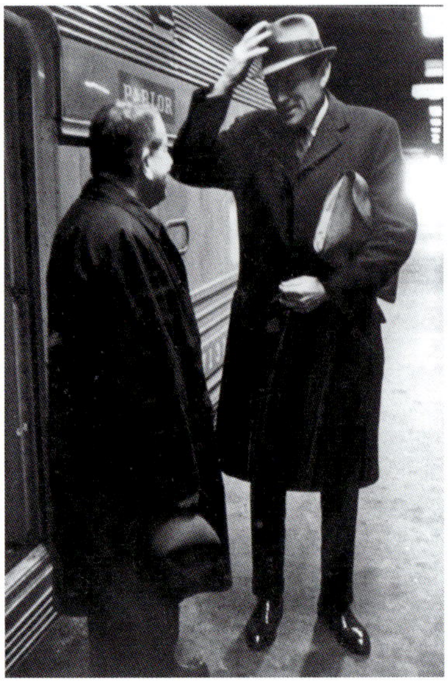

Ravdin with Gregory Peck

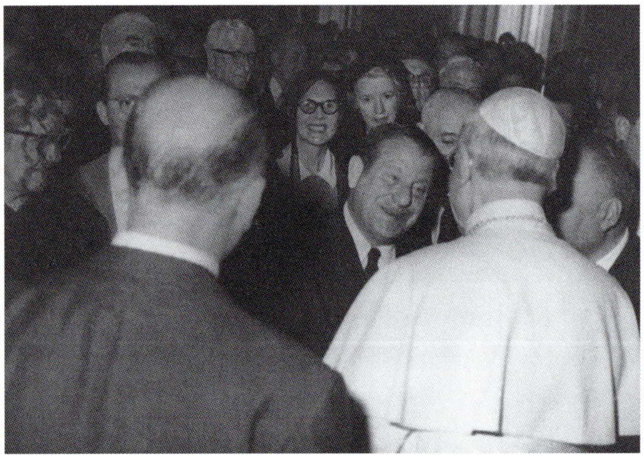

Ravdin with Pope Pius XII

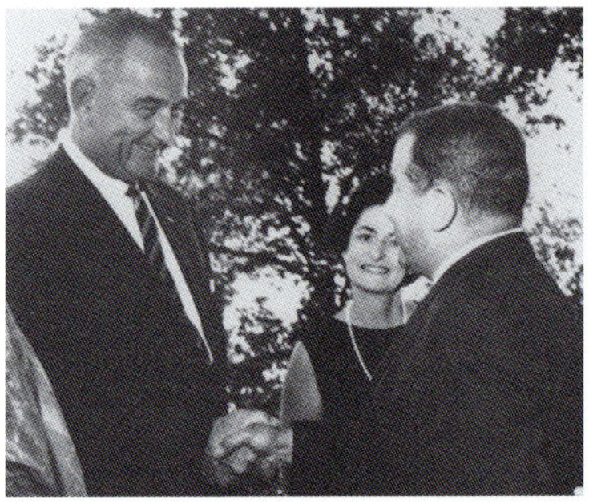

Ravdin, President Lyndon Johnson, and Lady Bird Johnson

ard Heaton, and Rav carried out a successful bypass procedure.[25] This and his subsequent friendship with Eisenhower increased public awareness of him. His frequent appearances with celebrities, such as Gregory Peck and the Pope, made him almost a cult figure. As winner of the Philadelphia Award, he was considered the city's best-known and most respected citizen.

Like the president, Rav's less-famous patients almost always did well, more because of his superb judgment than his technical skill. In the operating room, he was fast and somewhat unpredictable, impatient with his assistants, sometimes abruptly banishing them or scolding them for presumed infractions, only to reinstate them minutes later and praise them for reasons equally obscure.[26]

Outside the operating room, Rav was warm and his sense of humor often disarming. His residents and faculty simultaneously loved and feared him. In return, he protected and cherished them as though they were his own children, using his incredible political influence to foster their academic careers.

1951
A few months after the start of the Korean War, Ravdin resident, John Howard, and other MASH surgeons begin to repair arterial wounds rather than ligating them. This was against Army regulations based on earlier reports of bad results. At first, most of the sutured arteries thrombose because of unsuitable vascular clamps. Howard procures better clamps, and good results follow. President Eisenhower awards him the Legion of Merit. Howard is one of the Army surgeons considered the model for TV's Hawkeye

1953
Ravdin given honorary LLD from the University of Pennsylvania

1954
Strittmatter Award of the Philadelphia County Medical Society

1955
Ravdin promoted to major general

1956
With General Heaton, Ravdin operates on President Eisenhower for intestinal obstruction from regional enteritis

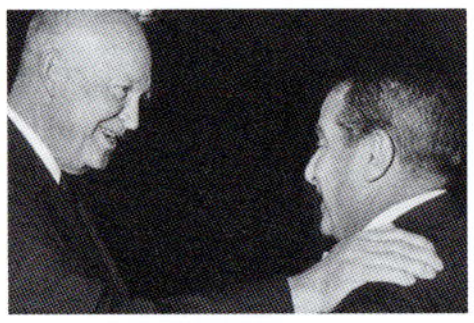

Eisenhower and Ravdin

The Professor's Lighter Side

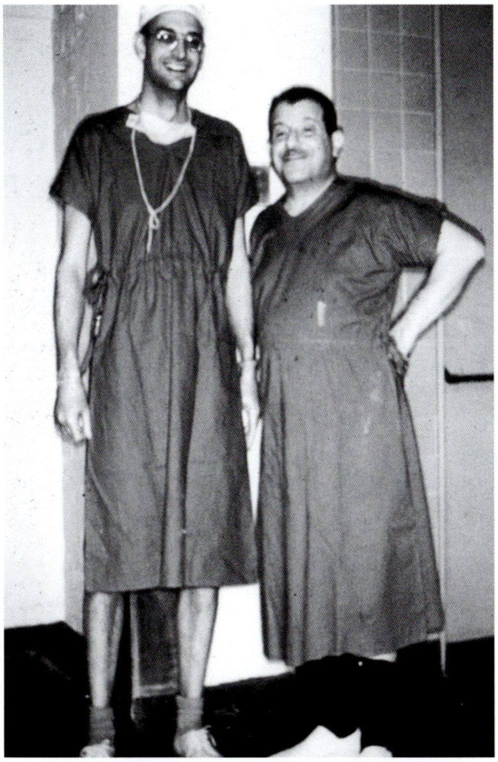

The laundry ran out of male scrub suits. Ravdin and Brooke Roberts are determined to operate anyway.

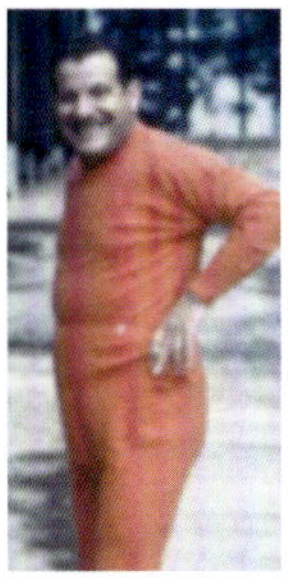

Clowning at his seaside retreat

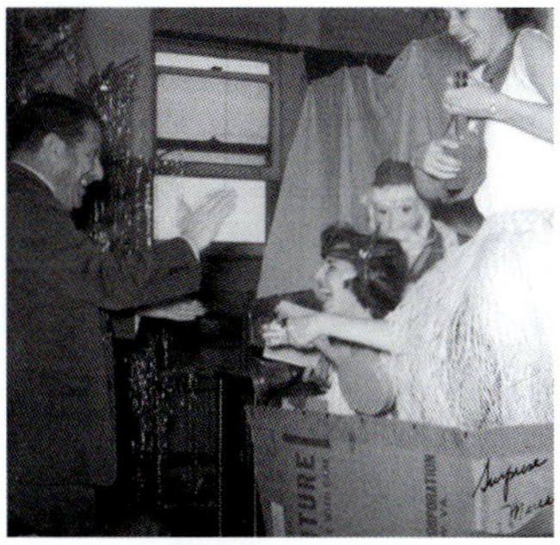

Christmas party for the nurses.

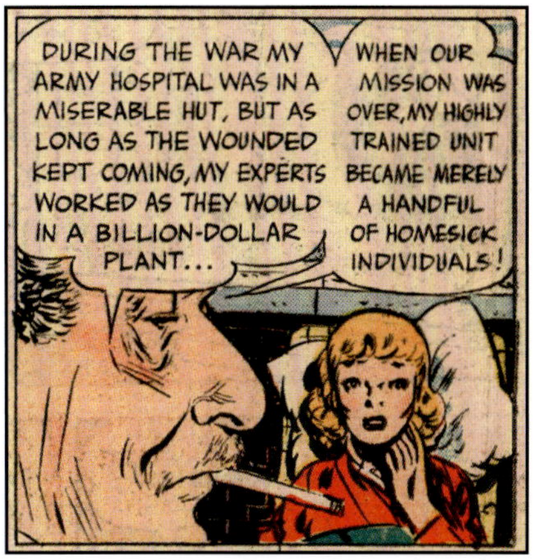

DURING THE WAR MY ARMY HOSPITAL WAS IN A MISERABLE HUT, BUT AS LONG AS THE WOUNDED KEPT COMING, MY EXPERTS WORKED AS THEY WOULD IN A BILLION-DOLLAR PLANT...
WHEN OUR MISSION WAS OVER, MY HIGHLY TRAINED UNIT BECAME MERELY A HANDFUL OF HOMESICK INDIVIDUALS!

Something of Rav's style was captured by the famous cartoonist, Milton Caniff, who featured "the professor" in an episode of his nationally syndicated comic strip, *Steve Canyon*.[27] For many years over coffee or cocktails with my fellow residents, I wondered what exactly it was that allowed this short, physically ordinary man to wield the power of a giant. Perhaps it was his aggressiveness, brilliant intellect, total confidence that he was right, self-discipline, a gift for command honed by military experience, cunning, charm, and occasional ruthlessness. He had a gift for remembering names, the capability to thrive on four or five hours of sleep, and to move rapidly through the other twenty hours, and a lifetime supply of his famous "grasshopper suppositories" he threatened to prescribe to speed up his slower associates.[28] All these had something to do with it. But underlying this was the uncanny ability to pick

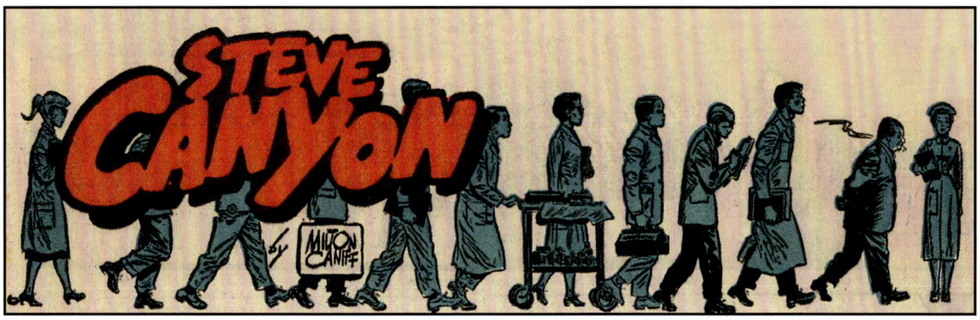

STEVE CANYON
by MILTON CANIFF

1956
Ravdin becomes fellow of Royal College of Surgeons of England

1957
Ravdin wins Philadelphia Award

1957
Ravdin is chairman of clinical standards committee on cancer chemotherapy at the NIH. He invites his former resident Bernie Fisher to attend a meeting to discuss creation of the Surgical Adjuvant Chemotherapy Breast Project (later NSABP).

Fisher does not want to attend, but later he is intrigued by breast cancer and multicenter randomized trials and becomes chair of NSABP. The outcome of his work is a revolution in treatment of breast cancer

1943–1960
Ravdin's hobbies include stamp collecting—some bought from FDR's collection

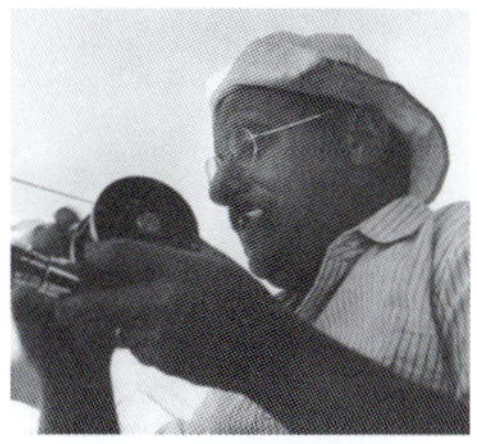

One of his hobbies

Other hobbies are cultivating hollies at his Bucks County retreat and deep-sea fishing.

At Christmas, Ravdin entertains his faculty, residents, and many other guests at his home on Delancy Street. The crowd is so large that invitation is by assigned shifts

1957 (October)
Cartoonist Milton Caniff stars Ravdin in his syndicated comic strip, *Steve Canyon*

1958–1959
President of American Surgical Association. Ravdin titles his presidential address: "A Surgeon and Something More"

1959
Jim Robinson, Ravdin's (and HUP's) first Black chief resident. He later becomes associate dean and director of minority affairs at Jefferson University Medical School

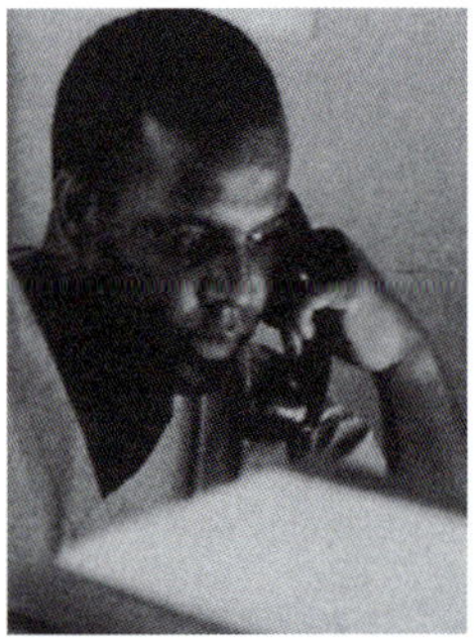

1960
Ravdin retires as chairman of surgery

1960–1961
President of American College of Surgeons

1960–1965
Ravdin is vice president of medical affairs at the University of Pennsylvania

the right person for a job, a colorful personality, sense of humor, and whatever it is that allows an occasional individual to be liked by many and respected by all. Call it leadership, call it charisma, I. S. Ravdin certainly had it.

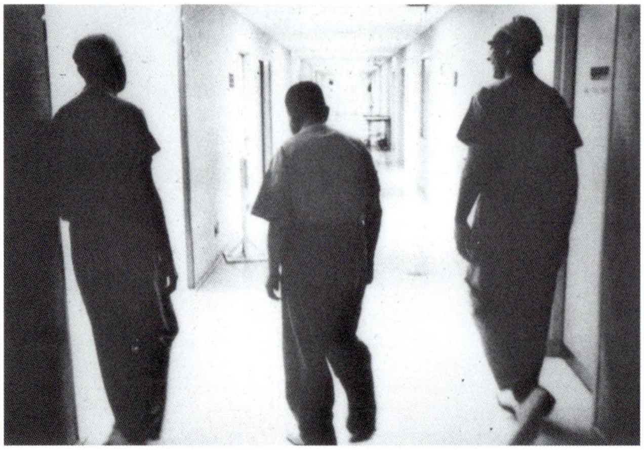

Walking reluctantly towards retirement.

After fifteen years as chairman, Dr. Ravdin arranged for Jonathan Rhoads to succeed him as Surgery's chairman and moved into the office of the university's vice president for medical affairs. There he concentrated on raising funds for buildings, which replaced more than half of the old University Hospital. One of these was appropriately named the I. S. Ravdin Institute.

Eventually, it became apparent that age and his incessant smoking were catching up with him. Although he was able to conceal angina and claudication by briefly pausing on rounds to tell one of his many stories, his conspicuously failing intellect and memory finally forced his retirement.[29]

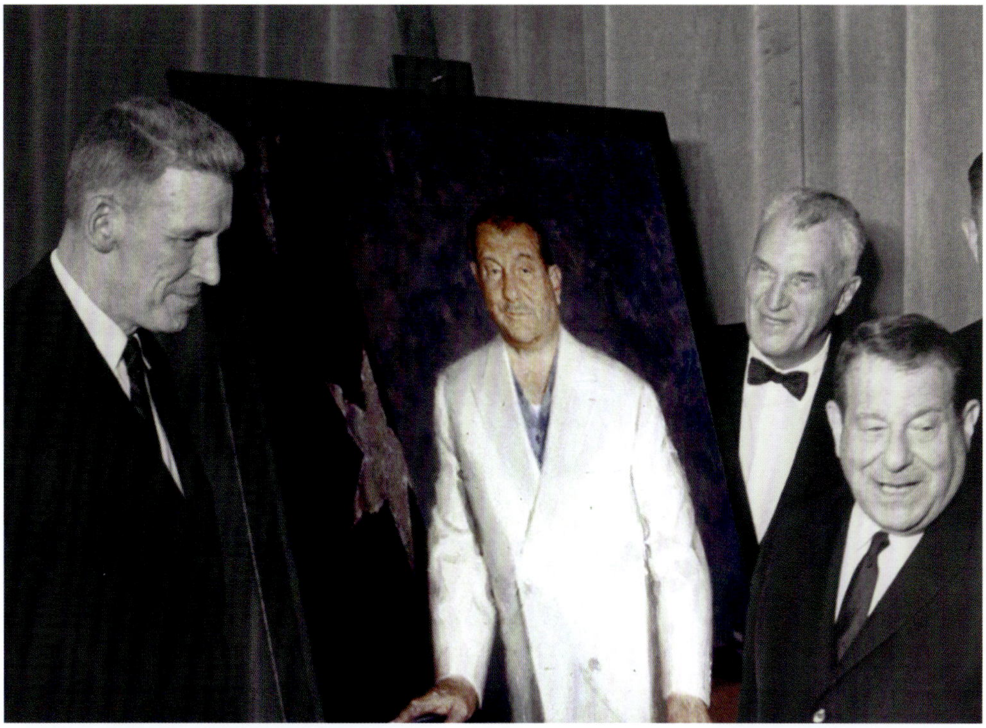

At portrait unveiling with University President Harnwell and Jonathan Rhoads.

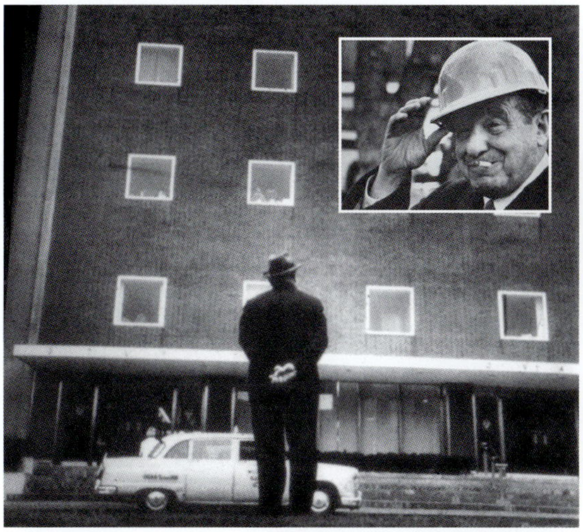

I. S. Ravdin looking at the building named after him.

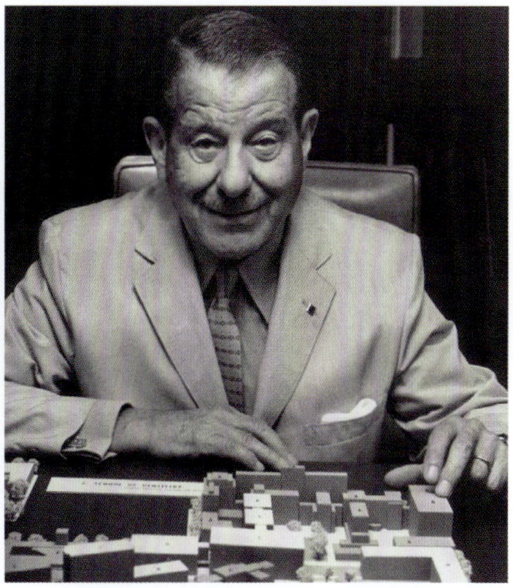

The university's vice president surveys a model of his empire.

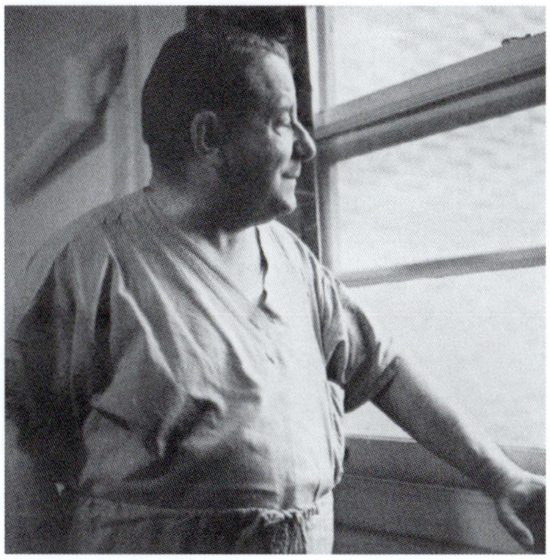

1962–1963
President of American Cancer Society

1962
Hollywood movie about Merrill's Marauders

1962
Ravdin Building opens

1963
Former Ravdin resident Jim Hardy, chair of surgery at the University of Mississippi, performs the world's first lung transplant

1963
Ravdin's oral history is compiled

1964
Ravdin's former resident Jim Hardy performs the world's first heart transplant. Without a suitable human donor, he uses a chimpanzee

1972
Ravdin dies

Ravdin's Chief Residents: The Finest Generation?

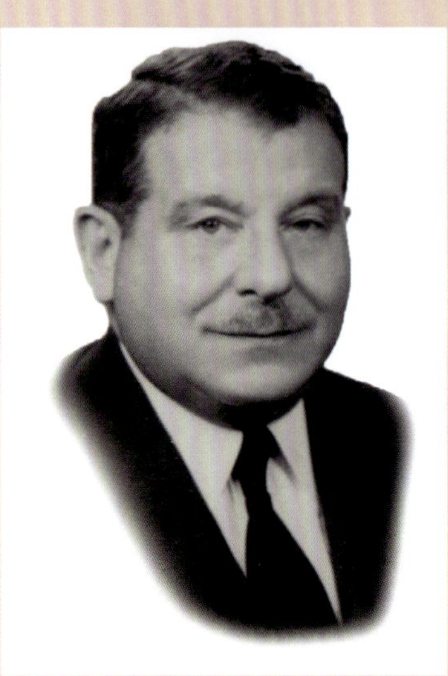

From the vantage of more than half a century, it is now easy to see that I. S. Ravdin was a transitional figure between the geheimrat clinicians of the last century and the modern scientific surgeon. His legacy was not the buildings he built, but the cohesive, modern, research-oriented department he created and the surgeons it trained. His influence was most easily recognized in the accomplishments of his 100 residents, many of whom became professors and a dozen who headed their own departments. Among this group was Jonathan Rhoads, whose stature eventually may have equaled or exceeded even that of his chief.

Because our archives of this era are sketchy, I was lucky to find the names of the thirty who survived Ravdin's pyramid to become chief residents at HUP during his fourteen years as chairman. They were the first generation at Penn to graduate from a real surgical residency. Earlier HUP residents were trained pretty much by preceptorship. In his oral history, Ravdin told the story of his residency's genesis.[30] In 1932, thirty-eight-year-old Ravdin accompanied Penn surgery chairman, Charles Frazier, to provide support for his chief during a visit to Johns Hopkins, where Frazier sought treatment for prostate cancer by the famous urologist Hugh Young.[31] After barely surviving a bloody operation, Frazier returned to Philadelphia with persistent urinary incontinence. Ravdin had used his time in Baltimore to learn about the Hopkins surgical residency from Hopkins's famous dean, William Welch. He returned to Philadelphia with the determination to install one like it at HUP.

In 1890, William Halsted had become chief of surgery at the new Johns Hopkins Hospital. Because the staff reporting to him were also new, Halsted encountered little opposition to installing a surgical residency based on his own priorities. In a classic publication, he revealed its essential elements: (1) a geographic, full-time department totally controlled by a single professor—himself; (2) over many years, graded responsibility of residents to their independence; (3) mandatory research experience of the residents; and (4) a specific intent to produce professors and teachers by emphasizing resident education rather than faculty practice and income.[32]

Within a short time, Halsted's system began to produce results. In his thirty-three years as chairman, his residency graduated only seventeen chief residents. Seven became department chairmen, and eleven started their own residency programs.[33] Of his fifty-five assistant residents, twenty became professors. Other universities took note of Halsted's residency system and began to copy it. Characteristically, Penn did not. A contingent of Penn faculty was sent to Hopkins to evaluate Halsted's residency. They decided not to copy it, preferring to stick with the traditional Penn system. As Osler said, nowhere is there more resistance to change than at the University of Pennsylvania. The traditional Penn residency system was continued. In it, each of the department's several autonomous professors selected and controlled his own separate residents. The emphasis was on faculty practice, not on resident education. There was no mandated research experience, no intent to produce professors, and none were produced.

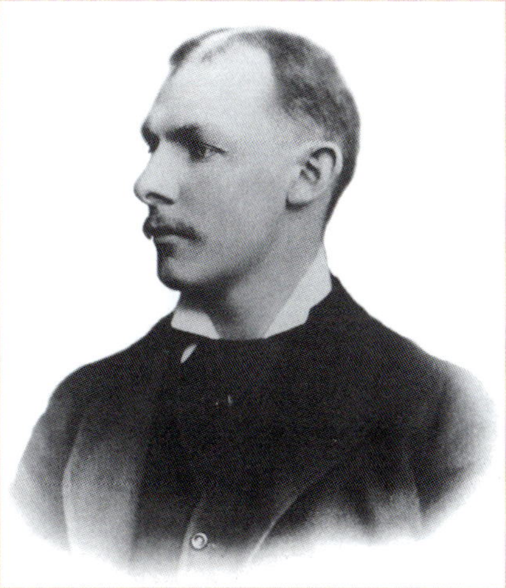
William Halsted

In 1946, when Ravdin became chairman, he got rid of HUP faculty surgeons other than those he had trained as residents or had commanded in India as a general in charge of World War II's 20th General Hospital.[34] Now he had the unchallenged power to make big changes. As he had planned to do since his visit to Hopkins with Frazier fourteen years before, he installed a Halsted-style residency at HUP with all of its essential elements: (1) a single all-powerful professor—himself; (2) graded responsibility of residents to independence; (3) mandatory research; and (4) an intent to produce professors. Just as it had in Baltimore, it worked. Of the thirty who survived Ravdin's pyramid to become chief residents at HUP, eight became university department chairmen. Of seventy others who had part of their training under Ravdin, many became university division chiefs or heads of surgery at community hospitals.

Many of his early residents had served under Ravdin in the 20th General Hospital. Others had followed General Patton as he chased the retreating Germans across Europe. After the war, Ravdin's requirement that his residents perform research encouraged them to explore fields that were new and become pioneers of cardiac surgery, vascular surgery, pediatric surgery, transplantation, and cancer chemotherapy. Profiled here are Ravdin's HUP chief residents. Maybe they were the greatest generation.

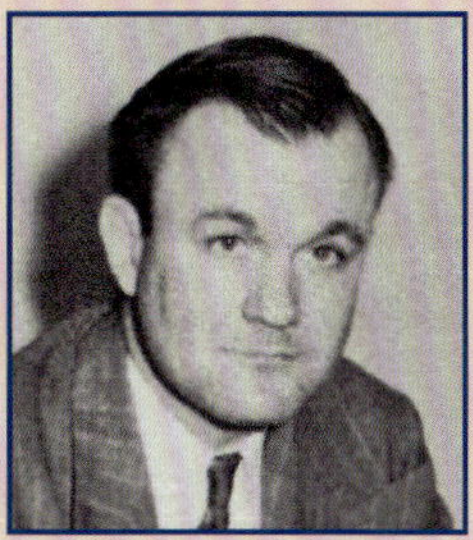

William T. Fitts Jr. (1947) Bill Fitts graduated as first in his class from Penn Medical School.[35] After his internship at HUP, he went with Ravdin to the 20th General Hospital where his work ethic and administrative skills made him his chief's favorite. Later as a Penn professor, he became prominent nationally, especially in the trauma field. Many predicted that he would become chairman when Ravdin retired in 1960, but this was precluded by Fitts's illnesses, including a bleeding duodenal ulcer. In 1972, Fitts eventually became Penn's surgery chairman by succeeding Jonathan Rhoads.

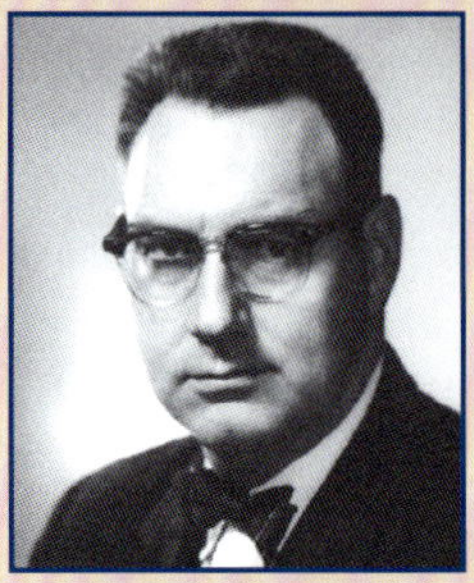

C. Everett Koop (1947) was the most famous of the group.[36] As a resident, Koop with Jonathan Rhoads managed the wartime skeleton Ravdin service at HUP while Ravdin was in India. Thus, although Koop's chief residency was under Ravdin, much of his training was under Rhoads. Ravdin appointed thirty-year-old Koop as chief of pediatric surgery at CHOP. He soon became the nation's foremost pediatric surgeon. Because of his well-publicized evangelistic and pro-life opinions, Koop was controversial as President Reagan's nominee for surgeon general. But Koop's outstanding performance in this role made him so famous that he become known as "America's Doctor."

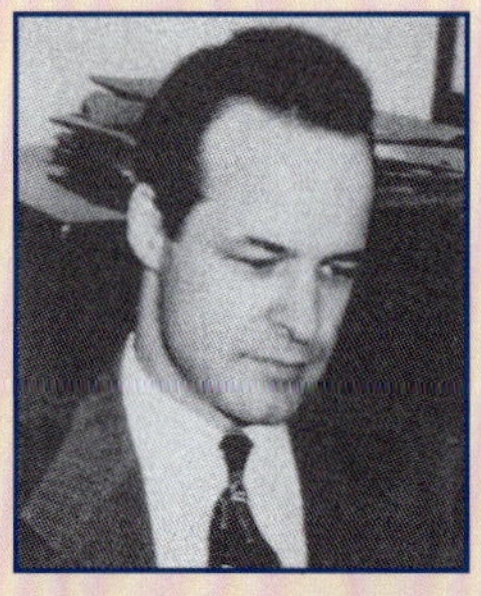

Charles K. Kirby (1947) A graduate of Cornell medical school, Kirby's excellent performance at the 20th General Hospital led to his appointment as a HUP resident and then as Julian Johnson's faculty understudy in cardiothoracic surgery.[37] A gifted researcher and writer, he probably had more to do than Johnson with designing and building HUP's first heart-lung machine and in coauthoring with Johnson the chest surgery textbook that became the field's standard. At age forty-nine, Kirby died suddenly from a massive coronary occlusion. We residents were convinced that Johnson's seemingly abusive dominance was responsible for Charlie's nervous mannerisms and perhaps for shortening his life. Frank Rosato and I did not know that Charlie had an identical twin. Sitting together at his funeral, we were startled when his twin brother walked in. Charlie's twin, a University of Washington internist not subjected to Johnson's sarcasm, lived comfortably another three decades.

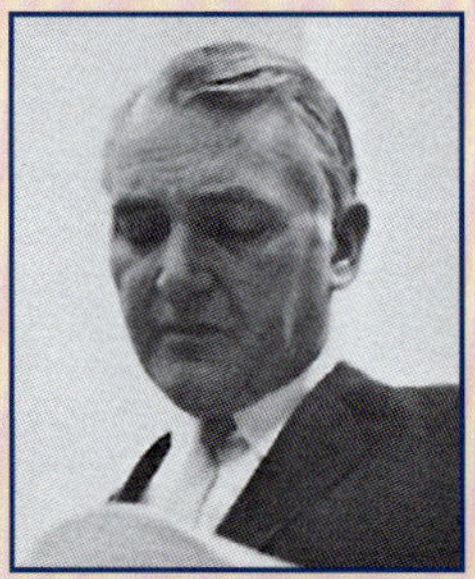

Cletus Schwegman (1948) After medical school and internship at Cincinnati, Clete was assigned to the 20th General Hospital where he worked with Robert Groff in neurosurgery, becoming particularly experienced and expert in hand surgery.[38] As a HUP professor, he became the "go-to" abdominal surgeon. His academic productivity may have been greater if he had spent less time as secretary of the American Board of Surgery. There, he was the terror of examinees. Actually, his generous personality caused him to fail fewer than other examiners. Around HUP, Clete had a swashbuckling image that was enhanced by his good looks, dapper wardrobe, and banter with the ladies. He took pride in extensively prepared lectures that he memorized and delivered in his impressively deep speaking voice. Ironically at age fifty, a laryngectomy for cancer reduced this to a whisper during the two remaining decades of his life.

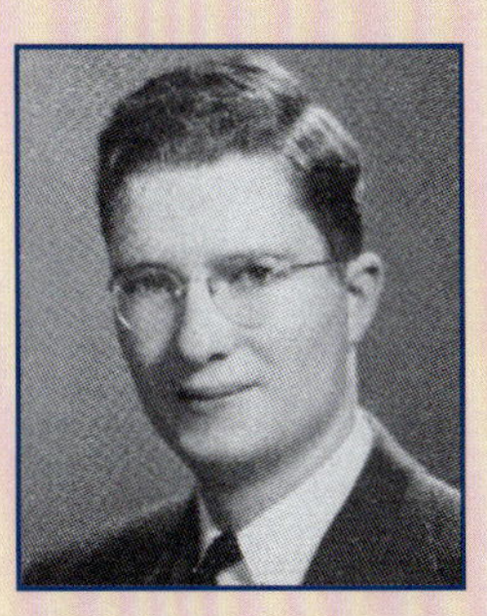

James D. Hardy (1949) After graduating from medical school at Penn, he became a medical resident.[39] During his Army service in World War II, he switched to surgery. Outstanding in research and a prolific author, known to his friends as the "boy wonder," he published the first of his twenty-three books while still a resident. He became the inaugural chairman of surgery at the University of Mississippi where he performed the world's first human heart and lung transplants. Despite Hardy's extensive preparation and research in animals, neither of these human recipients survived very long. But Hardy came closer than any other Ravdin resident to equaling his chief in honors and leadership positions of national surgical organizations, such as the presidencies of the American Surgical Association, the American College of Surgeons, and the Society of University Surgeons.

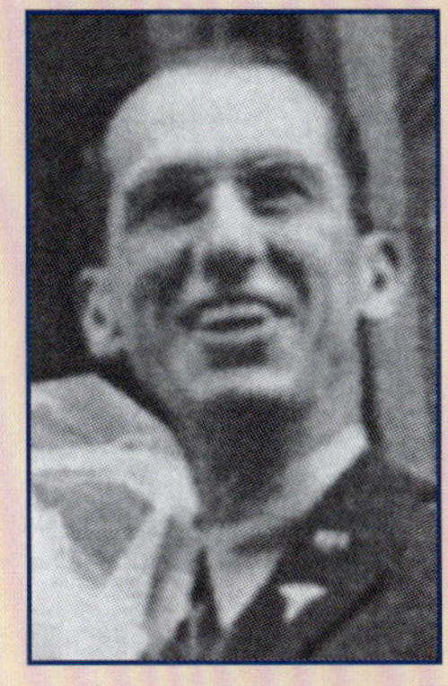

Archibald Fletcher (1949) has been completely forgotten at HUP. But from this collection of impressive careers, his was possibly the most striking.[40] Born in Taegu, Korea, where his father had established a missionary hospital, Arch came to the United States and graduated from Princeton University and Columbia medical school. During the war, he served in Europe with Patton's 3rd Army. Then, as a HUP resident, he studied blood substitutes with Doctors Rhoads and Hardy. After a year as an exchange resident in Montreal and HUP chief residency, he was sent by the Presbyterian Church to India where he helped found one of that country's major medical schools, Miraj Medical College. There, he became chairman of surgery and also director of the school's teaching hospital. From his autobiography, *To India and Beyond,* I learned more about his distinguished career. After visiting UCLA for two months, he designed and constructed a heart-lung machine and successfully performed the first open-heart operations in India. In 1977, he returned to the United States to teach surgery at the University of Washington. Spiritual wanderlust soon lured him back to missionary work in Kathmandu, Nepal, Cameroon, and India.

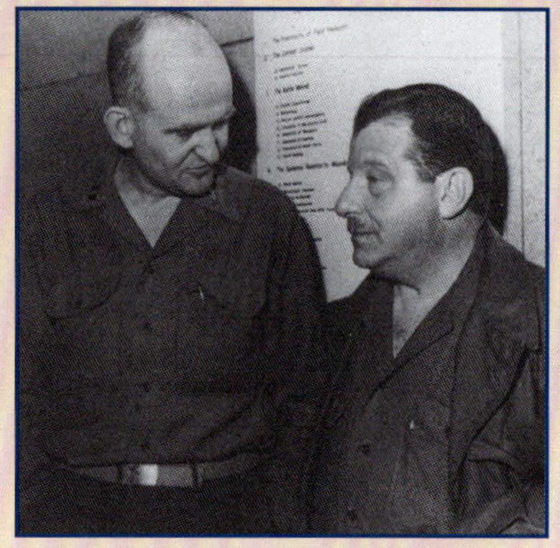

John Howard and Ravdin

John Howard (1950) After completing his HUP residency, he spent a short period at Baylor with Mike DeBakey.[41] John then briefly became chairman of surgery at Emory. During the Korean War, he directed the Army surgical research team (MASH), also establishing there a renal dialysis unit. For these accomplishments, President Eisenhower awarded him the Legion of Merit. He then returned to Philadelphia as chairman of surgery at Hahnemann (1958–63). In 1973, he followed Bill Blakemore to the Medical College of Ohio where John was a leading professor of surgery for thirty years. He was a renowned expert in pancreatic surgery, writing with Howard Reber (HUP chief resident 1970) the classic text on the pancreas that has remained the standard in the field.

James Walker (1950) During residency and for several years on the faculty, Walker was active in research with Dr. Rhoads. He won a prestigious Markle scholarship.

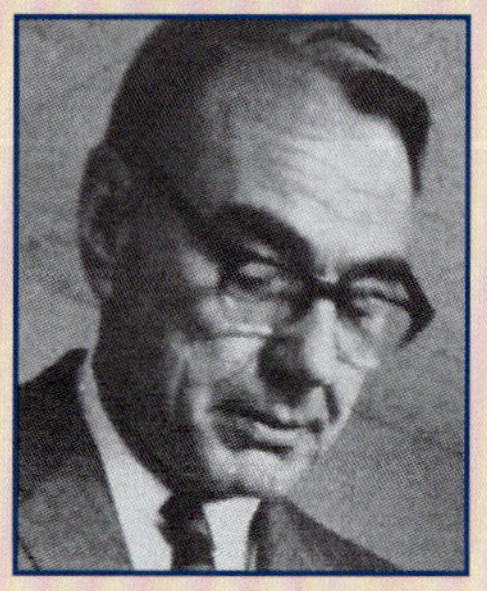

William Dyson (1950) After internship, "Dutch" Dyson served on a destroyer, carrying out anti-submarine warfare.[42] After residency, he was chief of surgery at Hazelton Hospital (1950–65). HUP residents were assigned to help him there with his huge practice. This became a much sought-after resident rotation. In 1965, Dyson developed an interest in psychiatry and returned to HUP where he completed a residency in that field and became a member of the psychiatry faculty. He directed HUP's first lithium therapy program for patients with bipolar disease. Also at HUP, he carried out a sizable practice in general surgery.

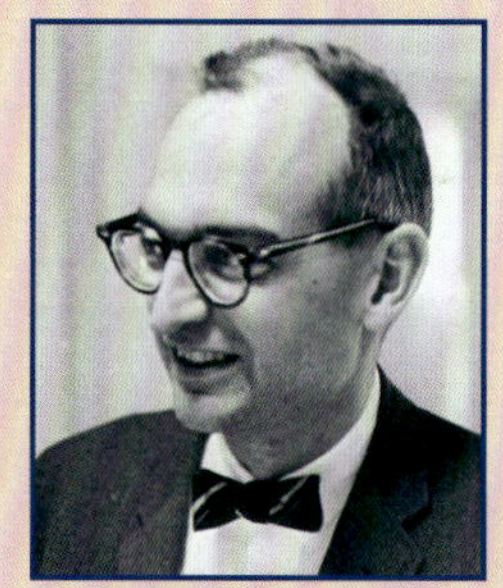

Brooke Roberts (1951) As a Penn student, Brooke won the school's Spencer Morris Prize as the top student in medicine.[43] After HUP residency and several years as Dr. Ravdin's understudy and clinical assistant, Ravdin placed him in charge of vascular surgery. At first, this field was nothing more than treatment of varicose veins, but as arterial surgery developed, Brooke became one of its important pioneers. With his medical colleagues, he was the first to describe and analyze the hemodynamic cause of subclavian steal syndrome. With his interventional radiology colleagues, he started one of the first programs in balloon catheter dilatation of stenotic artery lesions. His was one of the country's first vascular fellowships. During Len Miller's illness and absence, Brooke served as the department's acting chairman. At this crucial time, he managed the contentious transition of the John Rhea Barton Associates from a private practice partnership to a university department.

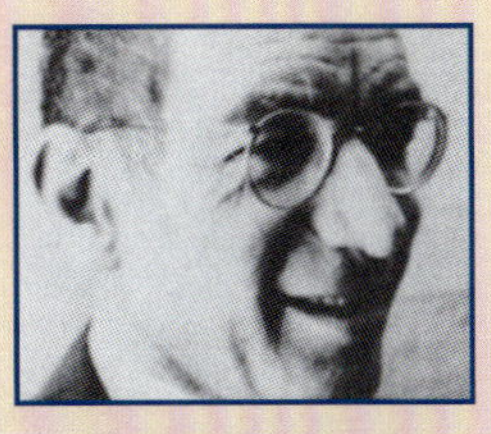

Nicholas Gimbel (1951) During residency and several years on the HUP faculty, Gimbel was an active researcher in burn therapy. He then moved to Wayne State where he became professor of surgery.

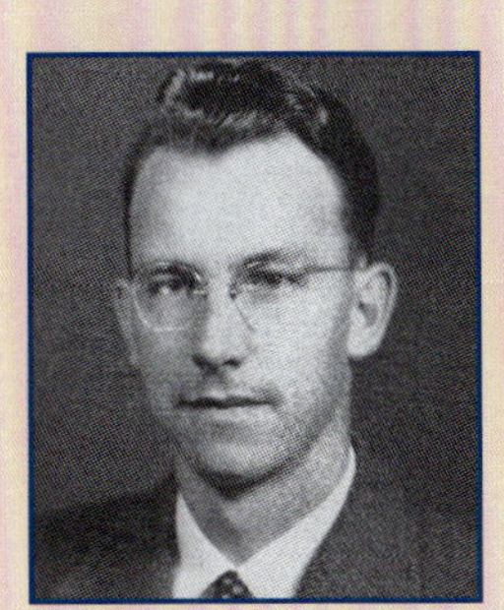

Harold Barker (1952) During World War II, my brother Hal served with the Army in England, Belgium, and Germany, sharing this experience with Jim Hardy and Archibald Fletcher.[44] Returning to Penn, he worked for a year as a research fellow in the Department of Pharmacology. After surgical residency and one year on the HUP faculty, he moved to New York as director of Columbia's new surgical metabolic unit and ICU. His research there was funded by NIH for twenty-two consecutive years. He also developed a large practice of general surgery and was very active in Columbia's teaching program. Becoming clinical professor of surgery in 1968, he was also Presbyterian Hospital's director of medical affairs in charge of developing new clinical programs.

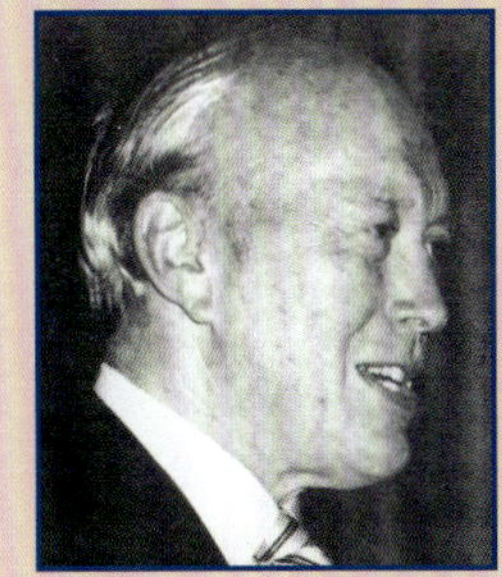

William Blakemore (1951) After residency, he was a fellow with Clarence Crafoord at the Karolinska Hospital in Stockholm from 1953–54. Returning to HUP, he brought the Seldinger equipment for catheterizing blood vessels. With Stanley Baum and Moreye Nusbaum, he was the first to identify and treat bleeding lesions in the GI tract by selective catheterization of mesenteric vessels.[45] After eight years on the HUP faculty, he was appointed in 1962 as chairman of surgery at Penn's Graduate School of Medicine and chief of surgery at Graduate Hospital. In 1972, he moved to Toledo where he served for ten years as surgery chairman at the Medical College of Ohio.

William Hagan (1952) Shortly after residency, William was killed in an automobile accident.

Robert Ravdin (1953) After graduation from Penn Medical School, I. S. Ravdin's son interned at Columbia before residency at HUP and appointment to the HUP faculty.[46] Much of his time was devoted to managing his father's practice, but he was also active in research. With internist Sylvan Eisman, he developed and headed HUP's first cancer

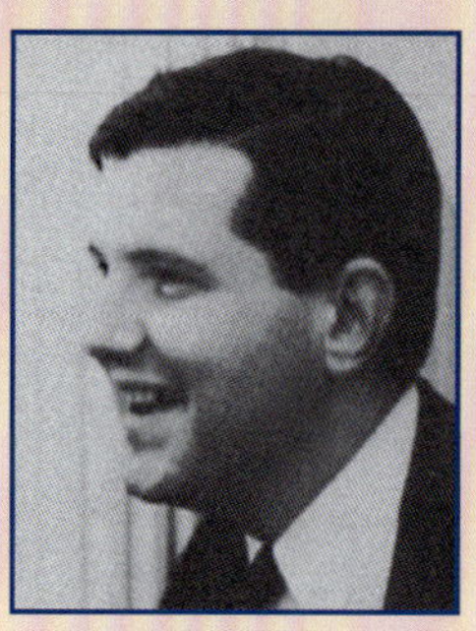

chemotherapy program, contributing many of the early patients to Bernard Fisher's National Surgery Adjuvant Breast and Bowel Registry. He was promoted to full professor in 1970 and two years later died from a massive coronary occlusion at age forty-nine. Bob Ravdin was an especially admired mentor and beloved friend of surgical residents. They raised the funding for an annual lecture in his name.

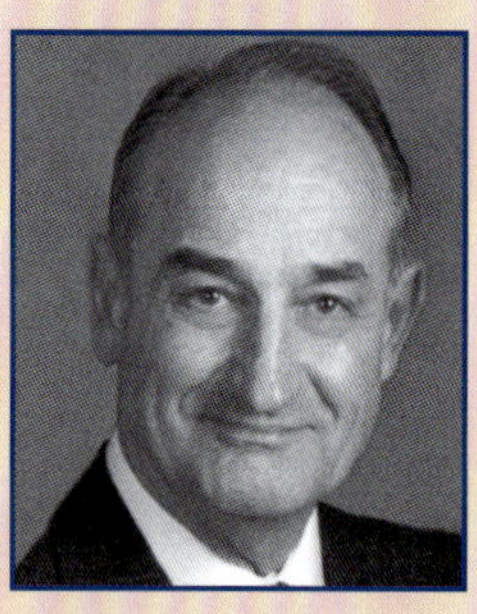

William DeMuth Jr. (1953) After residency, he was chief of surgery at Carlisle hospital for eighteen years.[47] Then in 1971, he was appointed professor of surgery at the newly founded Penn State Medical School at Hershey. He also served as chief of surgical services at the 376 Station Hospital in Japan. An expert in trauma, he studied the relationship between muzzle velocity of rifles and tissue damage. From 1977 to 1983, he was assistant dean for continuing education at Penn State.

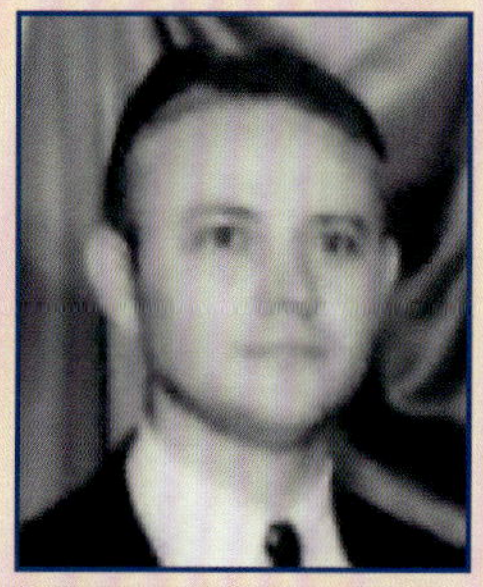

William C. Stainback (1953) After residency, he practiced at Bryn Mawr Hospital where he was chief of surgery (1962–78) and professor of surgery at Jefferson.

James Donald (1948), **Evan C. Reese,** and **Charles F. Rogers** (1954) appear in our archives only as names. If society members know more, I would appreciate hearing from them.

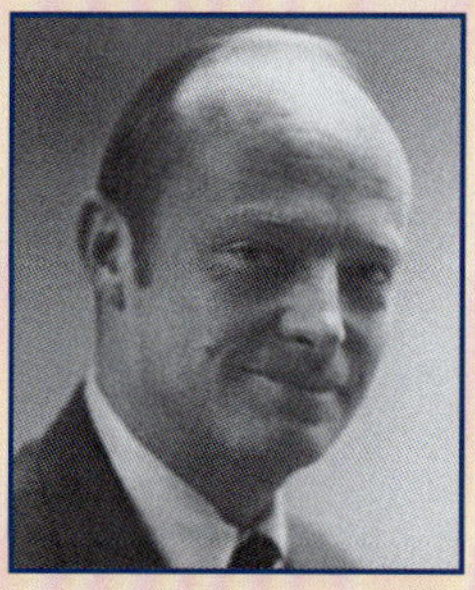

Julius Mackie (1955) Jack Mackie was the department's education officer from 1970 to 1980.[48] He was an exceptionally gifted clinical surgeon. Even after he was a full professor, much of his time was devoted helping Jonathan Rhoads conduct his huge practice, both in and out of the operating room. Without Jack, Dr. Rhoads could never have managed this along with his extensive travel and local and national leadership activities. In pre- and postoperative care, Jack was obsessively thorough, sometimes to the impatience of his residents. Jack's patients never complained about it. An example was Jack's discovery on late-night rounds of a tension pneumothorax that had developed in his colleague Clete Schwegman. Earlier that day, Clete had been operated on by another surgeon. Jack promptly stuck a needle in Clete's chest, saving his life.[49]

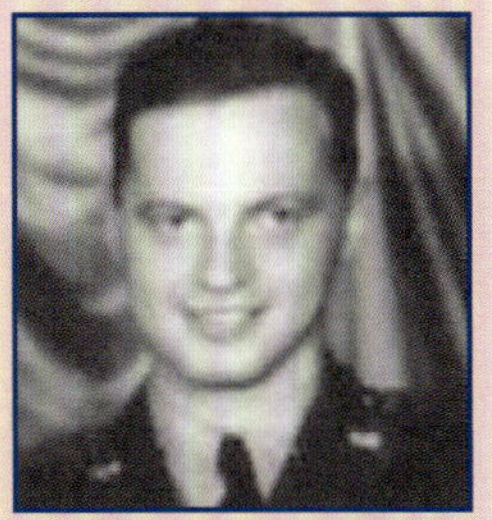

Henry Moss (1955) practiced at Albert Einstein and was professor of surgery at Temple. He also became president of the New York Academy of Science.

Theodore Shohl (1956) practiced in Los Angeles and in Anchorage, Alaska.

William Muir (1956) practiced in Long Branch, New Jersey.

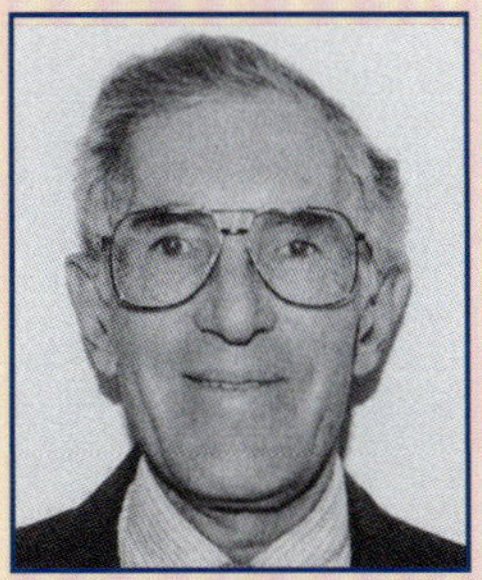

Gerald Peskin (1957) For ten years on the HUP faculty, Jerry was one of the most active in research and also the favorite mentor of the residents.[50] In 1967, he was recruited as professor of surgery at the University of Chicago and chief of surgery at Michael Reese Hospital. In 1971, he moved to California where he was chief of surgery at the San Diego Veterans Administration Hospital and professor at the University of California, San Diego. From 1984 to 1992, he was chief of surgery at St. Raphael Hospital in New Haven and clinical professor of surgery at Yale. In 1972, he moved back to California as professor of surgery at the University of California, Davis. There he was the teaching mainstay of Claude Organ's, and then Alden Harken's, surgical residency program at the University of California, San Francisco East Bay. In each of the institutions where he served, he was valued as the residents' friend and most valuable mentor.

Robert DeLong (1957) No information in the archives.

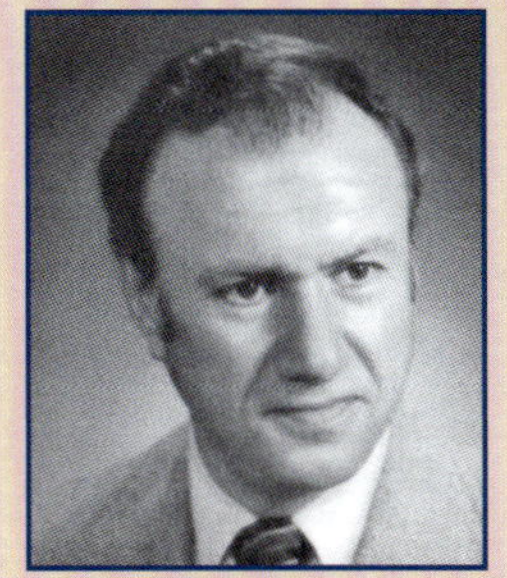

Marshall Orloff (1958) Marshall, the last survivor of Ravdin's chief residents, died at age ninety-one in 2018.[51] He received his BS, MS, and MD degrees from the University of Illinois as valedictorian of each class. After internship at UC San Francisco, Orloff completed his residency in general and thoracic surgery at HUP, interrupted by two years for service in Germany with the US Army (1953–55). Orloff then spent three years as assistant professor at the University of Colorado before moving to Los Angeles as chief of surgery at Harbor General and professor at UCLA. Four years later, he became the founding chairman of surgery at the University of California, San Diego's new school of medicine. He served in this role for the next sixteen years and continued at UCSD as a researcher and educator until his death in 2018. His research interests were portal hypertension, cancer immunology, obesity, and diabetes. He was president of the Society of University Surgeons in 1971 and in 2015 was named by the

Society of University Surgeons as its lifetime achievement awardee. His research was continuously funded by NIH for forty-eight years, perhaps a record, during which time he published over 450 scholarly articles, had forty different editorial appointments, and was visiting professor at ninety universities. He became best known for his advocacy of emergency portacaval shunts for patients bleeding from esophageal varices. This was controversial because his results were considerably better than those of others with this procedure and superior to other forms of therapy. His careful and well-documented follow-up of his patients was featured in multiple programs of the American Surgical Association. He attributed his superior results to meticulous follow-up and to his success in persuading his patients not to drink alcohol. Those who knew Marshall would not dispute this.

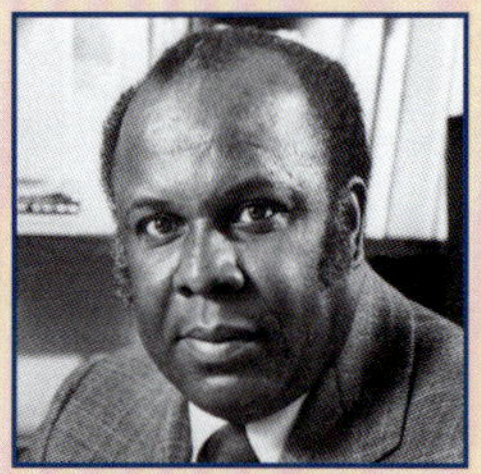

James H. Robinson (1959) Jim was HUP's first African American intern and Ravdin's first African American resident. After residency, he accepted an appointment as clinical professor of surgery at Jefferson where he was also associate dean for student affairs.

Donald Rochlin (1959) After residency, Rochlin was appointed to the faculty at UCLA where he developed an active practice and research program in oncology. He was one of the first to perform perfusion of isolated extremities with chemotherapeutic agents for treatment of metastatic melanoma. Unfortunately, he died an early death from lymphoma.

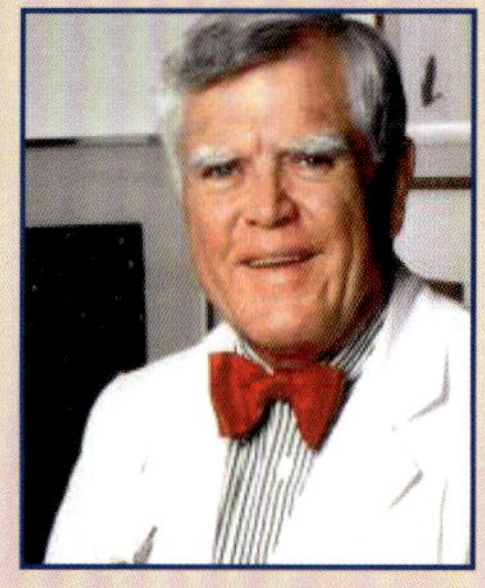

James C. Thompson (1959) was Ravdin's most colorful resident and one of the most distinguished.[52] He was not offered a HUP faculty position, perhaps because his exuberant personality was not an easy fit with conservative senior faculty. Instead, Jim accepted a position at Pennsylvania Hospital. There, isolated and very much on his own, he developed an NIH-funded lab, studying GI physiology. After three years, he moved to UCLA's Harbor General Hospital where his friend Marshall Orloff was chief. When Orloff moved to UCSD as chairman four years later, Thompson became chief at Harbor General and professor at UCLA. In 1970, Jim was appointed chairman of surgery at the University of Texas Medical Branch in Galveston, a job he kept for twenty-five years. There his studies of GI hormones and physiology maintained NIH funding continuously for forty-one years. He trained 130 research fellows from the United States and eighteen foreign countries. Of his 256 visiting professorships, seventy were abroad. Among his honors were the presidencies of the American Surgical Association and the American College of Surgeons and the Lifetime Achievement Award of the Society of University Surgeons.

But most would agree that it was Jim's personality, style, and sheer panache that set him apart. Marshall Orloff characterized him as outrageous, funny, bombastic, eloquent, sometimes inoffensively vulgar, charming, engaging, and never dull. Mark Ravitch, in his history of the American Surgical Association, added iconoclastic. I think Dr. Ravdin enjoyed Jim because Ravdin also had a quirky sense of humor. He would have seen Jim as a kindred spirit. Jim claimed that during his residency, Dr. Ravdin fired him at least eight or ten times (but always reappointed him within minutes). A dimension quite unusual for a surgeon was his interest and knowledge of nonmedical topics including literature, art, and music. Because of this, he valued his membership in the American Philosophical Society above almost any other of his many honors. Although he was a proud Texan by birth, childhood, and twenty-five years as chairman in Galveston, Thompson always said that his most important memories and loyalties were generated by his nine years at the University of Pennsylvania. Many of Dr. Ravdin's residents felt that same way. Jim epitomized the camaraderie that began with the Ravdin residents and which I believe persists at Penn.

Several important Ravdin residents finished their training while Ravdin was the Harrison Professor and before he became chairman of the department. Four such residents were Charles Johnston (later surgery chairman at Wayne State University), Harold Zintel, Doris Bender, and John Thomas.

Harold Zintel

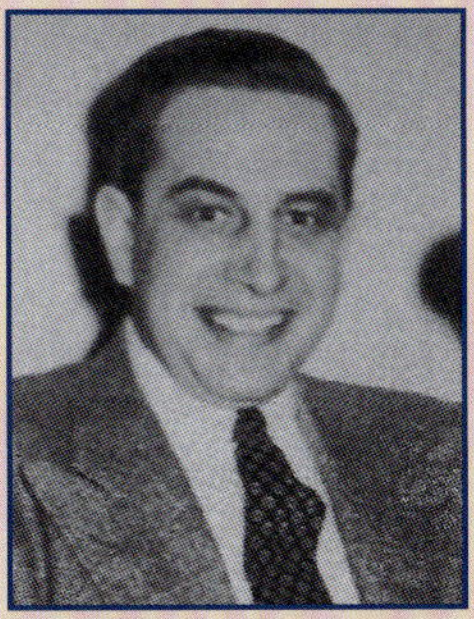

Harold Zintel graduated from Penn medical school in 1938 and, in 1940, began as a HUP resident under Ravdin.[53] During his first few years of residency, Ravdin recognized that he had unusually strong technical abilities. At this point, Ravdin left to command the 20th General Hospital for two years. During that time, Zintel remained a resident along with another Ravdin resident, Chick Koop. They, with junior faculty members Jonathan Rhoads and John Lockwood, managed Dr. Ravdin's busy HUP service in his absence. While Ravdin was still in India and before Zintel finished his final year of residency, Dr. Ravdin had decided to offer him a faculty position, which he did as soon as he returned to Philadelphia.

Ravdin rated Zintel as the best technical surgeon on his new geographic full-time faculty which, in the beginning, was comprised of Koop, Julian Johnson, Henry Royster, and Jonathan Rhoads. In fact, Ravdin believed that Zintel might be the best surgeon in the country,[54] citing as evidence of this his results of pancreatic resections which were far superior to those of Whipple. Zintel performed the first portocaval shunt in Philadelphia. In a series of 178 hypertensive patients, he evaluated treatment by sympathectomy and 95 percent adrenalectomy.[55]

Ravdin must have been greatly disappointed when, after a few years, Zintel left Penn to accept an appointment as chief of surgery at St. Luke's Hospital in New York. Zintel continued to be respected as one of the country's most proficient and productive academic surgeons.

Doris Harriet Bender

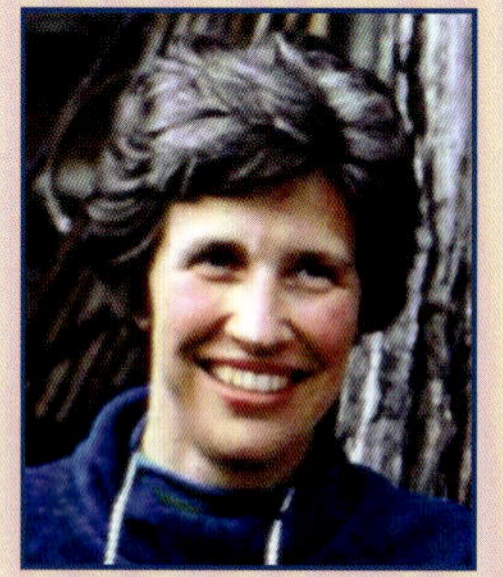

Never biased against women doctors, since he had married one himself, Dr. Ravdin had wanted to train a woman surgeon for years.[56] Doris Bender was his first. I. S. Ravdin's wife, Dr. Elizabeth Ravdin, essentially directed medical student education during World War II. She recommended Doris Bender as one of Penn's best medical students. After her HUP internship from 1944 to 1945, Dr. Ravdin brought her into his general surgery residency (1945–50). He later rated her performance as equaling or even exceeding that of his male residents. Midway through her residency, she fell in love with another Ravdin resident, James Maxwell. Ravdin advised them not to marry until they finished their residencies, fearing that otherwise Dorothy might not complete her training. They complied. Whether Doris Bender finished as chief at HUP cannot be ascertained from the department's archives. Toward the end of her residency, Ravdin writes she became proficient in pediatric surgery. Whether this was while she was still a general surgery resident is unclear. However, in his biography, Koop identifies her as his first pediatric surgery resident. He praises her for her technical skills and her resilience and loyalty to him during his difficult first years at CHOP, when the old guard there was attempting to block his leadership. Ravdin tells us in his autobiography that after her training, she and her husband went to Westmoreland Hospital in Greensburg, Pennsylvania, where they practiced for the rest of their professional lives. Ravdin believes she was the first pediatric surgeon in western Pennsylvania to whom many patients were sent from Pittsburgh before that city had a pediatric surgeon. She was the sixth woman surgeon to be certified by the American Board of Surgery. Ravdin also believed that she was the best woman surgeon in the country.

John Thomas

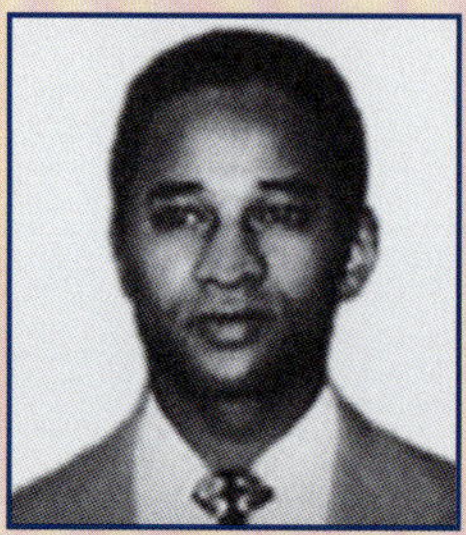

John Thomas graduated from Howard University School of Medicine in 1943. He obtained part of his residency and a Harrison Department Fellowship at HUP. He became director of surgery at Mercy-Douglas Hospital and for many years was on the faculty at HUP. In 1995, he died at age 76.

Timeline of Events During I. S. Ravdin's Career

1894	Ravdin is born in Indiana. His father, grandfather, and great-grandfather were physicians.
1914	Ravdin attends college and first two years of medical school at Indiana University.
1916	Army private Ravdin chases Mexican bandit Pancho Villa with George Patton and General Pershing.
1918	Ravdin graduates from Penn medical school, becomes HUP intern, and after only four months is promoted to chief resident.
1918	Spanish flu epidemic, with 50 to 100 million deaths worldwide. Philadelphia closes down, especially after the superspreader event of a bond drive in September. At its peak, there were more than 700 deaths per day in Philadelphia.
1918–1919	US enters World War I.
1918–1922	Ravdin has private surgery practice at Graduate Hospital and serves as assistant to George Muller.
1921	Ravdin marries Elizabeth Glenn, the first woman HUP intern.
1922	Ravdin is called back to HUP by Frazier, appointed department's executive director.
1927	A year of basic research for Ravdin in Edinburgh and London.
1928–1942	Ravdin combines HUP practice with research; becomes the department's director of research.
1933	Ravdin becomes secretary of Halsted Society and serves for thirteen years in this role.
1935–1942	John and Mary Gibbon make progress in the Harrison Department with their heart-lung machine.
1935	George Leib Harrison endowment of $2.7 million is at first intended for John Carnett's research, but when Carnett dies, it goes to support research in the Department of Surgery of the University of Pennsylvania.
1936	The endowment allows formation of the Harrison Department of Surgical Research, Ravdin becomes director, Ravdin becomes Harrison Professor of Surgery; there are now two professors at HUP: Eliason and Ravdin.
1936	George Muller leaves Penn to become chairman at Jefferson; becomes president of the American College of Surgeons in 1940.
1936	Frazier is operated on at Hopkins for prostate cancer, but soon dies of metastatic disease.

1936	While accompanying Frazier, Ravdin makes friends with Hopkins dean William Welch, who tells him about the Halsted residency.
1936	Ravdin is passed over as candidate for chairman of surgery. Eliason becomes John Rhea Barton Professor of Surgery. There are now two separate services and two professors and two separate residencies at HUP.
1937	American Board of Surgery is founded; mandates five-year surgical residencies.
1939	Jonathan Rhoads finishes his residency under Ravdin.
1939	Hitler invades Poland (Sept. 1); England and France declare war on Germany.
1940	France falls (June 22).
1940	Battle of Britain (July–Oct.).
1940	Ravdin develops acute cholecystitis and is operated on by Rhoads; Eliason and Whipple assist.
1941	Japanese bomb Pearl Harbor (Dec. 7).
1941	One day after the Japanese bomb Pearl Harbor, Ravdin is sent there to assess the treatment of casualties.
1942	Battle of Midway (June)—*USS Solace* treats wounded (see Chapter 13).
1942	Ravdin organizes the 20th General Hospital from HUP personnel.
1943	20th General Hospital arrives in Ledo (Mar.). Ravdin is commander.
1943	Mountbatten's eye injury is treated at 20th General Hospital (Mar.).
1943	Allies invade Sicily (July)—see Chapter 32.
1943	Quebec Conference—Roosevelt and Churchill plan to regain northern Burma (Aug.). Plan to send voluntary commandos (Merrill's Marauders).
1943	Marauders arrive at Ledo and begin 1,000 mile march (Oct.).
1944	D-Day (June).
1944	Paris liberated (Aug.).
1944	Market Garden (Sept.)—see Chapter 32.
1944	Marauders capture airfield at Myitkyina.
1944	Battle of the Bulge (Dec.).
1945	Ravdin promoted to brigadier general.
1945	Germany surrenders (May).
1945	Atom bomb at Hiroshima on Aug. 5. Japan surrenders Aug. 14.

1946	Returning from wartime service, Ravdin becomes John Rhea Barton Professor and Chairman of Department.
1950	Korean War begins (June)—see Chapter 32.
1955	Ravdin promoted to major general.
1956	Ravdin operates on President Eisenhower.
1957	Ravdin stars in episode of *Steve Canyon* (Oct.).
1958–1959	Ravdin is president of American Surgical Association.
1960	Ravdin retires as surgery chairman, becomes University's vice president for medical affairs.
1960–1961	Ravdin is president of American College of Surgeons.
1962–1963	Ravdin is president of American Cancer Society.
1972	Ravdin dies.

Notes

[1] Personal observation.

[2] *The Reminiscence of Isidor Ravdin,* Columbia University Oral History Collection, Part II, No 156. Isidor Ravdin, Saul Benison, Barbara Land, Columbia University Oral Research Office, New York Times Oral History Program (1971) p. 51.

[3] Cooper III, David Y and Ledger, Marshall A. *Innovation and Tradition at the University of Pennsylvania School of Medicine, An Anecdotal Journey* (Philadelphia: University of Pennsylvania Press, 1990) p. 168.

[4] *The Reminiscence of Isidor Ravdin,* p. 76.

[5] Ibid., p. 88.

[6] Cooper III, David Y and Ledger, Marshall A. *Innovation and Tradition at the University of Pennsylvania School of Medicine, An Anecdotal Journey,* p. 254.

[7] Shumacker, Harris B. *A Dream of the Heart, The Life of John H. Gibbon, Jr.: Father of the Heart-Lung Machine* (Santa Barbara: Fithian Press, 1999) pp. 128–129.

[8] Dudrick SJ, Wilmore, DW, Vars HM, and Rhoads, JE. Long-term Total Parenteral Nutrition with Growth, Development, and Positive Nitrogen Balance. *Surgery* (1968) 64:134.

[9] *The Reminiscence of Isidor Ravdin,* p. 136.

[10] Roberts, Brooke. *Memoir of I. S. Ravdin 1894–1972,* Transactions and Studies of the College of Physicians of Philadelphia (1974 Feb) 41(3), p. 238.

[11] Ibid., p. 237.

[12] Roberts, Brooke. *Memoir of I. S. Ravdin 1894–1972,* p. 238.

[13] *The Reminiscence of Isidor Ravdin,* p. 163.

[14] Ibid., p. 148. Ravdin forged a relationship with Heaton and other army doctors that would be important later in the war and when he was asked to share with Heaton the care of President Eisenhower.

[15] North, JP. The 20th General Hospital—I.S. Ravdin Commanding General. *Surgery* (1964 Oct) 56, p. 617.

[16] Hayden, John. Looking Back with the 20th General Hospital. Adapted from an article appearing in *Health Affairs* magazine of the University of Pennsylvania (Spring, 1984). https://cbi-theater.com/20th_gen_hosp/20gen.html.

[17] North, JP. *The 20th General Hospital – I. S. Ravdin Commanding General,* p. 622.

[18] *The Reminiscence of Isidor Ravdin,* pp. 193–195.

[19] Ibid., p. 199.

[20] Hayden, John. Looking Back with the 20th General Hospital, https://cbi-theater.com/20th_gen_hosp/20gen.html.

[21] *The Reminiscence of Isidor Ravdin,* p. 137.

[22] *The Reminiscence of Isidor Ravdin,* pp. 193–195. Ravdin would have found Eliason-trained Ferguson an acceptable faculty member, but Ferguson would not agree to a full-time salaried position.

[23] Personal observation.

[24] Rhoads, Jonathan. Memoir of I. S. Ravdin 1894–1972. *Transactions of Philadelphia Academy of Surgery* Vol XXXII (1969–75) p. 107.

[25] Ibid., p. 107.

The most accepted procedure would have been resection rather than bypass of the diseased segment of bowel. Ravdin chose to bypass, thinking this safer than resection. For years, Ravdin was criticized for his choice of treatment. He didn't care. Eisenhower recovered quickly and never had more trouble from his regional enteritis.

[26] Barker, Clyde F and Daly, John M, eds. *Jonathan E. Rhoads Eightieth Birthday Symposium* (Philadelphia: J. B. Lippincott Co, 1989) p. 76–77.

[27] Shea, John, IS Ravdin. Larger, and Smaller, Than Life. *Penn Medicine Magazine* (Summer 2015).

[28] Cooper III, David Y and Ledger, Marshall A. *Innovation and Tradition at the University of Pennsylvania School of Medicine, An Anecdotal Journey,* p. 256.

[29] Roberts, Brooke. *Memoir of I.S. Ravdin 1894–1972,* p. 239.

[30] *The Reminiscence of Isidor Ravdin,* pp. 113–117.

[31] *The Reminiscence of Isidor Ravdin,* p. 113.

[32] Halsted, William Stewart. *The Training of the Surgeon Bulletin,* Johns Hopkins Hospital (1904) XV: 267–275.

[33] Cameron, John. William Stewart Halsted, Our Surgical Heritage. *Annals of Surgery* (1997 May) 225 (5), p. 453.

[34] Personal observation.

[35] Miller, Leonard D. Memoir of William T. Fitts, Jr., M.D. *Transactions of the American Surgical Association* (1980) Vol 98, pp. 63–66.

[36] Ziegler, Moritz M. Memoir of Charles Everett Koop, MD, DSc 1916–2013. *Transactions of the American Surgical Association,* pp. 293–296. Hendren, W Hardy. In Memoriam: C. Everett Koop, MD, FACS. *Bulletin American College of Surgeons* (June 2013) Vol 98 No 6, pp. 74–76.

[37] Johnson, Julian. Memoir of Charles K. Kirby. *Transactions of the Philadelphia Academy of Surgery* (1970) Vol 31, p. 1–2.

[38] Barker, Clyde. Memoir of Cletus W. Schwegman. *Transactions of the American Surgical Association* (2007) Vol 126, pp. 392–394.

[39] Rhodes, Robert S. Memoir of James Daniel Hardy. *Transactions of the American Surgical Association* (2003) Vol 121, pp. 353–354. Hardy, James D. *The Academic Surgeon, an Autobiography* (Mobile, AL: Magnolia Mansions Press, 2002).

[40] Fletcher, Archibald G. *To India and Beyond, Memoirs of a Missionary Surgeon* (2005).

[41] Howard, John. Historical Vignettes of Arterial Repair, Recollections of Korea 1951–53. *Annals of Surgery* Vol 228 No 5, p. 716. Hagood, Carol Cook. John Howard '41: innovative leader, inspired scholar, mentor to many. *Southern Magazine* (Winter 2006). Barker, Clyde F and Daly, John M, eds. *Jonathan E. Rhoads Eightieth Birthday Symposium,* p. 24–30.

[42] The Class of 1937: In Memoriam William L. Dyson '37. *Princeton Alumni Weekly*.

[43] Barker, Clyde F. Memoir of Brooke Roberts. *Transactions of the American Surgical Association* (2003) Vol 121, pp. 372–373.

[44] Hardy, Mark. Memoir of Harold Grant Barker. *Transactions of the American Surgical Association* (2011) Vol 129, pp. 262–264.

[45] Nusbaum M, Baum S, Blakemore WS, Finkelstein AK. Demonstration of Intra-Abdominal Bleeding by Selective Arteriography. Visualization of Celiac and Superior Mesenteric Arteries. *JAMA* (1965) 191:389-390. doi:10.1001/jama.1965.03080050035009.

[46] Roberts, Brooke. Memoir of Robert Glenn Ravdin. *Transactions of the American Surgical Association* (1973) Vol 91, pp. 66–68. Rhoads, Jonathan. Robert G. Ravdin 1923–1972. *Transactions of the Philadelphia Academy of Surgery* Vol XXXII (1969–1975) pp. 109–110.

[47] Kauffman, Gordon L. Memoir of William E. DeMuth, Jr., M.D. *Transactions of the American Surgical Association* (2017) Vol 135.

[48] Barker, Clyde F. Memoir of Julius A. Mackie, Jr. *Transactions of Southern Surgical Association* (2004) Vol CXVI, pp. 355–356.

[49] See Chapter 31: A Collection of the Department's Educators.

[50] Barker, Clyde F. In Memory of Gerald W. Peskin, *Penn Surgical Society Newsletter (*Fall 2011) p. 11.

[51] Clary, Brian M. Memoir of Marshall J. Orloff, MD. *Transactions of the American Surgical Association* (2019) Vol 137. https://americansurgical.org/transactions/Fellows/Memoirs/MarshallJOrloff.cgi. Barker, Clyde F and Daly, John M, eds. *Jonathan E. Rhoads Eightieth Birthday Symposium,* pp. 49–61.

[52] Barker, Clyde F. James C. Thompson. *Proceedings of the American Surgical Association* (March 2010) Vol. 154 No.1. Barker, Clyde F and Daly, John M, eds. *Jonathan E. Rhoads Eightieth Birthday Symposium,* pp. 76–87.

[53] Koop, C Everett. Memoir of Harold A. Zintel. *Transactions of the American Surgical Association* (1993) Vol CXI, pp. 387–389.

[54] *The Reminiscence of Isidor Ravdin,* p. 342.

[55] Cooper III, David Y and Ledger, Marshall A. *Innovation and Tradition at the University of Pennsylvania School of Medicine, An Anecdotal Journey*, p. 298.

[56] Koop, C Everett. *Koop, The Memoirs of America's Family Doctor* (New York: Random House, 1991) p. 102. *The Reminiscence of Isidor Ravdin,* pp. 348, 349, 350.

CHAPTER 15
The Brothers Freeman

1895
Birth of Walter Freeman, pathologist, neurologist, and lobotomist

1903
Birth of Norman Freeman

1945
Walter Freeman invents prefrontal lobotomy

1950s
More than 5,000 lobotomies performed around the world

Ravdin's broad influence extended to other surgeons who had only part of their training under him. Norman Freeman was one of these. His history is important because he was America's first vascular surgeon, or at least the first one to limit his practice to that field. Much of his story is buried in Ravdin's oral history and can be found nowhere else.

Norman Freeman was born in Philadelphia in 1903. His was an unusual family. Norman's maternal grandfather was the dominant figure of his early years. His grandfather, W. W. Keen, was probably the nation's most famous surgeon at the time.[1] Keen succeeded S. W. Gross as Jefferson's chairman of surgery in 1889 and served in that position for twenty-three years. He was the first American surgeon to use antisepsis, and the first anywhere to succeed in removing a brain tumor. An even more interesting operation was his successful resection of a tumor from the jaw of President Grover Cleveland. This procedure was done in 1893 in a makeshift operating room on a yacht as it steamed up Long Island Sound. It was carried out in absolute secrecy to avoid precipitating financial panic if the public learned the president had cancer in a time of the country's financial instability.[2] The secret held for twenty-four years until Dr. Keen reported it in the *Saturday Evening Post*.

Another story of this medical family dynasty is that of Norman Freeman's older brother Walter, W. W. Keen's other grandson. This one would best be forgotten. Walter was a Penn medical student and pathology resident. After neurology training in Europe, he was appointed chairman of neurology at George Washington University. In 1945, he became famous (or infamous) for inventing prefrontal lobotomy.[3] Over the next twenty years, he performed this operation on over 3,000 patients. It was done with an ice pick inserted through the orbit and driven into the brain. The hypothesis for this rather horrifying experimental procedure was that destroying this part of the brain might calm disturbed or agitated psychiatric patients, making them easier to manage. This notion was based only on some animal experiments and anecdotal results in a few patients.

When Freeman proclaimed the operation's success, others followed his lead and, in the 1950s, performed about 5,000 more lobotomies around the world. At the time, there were no institutional review boards or antipsychotic drugs. No reliable data were collected. Some of the patients were helped, but many were left in a vegetative or childlike state. One of his unfortunate patients was the sister of President John F. Kennedy. About 490 of Freeman's patients died from the operation before he was discredited, stripped of his operating privileges, and stopped.

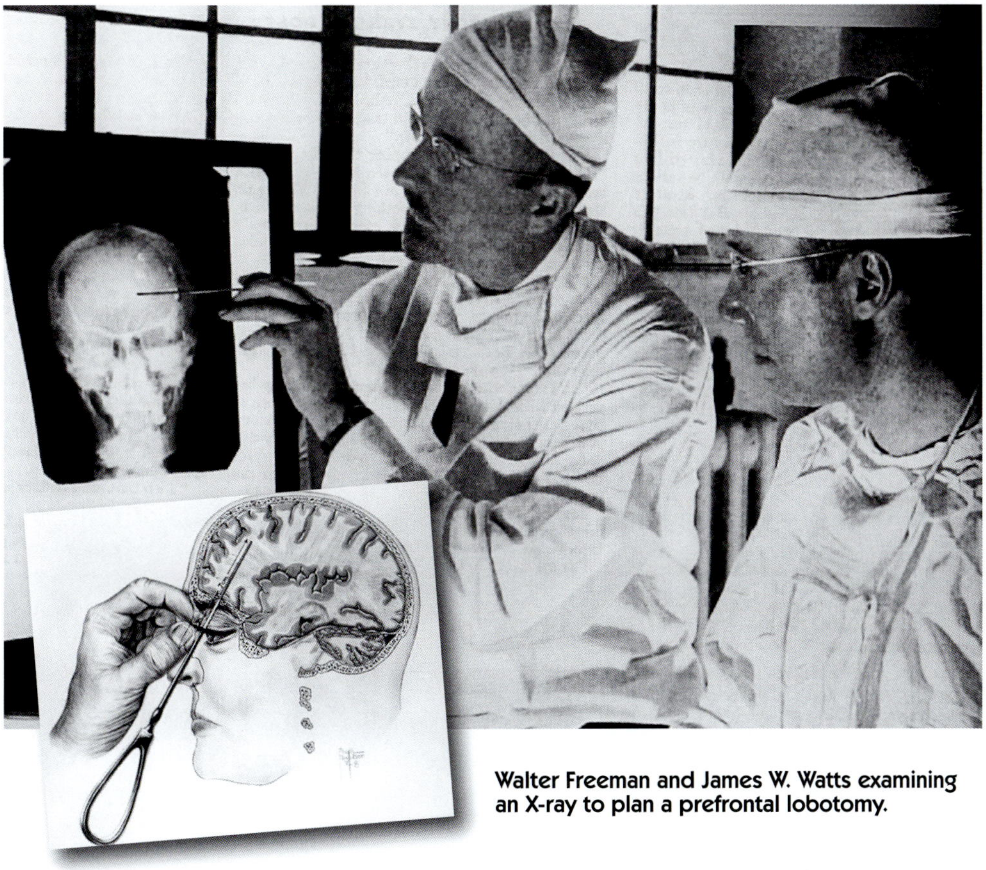

Walter Freeman and James W. Watts examining an X-ray to plan a prefrontal lobotomy.

The rest of this account is limited to the story of Walter's younger brother, Norman Freeman, a former member of Penn's department of surgery and the vascular surgeon who pioneered this specialty. He was educated at St. Paul's School and at Yale for college and medical school. He then came to HUP for a two-year internship under I. S. Ravdin. Ravdin was attracted by the intellect of the young man and, sensing his promise as a surgeon-scientist, arranged for him a two-year research fellowship in Harvard's Department of Physiology under the world-renowned Walter Cannon. Freeman studied the influence of the sympathetic nervous system on shock, blood loss, and the peripheral circulation, authoring with Cannon many highly regarded basic research papers. After this, he completed a surgical residency at Massachusetts General Hospital and two extra years there as a surgical fellow.

1945–1965
Four hundred ninety of Walter's lobotomy patients die from the operations. Many others are disabled.
He is discredited

1927
Norman Freeman MD, Yale

1927–1929
Norman Freeman, internship at HUP

1929–1931
Norman Freeman, research fellowship at MGH

1931–1934
Norman Freeman, surgical residency at MGH

1934–1936
Norman Freeman, clinical fellowship in surgery at MGH

1936
Norman Freeman appointed J. William White assistant professor of surgery and chief of vascular clinic at Penn

1943–1945
Norman Freeman is in India with the 20th General Hospital

In 1936, Ravdin acquired control of Penn's $2.7 million Harrison endowment. This allowed him to start building his own academic department. One of his first moves was to recruit the promising young Norman Freeman, whom he appointed as the J. William White Assistant Professor of Research Surgery.[4] Because of Freeman's strong interest and publication record in the vascular field, Ravdin appointed him chief of the vascular clinic and provided him with resources and space for a vascular lab for physiologic studies, possibly the first of its kind. For the next seven years as a member of Ravdin's surgical faculty, Freeman more than lived up to the expectations of his chief. He was extraordinarily productive both in clinical and basic research. His studies of peripheral blood flow demonstrated that during shock, blood flow to vital organs was protected. In other studies, he was one of the first to show that renal artery constriction resulted in hypertension. Ravdin was pleased with the progress of his golden boy despite the suspicion that Freeman was in an unrealistic hurry for advancement. Ravdin discounted gossip that Freeman was talking to his friends about himself as possibly replacing his chief.[5]

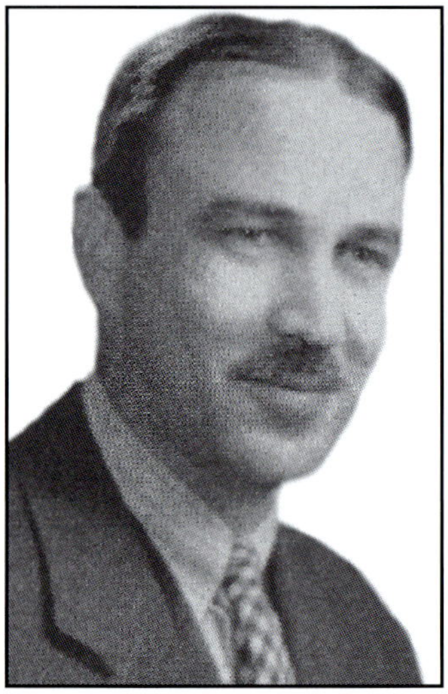

Norman Freeman Assistant Professor of Surgery at Penn.

In 1943, Ravdin took over 800 Penn doctors, nurses, and support staff to India where they built in the middle of the jungle World War II's largest and busiest military hospital, the 20th General. Major Norman Freeman was one of the most accomplished members of Ravdin's team. They cared for US and Chinese soldiers, including the legendary American commandos, Merrill's Marauders. These forces suffered incredibly high casualties as they struggled to drive the Japanese from northern Burma. They carved the Ledo Road through the jungle, mountains, and swamps to hook up with the Burma Road. This would be a crucial overland route to supply our Chinese allies. Otherwise, supplies could reach China only by dangerous flights over the Himalayas. The primitive and hazardous conditions were hardly ideal for conducting research, but Freeman succeeded in producing multiple papers based on studies done on wounded soldiers. One such report was of his treatment by sympathectomy of 114 patients with causalgia caused by gunshot wounds.[6]

Freeman's colleagues considered him a star. Heart surgeon Julian Johnson was his tent mate. Johnson, who was never given to hyperbole, remembered him as a superb technical surgeon, innovative, energetic, and driven to such an extent that he seemed happy only when working to the point of exhaustion, "at his best magnificent."[7] Freeman was also popular as a leader of a small jazz band.

Ironically, it was also during this time that the first seeds of Freeman's eventual professional demise can be detected. He and Ravdin, both uncompromisingly strong-willed, did not see eye-to-eye on Freeman's innovative approach to clinical research. Ravdin's autobiography does not detail the context of their disagreements, but he repeatedly accused Freeman of "using his patients as guinea pigs."[8] Perhaps it was only that Ravdin disapproved of Freeman using wounded soldiers as subjects for physiologic studies. But I have wondered about another area of possible conflict. Army regulations at the time, which General Ravdin, as the commander, would have been obligated to follow, dictated that arterial injuries be treated by ligation and not by repair. Unfortunately, this often resulted in amputation. I have only speculation for the idea, but I can't help wondering whether an experienced vascular surgeon as stubbornly independent as Freeman would balk over this mandate. Since all the principals are now dead, we will never know what the experiments were for which Ravdin criticized Freeman's use of "human guinea pigs." But the infraction was important enough to Ravdin that he resolved not to reappoint his previously favorite protégé to his postwar faculty at Penn.[9]

As World War II wound down and the 20th General Hospital closed, Freeman's reputation won him the appointment as chief of surgery at DeWitt General Hospital in Auburn, California, a US Army vascular center. There he pioneered vascular reconstructions, such as direct repair of AV fistulas, eighteen successful examples of which he reported to the American Surgical Association in 1946. The paper was discussed by Rudolph Matas who complimented Freeman on his "high degree of technical skill."[10]

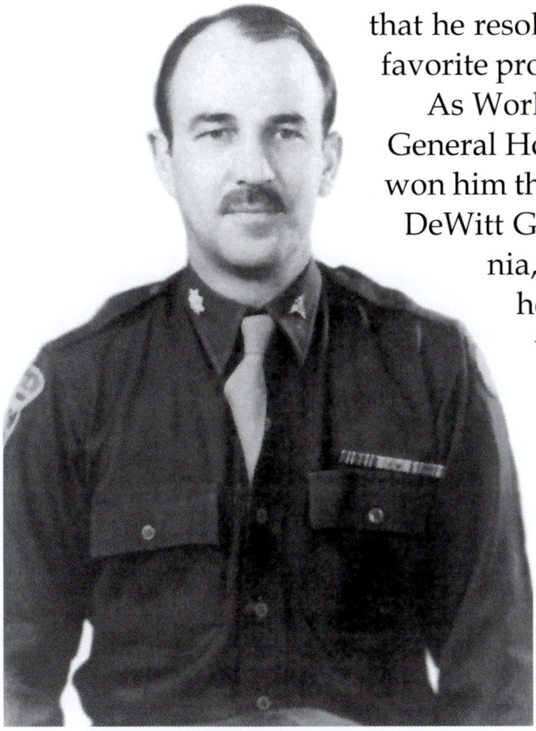

Norman Freeman

In 1946, Freeman, now forsaken by Ravdin, was recruited by Howard Naffziger to the University of California, San Francisco, as associate clinical professor and chief of the vascular clinic. Among Freeman's innovations at UCSF were establishment of the first noninvasive vascular lab and routine employment of arteriography.[11] Clinically active, he performed some of the first operations for coarctation of the aorta, patent ductus ligation, and Blalock shunts. He was also known as an unusually committed, effective, and popular teacher. Three future leaders of vascular surgery came under his influence, virtually becoming his trainees in the vascular field.[12] They were Jack

1943–1945
Norman Freeman performs research in 20th General Hospital. His disagreement with Ravdin prevents Freeman's postwar appointment at Penn

1945
Norman Freeman is Chief of Surgery at an Army Hospital in California

1946
Norman Freeman is Chief of Vascular Service at the University of California in San Francisco. Limits his practice to vascular surgery and advocates it as a distinct specialty

1948
Because of disagreement with his chief, Norman Freeman moves from UCSF to private hospital, continues research and studies in his vascular lab

1951
Norman Freeman performs the world's first resection of abdominal aortic aneurysm

1952
Norman Freeman performs first extra-anatomic bypass, right femoral to left femoral artery

Wylie, a surgical resident, and Rutherford Gilfillan and Frank Leeds, surgical fellows. After finishing their training, Wylie and Gilfillan joined Freeman as junior partners in his busy clinical practice.[13]

But before long, a familiar pattern recurred. Because of his temperamental personality and strongly held positions, he found himself at odds with Naffziger, his chief at UCSF. Naffziger offered to pay Freeman's salary for a year if Ravdin would take him back.[14] Ravdin refused, and Freeman then moved to Franklin Hospital, a private institution. During this time, Freeman performed several novel operations, which should have been sufficient to place him in the pantheon of vascular surgery. Unaccountably, they have been virtually forgotten. On February 26, 1951, Freeman performed the first resection of an abdominal aortic aneurysm.[15] A month later, Charles DuBost in France performed the same procedure, which ever since has been regarded as the world's first.[16] Even earlier, Freeman had resected an aortic aneurysm with restoration of distal blood flow with an iliac vein that had blown out, killing the patient.[17] Freeman's February 26 case also utilized an iliac vein to restore distal circulation, but this time he closed the arterial wall of the aneurysm over the vein. Further buttressing of the vein was provided by injecting blood between the vein and the shell of the aneurysm. A year later, the patient was alive and well.[18]

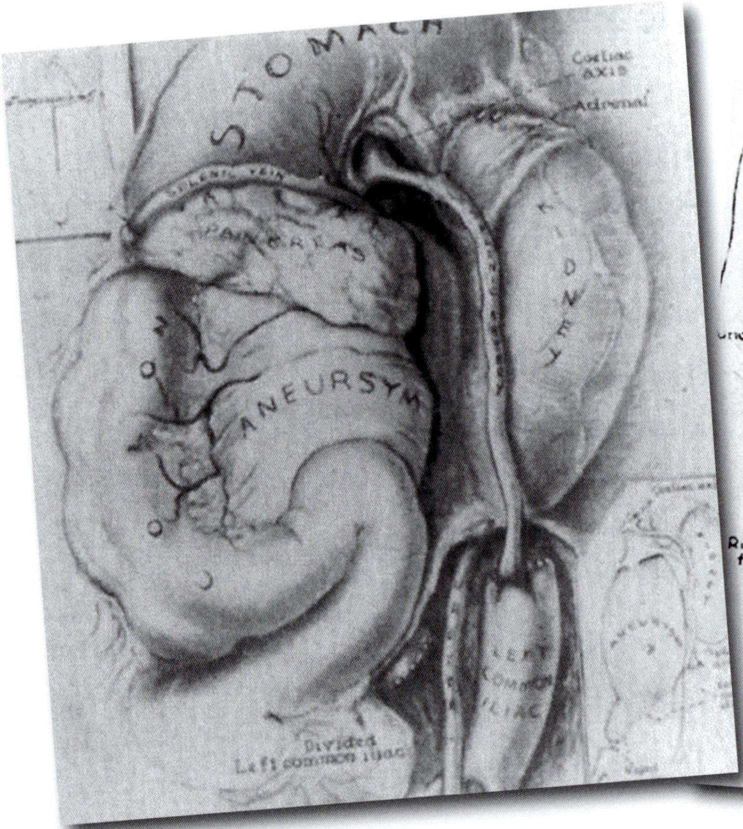

1951 Norman Freeman's resection of an aortic aneurysm, with restoration of blood flow by an iliac vein.

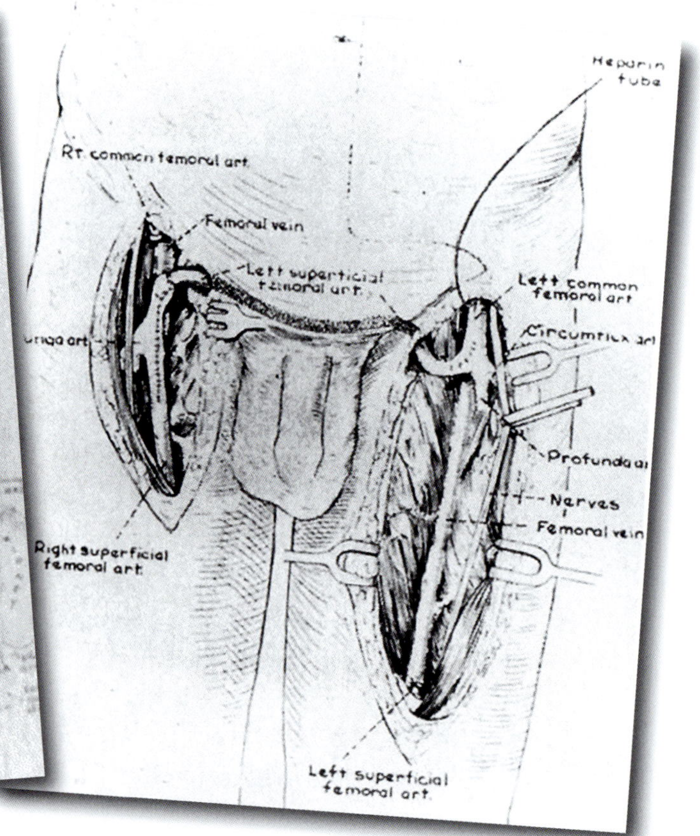

1952 first femoral-femoral bypass.

Other firsts by Freeman followed. In 1952, he performed the first renal endarterectomy, curing the patient of hypertension.[19] In the same year, he did the first extra-anatomic bypass (a femoral-to-femoral artery bypass).[20] These firsts made him highly respected by the few others in the vascular field at the time, such as Mike DeBakey who was fond of Norman and characterized him as capable and full of ideas.[21]

Perhaps of more lasting importance than Freeman's technical innovations was the influence of his vision of vascular surgery as a distinct, independent specialty.[22] Others like DeBakey and Blalock saw it as part of cardiac, thoracic, or general surgery. It seems likely that Norman's attitude was an important influence on his partner in practice, the young Jack Wylie, who is usually credited with the concept of vascular surgery as an independent entity with a dedicated fellowship, leading to special credentials.

Despite his many accomplishments, Freeman's unusual personality and erratic behavior consistently led to damaging conflicts. In retrospect, it is easy to recognize in him the symptoms of bipolar condition with which he was eventually diagnosed.[23] Before this entity or its successful treatment were understood, multiple periods of hospitalization caused Freeman's early retirement from surgical practice at age fifty-nine. With inactivity, his reputation in the expanding vascular field faded rapidly, forcing him to take clerical jobs. At age seventy-two, he died from heart disease, virtually forgotten and unheralded as America's first vascular surgeon.

Assuming that Dr. Ravdin's criticism of Norman Freeman was accurate and fair—that he treated his patients like guinea pigs—an odd sort of parallel exists between the Freeman brothers. Excessive or inappropriate use of human experimentation seems to have betrayed them both. At one extreme was Norman's brother, Walter, who was certainly guilty of using his prefrontal lobotomy patients as experimental subjects. At the other end of the spectrum, brother Norman's innovations worked out to the benefit of his patients and to the progress of vascular surgery. Unfortunately, neither of these talented Penn-trained doctors enjoyed a lastingly satisfying career.

1952
Norman Freeman performs the first renal artery endarterectomy

1962
Norman Freeman's health forces him to retire

1972
Death of Walter Freeman

1975
Death of Norman Freeman

Notes

[1] Darrach, William. William Williams Keen Memoir in Biographical Memoirs of Members of the American Philosophical Society. *Physicians Vol I 1787-1935,* edited by Barker and Starzl (Philadelphia: American Philosophical Society, 2013).

[2] Keen, WW. *The Surgical Operations on President Cleveland in 1893* (Philadelphia and London: JB Lippincott, 1928) pp.11–78.

[3] Caruso, JP & Sheehan, JP. (2017). Psychosurgery, ethics, and media: a history of Walter Freeman and the lobotomy. *Neurosurgical Focus FOC, 43*(3), E6. Retrieved Oct 12, 2021, from https://thejns.org/focus/view/journals/neurosurg-focus/43/4/article-pE6.xml

[4] Johnson, J. Obituary of Norman E. Freeman. *Trans American Surgical Association* (Philadelphia 1976) 94: 55-57.

[5] The Reminiscence of Isidor Ravdin, *Columbia University Oral History Collection* Part II No 156. Isidor Ravdin, Saul Benison, Barbara Land. *Columbia University Oral Research Office, New York Times Oral History Program* (1971) p. 128.

[6] Connolly, John E. Norman Freeman. The "First" American Specialist in Vascular Surgery. *J Vasc Surg* Vol 22 issue 2, p. 189.

[7] Johnson J. Obituary of Norman E. Freeman. *Trans American Surgical Association* (Philadelphia 1976) 94: 56.

[8] *The Reminiscence of Isidor Ravdin*, p. 128.

[9] Ibid., p. 129.

[10] Ravitch, Mark. *A Century of Surgery Vol I, 1880-1980* (Philadelphia and Toronto: J.B. Lippincott Company, 1981) p. 894.

[11] Connolly, John E. *Norman Freeman, The "First" American Specialist in Vascular Surgery,* p. 190

[12] Ibid., p. 189.

[13] Ibid., p. 189.

[14] *The Reminiscence of Isidor Ravdin*, p. 130.

[15] Connolly, John E. *Norman Freeman, The "First" American Specialist in Vascular Surgery,* p. 191.

[16] Ibid., p. 192. Dubost C, Allary M, Oeconomos N. Apropos du traitement des aneurysnes de l'aorte. *Mem Acad Chir* (1951) 77:381-3.

[17] Connolly, John E. *Norman Freeman, The "First" American Specialist in Vascular Surgery,* p. 191.

[18] Ibid., p. 192.

[19] Connolly, John E. *Norman Freeman, The "First" American Specialist in Vascular Surgery,* p. 192.

[20] Ibid., p. 192.

[21] DeBakey, Michael E., Blaisdell, F. William. The Society for Vascular Surgery: As I remember—An interview with Dr. Michael E. DeBakey. *J Vasc Surg* (1996) 23:1031-4.

[22] Freeman, Norman. Vascular Surgery, *California Medicine* Vol 68 No 1, pp. 43–44.

[23] Connolly JE. Personal reflections on the first 50 years of cardiovascular surgery. *J Am Coll Surg.* (2013) 217(2):358-373. doi:10.1016/j.jamcollsurg.2013.02.026.

CHAPTER 16

The Triumphs and Setbacks of a Revolutionary Cancer Surgeon

Bernard Fisher

1918
Fisher born in Pittsburgh

1943
MD, University of Pittsburgh

1944–1948
Intern and surgical resident at University of Pittsburgh

1950–1952
Fisher is research fellow and surgical resident at Penn

1953
Wins Markle Scholarship. Five years of research funding

In its 2017 obituary of Bernard Fisher, *The New York Times* praised him as one of the twentieth century's most important medical scientists.[1] Fisher spent almost his entire life in Pittsburgh. He was born there, went to college and medical school at the University of Pittsburgh, and after surgical residency there, served on that university's faculty for sixty-seven years, right up to the time of his death at age 101. Nevertheless, I always think of him as a HUP surgeon. The *Times'* extensive obit fails to mention that two of Fisher's most important years were spent not in Pittsburgh but in Philadelphia as a HUP surgery resident and research fellow in the Harrison Department. The *Times* does refer to a "former mentor" who played a pivotal role in Fisher's distinguished career but does not identify the mentor. It was I. S. Ravdin.

Some Ravdin residents spent no more than a few years with him. Yet his influence on their professional lives was crucial. In some cases, it shaped their entire career, as it did with Bernard Fisher. Of the Ravdin residents, Fisher's work probably had the greatest impact on modern surgical care. Not only did it improve treatment of one of the most common diseases; it also changed the entire field of medicine.

An important part of Ravdin's magic was his uncanny ability to recognize in young doctors those with a special gift for leadership. He also seemed to know, often before they did themselves, the particular field that would fit them best. Examples of this were his assigning Brooke Roberts to vascular surgery and Henry Royster to plastic surgery. In at least two other instances, Ravdin directed his trainees to enter a field quite different than the one they had chosen for themselves. One of these was C. Everett Koop, who asked Ravdin to make him head of cancer surgery at HUP. Denied, he was forced by Ravdin to settle instead for an appointment as chief of pediatric surgery. The other was Bernard Fisher, whose interest and highly successful early career were in transplantation, but he was induced by Ravdin to switch from transplantation to breast cancer research. In both these cases, Ravdin's intervention altered the future course of the field he chose for his trainees. Koop would dominate pediatric surgery, and Fisher would revolutionize the established treatment of breast cancer.

Fisher spent his two years at Penn as a HUP resident and in researching liver regeneration in rats. More importantly, he developed a lifelong relationship with Dr. Ravdin, who then helped him win a prestigious grant as a Markle Scholar in Medical Science. In its day, this was a big deal. Before the dominant importance of winning NIH RO1 grants, a Markle scholarship virtually identified the country's most promising young medical scientists. Each of the 100 US medical schools was allowed to submit as a candidate one young faculty member from any department. In an intense two-day interview process, twenty per year were chosen. They were generously funded by the Markle Foundation for the next five years. More important than the money, the Markle Foundation used its considerable influence with medical schools to lobby for and support the scholar's progress and promotions. Most Markle scholars became department chairs or deans.

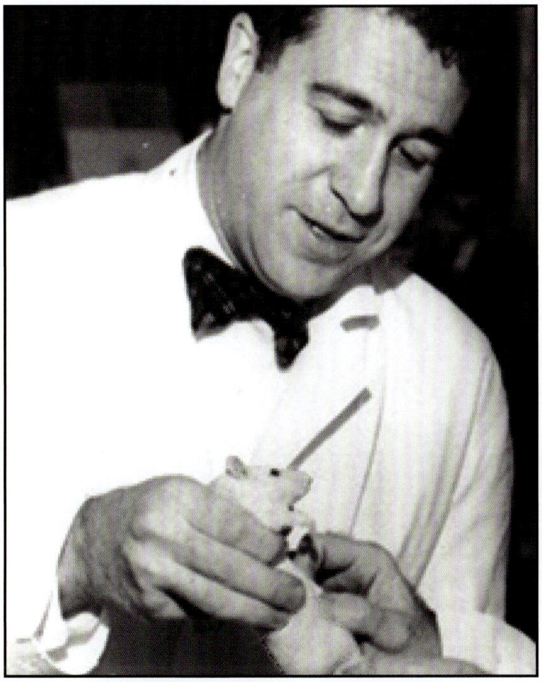

Bernard Fisher, research in transplantation.

The Markle scholarship allowed Fisher to return to the University of Pittsburgh in a favored status. He founded and directed Surgery's research program based on the model of Penn's Harrison Department. His research career flourished. He published dozens of well-regarded papers on work he had started at Penn and on transplantation biology, which he studied during a Markle-supported year in England. He performed one of the earliest human kidney transplants at a time when there were only a handful of transplant programs in the entire United States. Soon, Fisher was recognized as one of the most productive young leaders in the exciting new field of transplantation. He was well satisfied with this as the field in which he would spend his career.

Then one day, out of the blue, Fisher got a phone call from his old chief at Penn, Dr. Ravdin. He was invited to a meeting at the NIH. It was a meeting on breast cancer.[2]

As chairman of the Clinical Studies Panel of the Cancer Chemotherapy Service Center at NIH, Ravdin organized this meeting in 1957 to

1953–1954
At University of Pittsburgh, continues research in liver regeneration and transplantation

1955
Fellow in experimental surgery at Hammersmith Hospital in London. Research in transplantation

1956–1958
At University of Pittsburgh becomes director of surgical research. Continues to be most interested in transplantation

1957
Because he has no interest in cancer research, Fisher reluctantly attends Ravdin's meeting for organization of the National Surgical Adjuvant Breast and Bowel Project (NSABP)

Inspired by the NSABP meeting, Fisher begins to be interested in cancer research

1958
Fisher takes part in first NSABP trial of postoperative chemotherapy of breast cancer.
Research focus changes to cancer

1961
Fisher reports to American Surgical Association that chemotherapy delays recurrence of breast cancer

establish the National Surgical Adjuvant Breast and Bowel Project (NSABP). The purpose of the NSABP was to set up randomized clinical trials for study of chemotherapy in treatment of breast cancer.

Fisher was not at all pleased to get Ravdin's invitation. He was not the least bit interested in breast cancer or its treatment. Nor was he interested in clinical trials. But because General Ravdin was so persuasive, and at the time so powerful and so influential in academic surgery, Fisher interpreted the invitation almost as an order. He was afraid to decline. He felt that he had no choice but to participate, however reluctantly, in this meeting.

What happened then is one of the great stories of twentieth-century medicine. To his surprise, Fisher was intrigued with what he heard at the meeting. He learned that not much was known about the biology of breast cancer, nor was there much interest in understanding the disease. He later said that he was captivated by the mystery surrounding the phenomenon of tumor metastases. In addition, he was struck by the potential power of multicenter, randomized clinical trials, a concept that was quite new at the time.

Although Fisher remained interested in transplantation, he shifted the focus of his laboratory research to the biology of tumor metastasis. In 1958, he took part in the first NSABP trial in which data from twenty-three institutions compared radical mastectomy and a placebo with radical mastectomy and postoperative chemotherapy with Thiotepa. At the 1961 meeting of the American Surgical Association, Fisher, with I. S. Ravdin's son Bob and others, reported the results of this study. Chemotherapy had delayed early recurrence of breast cancer.[3] Fisher was hooked. By 1967, he become chairman of the NSABP, and during the succeeding decades, he led the clinical trials that would transform the treatment of breast cancer.

Surgical Adjuvant Chemotherapy in Cancer of the Breast:

Results of a Decade of Cooperative Investigation

Bernard Fisher,* M.D., Robert G. Ravdin,** M.D., Robert K. Ausman,*** M.D., Nelson H. Slack,† Ph.D., George E. Moore,†† M.D., Rudolf J. Noer,*† M.D.
(and Cooperating Investigators)

In 1957, under the auspices of the National Institutes of Health, Cancer Chemotherapy National Service Center, representatives of 23 institutions (Table 1) adopted a common protocol which was to determine the efficacy of administering chemotherapy

mals, as well as reports of the frequent presence of cancer cells in the circulating blood of patients with tumor.[4, 5] Thio-TEPA (Triethylenethiophosphoramide), because of its effectiveness in palliation of mammary cancer, was at that time deemed the drug

Fisher's own laboratory experiments studying tumor metastasis in rats and the results of his NSABP clinical trials caused him to question the dogma that for a century had dictated treatment of breast cancer—the Halsted radical mastectomy. That treatment was based on the premise that radical or ultra-radical resection was the logical way to treat breast cancer since this disease surely must spread from the tumor's original site by predictable extension along anatomical planes. Thus, the more tissue surrounding the tumor that could be removed, the greater would be the chance of stopping the cancer.

It was heresy to suggest otherwise, but Fisher advanced the alternative hypothesis that breast cancer was a systemic disease in which tumor cells were likely to have disseminated throughout the body by the time of diagnosis. If this were so, he argued at meeting after meeting that more extensive regional therapy would not improve survival and radical mastectomy should be abandoned. This was such an extremely unpopular position that many considered it malpractice. He was criticized, even vilified, by many of his surgical colleagues. Fisher's persona did not help him.[4] He had a direct approach that helped him accomplish things but not to make friends. He was characterized by some as brash and by others as arrogant. Some were simply bored by the repetitiveness of his message.

But by the late 1960s, Fisher's hypothesis was supported by the results of his NSAPB trials that found radical mastectomy no more effective than simple mastectomy or even lumpectomy.[5] Many surgeons, set in their ways, greeted these findings with skepticism, arguments, resistance, and personal antagonism for Fisher. But Fisher's data were so persuasive that they eventually demanded universal acceptance of his concept. Over the next two decades, the Halsted radical mastectomy was pretty much abandoned.

Other clinical trials by Fisher demonstrated that postoperative chemotherapy and hormonal therapy with the antiestrogen tamoxifen would improve survival and could even prevent the disease in high-risk women. Then Fisher became widely praised, heralded as a hero for sparing breast cancer victims from the disfiguring impact of radical mastectomy, while also improving their survival. Multiple awards came to him, including election to the Institute of Medicine of the National Academy of Sciences, presidency of the American Society of Clinical Oncology, and in 1985, the Lasker Award, often regarded as the American Nobel Prize.

Then the roof fell in. Once again, Fisher's life was turned upside down. In 1990, one of his statisticians noticed a discrepancy in the chart of an NSABP patient being treated by a researcher in Montreal. This researcher admitted that he had falsified data to get unqualified patients into the lumpectomy trial. After removing the falsified entry, Fisher reanalyzed the data, finding that the results were hardly changed and still

1967
Fisher becomes chairman of NSABP

In the late 1960s, NSABP studies show that simple mastectomy is as effective as radical mastectomy in treatment of breast cancer

1985
Fisher is widely praised, wins Lasker Award. Elected member of National Academy of Medicine

1990
One of Fisher's collaborators is discovered to be falsifying data. Outcome of NSABP study is not affected, but Fisher is blamed

1994
NIH fires Fisher from NSABP. University of Pittsburgh also punishes him

1994
Fisher sues NIH and Pittsburgh for unfounded accusations

1997
After three years of investigations, Fisher is found innocent of any misconduct, gets apology from NIH and University of Pittsburgh, as well as $2.75 million in damages to his reputation

valid. He notified the federal officials at the granting agency, the National Cancer Institute. But federal investigators were not satisfied; they accused Fisher of delaying the notification and found problems of misconduct at some of Fisher's other sites. They cited sloppy paperwork in some of the more than 500 centers from which Fisher was collecting data. By 1994, the criticism became front-page news. Accused of publishing false data, Fisher was summarily fired by NIH as head of the NSABP and, if that wasn't bad enough, also punished by his own institution, the University of Pittsburgh, which totally failed to support him.[6] According to a feature article in the *Philadelphia Inquirer,* the once overconfident, even arrogant Fisher now appeared to be a subdued, if not broken man. His reputation was ruined. Fisher himself said his life had been spoiled.

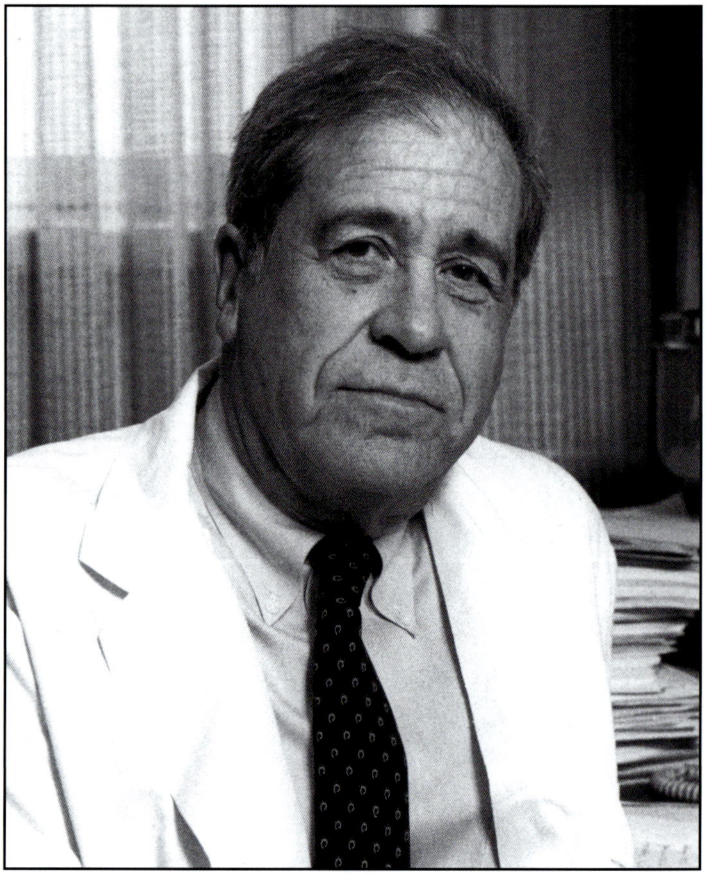

Bernard Fisher, criticized and fired by NIH and the University of Pittsburgh.

But this phase was brief. A more passive or shy individual might have been finished by this attack by the powerful NIH and by his own institution, but not Fisher. Even his enemies agreed that he was tough. Refusing to grovel, he fought back, bringing suit against both the NIH and the University of Pittsburgh for unfounded accusations and for ignoring due process.[7] After three painful years of an investigation by the Federal Office of Research and a congressional committee, Fisher was found innocent of any scientific misconduct. Six weeks before the case was to go to trial, Fisher settled for an apology from both the NIH and the University of Pittsburgh, as well as a $2.75 million award for damages to his reputation plus $300,000 for legal fees. To the extent possible, Fisher was satisfied with this outcome. His former honored status at Pittsburgh was restored, in fact, upgraded.[8] He was appointed to a distinguished professorship. An endowed chair was named for him (HUP 1993 Chief Resident David Bartlett was the first incumbent). He was again considered a hero.

And yet, a reputation once tarnished is difficult to restore completely. When I called Dr. Fisher ten years later, asking him to write a letter of support to the Lasker Foundation for his colleague, Tom Starzl, he was at first reluctant, fearing that a letter from him might have negative influence. He believed that the Lasker Foundation was still critical of him because of the NSABP data scandal. Fortunately, he eventually wrote the letter, and Starzl got the Lasker Award.

Bernard Fisher is now fully credited with transforming treatment of breast cancer, sparing its victims the disfigurement of radical mastectomy while also saving lives. Less widely recognized is that through his hypothesis and studies, he advanced the understanding of metastasis of other tumors. As important, perhaps, was the influence of his pioneering role in the use of multicenter, randomized clinical trials as the foundation of what we call evidence-based medicine. Finally, he was a role model for the surgical scientist, bringing hypotheses from his laboratory work to the decisive test of clinical trials.[9]

The New York Times, in its obit, forgot about Fisher's important years at Penn. While researching and writing this chapter, I was surprised to find that few of our residents and faculty knew anything about them. But Bernard Fisher never forgot them or how much he owed to Penn and to Dr. Ravdin. In biographical sketches, Fisher always documented his time as a HUP resident and spoke of it with pride. Certainly, he was one of our finest.

1998–2017
Fisher is honored for his seminal role in changing treatment of malignant diseases and demonstrating the value of clinical trials

2009
Jacobson Innovation Award of American College of Surgeons

2019
Death of Bernard Fisher at age 101

Bernard Fisher, reputation restored.

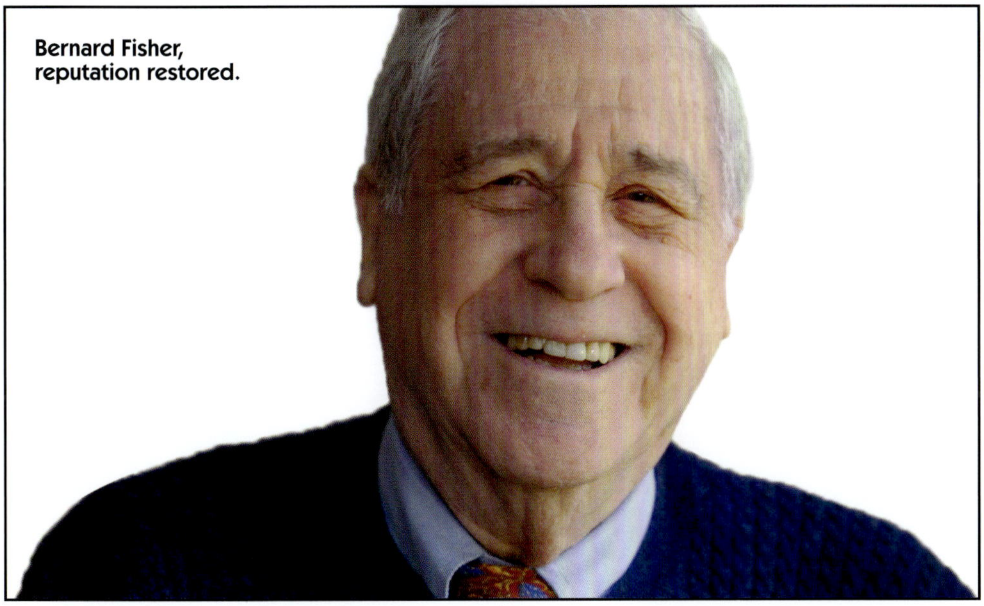

Notes

[1] Gellene, Denise. Dr. Bernard Fisher, Who Revolutionized Breast Cancer Treatment, Dies at 101. *The Philadelphia Inquirer.* (19 Oct 2019).

[2] Kate Travis. Bernard Fisher Reflects on a Half-Century's Worth of Breast Cancer Research. *JNCI: Journal of the National Cancer Institute,* Vol 97, No 22 (16 November 2005) pp. 1636–1637.

[3] Fisher B, Ravdin RG, Ausman RK, et al. Surgical Adjuvant Chemotherapy in Cancer of the Breast: Results of a decade of cooperative investigation. *Ann Surg* 168; 337–356 (Sept 1968).

[4] Ibid.

[5] Fisher B, Anderson S. Conservative surgery for the management of invasive and noninvasive carcinoma of the breast: NSABP trials. National Surgical Adjuvant Breast and Bowel Project. *World J Surg*. (1994) 18(1):63–69.

[6] Davidson, Nancy. Bernard Fisher, MD: In Memoriam (1918–2019). *Cancer Research* (1 January 2020) 80:3–4.

[7] Ibid.

[8] Bernard Fisher, MD, Pioneer in Breast Cancer Research, Dies at 101. *PittWire* (October 21, 2019)

[9] Ibid.

CHAPTER 17

PhDs: The Past and Future of a Surgery Department

The death of David Cooper in 2013 reminded me of a bygone era when the Harrison Department of Surgical Research was largely staffed by a cadre of full-time basic scientists who had been recruited by Dr. Ravdin, and subsequently by Dr. Rhoads, to conduct the department's research. Dave Cooper was almost the last surviving member of this group.

In 1927 as a young surgeon, Dr. Ravdin had decided during a year of laboratory research in Scotland and in England that collaboration with professional scientists was almost essential for clinical surgeons to be productive investigators. In 1935, George Leib Harrison's bequest of $2.7 million for support of the department's research allowed Ravdin to fund basic scientists. His plan went beyond hiring research collaborators for the department's practicing surgeons. In characteristic exuberance, he decided that as the department's director of research, he would develop his own basic science departments in disciplines such as biochemistry, microbiology, physiology, and so forth. In most instances, his scientists, instead of collaborating with the department's surgeons, conducted their own independent research. But Ravdin saw to it that his department always got the credit since their appointments were in Surgery.

Under Dr. Ravdin's chairmanship, and later during Dr. Rhoads's, this group of fundamental investigators grew to a large number. Older members of the department will recognize the names of many of these scientists: Otto Rosenthal, K. C. Tsou, Sidney Levin, Henry Parkins, Harry Vars, Benjamin Miller, Heinz Schleyer, Henry Sloviter, Rudi Eisenhart, Adair Rogers, Elizabeth Miller, Joe Touchstone, Sidney Wolfson, and David Cooper. Only Cooper and Wolfson had any surgical training, but all of these researchers had primary or secondary appointments in Surgery. Surgery also had the continuing responsibility for their funding.

In several instances, this model paid off handsomely. These included David Cooper's important studies of cytochrome P-450 enzymes (in which Otto Rosenthal, Heinz Schleyer, Shakunthala Narasimhulu, and

Sidney Levin all collaborated). Another example was the landmark study in total parenteral nutrition by Drs. Rhoads and Dudrick. A crucial role in the TPN work was played by the department's biochemist Harry Vars, who concocted the complex nutritional solutions the dogs received intravenously. Even more importantly, he devised the harness the dogs wore to protect the central lines necessary for chronic IV therapy.

Also, during the 1960s, Adair Rogers, one of the department's scientists, was trying with Kirkley Williams, a faculty surgeon, to develop a fully implantable artificial heart. In parallel work, Bill Pierce, as a student and surgical resident, was doing his pioneering work with a blood pump, which years later culminated in his successful mechanical heart, now in clinical use.

In time, the effectiveness of this research model began to decline. During the 1970s and 1980s, extramural grants became more difficult to sustain while the department remained responsible for supporting its aging basic science faculty. Eventually, the department's basic scientists retired or moved into the preclinical departments of their fundamental disciplines. By the 1990s, only a few tenured ones remained in the Department of Surgery.

Dr. Ravdin's conviction that surgeons need collaboration with basic scientists is even more valid today in the era of molecular biology than it was in his time. But it probably needs to be accomplished by a different model.

A few of the department's clinical surgeons have had PhDs, for example, Drs. Naji, Drebin, Markmann, Shaked, and Porrett. Recently, with the help of funding by the Measey Foundation, the department has encouraged residents to obtain master's degrees or PhDs. The first PhDs in this new program are Ian Folkert and Anna Garcia.

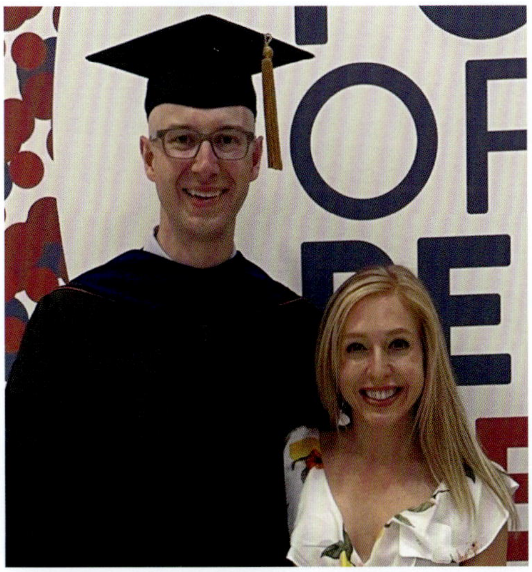

Ian Folkert and his wife, Dr. Hilary Bollman, at his graduation from the PhD program.

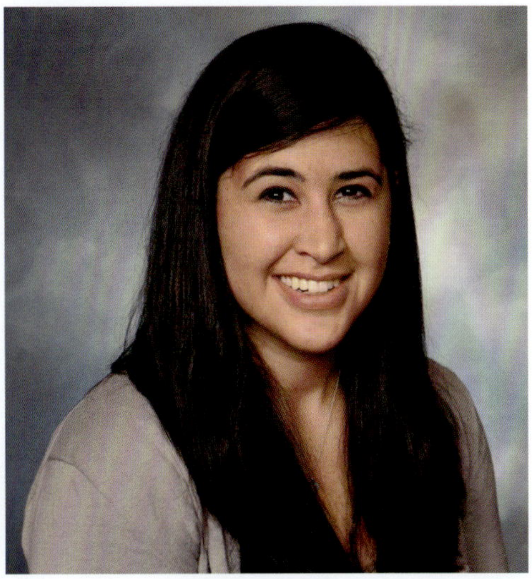

Anna Garcia

CHAPTER 18

Epitaph for a Legendary Bully and Gifted Teacher

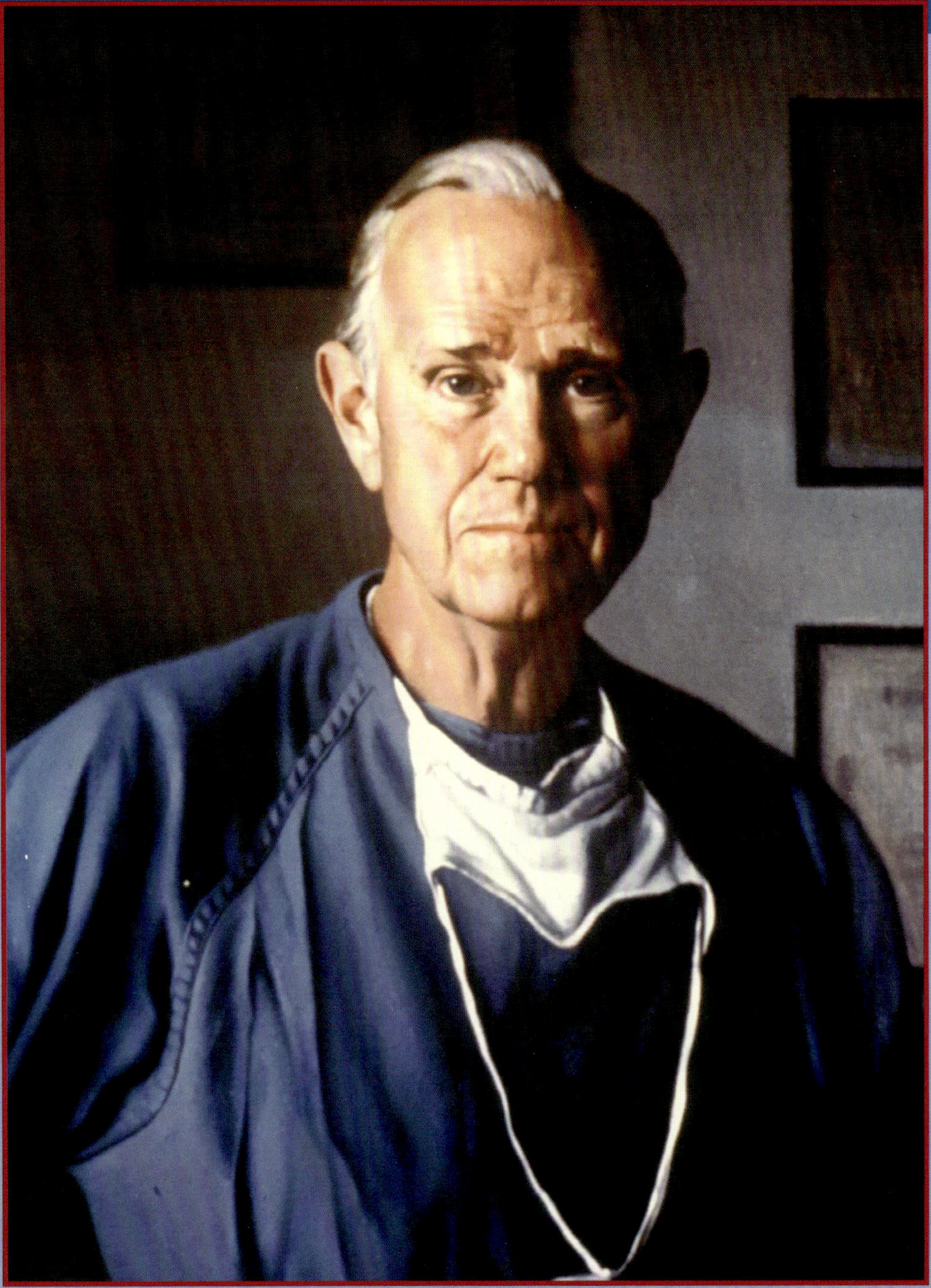

Julian Johnson (1906–1987)

1931
MD, University of Pennsylvania

1932–1939
Internship and residency under Eliason

1942–1945
Member of Ravdin's 20th General Hospital in India

In the 1960s, HUP was an environment incredibly rich in unusual personalities, some of which belonged to the major figures in American surgery. Examples of this were I. S. Ravdin, Jonathan Rhoads, Bill Fitts, Bugs Lehr, and C. Everett Koop. Among these memorable individuals, Julian Johnson was, for most surgical residents, life's most unforgettable character. His name was Julian, but we residents called him J. J., although never to his face. He was also called by some the meanest man in the world.

When Ravdin returned from India in 1945 to become department chairman, he got rid of any dissenters and all ex-HUP residents who had trained under Eliason or other chairmen. Julian Johnson, an Eliason resident who had served under Ravdin at the 20th General Hospital, was the one exception. Johnson and Jonathan Rhoads became Ravdin's partners in the new department, which was actually just a private practice that the three of them owned. Later, other faculty were hired, but none ever had the same status as Ravdin, Rhoads, and Johnson.

When visiting professors delivered the annual Julian Johnson Lecture, they praised Johnson as a founder of cardiac surgery, a field that he helped start as soon as he finished his HUP residency in 1939. As is customary, especially with the passage of time, they recalled only his virtues. The blemishes were forgotten. I think Dr. Johnson would have been disappointed, as I was, that nothing was said about him as a man. Though celebrated for his accomplishments, this was a man full of blemishes but unapologetic or possibly even proud of them. He was a man feared by many and detested by some but seemingly content with his motives, actions, and impact. This enigmatic surgical icon's role in establishing Penn's modern department of surgery was as crucial as that of its other two founders, Ravdin and Rhoads. It would be satisfying, though nigh impossible, if I could set the record straight and balance the virtues with the blemishes to capture his persona.

1963 (June 15)
Johnson pictured on cover of *Saturday Evening Post*

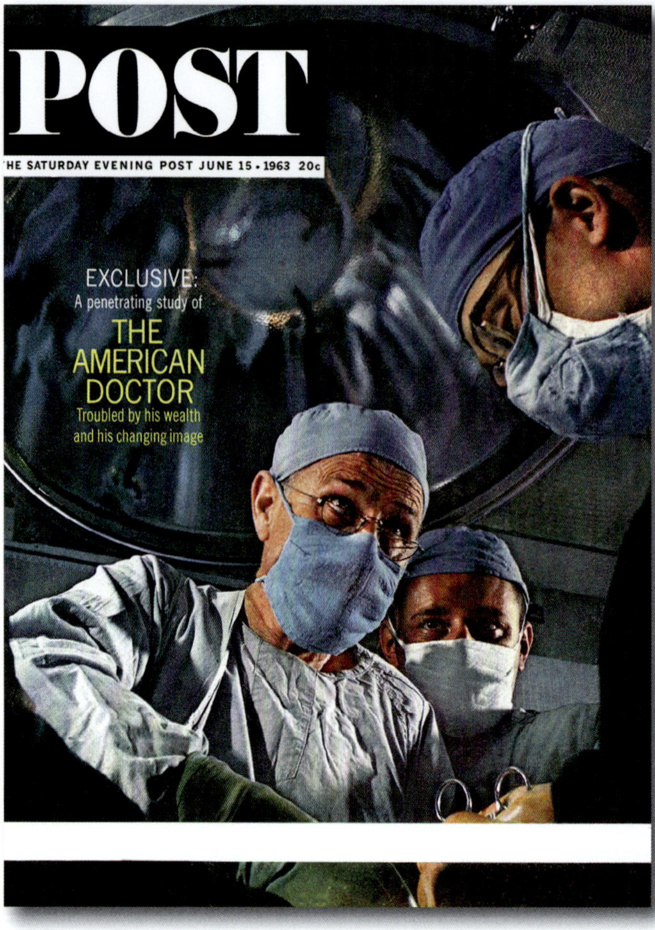

From a safe vantage point, beautiful to watch—the Roger Federer of surgery.

While seeking illustrations for this memoir, I remembered that over fifty years ago, the *Saturday Evening Post* featured Julian Johnson on its cover.[1] For a short time, this magazine cover had been tacked to the bulletin board in the doctors' dressing room—until one of Johnson's many detractors angrily took it down and tore it up. Since the picture had no caption, my wife wondered how I could recognize the masked figure. Once transfixed by staring into those penetrating blue eyes, there was no mistaking him.

As I studied the image, long-forgotten memories came flooding back. To stand opposite Dr. Johnson at the operating table as he looked over his half glasses at you and hummed "Red River Valley" (which he tended to do if the blood loss was large) could produce a type of anxiety seldom experienced, the twinges of which I sometimes think I can still feel. The only thing more frightening than helping him on a tough case was to help him on an easy case, which would allow him the leisure to teach the junior residents by quizzing them on surgical anatomy. Recently, I took my copy of Johnson and Kirby's *Surgery of the Chest* off my bookshelf. It opened spontaneously, just as it did fifty years ago, to the section on the anatomy of the pulmonary veins. This was Dr. Johnson's favorite quiz subject, and if you made a mistake, he would say, "Doc, maybe you better drop out and look that up." You would then have the embarrassing assignment of leaving the operating room to review anatomy.

This was a painful teaching style, but I now realize that it was one of the things that, while I was a resident, made for a more personal relationship with J. J. than I had with other attendings. Maybe he cared more than others whether we were learning something as we helped him. True, many of the interpersonal exchanges generated something between uneasiness and terror but filtered now through half a century (including five years as his resident and ten as his faculty colleague), other exchanges were distinctly positive.

1959–1964
Barker's HUP residency, much of it under Johnson

Summers of
1962 & 1964
Barkers house-sit for Johnsons

Although Johnson could be sarcastic or downright mean, he usually had a reason. Most often, it was his determination not to have a patient die on his watch, at least not unless he had driven himself and his staff to their limits to prevent it—not such a bad attitude for a surgeon. In spite of these efforts, many patients died in those early days of cardiac surgery. For example, of Johnson's first dozen patients to undergo open-heart operations, fewer than half survived. Many of the deaths took place on the table. Sharing these painful experiences forged close friendships among the residents on his team. Sometimes (especially when a sick patient got better), the comradery even extended to include "the old man."

Outside of the hospital, this seemingly sadistic taskmaster was a different person. At the end of each three-month rotation, he entertained his house staff team and spouses for dinner in his elegant house in Gladwyne. No other attending did this. On these informal occasions, residents were surprised to find him disarmingly gracious. He even exhibited some homespun humor and told folksy stories reflecting his background as the son of a Baptist minister growing up in a small farming town in Kentucky. The spouses could not believe this soft-spoken Southern gentleman was the monster they had heard about.

Dr. Johnson and his wife always took a month's summer vacation, usually traveling in Europe. Residents would be invited to stay in their house. Dode and I did this twice. We were delighted to leave our non-air-conditioned apartment in West Philadelphia, but distinctly uneasy about the consequences if our two-year-old son should break something. Once, I spilled some ink on the Johnson's expensive bedspread. When I confessed, vowing to replace it, the offer was refused with a gentle smile.

As I progressed through the residency while keeping my guard up, I increasingly valued my relationship with this enigmatic character. I also realized that I was learning as much about surgery (maybe more) by watching this master surgeon operate as I learned from other, well-liked attendings as they patiently helped me struggle through operations.

J. J. was almost an exact contemporary of Jonathan Rhoads, but these two giants could hardly have been more different. J. J. was one year older and finished his HUP residency one year before Rhoads. Fifty-five years later, in writing his colleague's obituary, Rhoads recalled that, as an intern,

1939
Johnson finishes residency, is assigned to head the department's thoracic surgery program. His thoracic training is limited to two weeks in Boston, observing chest operations

1942–1945
Johnson serves under Ravdin on staff of 20th General Hospital in India

1945
World War II ends. Ravdin appoints Johnson chief of cardiothoracic surgery at HUP

1951
Johnson performs closed surgery of heart valves

he had helped Johnson, a first-year resident, do a thyroidectomy. He observed that Johnson, "did a smoother and better operation than most of the senior surgeons I had assisted. He had, in fact, extraordinary coordination of mind and body . . . his hands seemed to carry out almost automatically the instructions of his brain."[2] My assessment of his operative skill was not as analytic as Rhoads's, but I know I never saw anyone as good. Virtually everyone who saw him agreed. The dichotomy in the native talents of Rhoads and Johnson was probably magnified by Johnson's residency training under Eldridge Eliason, who emphasized technical proficiency, while Rhoads's chief, I. S. Ravdin, focused on surgical physiology and basic laboratory research.

After finishing his residency in 1939, Johnson was appointed to the HUP staff. He was assigned to develop thoracic surgery, at the time a field limited in Philadelphia to treatment of patients with emphysema and lung abscesses. Johnson's training in the new specialty was meager, being limited to two weeks in Boston where he observed a few lung operations performed by Edward Churchill at MGH and Richard Overholt at the Lahey Clinic.

Johnson later said he had never witnessed any of the modern thoracic and cardiovascular procedures he subsequently performed before doing the operations himself. He was truly a self-trained thoracic surgeon. Yet quite soon, Johnson was able to publish that in his first twenty pneumonectomies, there was only one death, a far better record than anyone else had reported up to that time. Evarts Graham, in discussing the paper at a national meeting, predicted that as this young surgeon accumulated more cases, his results would get worse. But they never did.

Only months after J. J. joined the HUP faculty, World War II began with Hitler's invasion of Poland. After enlisting in the Army, Johnson served from 1942 to 1945 in India as a member of General I. S. Ravdin's 20th General Hospital. There, he managed the treatment of over 300 patients with thoracic trauma, most due to small arms fire or shrapnel from mines, bombs, or grenades. Despite the challenges of jungle warfare, primitive facilities, and associated injuries, the overall mortality of his patients was a remarkably low 7.4 percent.

Johnson returned to HUP in 1945, just as Dr. Ravdin became chairman of surgery. At once, Ravdin appointed the young Julian Johnson as chief of cardiothoracic surgery, a position he held until his retirement in 1973. Early in his faculty career, he conducted basic research in thyroid and biliary physiology. He also designed and built a defibrillator and reported four successful resuscitations from ventricular fibrillation.

His early clinical activity was in thyroid, pulmonary, and esophageal surgery. In 1951, his practice expanded to include closed procedures on heart valves damaged by rheumatic fever. He also began a congenital heart surgery program at the Children's Hospital of Philadelphia. Soon after John Gibbon's first successful use of cardiopulmonary bypass in 1953, Johnson initiated open-heart surgery programs at HUP and CHOP. The early results of cardiac surgery were discouraging. Johnson first treated aortic stenosis with a mechanical dilator inserted through an incision in the left ventricle and manipulated blindly to force open (or fracture) the aortic valve. Of 161 patients, fifty-one died. After cardio-pulmonary bypass allowed an open approach, he decreased the mortality to 20 percent. Yet with the open-heart approach to mitral valve disease, more than half of his first dozen patients died, many on the table. These early results were adversely influenced by Johnson's conviction that new operations should be offered only to very high-risk patients whose advanced heart failure left them no options to surgical treatment, however risky. He was critical of other heart surgeons, who in those early days because of concern over their own statistics, operated on good-risk patients who J. J. thought could have waited until more experience accumulated. Nevertheless, in 1964, Johnson and his associates (including Charles Kirby and Gordon Danielson), after accumulating substantial experience, were able to report a combined series from the two institutions of 100 consecutive open-heart operations with a remarkably low mortality of 10 percent. For the rest of his career, Johnson's surgical results were always among the best.[3]

1953
Johnson starts open-heart surgery at HUP. Mortality is high

1964
Report of 100 open-heart operations at HUP with low mortality (10%)

Johnson is considered best at HUP in general surgery as well as chest surgery

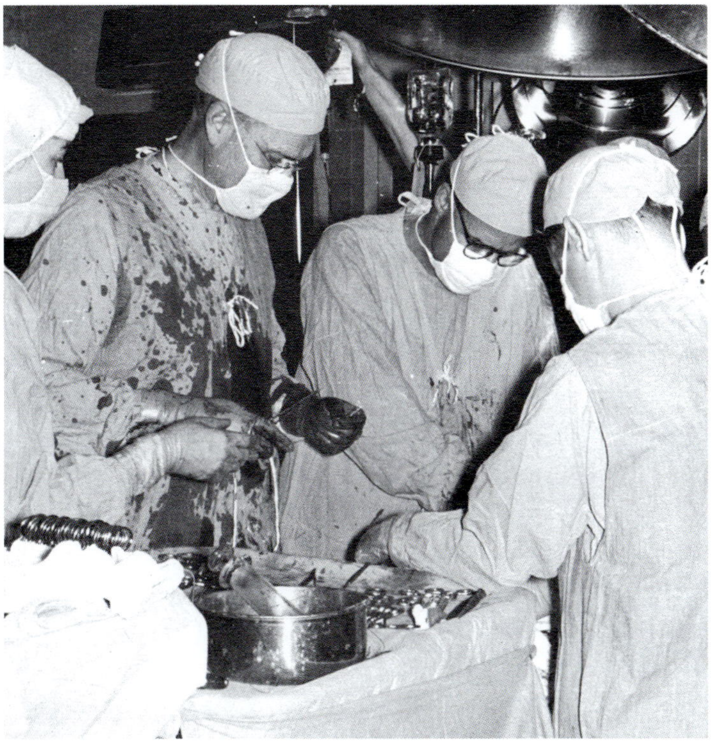

Early days of open heart surgery

Throughout his career, Johnson continued to do a substantial amount of general surgery and to head one of the department's two general surgery ("ward") teaching services. His versatility needed no justification. In fact, there was general agreement that J. J. could operate circles around other general surgeons, being faster and surer on gastrectomies, thyroidectomies, resection of aortic aneurysms, or what have you, than other accomplished surgeons who claimed to be specialists in these procedures. An example of the confidence he had in his powers was that he chose himself as the best surgeon to operate on his wife for her peptic ulcer. Although Dr. Ravdin was also present as the nominal operator,

1955
Vice president American Surgical Association, president of the American Association of Thoracic Surgery

1958
Publication of Johnson and Kirby's *Surgery of the Chest.* Through multiple editions, it is a standard

1962
President of Society for Vascular Surgery

1971
Johnson is founding member of American Board of Thoracic Surgery

J. J. asked him to drop out before the case was finished, telling his chief that he would finish the operation since he had "more recent experience."

As one of the first members of the American Board of Thoracic Surgery, he maintained that "thoracic surgeons should be general surgeons and something more, not something less," staunchly opposing the subsequently inevitable movement to forgo the requirement that thoracic surgeons pass the general surgery board exam before they were eligible for the thoracic board.[4]

Unlike Dr. Rhoads, Johnson's propensity was for clinical surgery, rather than basic research or achievement of prominence in surgical politics. Despite this, he was an accomplished and highly regarded academic surgeon. His early research and publications dealt not only with cardiac surgery and physiology, but with a variety of other topics, including peptic ulcer disease, the function of the superior laryngeal nerves, the effects of biliary obstruction, the influence of diet on the liver, and even treatment of fractures. Soon after John Gibbon's breakthrough success with cardiopulmonary bypass, Johnson, with his junior faculty member Charles Kirby, perfected in the laboratory the pump oxygenator necessary to start HUP's open heart surgery program. He was probably best known for the book he published with Kirby on *Surgery of the Chest.*[5] It became the standard in the field, and subsequently went through many editions and coauthors, including his young colleagues and trainees John Waldhausen, Bill Pierce, and Horace McVaugh.

Johnson's talents and accomplishments were well recognized nationally and internationally. He soon became a prominent member of all the important surgical societies including the Society of University Surgeons, the American Surgical Association, the Society of Clinical Surgery, and the International Surgical Group. He was elected vice president of the American Surgical Association (1955), president of the American Association of Thoracic Surgery (1962), president of the Society for Vascular Surgery (1960) and president of the Philadelphia Academy of Surgery (1970).

Ironically, much better known at HUP than Johnson's accomplishments and honors, and perhaps more interesting, was his dark side. As Dr. Rhoads put it in writing Johnson's obituary, "he was never soft in his dealings with residents . . . for some, he was almost too much of a disciplinarian."[6] Dr. Rhoads could never call a spade a spade.

Ernie Rosato, in a retrospective tribute to J. J., tried to excuse J. J.'s negative dealings with residents as "fueled by the frequent failures during the pioneering days of heart surgery," this being "the reason he drove himself and his protégés so hard, many finding him too harsh." Maybe so, but like Rhoads, Ernie was far too generous.

In fact, Dr. Johnson could be a real son of a bitch, a moniker he sometimes actually used for himself. He consistently struck terror into the hearts of junior residents and kept even the most seasoned of his trainees on edge. He was not a shouter, but his sarcasm cut to the quick. He called students, interns, and residents "Doc" or "Son," but his relationship with them was anything but filial. In an era when senior surgeons (perhaps especially cardiac and neurosurgeons) were not expected to coddle their trainees, he was an outlier. From his residents, he expected no less than fanatical devotion to his patients, hard work to the point of their exhaustion, and detailed accuracy and truthfulness. Pity the poor resident he caught cutting corners, trying to make up a lab value, or attempting to cover up a mistake. These were unforgivable sins. For lesser offenses in the OR, such as falling asleep, mismanaging a retractor, or clumsiness in tying a knot, a sharp reprimand or rap on the knuckles would suffice. A mistake on an anatomy quiz was only one of a number of things that warranted abrupt dismissal from the OR.

Even the best residents were susceptible to such treatment. One (who later became department chairman) arrived late in the OR one day and found J. J. himself prepping the patient and then inserting a foley catheter. When this resident tried to make amends and take over these preparations, J. J. brushed him aside and said, "Len, I'm not going to say anything about this now because I've got four years to make it up to you." Another HUP faculty surgeon, remembering his unhappy experience as a resident on the Johnson service, confided to a friend during a memorial service for J. J. that he only showed up to be sure the old devil wasn't coming back.

There are a plethora of such stories that his residents loved to tell, but I believe it is more important to document that there was another side to this unusual character. If you could get beyond the fear generated by Johnson's reputation and observation of his treatment of residents who failed to measure up to his expectations, there was quite a lot to J. J. on the positive side. Those interested in this side of the story—the minority view of J. J.—and more about why I came to love the old SOB should read on.

In an odd way, the relationship that evolved between Johnson and his residents was more intense and personal than with other, more aloof senior faculty members. You always knew where you stood with him. He was quite predictable once you learned his relatively straightforward routines and what he expected of you, which was common sense and, in addition, total dedication to patient care to the limit of your endurance, even after a series of consecutive nights without leaving the hospital or sleeping. Residents who got into trouble were those who couldn't master his routines, thinking that perhaps they should modify them or suggest improvements.

For residents, working for Dr. Johnson was an experience that could be divided into three stages. The first stage was that of total intimidation. For example, a favorite story of a future chairman of surgery at another school was that of having Dr. Johnson patiently watch him, as a resident, close a skin incision after a long operation. Dr. Johnson then, being dissatisfied with the quality of the skin closure, without saying a word, cut out every last suture and reclosed the wound himself, to emphasize how it should be done.

Another traumatic setting at this stage of the residency was "night report," at which time the junior resident on the service had the assignment of telephoning Dr. Johnson to report on the postoperative patients. At the slightest suggestion that the resident was not in total command of the situation, Dr. Johnson would say, "Son, maybe you better have a doctor call me." By doctor, he meant the chief resident, his junior faculty colleague, or one of the two senior cardiologists that Dr. Johnson paid with his personal funds.

These were unquestionably traumatic experiences, but generally speaking, after the first month or two on the Johnson service, a resident began to feel more comfortable, his anxiety declined to a subliminal level, and it was apparent that he had entered "stage 2." He had learned the routine. During night report, he knew that Dr. Johnson preferred to hear only the vital signs, the hemoglobin, and the number of cubic centimeters of blood in the chest drainage bottle. Additional information was volunteered by a junior resident only with some risk since Dr. Johnson expected any significant problem to be checked out and reported by his senior resident. Thus, for the junior resident who understood Dr. Johnson's system, the job was easy, at least it was if he understood that Dr. Johnson also expected total devotion and, if necessary, the expenditure of the last ounce of energy in behalf of his patients. If you didn't weaken, you could complete "stage 2."

It was also likely that by then, you had been invited to the Johnsons' for dinner, and you found that your wife considered Mary Johnson a lovely friend and Dr. Johnson himself, who was always gracious socially, to be an old softy. So your wife didn't believe any of the stories you had told her about the Johnson service. Residents at this stage of their training would sometimes say that the old man had mellowed. This was never true. A few days before he died, Julian reminded me with thoughtful pride that he always ran "a tight ship." Some undiscerning senior residents found out to their dismay that he still had his eye on them at this stage. He hadn't mellowed or changed. He was just as disciplined as ever. You had changed.

You may not have realized it, but you had learned his system. Because of this, he knew he could rely on you, and you had become "one of his boys." Although he seldom, if ever, addressed a compliment directly to you, you sometimes overheard his hallway conversation with another faculty member or consultant as he bragged about the quality of his residents and what good care they took of his patients. This affected a tremendous esprit de corps.

By this time, you were probably the chief resident on his service, and you were now ready for "stage 3," one of the more valuable learning experiences I've had in surgery. Dr. Johnson's extensive and varied surgical practice constituted a major resource of teaching material. He was a superb teacher of surgery in the style of that day. You learned from him entirely by watching him operate. This, however, was an important and virtually unique experience since there were many, including some of America's senior surgeons, who said that he might be the finest technical surgeon in the world at that time.

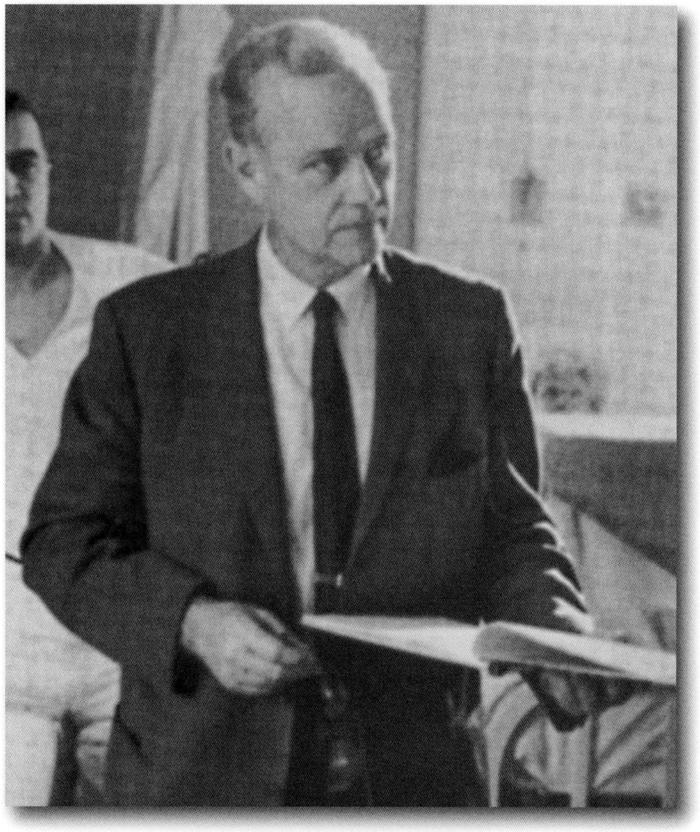

On rounds with Julian Johnson,
a sight to make the hairs on the back of your neck stand up.

It was also of great value to observe his pre- and post-op care. During "stage 3," Dr. Johnson would confide strategy and reasoning on patient care. His approach to surgical treatment, both operative and nonoperative, was beautifully direct and effective. He often said, "You don't have to be a PhD to be a good surgeon"; in fact, he preferred the residents with outstanding practical skills to those more attracted to research, whom he denigrated as "salt-water surgeons."

Occasionally, he would let his guard down and reveal his compassion by confiding, after seeing a particularly high-risk patient preoperatively, "I'd rather take a beating than operate on that patient because the risk is so great." Quite often he would say, "I am not quite sure what to do in this situation, but I know what my old chief, Eli, would do, so I think I'll do that." And just as Johnson knew what Dr. Eliason would do, the residents found they knew what J. J. would do in almost any circumstance. They had learned his way, and it was a good way.

Mentioned earlier was the possibility that Johnson's negative dealings with residents stemmed from well-concealed anguish over the many patient deaths during the early years of cardiac surgery. Maybe this did have something to do with it. If so, it would help to explain his surprising early retirement. Unlike Dr. Rhoads who never retired, when Johnson turned sixty-six, still in full command of his powers, he walked out of the hospital and never came back.

Until then, it had seemed to us that he lived only to operate. As it turned out, he was devoted just as much to the avocations he had ac-

1972–1987
Johnson retires. Fifteen years of duck hunting and gardening

1987
Johnson dies

quired during his small town Kentucky childhood, but by necessity had neglected during his professional career. Now, besides spending time with his wife and daughter, perhaps because his father was a minister, J. J. became an elder in the Baptist church and later in his wife's Presbyterian church. But during his fifteen-year retirement, he spent most of his time working on his hobbies. He was deeply interested in farming, gardening, and hunting. His boyhood reputation as a crack shot had been enhanced during World War II when he shot and killed a leopard that was terrorizing the staff on the grounds of the 20th General Hospital in India. In his retirement, he delighted in maintaining a huge vegetable garden on the grounds of his Gladwyne home and another on his farm in southern Jersey. There, with a few friends including two cronies from 20th General Hospital days (Paul McCray and Sergeant Pepper), he would spend weeks at a time living in his hunting cabin on the Delaware Bay, cooking the meals for the group, raising fresh vegetables, and above all, whenever possible, shooting ducks.

Who can know what Julian Johnson's motivation may have been. Was he really a vicious and unrepentant SOB, as many thought? Or was he a misunderstood but dedicated teacher—or both, or something in between? Did he take pride in the important role he had played in training a generation of accomplished HUP surgeons? Or was he consumed by and content with his own remarkable skills and accomplishments? His interpersonal style left a lot to be desired, but few if any could duplicate his moves in the operating room. It was an education to try.

Subsequent generations of HUP residents are poorer from not having the chance to fear and learn from this inscrutable master surgeon. Was he misunderstood or understood too well? Those who had the privilege of being his trainees and colleagues still think about him and wonder.

Notes

[1] *Julian Johnson operating.* "The American Doctor." *Saturday Evening Post* (June 15, 1963). Cover photograph. The Saturday Evening Post cover © SEPS licensed by Curtis Licensing Indianapolis, IN

[2] Rhoads, Jonathan E. Memoir of Julian Johnson. *Transactions of the American Surgical Association* 1988, Vol. 106, p. 302.

[3] L. Henry Edmonds. Memoir of Julian Johnson. *Journal of Thoracic and Cardiovascular Surgery* Vol 96 (4) (Oct 1988) pp. 515-517.

[4] Johnson J. A Surgeon and Something More. *J Thorac Cardiovasc Surg.* (1963) 46:141-149.

[5] Kirby, Charles K. and Johson, Julian. *Surgery of the Chest* (The Year Book Publishers: 1952).

[6] Ibid.

CHAPTER 19

Colossus of 20th-Century Surgery

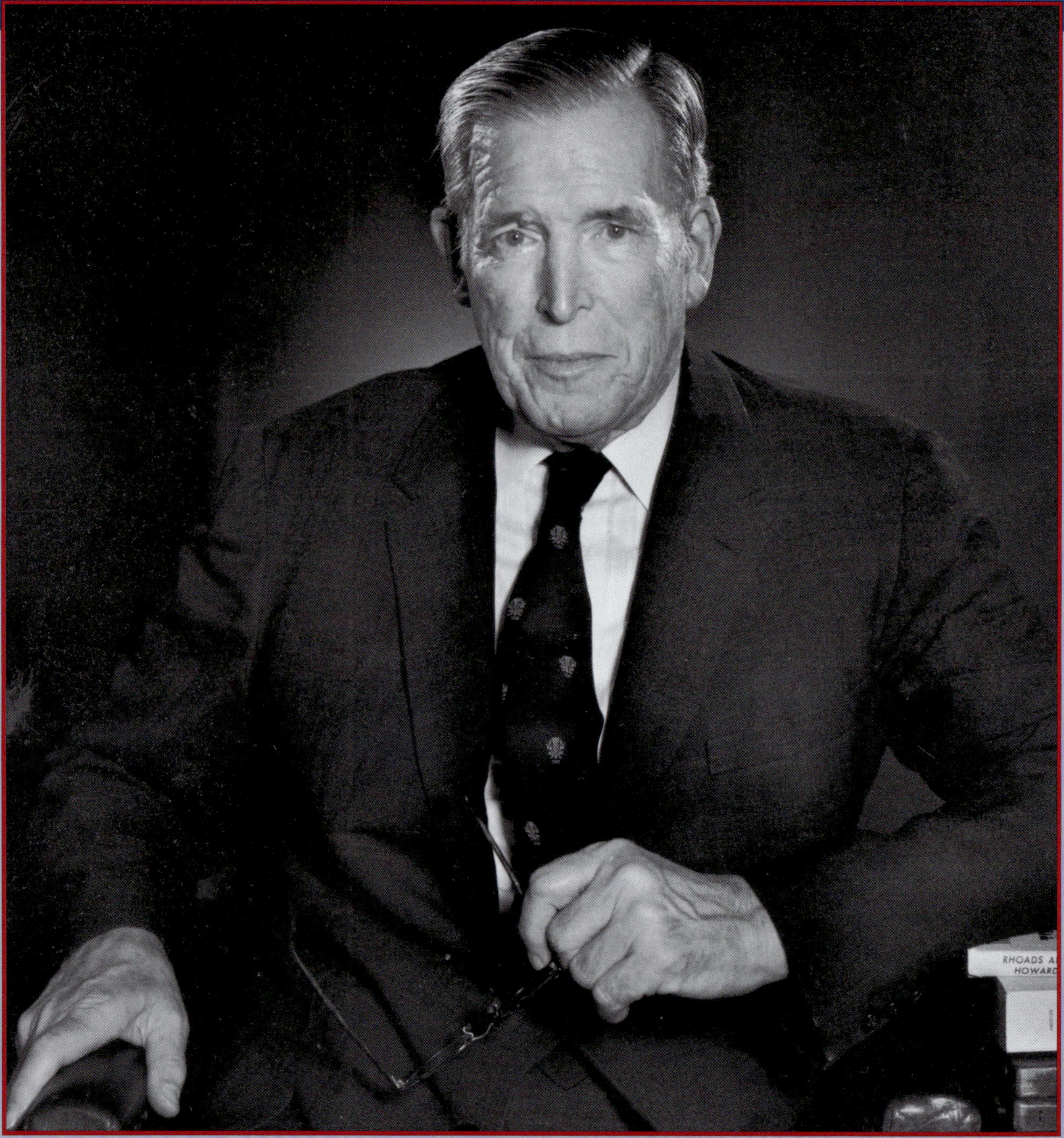

Jonathan E. Rhoads (1907–2002)

JRB Professor and Chairman of Surgery (1960–1972)

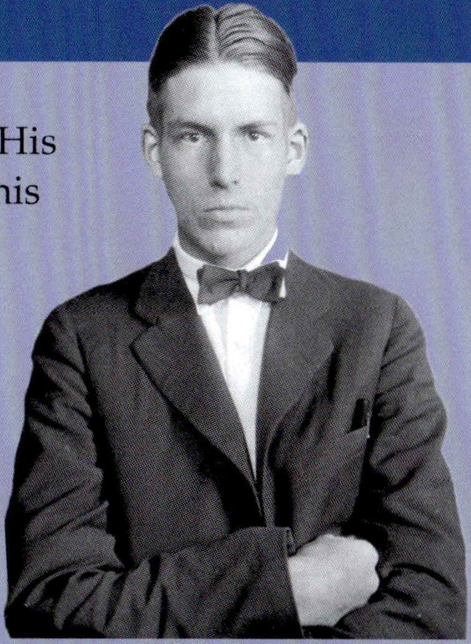

Young Jonathan Rhoads

1912–1924
Elementary education at Westtown (a Quaker school)

1928
Senior at Haverford College

1932
Graduation from medical school at Johns Hopkins

1932–1934
Two-year internship at HUP

1936
Marries his medical school classmate Terry Folin

1939
Finishes five-year general surgery fellowship under Ravdin

Jonathan Rhoads was born on May 9, 1907. His father Edward was a physician who served his internship under D. Hayes Agnew and William Osler at the Hospital of the University of Pennsylvania, the nation's first University Hospital, which had opened in 1874.[1]

At Haverford College, the young Jonathan was Phi Beta Kappa and a track star, excelling in the pole vault, an event in which he was undefeated in intercollegiate competition. While he was in medical school at Johns Hopkins, he met his classmate and future wife, Terry Folin, whose father Otto was the professor of biochemistry at Harvard.[2] After graduation in 1932, Jonathan accepted an internship at HUP and Terry one at Yale. He credited her with the predominant role in raising their six children, for which she gave up a promising career in pediatrics.

During Dr. Rhoads's surgical training at HUP (1934–39), Eldridge Eliason was the official department chairman, but his mentor was another senior faculty member, I. S. Ravdin. Ravdin was head of the Harrison Department of Surgical Research and in addition, had an independent clinical service with its own separate staff of residents, one of whom was Rhoads.

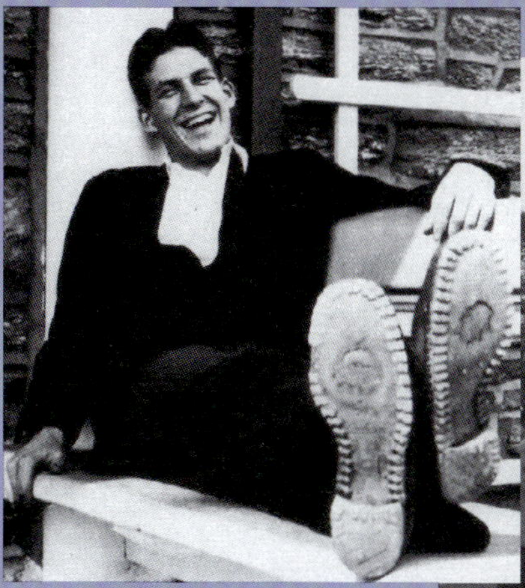

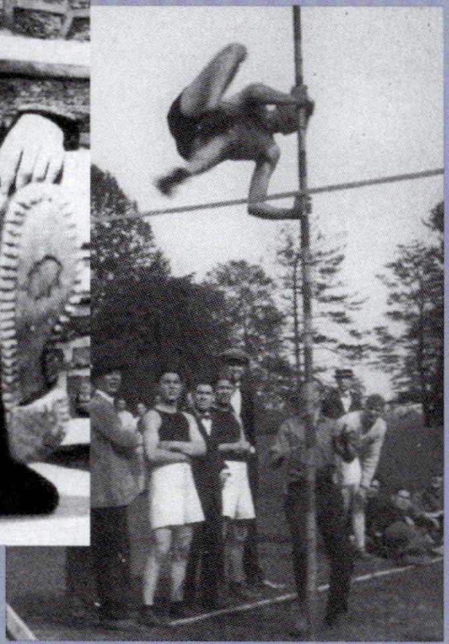

A few months after Rhoads finished his residency, Ravdin became acutely ill with cholecystitis. Dr. Alan O. Whipple,

1940
I.S. Ravdin's gallbladder attack. He chooses young Rhoads to operate on him

Ravdin said he chose Rhoads as his surgeon to promote his career, but it is hard to believe that he wasn't just teasing his close friend, the famous Professor Whipple. He didn't like Eliason and wouldn't have worried about offending him

Always conservative, Ravdin instructed his surgeons to decompress the gallbladder with a tube rather than remove it which was a more commonly advised procedure. Ravdin recovered quickly and never had more trouble with his gallbladder that was never removed

Columbia's chairman, was summoned from New York to see him. Expecting to operate, Whipple arrived with a bag of his instruments only to be informed that he would be assisting the virtually unknown Jonathan Rhoads, whom Ravdin had chosen to do the operation.[3]

Chosen to operate

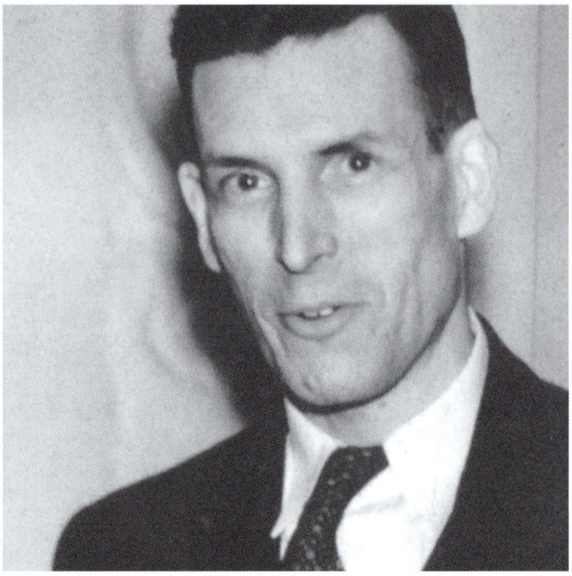

Whipple and Eliason were relegated to the role of assistants during the operation, a cholecystostomy. Ravdin insisted that the procedure be performed under spinal anesthesia so that he could direct the operation. Ravdin's kibitzing throughout the procedure added to Whipple's visible annoyance with this arrangement. Finally, Whipple exclaimed, "Rav, scrub up or shut up."[4]

The Annoyed Assistants

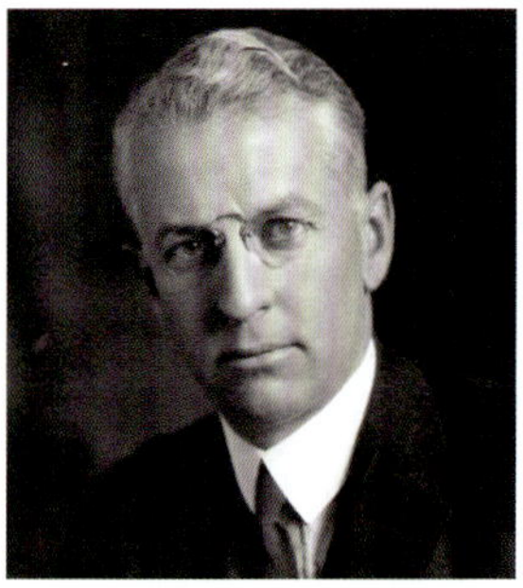

Eldridge Eliason
Penn's Chairman

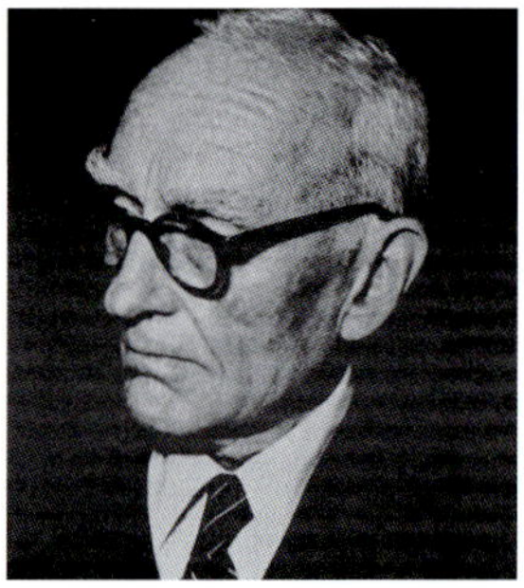

Allen Whipple
Columbia's Chairman

Rhoads later reviewed his productive early years at Penn,[5] where he remained for his entire career: "We began using Wangensteen Suction to decompress obstructed bowel in 1933 or '34 and with William Osler Abbott participated in defining the use of the Miller-Abbott tube. We operated on the first cases of Crohn's disease in 1933 and I believe the first islet cell adenoma of the pancreas about 1936. We attempted to autotransplant slices of it into the rectus muscle of a diabetic and to get the cells to grow in tissue culture. We got sulfanilamide in 1936, sulfadiazine by 1938, Vitamin K in 1938. I set up the Quick test for prothrombin in 1938 and personally ran all the prothrombins. About 1935, I did the first four peritoneal dialyses for uremia that were done in the Philadelphia area [probably the first anywhere]. We studied the effect of hypoproteinemia on wound healing and later its effect on hemorrhagic shock.

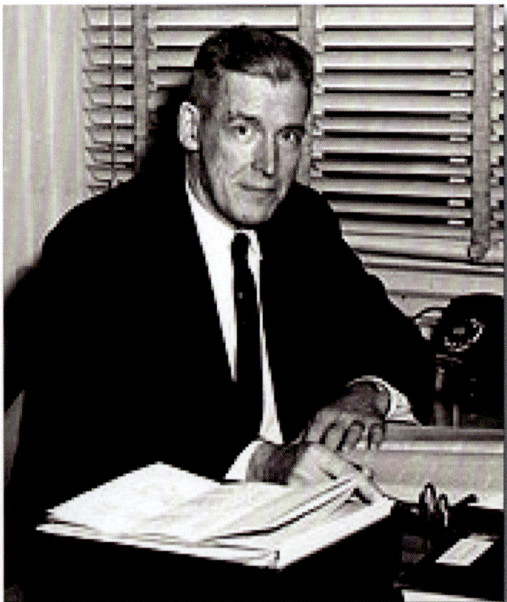

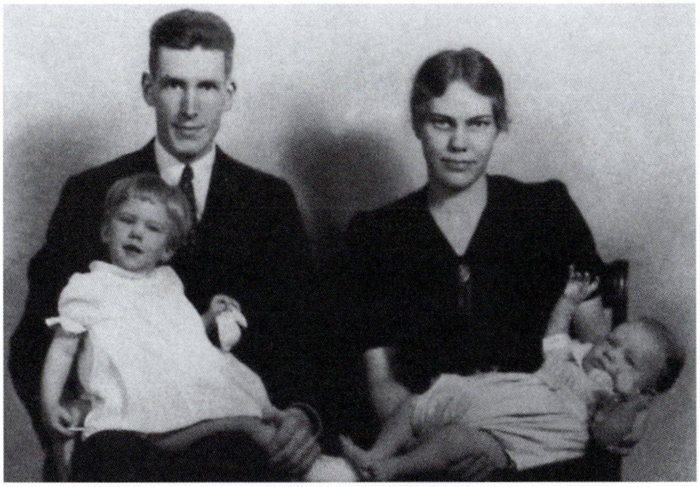

Jonathan and Terry Rhoads in 1938 with their children, Margaret and Jonathan Jr.

I studied blood coagulation, demonstrating that the prothrombin fell rapidly in the hepatectomized dog."

Rhoads's bibliography, from its first entry in 1935 to the last of his nearly 400 papers written in 2001, virtually charts the evolution of modern surgery.[6] His most important contributions were in the fields of nutrition and cancer. He wrote on pancreatic, gastric, colon, and breast cancer and on a tumor marker for liver cancer. He was a pioneer in the study of coagulation and the use of vitamin K and Coumadin. During his early career, he was a recognized expert on shock and burns. He was one of the first to use the sulfas for burns and peritonitis. Streptomycin became available just at the time he was diagnosed with advanced tuberculosis in 1946. Experience with damage to his own eighth nerve helped to define the toxicity of this drug. Although it cured his disease, it unfortunately left his balance impaired,[7] forcing him in his declining years to use a walker. Other subjects of his reports were thyroid and parathyroid disease, parotid tumors, portal hypertension, intestinal obstruction, hernia, biliary surgery, wound healing, inflammatory bowel disease, and pediatric surgery.

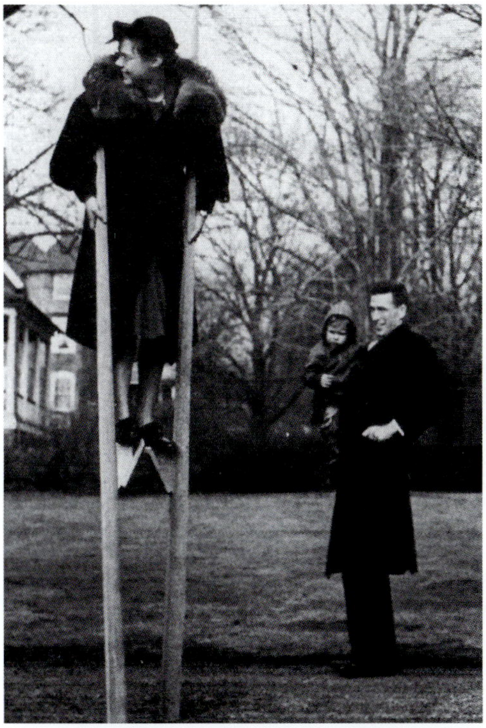

Send in the clowns—Terry in mid-air, Jonathan on the ground, 1942 (Apologies to Stephen Sondheim)

During World War II when Ravdin left HUP to command the 20th General Hospital in India, he left Rhoads in charge of his large service with only a skeleton crew of residents (including C. Everett Koop) to help him. After the war, I. S. Ravdin returned to HUP as department chairman. Rhoads settled into a role as second-in-command. This gave him the opportunity to focus on research and also to serve as provost of the University of Pennsylvania until 1959, when he succeeded Ravdin as chairman.

1935–1956
Rhoads was frequently ahead of his time. He carried out a hemodialysis in 1935, possibly the first. Because the patient died, Rhoads performed no more dialyses, but this case probably stimulated Willem Kolff, who is credited with pioneering this field

In 1936, he attempted a pancreatic islet cell transplant. Forty years later, this type of cellular transplant was successful in treatment of diabetes

1946
Rhoads is diagnosed with advanced tuberculosis and is hospitalized and out of work for almost a year

1956–1959
While he is University provost, an officer of Surgery's most important scientific societies, and writing the standard surgery textbook, Rhoads operates all day every Saturday to maintain control of his clinical practice

1959–1972
Chairman of Penn's Department of Surgery

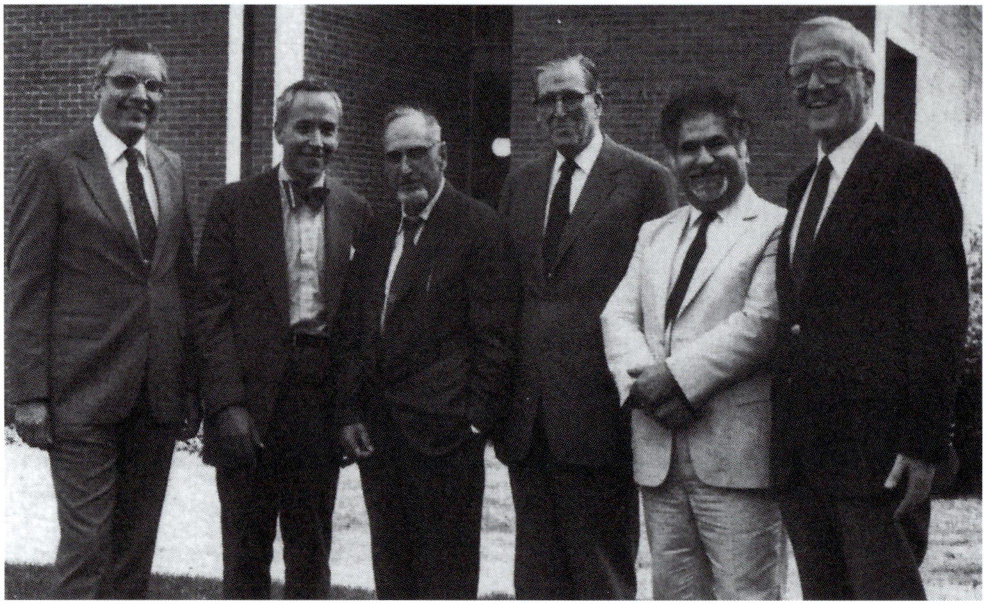

University of Pennsylvania provosts: (left to right) Curtis Reitz, Thomas Ehrlich, David Goddard, Jonathan E. Rhoads, Vartan Gregorian, and Elliot Stellar

From 1959 to 1972, Rhoads served as John Rhea Barton Professor and Chairman. During this period, he kept a number of other balls in the air.[8] In addition to departmental administration and his busy clinical practice, he was almost simultaneously president of the American College of Surgeons, president of the American Surgical Association, president of the American Cancer Society, chairman of the Board of Managers of Haverford College, and a member of the Residency Review Committee, the American Board of Surgery, the National Research Council, and the Philadelphia School Board. In addition, he was the editor of the *Annals of Surgery* and coauthor of the most widely read standard surgical textbook.

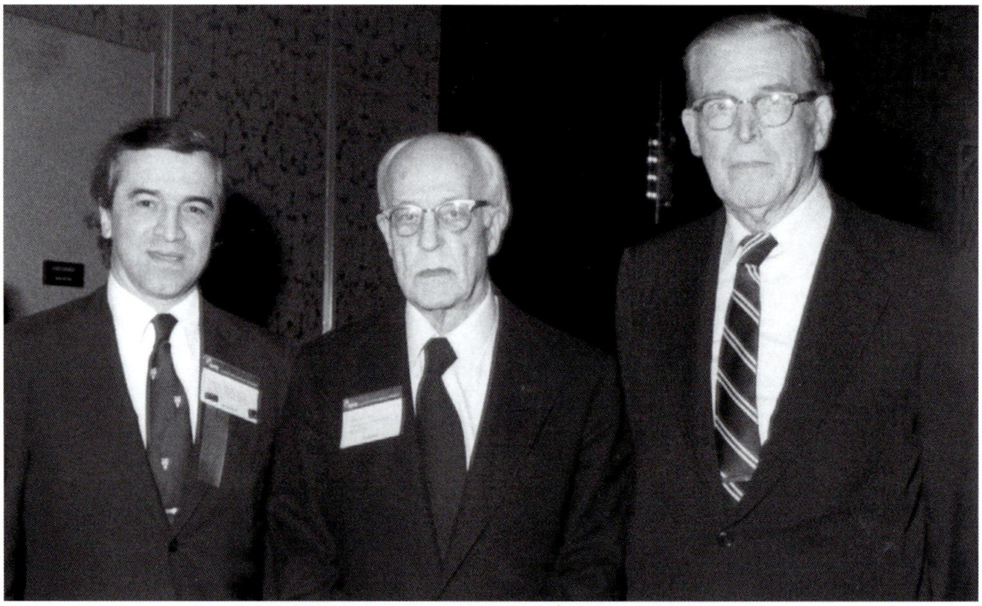

The team that developed Total Parenteral Nutrition (TPN)
Stan Dudrick, Harry Vars and Jonathan Rhoads

It was also during this time that Dr. Rhoads made his great research contribution—the development of total parenteral nutrition. The origin of his focus on nutrition was the long-term interest of Dr. Ravdin in this topic.[9] Together they had investigated the delayed gastric emptying seen after gastroenterostomy in malnourished patients and in dogs which they plasmaphoresed to produce hypoproteinemia. These studies were the stimulus for identifying appropriate diets and methods of dietary delivery to malnourished patients who were unable to eat.

1966
Landmark success of total parenteral nutrition

1966
Total parental feeding allows puppies to grow as well as oral feeding

1976
Philadelphia Award to Rhoads

In attempts to utilize the intravenous route for nutrition, several limitations were encountered. One was the volume of fluid necessary to provide adequate caloric intake without precipitating pulmonary edema. But if the concentration of the glucose solution was increased to provide more calories in smaller volumes, the infusate irritated and thrombosed peripheral veins.

The problem of delivering large volumes of hypertonic parenteral nutrients was taken to the laboratory. The crucial experiment was performed by Dr. Rhoads's research fellow, Stanley Dudrick, with the assistance of Harry Vars, the department's biochemist, who devised the formula of nutrients and a method of continuous intravenous infusion in puppies. These experimental animals, which received all of their nourishment parenterally via a catheter in the superior vena cava, were shown to grow as normally as those fed by mouth.[10]

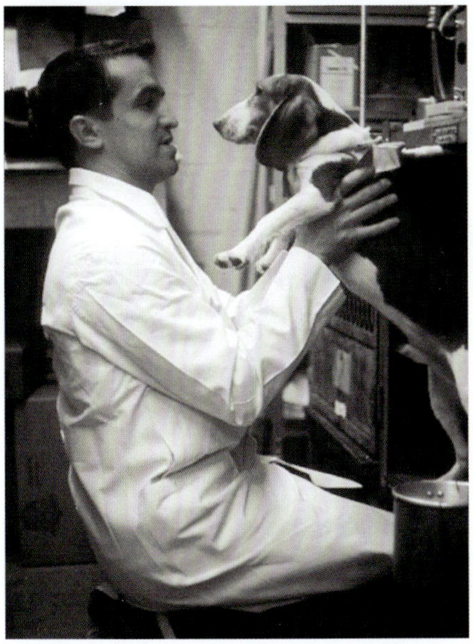

Stan Dudrick devotes his full time to care of the pups.

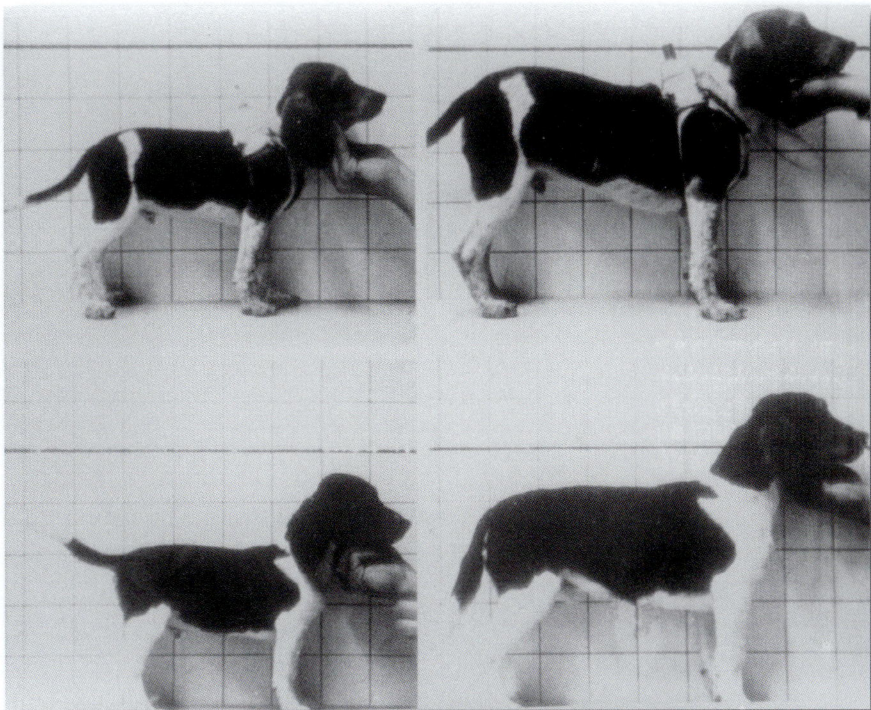

Puppies on IV feedings (top row) grow as well as their littermates fed normally (bottom row).

Because of the hyperosmolality of the parenteral solution, its delivery into peripheral veins of humans caused clotting and sclerosis. To solve the problem, Dudrick adopted a technique described by Aubaniac, a

1976–1984
President of American Philosophical Society

1960–1980
Rhoads is statesman of medicine and surgery

1980
A position he particularly enjoyed was as a member of the committee to chose the winner of the annual Sloan Kettering Prize. One of the perks was an annual loan of a new automobile of his choice. A lover of fast cars, he chose a variety ranging from a Porsche to an armored Hummer. Over the course of his career he acknowledged six crashes. Very few would ride with him a second time

French army surgeon, in which the subclavian vein was punctured percutaneously to gain access to the large central veins where high blood flow generally prevented clotting.[11] Thus, he succeeded in infusing highly concentrated solutions of glucose and large amounts of protein without causing venous thrombosis. Soon after this, Doug Wilmore and Dudrick successfully treated an infant with atresia of the jejunum, ileum, and distal colon.[12] Nourished entirely by vein, this baby not only gained weight but grew normally. As a result of these landmark reports, intravenous hyperalimentation was rapidly accepted and employed around the world. The success of these classic experiments in 1966 was the culmination of Dr. Rhoads's lifetime scientific obsession with perioperative nutrition. Francis Moore, the emeritus chief of the Peter Bent Brigham Hospital, ranked it with the most important scientific contributions ever made by a surgeon.[13]

As a statesman of science and medicine, Dr. Rhoads was known for his record of service to the National Research Council, the Public Health Service, Congress, and the Veterans Administration and as a consultant to several US presidents. His most important influence on behalf of federal support of cancer research came from membership on the panel of consultants on the conquest of cancer, whose recommendations led to the National Cancer Act of 1971.[14]

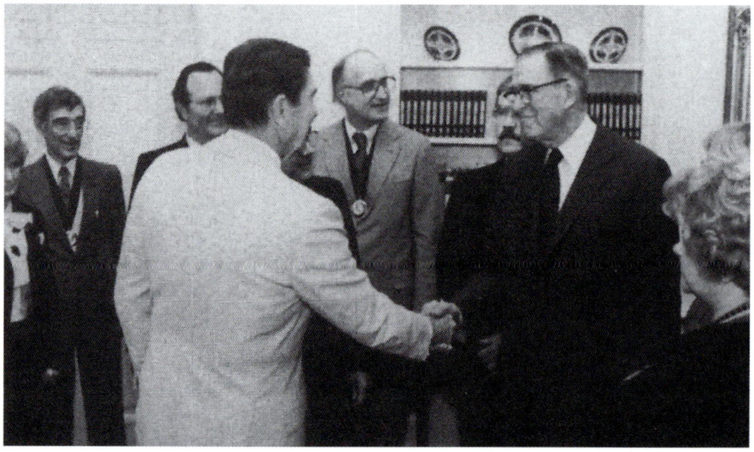

Jonathan Rhoads shaking hands with President Ronald Reagan

The esteem with which his colleagues regarded Dr. Rhoads was evidenced by the number of professional society officerships he held.[15] Those of which he was president or chairman included: the American College of Surgeons; American Cancer Society; American Philosophical Society; American Surgical Association; Society of Clinical Surgery; Society of Surgery of the Alimentary Tract; Surgical Infection Society; and Society of Surgical Chairmen. Many special awards came to him[16]: the Distinguished Service Award of the American Cancer Society; the Joseph Goldberger Award of the American Medical Society for Clinical Nutrition (with Stanley Dudrick); the Citation of the Association for Academic Surgery; the Roswell Park Medal; the American Cancer Society National Award; the Papanicolaou Award; the Medallion for Scientific Achievement and the Flance-Karl Award of the American Surgical Association; the Distinguished Service Award of the American Trauma Society; the Prix de la Société Internationale de Chirurgie; an Honorary Benjamin Franklin Fellowship of the Royal Society of Arts; the American

Medical Association's Sheen Award for Scientific Accomplishment; the Franklin Medal of the American Philosophical Society; the Medallion of the Surgeon General; and the Cosmos Club Award. Surgical colleges of nine nations honored Dr. Rhoads with memberships, and ten universities awarded him honorary degrees. Among the latter was the first Doctorate of Medical Science ever awarded by Yale. Its citation would have been an appropriate epitaph: *Jonathan Rhoads, Physician, Scientist, Educator, Editor, Civic Leader, Statesman and President of the American Philosophical Society, you are considered to be a clone of Benjamin Franklin, the founder of the University of Pennsylvania 250 years ago.*[17]

Dr. Rhoads's breadth extended well beyond the scope of the medical profession.[18] In addition to his service as provost of the University of Pennsylvania (1956–59), he served on the Board of Public Education of the city of Philadelphia and was on the trustee or executive committees of Bryn Mawr College, the Westtown School, and Haverford College. He served on the Council of the American Academy of Arts and Sciences.

Rhoads was perhaps even more proud of his record as an educator than of his research and honors. During his twelve years as department chairman, his residency program graduated sixty-two surgeons who have served as faculty members in thirty-four different medical schools, twenty-eight as full professors and eleven as departmental chairman.

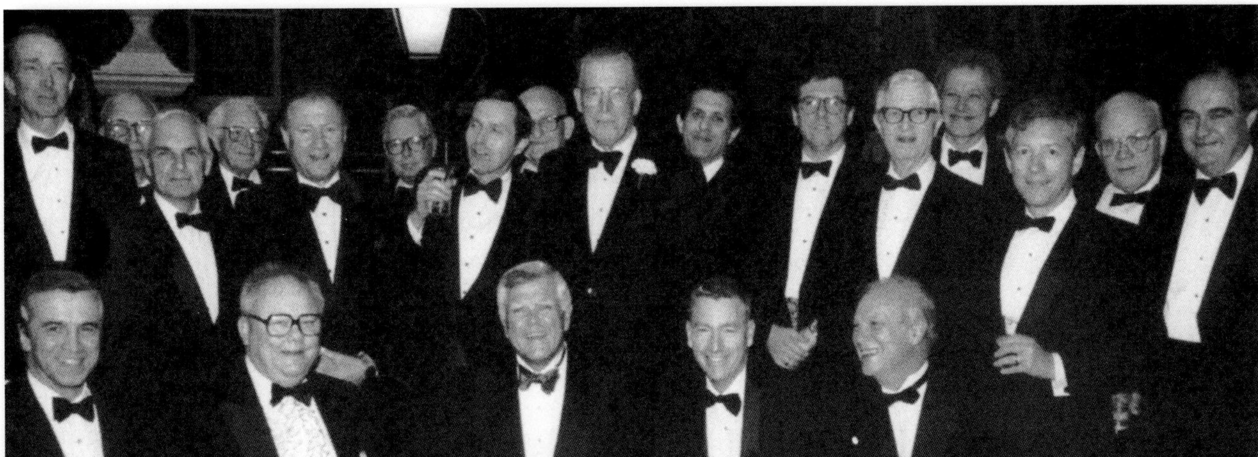

Jonathan Rhoads 80th birthday symposium speakers. Sadly, Rhoads's wife Terry died three days later.

1987
At his festschrift marking Rhoads's eightieth birthday, nineteen of America's leading surgeons speak, all of them trained by Ravdin or Rhoads. Almost 400 guests celebrate at a dinner the night before

Three days later, his wife Terry dies

1990
Marries Kitty Goddard, widow of past provost David Goddard

1990
Honorary degree from Yale, one of a total of ten honorary university degrees

After finishing as department chairman at age sixty-five, Dr. Rhoads pursued an active professional career for another three decades. Although he stopped operating at eighty, his other activities never decreased. His friend Wally Richie once speculated that he had made a pact with the devil that he could live forever if he continued to attend every meeting of his 139 professional societies.[19] This was apparently not true since he did attend all of the meetings, never accepted emeritus status, and continued to travel and work productively until a few weeks before his death at age ninety-four.

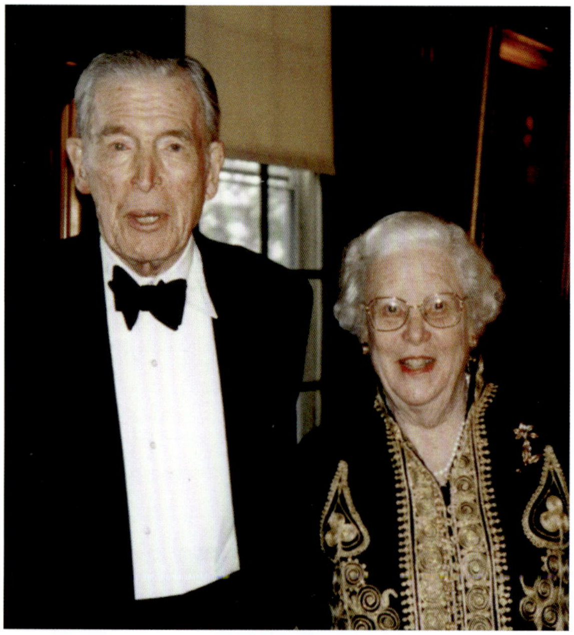

Jonathan and Kitty Rhoads

In 1987, Dr. Rhoads's marriage of fifty-one years ended with Terry's sudden death from heart failure. In 1990, he married Kathryn Evans Goddard. Kitty, like Terry, was a pediatrician and was the widow of David Goddard, who succeeded Rhoads as provost of the University of Pennsylvania. This prompted the comment by one wag that he only married pediatricians while she only married provosts. At the wedding, Rhoads admitted that he and his seventy-four-year-old bride were cousins but said with a twinkle in his eye that they were not worried about consanguinity.[20]

Dr. Rhoads was widely known during his early professional career and through the period of his chairmanship for his wisdom, self-discipline, and capacity for work, qualities that no doubt helped him to become such a successful academic surgeon. But the emphasis on these serious traits made him seem somewhat austere and aloof to his residents and young colleagues. In contrast, during his later decades when he was relieved of the pressures of the chairmanship, it became clear that the reserved persona for which he had been so well known was probably a well-studied façade.[21] As a college student, he had been known by his friends as a disruptive practical joker.[22] During a summer trip to Europe, his impulsiveness led him to jump in and swim the Bosporus (from Asia to Europe). Later, as he navigated the more treacherous waters of academic and political life, he found that a steadier style was necessary. During that time, his playful or unpredictable side was rarely seen. Only occasionally was there a glimpse of it, such as when he got behind the wheel of a fast automobile. He acknowledged six crashes, and very few would ride with him a second time.[23]

During the last three decades of his life, after the austere façade of his middle years faded, it seemed to his disciples that he became almost a different person. His humor was always dry, but there was no longer any missing it. While he had been considered a dull speaker, he now became an entertaining after-dinner raconteur and so sought after as a visiting lecturer that sixty-two of his sixty-eight visiting professorships came after his department chairmanship.[24] He also turned his giant intellect to cataloging a library of jokes (many of them ribald) and one liners that he would pull off with perfect timing.

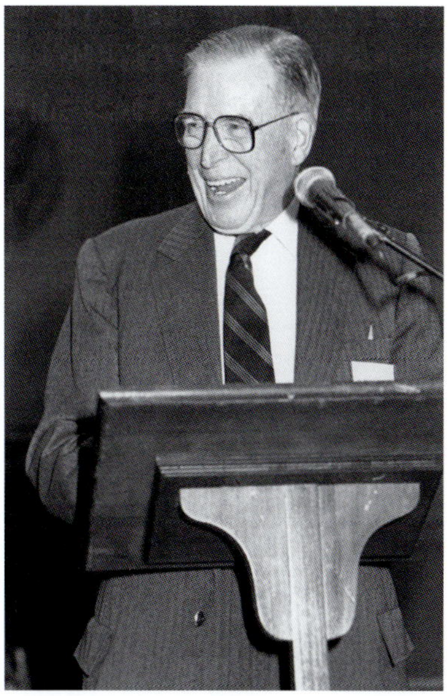

1992–2002
He catalogues a library of jokes and one liners that he pulls off with perfect timing

1997
At age ninety, Rhoads is still active, traveling, speaking, and serving on committees

To the end of his life, Dr. Rhoads was a master committee man and administrator. After he could no longer call on the intrinsic power of chairmanships and presidencies, it was an educational experience to watch him work his magic at a scientific meeting or even more so in a committee or board meeting. One will never know whether it was a humorous con on his part that he would appear to be sleeping throughout a lengthy presentation at a scientific conference or committee meeting

The colossus at the opening of HUP's Rhoads Pavilion (1994).

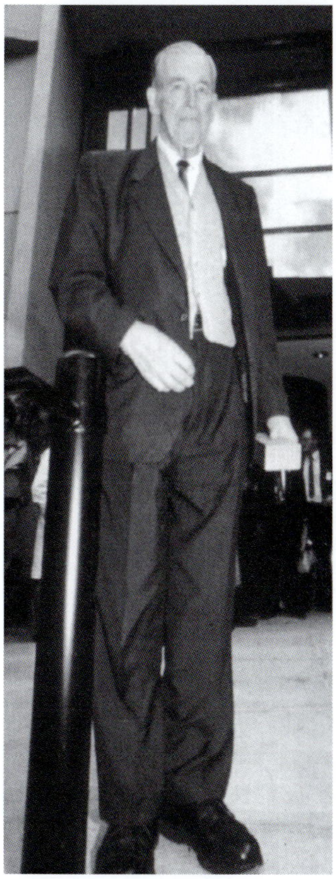

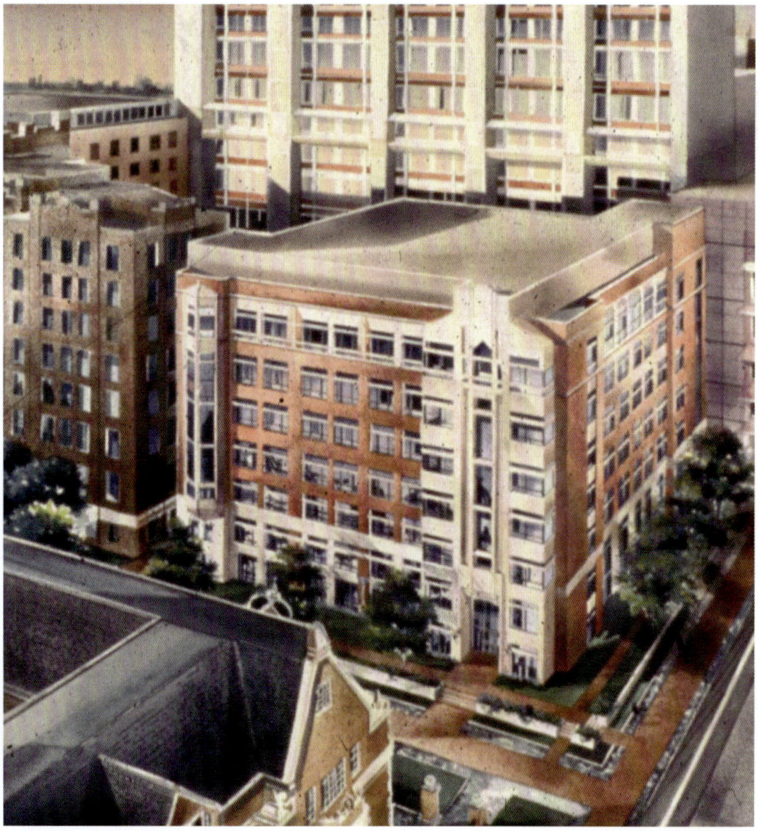

2002
Rhoads dies at age ninety-four

debate. Then at the appropriate moment, he would "awake" with a start, ask the perfect question, or summarize the pros and cons of the debated issue in such a way that he got the decision he was after. I think he knew exactly what he was doing. He was never asleep![25] Many of his disciples have tried to copy this maneuver as well as other aspects of his remarkable career—but rarely with success. Jonathan Rhoads was unique.

During his final illness from gastric cancer, Dr. Rhoads's courage and consideration for others were apparent. He had decided that whatever the cost in personal comfort, he would continue for as long as possible to be useful to his family, his institutions, and his colleagues. He carried on with a virtually full schedule of meetings, travel, and correspondence until a few days before his death. It was especially fitting that the extension of his life by several months (which he greatly valued) was made possible after he could no longer eat by total intravenous nutrition,[26] a treatment he and his colleagues had devised. It was also appropriate that his last days were spent in the hospital pavilion which the University of Pennsylvania had named for him[27] and that he was under the care of a group of physicians which included members of his department and his own family.

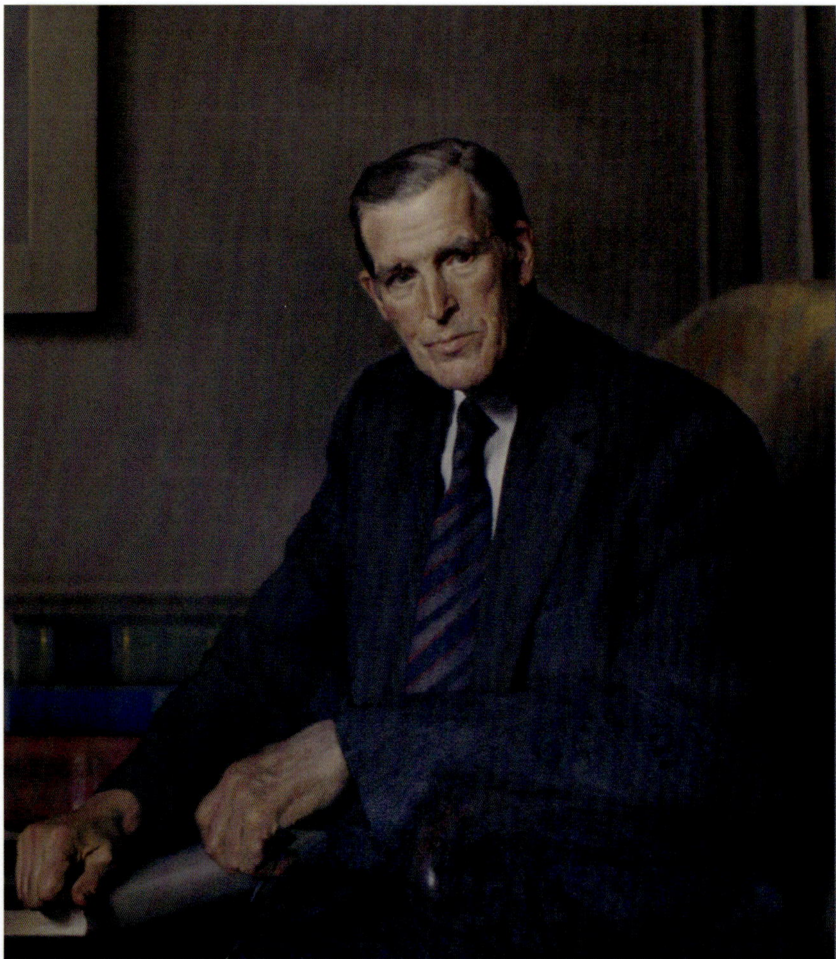

Timeline of Events During the Career of Jonathan Rhoads

1927	During college vacation, Rhoads tours Europe and swims the Bosporus.
1928	Rhoads graduates from Haverford College, is star of the track team.
1932	Rhoads obtains his MD from Johns Hopkins.
1936	Rhoads marries his medical school classmate, Terry Folin.
1933–1934	Rhoads serves two-year rotating internship at HUP.
1934–1939	Rhoads has surgical fellowship under I. S. Ravdin.
1935	Rhoads does research on intestinal obstruction with Miller-Abbott tube and early use of sulfanilamide; carries out peritoneal and hemodialysis, perhaps the first.
1936	Department receives $2.7 million Harrison endowment for research.
1936	Frazier dies; Eliason appointed chairman.
1937	American Board of Surgery founded.
1938	Rhoads studies vitamin K and coagulation system.
1939	Rhoads finishes HUP residency; research in shock and burns.
1940	Rhoads operates on his chief, I. S. Ravdin, for cholecystitis. Eliason and Whipple assist.
1940–1942	At Ravdin's suggestion, Rhoads becomes Walter Estell Lee's assistant and spends most of his time at Graduate Hospital.
1941–1945	The United States participates in World War II.
1943–1945	Ravdin is in India as commander of 20th General Hospital.
1942–1945	As a Quaker, Rhoads declines Army service. Is declared essential to HUP, serves in the "Battle of Spruce Street." In charge of Ravdin's 100-bed service with only residents Zintel and Koop to help him.
1946	Ravdin returns from military service and becomes John Rhea Barton Professor and Chairman; gets rid of faculty trained by Eliason except for Johnson who was with him in India; revises HUP surgical residency to emulate Halsted's.
1946	Rhoads is diagnosed with advanced tuberculosis, hospitalized for most of a year, eventually cured by streptomycin.
1946–1960	Nutrition research with Ravdin and series of HUP residents.
1956–1959	Rhoads is University provost.
1960	Ravdin becomes vice president of the University, Rhoads succeeds him as chief of surgery.

1960–1972	As chairman, Rhoads trains sixty-two residents, eleven become chairmen of university departments.
1960–1972	Rhoads is elected president of American College of Surgeons, American Surgical Association, American Cancer Society, and most surgical societies.
1966	Success of hyperalimentation studies by Rhoads, Dudrick, Vars, and Wilmore.
1966	Ravdin suffers memory loss, retires.
1972	Rhoads retires as chairman of surgery; succeeded by William Fitts.
1976–1984	President of American Philosophical Society.
1987	Eightieth birthday symposium, his wife Terry dies suddenly three days later.
1990	Marries Kitty Goddard.
2002	Death from gastric cancer at age ninety-four.

Notes

[1] Rombeau, John and Muldoon, Donna. *Quaker Sense and Sensibility in the World of Surgery* (Philadelphia: Hanley and Belfus Inc: 1997) p. 7.

[2] Ibid., p. 72.

[3] Ibid., p. 115.

[4] Conversation with Bob Ravdin.

[5] Barker, Clyde F. Jonathan Rhoads, MD. *Annals of Surgery* (2002 May) 235 (5) p. 741.

[6] Ibid., p. 741.

[7] Ibid., p. 741.

[8] Barker, Clyde F. Jonathan E. Rhoads, 9 May 1907 · 3 January 2002. *Proceedings of the American Philosophical Society,* vol. 149, no. 3, American Philosophical Society (2005) p. 435.

[9] Barker, Clyde F. Jonathan Rhoads, MD. *Annals of Surgery*, pp. 741–742.

[10] Barker, Clyde F. Jonathan E. Rhoads, 9 May 1907 · 3 January 2002. *Proceedings of the American Philosophical Society*, p. 434.

[11] Barker, Clyde F. Jonathan Rhoads, MD. *Annals of Surgery*, p. 742.

[12] Wilmore, DW and Dudrick, SJ. Growth and development of an infant receiving all nutrients exclusively by vein. *JAMA* 203: 142, 1968.

[13] Barker, Clyde F and Daly, John M, eds. *Jonathan E. Rhoads Eightieth Birthday Symposium* (Philadelphia: J. B. Lippincott Co, 1989) pp. 249–250.

[14] Barker, Clyde F. Jonathan E. Rhoads, 9 May 1907 · 3 January 2002. *Proceedings of the American Philosophical Society*, p. 435.

[15] Barker, Clyde F. Jonathan Rhoads, MD. *Annals of Surgery*, p. 742.

[16] Ibid., p. 742.

[17] Barker, Clyde F. Jonathan E. Rhoads, 9 May 1907 · 3 January 2002. *Proceedings of the American Philosophical Society*, p. 436.

[18] Ibid., p. 436.

[19] Conversation with Wally Richie.

[20] Conversations with Jonathan Rhoads.

[21] Barker, Clyde and Warshaw, Andrew. Jonathan E. Rhoads, 1907–2002. *Surgery* (2003) 133:133–4.

[22] Ibid.

[23] Barker, Clyde F. Jonathan E. Rhoads, 9 May 1907 · 3 January 2002. *Proceedings of the American Philosophical Society,* p. 437.

[24] Barker, Clyde F. Jonathan Rhoads, MD. *Annals of Surgery,* p. 744.

[25] Barker, Clyde and Warshaw, Andrew. Jonathan E. Rhoads, 1907–2002. *Surgery* (2003) 133:133–4.

[26] Barker, Clyde F. Jonathan Rhoads, MD. *Annals of Surgery,* p. 744.

[27] Ibid., p. 744.

CHAPTER 20

HUP Chief Residents During Dr. Rhoads's Chairmanship: A Generation of Leaders

Despite Jonathan Rhoads's prominence as a clinician, administrator, and surgical scientist, his impact as a mentor of young surgeons was probably more important. During his twelve years as a department chairman, his residency program graduated sixty-two surgeons who would serve as faculty members in thirty-four different medical schools, twenty-eight as full professors and eleven as department chairmen.

1959–60 **Davis, Arnold V. O.**

Dexheimer, Frank R. BA University of Missouri; MD University of Pennsylvania; practiced in his hometown of Columbia, Missouri; died 2012.

Gyorgy, Tilbert R. BA Dartmouth University; MD Harvard Medical School; assistant chief of surgery at the Veteran's Administration Hospital at Togus, Maine, for ten years. Commander in the US Naval Reserve. Father was chief of pediatrics at HUP and won National Medal of Science for discovery of eight vitamins. Died 1978.

Muir, William R. MD Columbia University; practiced in Lumberton, New Jersey; founder of residency program at Burlington County Memorial Hospital and for twenty-five years chair of department of surgery; in retirement, served in Indian Health Service in Shipwreck, New Mexico; died 2021.

Orr, Jack T. MD Columbia University; chief of surgery at Danbury Hospital (CT); started and directed residency program; died 1992.

Wolferth, Charles C. Jr. BA Yale University; MD University of Pennsylvania; all but a few months of residency was under Ravdin. Important trauma surgeon; spearheaded law that created Pennsylvania trauma system's foundation that monitored hospitals' quality of trauma care; this foundation served as a model for the other states;

president of Philadelphia Academy of Surgery and the Philadelphia chapter of the American College of Surgeons; chairman of surgery at Hahnemann University Hospital, Graduate Hospital, and Presbyterian Hospital. Died 2005.

Akin, John M. Jr. Like his father, a graduate of Penn Medical School; an exemplary HUP resident, Julian Johnson bragged that John lost thirty pounds while on his service. Returned to his native Birmingham where he became president of the County Medical Society, vice president of the Medical Association of Alabama, and president of the Birmingham Academy of Medicine. Clinical professor of surgery at the Medical College of Alabama and for fourteen years, program director of the Baptist Health System residency. Died 2013. **1960–61**

Hood, Frederick R. Jr. Born in Oklahoma of Cherokee ancestry; graduated from Oklahoma University; MD University of Pennsylvania; interned at University of Michigan; practiced general and thoracic surgery in Oklahoma and Anchorage, Alaska; died 2011.

Inouye, William Y. MD University of Pennsylvania; invented coil dialyzer that served as model for Kolff's; important HUP faculty member; see Chapter 34; died 1985.

Light, Harry G. MD Jefferson University; practiced in New Jersey; died 2017.

Patterson, Lewis T. MD University of Pennsylvania; chief of surgery at Harrisburg Hospital; for many years, highly regarded mentor of HUP residents rotating on his service. His wife, Phyllis, was I. S. Ravdin's scrub nurse.

Smart, Charles R. Born in Ogden, UT; graduate of University of Utah and Temple Medical School; at seventeen, enlisted in Army, serving during World War II; worked as cowboy breaking wild horses on ranch of a distant cousin of mine in Idaho, married his boss's daughter, Dorothia Sharp; oncology fellow and faculty member at UCLA; ten years as chief of surgery at LDS Hospital in Salt Lake City; five years as director of Cancer Division of ACS; grandfather of Elizabeth Smart (kidnapping victim). Died 2006.

Danielson, Gordon K. Julian Johnson's first postresidency fellow. After fellowship at the Karolinska in Stockholm, HUP faculty member for two years. Markle Scholar. Succeeded Frank Spencer as chief of cardiac surgery at University of Kentucky. In 1967, recruited to the Mayo Clinic where he became chairman of cardiovascular surgery. Performed the Mayo Clinic's first coronary artery bypass procedures. Recipient of many awards and author of 800 publications. Died 2017. **1961–62**

Johnson, LeRoy L. MD University of Kansas; practiced general and vascular surgery in Ames, Iowa; two years research on portal hypertension with Jerry Peskin; rated as best HUP resident; declined HUP faculty offer; died 2015.

Kessler, Frederick B. Hand surgery fellowship in New York City with William Littler at Rosefeld Hospital; clinical professor of surgery at Baylor; founded hand fellowship at St. Luke's and Texas Children's Hospital; trained 140 hand surgeons in Houston.

Nightingale, David S. Practice of general and thoracic surgery in Louisville, Kentucky.

Timmis, Hilary H. As HUP resident, did research with Blakemore on artificial heart valves. Recruited by Jim Hardy to University of Mississippi; was prominent member of Hardy's faculty and coauthor on many publications on the first heart and lung transplants and other pioneering heart and vascular surgery. Later moved to his native Michigan where he practiced cardiac surgery at Beaumont Hospital in Royal York. Died 2018.

1962–63 **Barnes, Anne U.** Practiced general surgery in Philadelphia for forty-four years; professor of anatomy at Drexel University. Died 2012.

Berggren, Ronald B. BA Johns Hopkins University; MD University of Pennsylvania; director of division of plastic surgery at Ohio State University Medical Center and Nationwide (Columbus) Children's Hospital.

Crichlow, Robert W. BA Haverford College; MD University of Pennsylvania; assistant to associate professor at University of Pennsylvania (1963–1972); chairman of department of surgery at Dartmouth (1980–1995); largely responsible for establishment of Dartmouth as a four-year MD-granting school; president of New England Surgical Society and Eastern Surgical Society; died 2012.

Heisterkamp, Charles A. Graduate of Penn Medical School, finished HUP residency as chief at Lancaster General Hospital. During Vietnam War, commanded surgical research team of the Walter Reed Army Institute of Research at a mobile research hospital. Established and directed the biomedical engineering program in the research and development command of the US Surgeon General where he set up national trauma treatment protocols. Served as commander of the 103rd Medical Battalion of the 28th Infantry Division. Consultant on computers for the Australian and Canadian governments. Chairman of the emergency medical council in Lancaster County and medical commander of the Lancaster County civil defense during the Three Mile Island crisis. Died 2012.

Jannetta, Peter J. HUP general surgery resident, UCLA neurosurgery fellowship; devised cure of tic douloureux; chairman of neurosurgery at University of Pittsburgh (1971–1996); see Chapter 34; died 2016.

Nelson, Harry M. Jr. BA Carlton College; MD Wayne State University; Brooke Roberts' first vascular fellow; practiced vascular surgery in Norristown, Pennsylvania; president of Eastern Pennsylvania Chapter of the American College of Surgeons. Died 2013.

Barker, Clyde F. Chairman of department of surgery, University of Pennsylvania (1983–2001); see Chapter 27. **1963–64**

Hardesty, William H. MD University of Pennsylvania; practice of general and vascular surgery in New Jersey and Yardley, Pennsylvania; died 2020.

MacVaugh III, Horace CT fellowship with Julian Johnson; After several years as Johnson's successor, left HUP to direct CT programs at Lankenau and then Graduate Hospital; died 2021.

Miller, Leonard D. Chairman of department of surgery, University of Pennsylvania (1975–1978); see Chapter 23. Died 1997.

Myint, Maung Kyaw. Finished HUP residency at Jeanes Hospital. CT fellow UCLA; Practiced thoracic surgery in LA. Highly ranked nationally in tennis at 90.

Hartzell, George W. Practice at Lehigh Valley Medical Center, Allentown, Pennsylvania. **1964–65**

Johnson, Charles J. Assistant professor, University of Wisconsin; died 2012.

Spagna, Paschal M. CT fellowship under Julian Johnson; Chief of CT surgery at Graduate Hospital; died 1992.

Talman, E. Armistead Native of Virginia, graduate of University of Virginia medical school. Practiced in Richmond, clinical professor of surgery at Medical College of Virginia. President of Virginia Surgical Society and Eastern Surgical Society; died 2018.

Hamilton, Ralph W. Plastic surgery training under Henry Royster. HUP faculty for twenty-nine years, professor and associate chief of division. With Bugs Lehr, did research on organ preservation by freezing. Expert in head and neck cancer surgery as well as in cosmetic and reconstructive surgery; died 2019. **1965–66**

Nance, F. Carter. MD University of Tennessee; long-term professor at LSU; nationally prominent trauma surgeon; later chairman of surgery at St. Barnabas in New Jersey; president of Association of Surgery for Trauma.

Reis, Robert L. After HUP residency and CT fellowship, served as senior surgeon and deputy chief of cardiac surgery at NIH. Then chief of cardiothoracic surgery at the University of Kansas, where he developed one of the first artificial heart valves. In 1976, moved to Coral Gables, Florida, and started the cardiac surgery program at Cedars Medical Center (now University of Miami hospital). Died 2021.

Rosato, Francis E. Chairman of surgery at Eastern Virginia University (1975–78) and then chairman at Jefferson (1978–2000); died 2006.

1966–67 **Dudrick, Stanley J.** With Rhoads, developed parenteral hyperalimentation; Distinguished Graduate Award of the department of surgery; see Chapter 35; died 2020.

Jones, Rayford Scott. BA University of Texas, MD University of Texas Medical Branch; chairman of surgery at University of Virginia (1982–2001); president of ACS and American Surgical Association; Distinguished Graduate Award of the department of surgery; see Chapter 35.

Kaplan, Edwin L. BA and MD University of Pennsylvania; professor at University of Chicago. World-respected endocrine surgeon. President of American Association of Endocrine Surgeons, Chicago Surgical Society, and Metropolitan Chapter of the American College of Surgeons.

Noto, Joseph A. General and thoracic surgery practice in Damascus, Oregon, and Asheville, North Carolina.

Weiner, Leonard J. After HUP residency, spent a year as a transplantation research fellow at the Wistar Institute with Rupert Billingham. Faculty at Louisville, Kentucky in plastic surgery. The university has endowed a chair of plastic surgery in his name.

1967–68 **Boruchow, Irwin B.** Graduate of Wharton School in 1954; MD Georgetown University 1962; CT training at the University of Florida. Assistant professor of surgery at the University of Florida and chief of CT surgery at the VA hospital in Gainesville; from 1973, practiced CT surgery at St. Francis Hospital and Mt. Sinai Medical Center in Miami. Died 2009.

Curreri, P. William. As a resident, was influenced by Bill Fitts to enter the trauma field. For several years at the US Army burn unit in San Antonio, worked under Basil Pruitt and John Moncrief; moved to the University of Texas where he worked with Tom Shires in the trauma unit, later following him to Seattle and Cornell. As a trauma and burn surgeon, became prominent for metabolic studies. President of the American Association for the Surgery of Trauma and winner of the Curtis Artz Award from the Trauma Society. Served as president of the Society of University Surgeons. Chairman of surgery of the University of South Alabama, in Mobile. In the last part of his career, became the chairman of Stratagem Inc., a company that consulted and helped academic surgery programs.

Neiby, C. Paul. Practice in Sierra Madre, California.

Rosato, Ernest F. MD University of Pennsylvania; chief of GI surgery at HUP; see Chapter 33. Died 2012.

Tyers, G. Frank Professor emeritus department of surgery University of British Columbia, former head of the divisions of CT surgery at BC Children's Hospital and British Columbia Institute of Technology. Surgical training at HUP and CHOP, and CT surgical residency at Toronto General Hospital. Expert on treatment of arrhythmias, cardiac pacing, and electrophysiology. Pioneer of biventricular pacing and telemetry systems for implantable cardiac devices. Associate professor at Penn State University Medical Center, professor and head of CT surgery at University of Texas Medical Branch; professor and head of division of CT surgery at the University of British Columbia; member of twenty-seven national and international academic societies, including the American Surgical Association. Authored 230 papers and twenty-six books.

Vibul, Santi. Practice of CT surgery in Evansville, Indiana.

Berkowitz, Henry B. During residency, highly regarded research on angiotensin with Leonard Miller; vascular fellowship with Brooke Roberts; gifted surgeon with largest vascular surgery practice at HUP; later, chief of vascular surgery at Presbyterian Hospital. **1968–69**

Copeland III, Edward M. MD Cornell University; chairman of department of surgery at the University of Florida (1982–2003); president of Society of Surgical Oncology and Halsted Society; president of American College of Surgeons; chairman of the American Board of Surgery; Distinguished Graduate Award; see Chapter 35.

Hanson, Victor A. MD University of Pennsylvania; practice of surgery in Atlanta, Georgia.

Knecht, James W. Graduate of the University of Chicago where he earned a BS and was a member of the fencing team. MD University of Chicago as Alpha Omega Alpha (AOA). Practiced general and vascular surgery in Monmouth County, New Jersey, for fifty-five years and was chairman of surgery at the Jersey Shore University Medical

Center. He played the violin for the Monmouth Symphony Orchestra for forty-six seasons. Died in 2017.

Park, C. Dick. Graduate of Penn Medical School, HUP residency, CT fellowship under Julian Johnson. HUP and CHOP faculty (1970–1973). Practiced CT surgery in Tidewater region of Virginia for thirty-seven years until death in 2016.

Pierce, William S. As a Penn medical student, HUP resident, and CT fellow, built his first models of an artificial heart. In 1970, appointed to faculty of Penn State University where he designed and built the most advanced artificial pump in the world, approved by the FDA in 1980 and in 1985, successfully applied as a bridge for cardiac transplantation. Also developed fully implantable pump named the Lionheart, first implanted in patients in 2001. Member of all important surgical societies and the National Academy of Medicine. Among his many awards are the Jacobson Innovation award of the American College of Surgeons and the Distinguished Graduate Award of the Penn School of Medicine.

1969–70 **Diaco, Joseph F.** Sports medicine expert; surgeon for Tampa Bay Buccaneers.

Lundy, Barbara S. Did research with Bugs Lehr during residency.

Noble, Raymond. Practiced in Wilmington, Delaware.

Reber, Howard A. Professor and head of GI surgery at UCLA; Distinguished Graduate Award of department of surgery. See Chapter 35.

Saik, Richard P. Prominent colleague of Marshall Orloff at UCSD in his emergency portacaval shunt program; practice in La Jolla, California.

1970–71 **Appel, Sidney D.** Participant with Bugs Lehr in kidney-freezing research; practice in Georgia.

Attkiss, Michael J. Practiced at North Shore University Hospital. Member of teaching faculty at Cornell Medical College and Albert Einstein College of Medicine.

Finnegan, James After second year residency, volunteered for Marine Corps as combat surgeon in Vietnam. During the enemy siege of Khe Sanh, he commanded a surgical team which treated 2,500 wounded Marines; sustained shrapnel wounds, and was awarded Purple Heart and Bronze Star with combat V for valor; returning to HUP, finished residency and CT fellowship under Julian Johnson; subsequently served as chief of CT surgery at Medical College of Pennsylvania, St.

Agnes, and Crozier Chester Medical Center. Died from metastatic melanoma in 2013.

Noone, R. Barrett. MD 1965 University of Pennsylvania; after general surgery training, completed plastic surgery residency at HUP; Past chair of department of surgery at Bryn Mawr Hospital; first chair of plastic surgery at Main Line Health; first executive director of the American Board of Plastic Surgery; more than 100 publications including two books; 2013 Honorary Award of the American Association of Plastic Surgeons; 2012 Trustees Special Achievement Award from the American Society of Plastic Surgeons.

Perloff, Leonard J. BA and MD University of Pennsylvania; Prominent HUP faculty. See Chapter 33. Died 1993.

Seltzer, Murray H. MD University of Pennsylvania; breast cancer research HUP 1968–69; Major in US Army Medical Corp, Fort Dix, New Jersey, 1971–73; clinical professor of surgery at University of Medicine and Dentistry of New Jersey 1986–2010; medical director of the breast center at St. Barnabas Medical Center 1997–99; chairman surgery section Medical Society of New Jersey 1982; president of American Society for Parenteral and Enteral Nutrition 1980–81; faculty member Rutgers; sixty-three peer-reviewed articles; numerous chapters, abstracts, and other contributions.

Staroscik, Rudolf N. Prominent Penn faculty mentor of residents as chief of surgery at Jeanes Hospital.

Wilmore, Douglas W. With Dudrick, Rhoads, and Vars, pioneered TPN (see chapter 34); After several years at the US Army Institute of Research in San Antonio, moved to Boston and became highly regarded for classic publications on glutamine and other metabolic studies as Harvard's Frank Sawyer Professor at the Brigham. President of Society of University Surgeons. Member of American Academy of Medicine, Society of Clinical Surgery, and many important surgical societies. Retired to Kauai, Hawaii, where he continues to study the effects of pesticides.

Agnew, Robert F. Practice in Fargo, North Dakota. **1971–72**

Allen, Terry R. Vascular training and faculty at Vanderbilt.

Coller, John A. Colorectal surgeon at the Lahey Clinic.

Friedman, Jerald N. MD Tufts University; practice of general and vascular surgery in Easton, Pennsylvania. Died 2017.

Long III, James M. Faculty at University of Texas Medical School at Houston.

Lynch, Dennis J. MD Georgetown University; fellowship in plastic surgery at HUP. Past chairman of department of surgery at Texas A&M and Scott White Clinic, Temple, Texas.

Nicholas, Gary G. Vascular fellow with Brooke Roberts. After ten productive years at Penn State, Hershey, as chief of vascular surgery, moved to Allentown's Lehigh Valley Hospital as director of surgical education. Died 2007.

Silberman, Howard. HUP transplant fellowship; professor and long-term faculty at USC in Oncology Division. One of my earliest transplant fellows.

CHAPTER 21

Graduate Education for Surgeons: Failure of a Worthy Experiment

From 1919 to 1964, the University of Pennsylvania carried out an interesting experiment in medical education. The department of surgery was very active in this. The Graduate Hospital played a vital role in the development of several of the department's important leaders.

The University's self-serving interpretation of the 1910 Flexner report was that, unlike many of the medical schools of the day, Penn was just fine. Closer examination indicated that this was not true. Penn was not specifically criticized but received no praise for its academic and research programs.[1] The University's provost, Edgar Fahs Smith, conceived a response to Flexner's implied critique. His idea was to provide a course for additional didactic teaching of medical school graduates.[2] He anticipated that with further education, especially in the basic sciences, young Penn doctors would be attracted to research and that this would strengthen Penn's academic image. Although it was not the reason for Smith's proposal, it happened that when the Graduate School came to fruition in 1919, it was just in time for the re-education of doctors returning from World War I, especially if their medical school education had been abbreviated by their military service. It was also a time when there were not enough positions in residency programs to accommodate the backlog of candidates applying. Popularity of the course was further enhanced by the willingness of the government to pay for tuition through the GI Bill and agreement of the specialty boards to count time in the Graduate School course toward accreditation.

The curriculum for the two-year Graduate School course was designed by Julius Comroe.[3] It was organized not around departmental silos but instead around organ systems and how basic science explained their physiology and diseases. The faculty was made up of experts from the basic sciences and from clinical disciplines, including surgery. Those who took the course evaluated it as superb. Other medical schools such as Case Western Reserve copied it for their basic medical school curriculum.

The greatest success of the Graduate School course occurred during the periods following World War I and World War II. At its peak, 300 students enrolled, most of them returning veterans. The quality of the course was enhanced by the excellence of the faculty which approached and, in some areas, exceeded the quality of the undergraduate medical school.

Several of the Graduate School faculty were superstars. Julius Comroe was chief of the Graduate School's department of physiology and pharmacology, a position this scientific prodigy had acquired at age thirty-five. Comroe obtained his MD from Penn in 1934 as first in his class. After his HUP internship in 1946 to 1947, he planned to train in surgery. Unfortunately, an infection in his eye and its delayed treatment led to loss of the eye, ending his ambition for surgery.[4] In 1946, he joined Carl Schmidt's Department of Pharmacology. There he worked with the department of surgery's Robert Dripps, producing many classic papers in heart and lung physiology.[5] With Carl Schmidt, he also did important work defining the pressure and chemo receptors of the carotid body.[6] In 1957, as the Graduate School lost support, Comroe moved to the University of California at San Francisco as head of its Institute for Cardiovascular Diseases. He helped convert this somewhat unimportant new school to its present stardom.

Seymour Kety was another Graduate School faculty star.[7] He devised a method for measuring cerebral blood flow. After college and medical school at Penn, he interned at Philadelphia General Hospital in 1940. He was renowned as a superb teacher who could make any topic and its story sound like a marvelous adventure. Several times, Penn medical students dedicated their yearbook to him. His first research was in discovering a cure for lead poisoning by administrating citrate, which after chelation, allowed elimination in the urine.[8] He then became interested in genetic factors of schizophrenia. In 1961, his innovations in this area were so spectacular that he was named chairman of psychiatry at Johns Hopkins.[9] Having never trained in psychiatry, he found this experience unrewarding and resigned after a year. Returning to his research on cerebral circulation with Carl Schmidt in the department of pharmacology, in 1999 he received the Lasker Award.

In 1916, a clinical facility for the Graduate School faculty had been built. It turned out to be one of Philadelphia's most important major hospitals of the next several decades. Located at Lombard Street between 18th and 19th Streets, it eventually had 497 beds.[10] Its surgical staff was a mixture of young doctors just starting out and seasoned practitioners like Walter Estell Lee, who had the largest surgical practice in town. In surgery, the Graduate Hospital staff was used something like a farm team. When Dr. Ravdin finished his residency in 1918, he was sent by John B. Deaver for seasoning at the Graduate Hospital as George Muller's assistant.[11] After several years of this experience, Frazier called Ravdin back to HUP as his right-hand man. When Jonathan Rhoads finished his residency in 1939, he was sent by Ravdin for three years at Graduate Hospital as Walter Estell Lee's assistant.[12] He was then called back to HUP to manage the Ravdin service during World War II while Ravdin was in India.

Many other prominent surgeons practiced at Graduate Hospital or at least had appointments on the Graduate School faculty and gave lectures in its course. Those who served in turn as chairman of the Graduate School's department of surgery included Walter Estell Lee, Herbert Hawthorne, William Erb, Kraeer Ferguson, and George Muller. Robert Groff was chief of neurosurgery at Graduate and then came back to HUP as chairman of the department. John Carnett was director of HUP's World War I Army hospital in France. After being denied a faculty position at HUP by Deaver, he became chairman of surgery at Graduate.[13] Isadore Cohn, Charles Wolferth, and Paul Nemir also worked at Graduate. Bill Blakemore became chief of surgery at Graduate Hospital, leaving HUP with the understanding that when Dr. Rhoads retired, he would become the medical school's chairman of surgery.[14] This never happened, but while he was at Graduate, Blakemore participated with Moreye Nusbaum and radiology's Stanley Baum on the breakthrough studies with catheterization of mesenteric arteries to stop bleeding.[15] This turned out to be the birth of endovascular surgery.

After its peak during the post-World War II era, enthusiasm for the Graduate School and its hospital gradually waned. The backlog of war veterans requiring residency positions dropped. The largest number of students then became foreign graduates rather than US veterans, diminishing the support of the medical school administrators and faculty.

In the early 1950s, specialty boards withdrew their approval of credit given for the Graduate School's courses. Grants became more readily available for basic scientists in the undergraduate medical schools where research was booming. Advanced clinical and basic science training were done in residency programs in hospitals connected to undergraduate medical schools. Time seemed to have passed the Graduate School by. It won a reprieve by attracting more foreign students, but because of language difficulties, this reprieve was short-lived. The upshot was that in 1964, the faculty of the Graduate School was officially merged with that of the undergraduate medical school, and the famous Graduate School course ceased to be given.[16]

Graduate Hospital remained open for several decades. Chiefs of surgery in this era included Penn-trained Charles Wolferth and Paul Nemir. The hospital began to lose money and in 1979, it was spun off from university ownership.[17] From 1997–98, the hospital was a member of Pittsburgh's Allegheny Health System. In 1998, it was acquired by Tenant Health Systems, which in 2007, sold it to Penn that now uses it as the Rittenhouse Rehabilitation Center with its fifty-eight beds operated by Good Shepherd Penn Partners. In addition, it houses a center for outpatient surgery.

Notes

[1] Flexner, Abraham (1910). *Medical Education in the United States and Canada: A Report to the Carnegie Foundation for the Advancement of Teaching* Bulletin No. 4. (New York City: The Carnegie Foundation for the Advancement of Teaching) p. 293.

[2] Cooper III, David Y and Ledger, Marshall A. *Innovation and Tradition at the University of Pennsylvania School of Medicine, An Anecdotal Journey* (Philadelphia: University of Pennsylvania Press, 1990) pp. 169–170.

[3] Ibid., p. 172.

[4] Ibid., p. 270.

[5] Ibid., p. 265.

[6] Ibid., p. 266.

[7] Ibid., p. 270.

[8] Holzman, P, Kety, Seymour S. 1915–2000. *Nat Med* 6, 727 (2000). https://doi.org/10.1038/77435.

[9] Seymour Kety. *Harvard Square Library* (23 Feb. 2022); adapted from an essay by Louis Sokoloff in Biographical Memoirs. https://www.harvardsquarelibrary.org/biographies/seymour-kety/#:~:text=In%201961%2C%20Seymour%20accepted%20the%20position%20of%20chairman,achievements%20gained%20him%20enormous%20international%20recognition%20and%20acclaim.

[10] Cooper III, David Y, and Ledger, Marshall A. *Innovation and Tradition at the University of Pennsylvania School of Medicine, An Anecdotal Journey*, p. 170.

[11] The Reminiscence of Isidor Ravdin, *Columbia University Oral History Collection*, Part II No 156. Isidor Ravdin, Saul Benison, Barbara Land, Columbia University Oral Research Office, New York Times Oral History Program (1971) p. 69.

[12] Rombeau, John, and Muldoon, Donna. *Quaker Sense and Sensibility in the World of Surgery* (Philadelphia: Hanley and Belfus Inc: 1997) p. 113.

[13] Memoir of John Berton Carnett. *Transactions of the Philadelphia Academy of Surgery* 1932–33, Volume XXVI, p. xxxiv–xxxivi.

[14] Personal recollection.

[15] Baum, S, and Nusbaum, M. The control of gastrointestinal hemorrhage by selective mesenteric arterial infusion of vasopressin. *Radiology*, 98(3), (1971) 497–505. https://doi.org/10.1148/98.3.497.

[16] Cooper III, David. Y, and Ledger, Marshall A. *Innovation and Tradition at the University of Pennsylvania School of Medicine, An Anecdotal Journey*, p. 173

[17] Ibid., p. 173.

CHAPTER 22

The Right Man at the Wrong Time

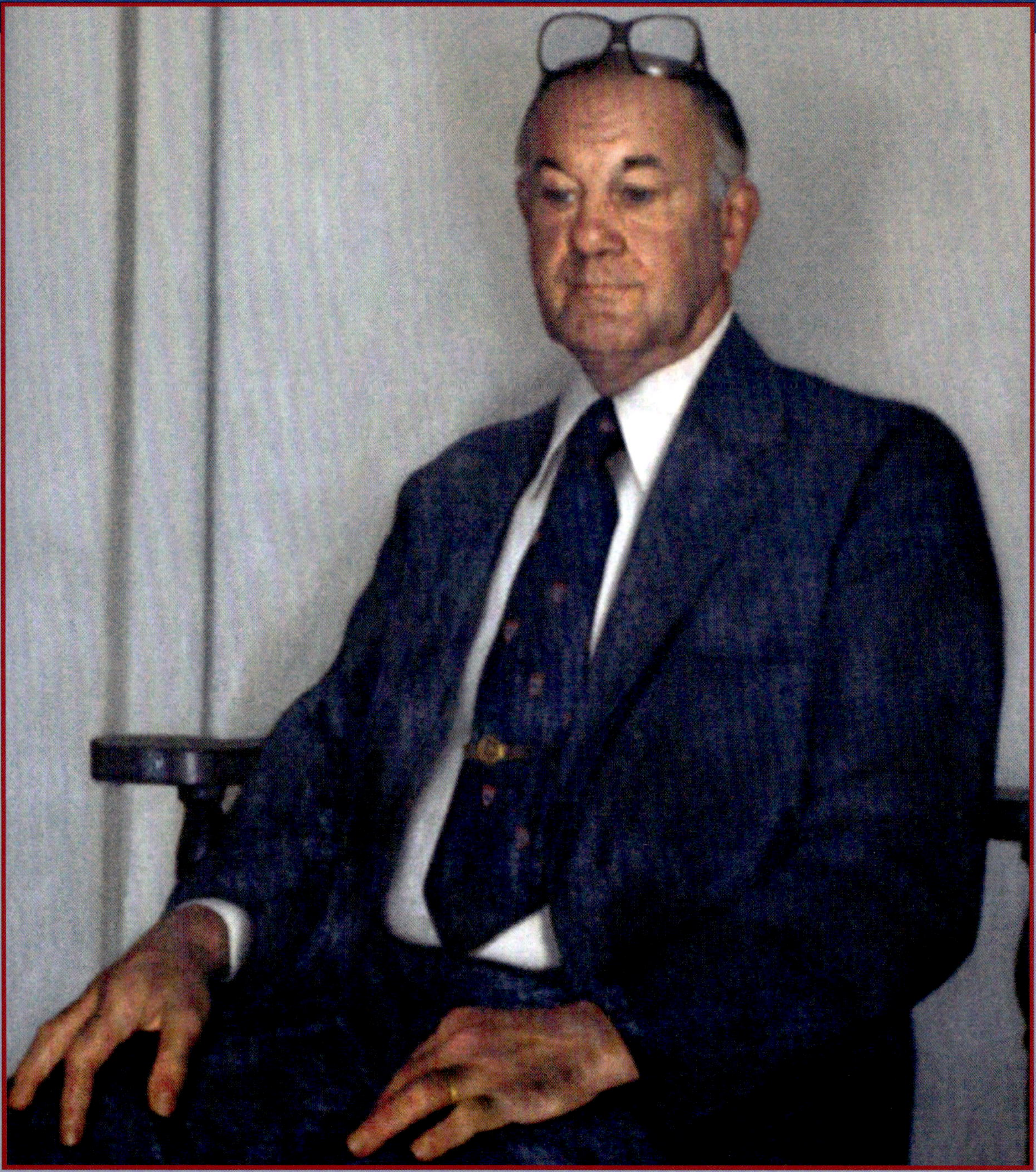

William T. Fitts Jr. (1915–1980)

JRB Professor and Chairman of Surgery (1972–1975)

William Thomas Fitts Jr. was born in Jackson, Tennessee, on October 6, 1915. His father was a distinguished internist in Jackson, and at first, Bill aimed to follow in his footsteps. At Penn Medical School, he was class president and graduated at the top of his class. At the outbreak of World War II, Bill was finishing a two-year rotating internship at HUP. He became an officer in the 20th General Hospital, the University of Pennsylvania unit serving in India near the border of enemy-held Burma. The hospital's task was to support the planned invasion of Japanese-held Burma, which was being undertaken to restore a land supply route from India to Allied forces in China, otherwise only reached by treacherous flights over the Himalayas. The hospital began as a collection of bamboo huts surrounded by jungle. It eventually grew to 289 buildings with 2,500 beds. It was the largest military hospital of World War II and admitted 73,000 patients. It provided a wealth of clinical material, especially in trauma.[1]

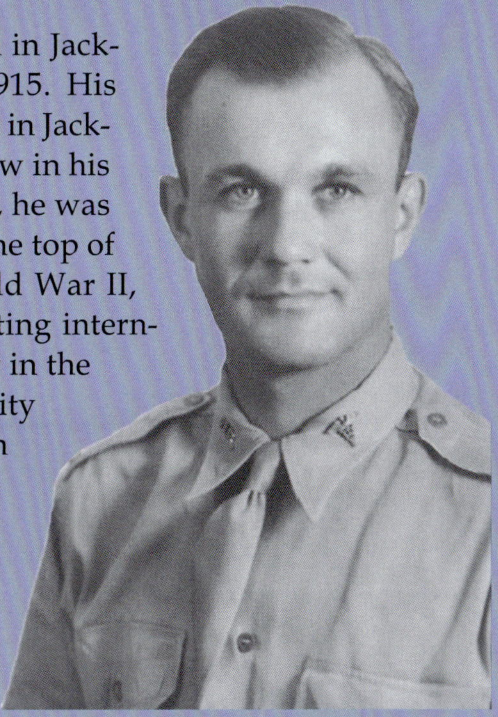

Bill Fitts, Officer in 20th General Hospital.

1915
Fitts born in Jackson, Tennessee

1940
MD at Penn, first in his class

1942–1945
As member of Ravdin's 20th General Hospital in India is assigned to orthopedic service

Bill's assignment to the hospital's surgical service was not particularly to his liking, because before being called into the Army, he had been accepted for a medical residency at the Mayo Clinic. His assignment to the hospital's orthopedic service was fortunate because Bill learned a great deal about trauma and shock. This experience and the close relationship he developed with I. S. Ravdin, the hospital's commanding general, changed his direction to a surgical career and a lasting special interest in

1947
Finishes surgical residency under Ravdin and appointed to Penn faculty

1956–1959
Jonathan Rhoads becomes provost of the university. Speculation that Fitts might be the next chairman of surgery

trauma and fractures.[2] Ravdin, although often given to hyperbole, was probably correct when he stated that while in India, Dr. Fitts had done more onlay grafts for delayed union of the tibia than any surgeon in the United States.

After the war, Bill returned to HUP where he finished his surgical training under Ravdin (who had become department chairman) and began his career-long appointment to the Penn faculty. Fitts may have been the most important member of the team recruited by Ravdin to help him develop a modern department of surgery. He was probably the smartest, hardest-working, and most versatile of this cadre. He seemed to be Dr. Ravdin's foremost assistant, and as Rav approached retirement in the late 1950s, it was rumored that he might be the next chairman. The other candidate for the job was the austere Jonathan Rhoads—more accomplished, but at age fifty-three, yet to achieve legendary status, and less popular than charismatic, forty-five-year-old Fitts. In addition, Rhoads had recently accepted an appointment as provost of the university, suggesting that he had moved upstairs and might be positioned to become president of the university instead of just a department chair.

Residents and young surgical faculty rooted quietly for Fitts to win the job. He was everybody's friend. Early in my residency, my wife and I were neighbors of Bill and Barbara Fitts in West Philadelphia. We became friends and stayed in their house to look after their three young children and skittish dog while they were away at meetings of the American College of Surgeons and the trauma society. This sort of relationship with the Fittses was nothing special or limited to us. Bill Fitts was easily the most informal and unpretentious member of the faculty. A typical illustration was the good-natured enthusiasm with which Fitts gabbed with everybody in his broad southern accent about his wager with the similarly portly plastic surgery chief, Bugs Lehr, over which of them could lose the most weight by a prescribed date. Fellow faculty members and residents placed bets on the outcome as these two strived to outdo each other by sneaking large doses of Lasix as the deadline of the contest approached.

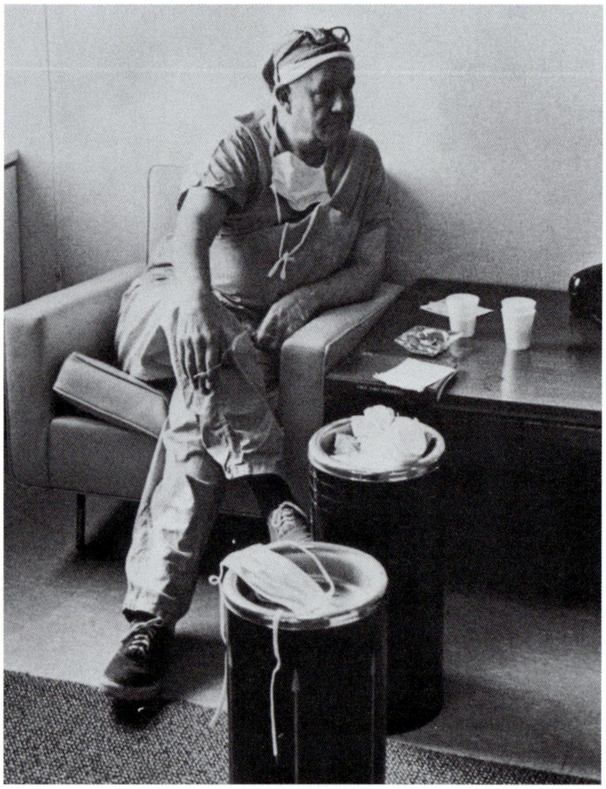

Bill Fitts: unpretentious scholar.

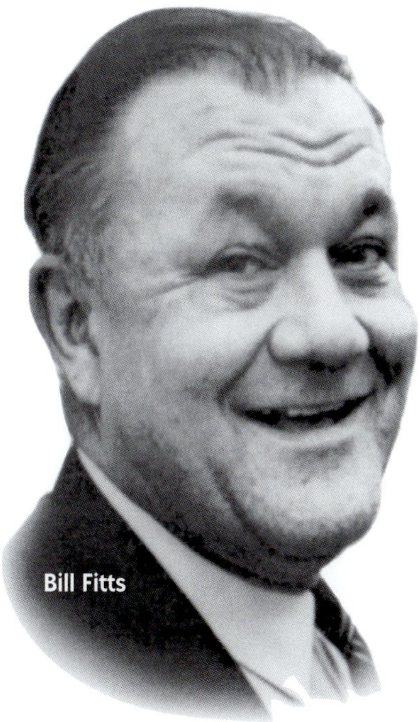

Belying the façade of his homespun personality, the enigmatic Fitts was an intellectual giant, who had graduated at the top of his class in every school he attended, including Penn's medical school. He had an encyclopedic knowledge of not only medicine and surgery, but outside of his professional field as well. In writing a memoir of Fitts, Len Miller commented that he used language well, an understatement since Fitts had served as a consultant to the publishers of the third edition of Webster's International Dictionary. Because Miller also used language well, I found it impossible to improve on his attempt to capture the essence of the man in the following paragraph, which is reproduced here with only minor changes as it appeared in the *Transactions of the American Surgical Association*.

1960
The paradoxical Bill Fitts is considered a candidate for surgery department chair

1960
Fitts is disabled by illness. Jonathan Rhoads appointed chairman of department of surgery

> Bill Fitts had a many-sided, often paradoxical personality.[3] Sometimes garrulous, a yarn-spinner with the best, he could also be the most silent and reflective of men. Every intern who at the operating table sought to earn points by pointing to a tiny bleeder knew how sharply reproachful he could be, yet gentleness and generosity were at the core of him. Some saw him as rustic and provincial in demeanor, but in truth, he was a scholar of considerable depth and breadth. Books were his primary outside interest, and he would often methodically pile up all the books he could find on a subject, anything from big city political bosses to Native American dialects, and read them voraciously, one after the other. The most informal and unpretentious of men, he had an innate sense of propriety and appreciation for style that allowed him to fit in anywhere. As a clinical surgeon, he was a model of confidence and determination outwardly, yet constantly gnawed at by questions of diagnosis and treatment until satisfied that his course was correct.

As Ravdin approached retirement, Fitts became a rising force in the department. He even began to assume some of Ravdin's administrative tasks. Many believed Fitts was slated for the chairmanship and would be ideal. But in 1960, when Ravdin stepped down, Fitts had become temporarily disabled by a series of illnesses, including a near-fatal hemorrhage from a long-standing duodenal ulcer. Fitts, the popular candidate, was unavailable. Instead, Jonathan Rhoads resigned as provost, returned to surgery full-time, and was appointed chairman. But read on; the story wasn't over yet.

1960–1972
Jonathan Rhoads's chairmanship

1964
Fitts wins Lindback Award

1965
Fitts is elected president of American Society for Surgery of Trauma

1968–1973
Editor of *Journal of Trauma*

1968–1973
Alfred Gellhorn is dean

1970
In Scudder Oration, Fitts criticizes trauma care in the United States and proposes model of a trauma team

Twelve years later, when Rhoads finished his term as chairman, turbulent circumstances in the medical school afforded sixty-year-old Bill Fitts another shot at heading the department. The multiple factors allowing him to reemerge as a possible chairman in 1972 are detailed in Chapter 24. During Rhoads's years as chairman, Fitts's national stature had increased, making him, in some ways, a more attractive candidate for the chairmanship than before. Also on the positive side were his undiminished popularity, the unsuccessful effort of an unpopular dean to attract outsiders as chairman during this turbulent period, and the relative inexperience of other young, local candidates like Miller and me. On the negative side were only Fitts's advanced age and his fragile health.

During Rhoads's chairmanship, much of the enhancement in Fitts's reputation had come from his substantial activities in the trauma field. His continuing interest in trauma led him to active participation in the American College of Surgeons' Trauma Committee,[4] first as chairman of the Regional Trauma Committee, later as a member of the National Committee on Trauma, and afterward, as its vice-chairman. He also became extremely active in the American Association for the Surgery of Trauma and was elected to all of the offices in the Association, serving as secretary, vice president, and president. He also became editor of the *Journal of Trauma* in 1968 and transformed it to a monthly journal, greatly expanding its circulation and scope. In 1975, the Association established an annual lectureship in his honor. He was also one of the founders of the American Trauma Society and rejuvenated its activity and effectiveness when he became president in 1972. The National Safety Council awarded him its Surgeon's Award for Distinguished Service to Safety in 1971.

Before the idea's time had come, Fitts challenged and rebuked his colleagues about the state of trauma care in the United States. At the 20th General Hospital, Fitts had observed the quality of care that could be delivered in even the most hostile of environments. In contrast, Fitts rated trauma care in the United States as unacceptable. In his 1970 Scudder Oration on Trauma, Fitts called attention to this problem: "with the exception of those wounded by enemy action, we are failing to provide adequate care for our injured . . . Treatment of trauma in this country is unique in that existing competence is more poorly applied than in the treatment of any other disease."[5] More bluntly, he once stated that a person had a better chance of surviving injury in the rice paddies of Vietnam than on the streets of West Philadelphia.[6] He criticized the fragmentation of trauma care and stressed the need for a team approach, regionalized trauma centers, specialized training in trauma and critical care, shock and trauma research, and a dedicated critical care service. His influence helped in eventually bringing these things to pass.[7]

With Dr. Oscar Hampton, Dr. Fitts wrote the four chapters on fractures in each of the four editions of Lippincott's *Textbook of Surgery*. He and Dr. Hampton also published a monograph on the open reduction of fractures. He published 150 scientific papers, which had a substantial impact on surgical practice not only in trauma, but also on the treatment of breast cancer and inflammatory and malignant disease of the gastrointestinal tract, areas in which Dr. Fitts possessed a wealth of surgical experience.[8]

1972–1975
Fitts becomes John Rhea Barton professor and chairman of department of surgery

In addition to his many contributions to trauma care and research and his reputation as a surgeon with superior judgment and skill, Bill was a superb teacher with a unique impact on those he taught.

Fitts was elected to membership in all of the important surgical societies and organizations including the American Surgical Association, the Society of University Surgeons, the Halsted Society, the Society for Surgery of the Alimentary Tract, the Eastern Surgical Society, the Pan-Pacific Surgical Association, the Allen Whipple Society, and the Southern Surgical Association, for which he had a special fondness.[9]

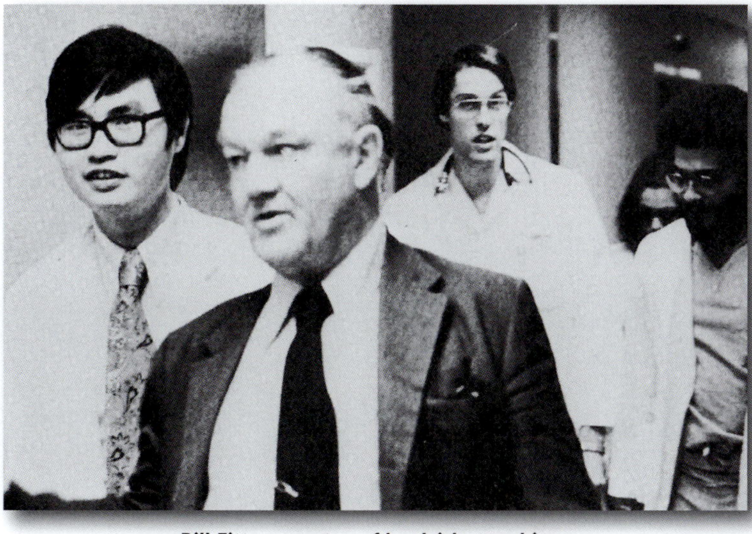

Bill Fitts—master of bedside teaching.

Whatever the determining factor was, Fitts was appointed surgery chairman in 1972, to the enthusiastic approval of the residents and most of the faculty. But unfortunately within weeks, it was evident that he was severely compromised by the pressure being directed at him to bring the surgery department into the medical school's consolidated practice plan that was being formed. Fitts's senior colleagues in surgery were adamantly opposed to this, anticipating that it would be the end of surgery's independence and might result in the department's practice income being tapped to support the school and needy departments. Twelve years earlier, as a younger, healthier chairman, I think Fitts could have handled this situation in stride. But weakened by age and illness at this stage, the unpleasantness of the surrounding conflict was too much for him. Within three years of his appointment as chairman, he chose to resign. To me, it seemed a case of the right man at the wrong time.

1980
While in presumed good health, sudden death from mesenteric thrombosis

In spite of this disappointment and several other misfortunes, including the sudden death of his wife, Bill Fitts again became active and productive. In fact, relieved of the responsibility of the chairmanship, he was restored to his usual cheerful, even ebullient, self. For the rest of his life, he remained an effective and valued member of the department of surgery, a beloved and unforgettable character.

At this stage, he also had time to enjoy and take pride in his family. In 1942, Bill had married Barbara Willits, whose father was dean of the Wharton School. They had three children, Barbara and Michael, both lawyers, and Austin, highly successful in the business world. Michael served as dean of Penn's Law School and is now president of Tulane University. After Barbara died, Bill married Stella White in 1976. Bill had known Stella since childhood. In fact, he was Stella's babysitter at a tender age, when their fathers both were training at the Mayo Clinic—her father in surgery and his father in medicine.

Bill's contributions to Penn extended well beyond its department of surgery. His list of important university committee assignments and chairmanships was extensive.[10] In 1979, the university reciprocated by honoring him with an Alumni Merit Award, the highest honor it can bestow on one of its own. In the same year, Union University, his alma mater, gave him its Distinguished Service Award.

One of Bill's last major undertakings was in connection with the "Campaign for the '80s" to raise $255 million for the University of Pennsylvania. He headed, at first, the department's fundraising efforts, and then the successful drive for the university as a whole. Ironically, in the week it went over the top, death came to Fitts with unexpected suddenness on June 17, 1980, from a mesenteric artery thrombosis.

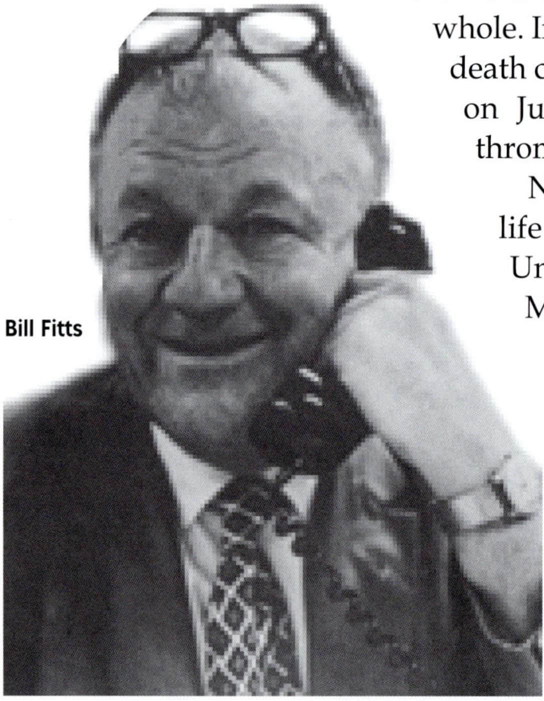
Bill Fitts

Nearly a thousand people from all walks of life attended Bill's memorial service at the University Museum on June 30th, 1980.[11] Many of his university faculty colleagues were also patients of his. One of the speakers was such a patient, a distinguished professor of economics. He summed it up best when he said, "Others will esteem Bill as a colleague, teacher, and eminent surgeon. I speak from the other side of the operating table, as the 'patient anonymous' who gives purpose and poignancy to the science of medicine. I am among the untold numbers who live because of Bill's superb skill, tender compassion, and unswerving dedication to his life-assisting mission."

Notes

[1] North, JP. The 20th General Hospital—I.S. Ravdin Commanding General. *Surgery* (1964 Oct) 56: 614–623.

[2] Miller, Leonard D. Memoir of William T. Fitts, Jr., M.D. Transactions of the American Surgical Association (1980) Vol 98 p. 64.

[3] Ibid., pp. 65–66.

[4] Ibid., p. 64.

[5] Schwab, C William. Scudder Lecture: Winds of War: Enhancing Civilian and Military Partnerships to Assure Readiness: White Paper. *Journal of the American College of Surgeons* Vol 221 No 2 (August 2015).

[6] Kim PK, Nance FC, Nance ML, Schwab CW. William T. "Billy" Fitts Jr, MD: An AAST Visionary. *J Trauma* (2007) 63(1):221–227. doi:10.1097/TA.0b013e31806842d9.

[7] Personal communication.

[8] Miller, Leonard D. *Memoir of William T. Fitts, Jr., M.D.* p. 65.

[9] Royster, Henry P. William Thomas Fitts, Jr. 1915–1980. *Transactions of the Southern Surgical Association* (1980) Volume XCII pp. 297–298.

[10] Miller, Leonard D. *Memoir of William T. Fitts, Jr., M.D.* p. 65.

[11] Miller, Leonard D. *Memoir of William T. Fitts, Jr., M.D.* p. 66.

CHAPTER 23

A Master Teacher Delays the Demise of the Halsted-Ravdin Residency

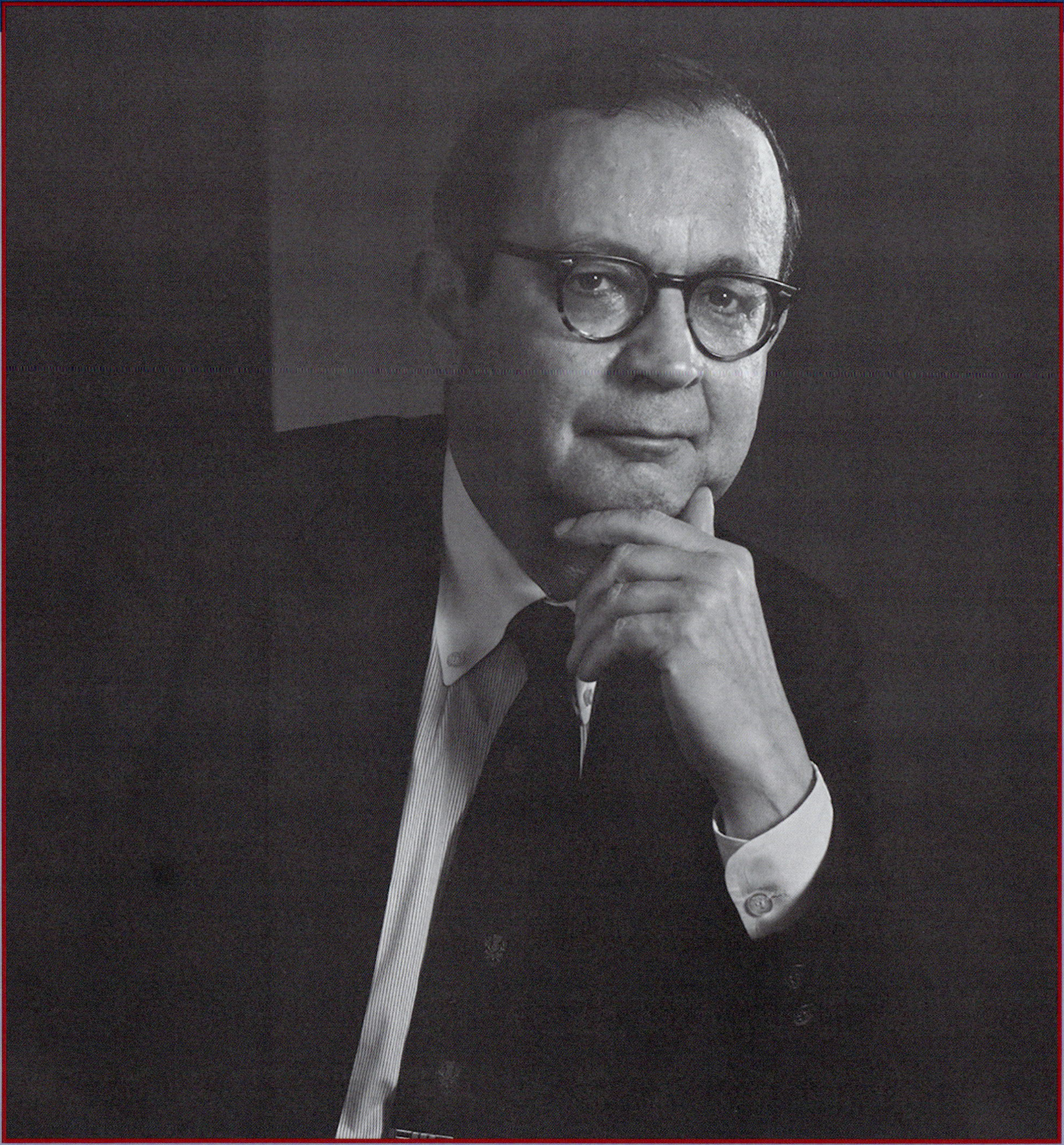

Leonard D. Miller (1930–1997)

JRB Professor and Chairman of Surgery (1978–1981)

Buried in the department's archives is the story of the ironic failure of this brilliant, broadly accomplished surgeon-scholar to succeed as chairman. While a student, resident, and to the midpoint of his distinguished career, everything was working for him. His research was thriving. Students and colleagues recognized him as the department's and even the medical school's best teacher. His broad and detailed knowledge of surgery and medicine were second to no one else's. His talent even extended to administrative and political skills. The only soft spot was a never-explained reluctance to operate. This was not widely recognized or else was considered an idiosyncrasy of minor importance until he became chief of surgery.

1930
Miller's birth in Jersey City, New Jersey

1951
BA at Yale

1955
MD at Penn

It was hard to understand. He was well and fully trained as a surgeon, and throughout his career, he maintained a detailed knowledge of operative technique with all its advances and nuances. At the operating table, he often stood behind his residents. From there, if necessary, he advised or instructed them. He was a very effective teacher of technical surgery. But he never scrubbed or played an active role in the operation. And he never operated himself. Why, we will never know.

Leonard Miller was born July 8, 1930, in Jersey City, New Jersey.[1] After early education in the Jersey City public schools, where he was a distinguished scholar and an All-City high school basketball player, he attended Yale University, graduating in 1951. At Penn's medical school, he was president of his class and editor of the yearbook, graduating in 1955. After internship and a year of surgical residency under I. S. Ravdin at the Hospital of the University of Pennsylvania, he served from 1957 to 1959

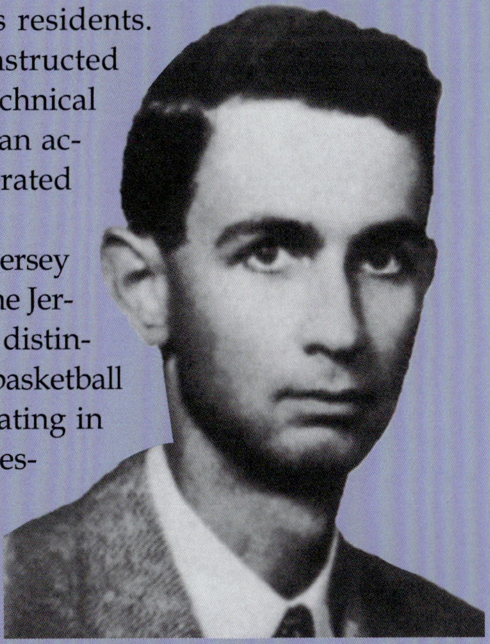

Leonard Miller

1957–1959
Interruption of HUP residency. Commander of Air Force Hospital in England

1964
Finishes HUP residency

1964–1976
Acts as Fitts's assistant

1969
Promoted to full professor

1976–1978
Acting chairman of surgery

1978
John Rhea Barton Professor and chairman of department of surgery

1981
Becomes ill and resigns as chairman. Thereafter devotes himself to education

as a captain in the US Air Force and as chief of the surgical service and commander of a large Air Force hospital in England. After returning to the University of Pennsylvania and completing his surgical residency under Jonathan Rhoads in 1964, he was appointed to the faculty and became a full professor only five years later. During this period, he was Dr. Fitts's clinical associate, essentially functioning as his assistant. When Fitts became chairman in 1972, Miller managed many of the department's administrative tasks. Then in 1975, as Dr. Fitts's health induced him to resign, Miller became for two years acting chairman of the department. He soon fell heir to the turbulence that had plagued the brief Fitts tenure.[2]

Whether those who were determined to bring surgery into the school's consolidated practice plan (CPUP) saw Miller's reluctance to operate as a sign of his vulnerability, we will never know. But from the time of his official appointment as chairman in 1978, his adversaries progressively increased the pressure for surgery to join CPUP. Surgery's powerful senior faculty, including Jonathan Rhoads, were strongly opposed to this because of their commitment to the financial independence of the department and its emphasis of clinical practice. Miller found himself at the center of a conflict that had threatened to tear the medical school's faculty apart and had already caused his predecessor, Bill Fitts, to resign. The signs of stress became obvious in Miller's demeanor and seemed a likely factor in a clinical depression that followed, causing him to resign after only three years as chairman. It was an outcome this gifted academic surgeon did not deserve.

Fortunately, Miller's resignation as chairman was not the end of his otherwise stellar career. In fact, he probably achieved more subsequently as an educator than if he had remained chairman. In measuring a man's career, it is interesting to reflect on the extent to which he may have accomplished his goals. During his entire professional life, Len's greatest commitment was to education. As he began his faculty career, he set forth his professional goals in a career development grant application, which is preserved in the archives of the department of surgery. It could have served as his epitaph. He wrote:

> I hope the coming years will bear evidence of the realization of some, if not all, of my fundamental aims. The three cornerstones upon which Penn's Medical School was built listed in their order of importance are: teaching, research, and the care of patients. I am intent upon devoting myself primarily to teaching and research. Teaching is the aspect of medicine that satisfies me most fully. However, I am unwilling to give up the care of surgical patients because a surgeon cannot adequately teach completely from the printed page. My first experience with teaching came in 1951. I took a position with an inter-denominational church group called the East Harlem Protestant Parish. East Harlem is a remarkably

> overcrowded, slum-infested area of New York City which has the highest tuberculosis and narcotics addiction rate of any neighborhood in the country. There, I worked, lived with teenagers and taught informal sessions in the natural sciences . . . I had several other duties including getting the children out of the city into summer camps. My own purposes were humanistic rather than evangelical, but the experience left a deep impression on me. Small steps forward with these youngsters were large triumphs to me.

1981–1997
Miller consistently wins the most teaching awards from students and residents

1981–1997
Miller is chief of the residents' ward service and recognized as their most important mentor

One can easily imagine what Len must have meant to the teenagers in East Harlem. Although HUP and Penn's medical school are quite different venues, his style as a teacher never changed much. His approach was, in fact, almost evangelical. After finishing his tour as department chairman, Len took on the responsibility as chief of the teaching service. For the next fourteen years, he closely supervised the patients on this "ward" service by attending all the residents' operations, including those at night and on the weekends. Students and residents schemed for a place on his teaching service, his quiz sections, and his other classes. Like the Harlem teenagers, Len viewed their small steps forward as major triumphs. He was recognized with many awards: a Lindback Award; an honorary faculty membership in AOA; designation as the best clinical teacher by the medical school classes of 1992, 1993, and 1996; and, by the surgical residents, five times as their best teacher of the year. His national recognition as an educator was confirmed by his appointment as chair of the Surgical Education Committee of the Society of University Surgeons. Len truly accomplished the goals as a teacher he had set for himself in 1964.

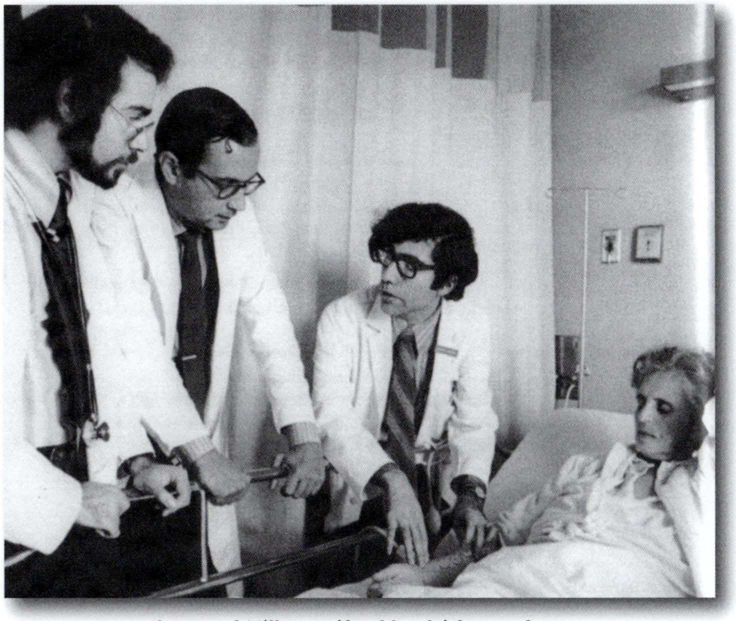

Leonard Miller—gifted bedside teacher.

During his thirty-three years as a faculty member, Len assumed many important administrative roles. He served as chair of the medical board of the Hospital of the University of Pennsylvania. He also chaired the steering committee of the Medical Faculty Senate, and the admissions committee of the School of Medicine. He was the J. William White Professor of Surgical Research from 1970 to 1978. After several years as

1972–1983
Miller is director of Harrison department of surgical research

acting chairman of the department of surgery, he succeeded William T. Fitts Jr. as John Rhea Barton Professor and chairman of the department of surgery in 1978 and served in this role until 1981.

During his early career, Len was productive in basic research. The scope and success of a researcher is often determined by those he chooses to collaborate with or mentor. For Len, individuals in these categories included a remarkably large group: Jonathan Rhoads, Brooke Roberts, John Murphy, Jerry Peskin, Carter Nance, Clyde Barker, Bill Fitts, Stan Dudrick, Peter Kuo, Claude Joyner, Henry Berkowitz, Harold Itskovitz, Ted Copeland, Frank and Ernie Rosato, Scott Jones, Frank Oski, Maria Papadopoulos, Harvey Sugarman, Lena Mela, Saul Winegrad, Bob Forster, John Senior, Cleon Goodwin, and Frank Brooks, with whom he worked for a year in the department of physiology. From 1972 to 1983, Len was director of the Harrison department of surgical research. His research contributions, which led to more than 100 publications, were significant in several different areas, which included blood flow to the kidney, the renin-angiotensin system, and the impact of shock on oxygen transport and mitochondrial function. He was director of the department's NIH-funded shock and trauma unit from 1967 to 1972. His major clinical research interests were cancer of the large bowel, portal hypertension, and the use of portacaval shunts.

Len was elected to membership in many distinguished medical and scientific societies including the American Physiological Society, the Society of University Surgeons, the American Surgical Association, the Surgical Biology Club I, and the Halsted Society. For many years, he was a member of the editorial board of the *Annals of Surgery*. He also edited with HUP residents, Ed Savage and Steve Fishman, a book on the essentials of basic science in surgery.

For more than forty years, Len Miller was an important force at the University of Pennsylvania and especially in its department of surgery. Even as a resident, he was recognized by medical students and junior residents as the department's best teacher. Later, his teaching skills would become almost legendary. He was more broadly knowledgeable about surgery than anyone I can remember, and he was eager and effective in sharing this knowledge.

Len Miller: surgical scientist.

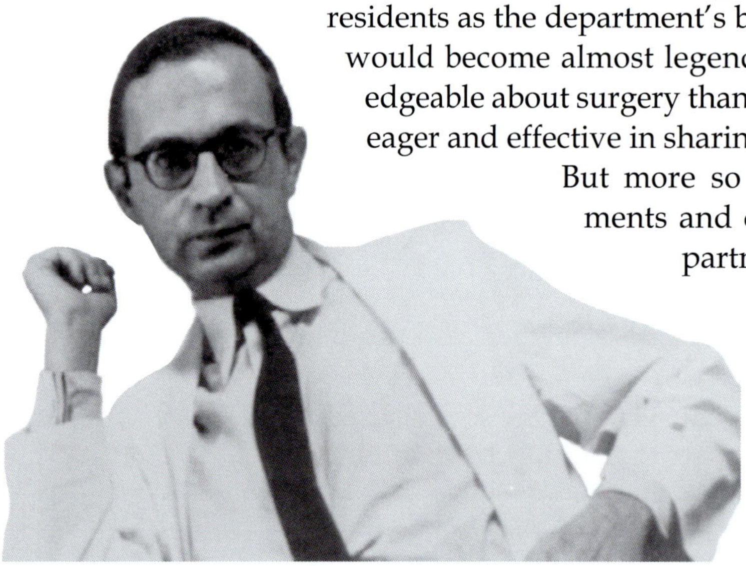

But more so than his professional accomplishments and contributions to his school and department, it was Len's personal qualities which endeared him to his students and colleagues. His quirky sense of humor was frequently exhibited with an inimitable laugh that can never be forgotten by those who knew him.

Over the last decade of his life, and particularly in his last illness, he exhibited great courage and resilience. This was apparent first in his return to an active role in the department after the disappointment of being forced by his health to give up the chairmanship he had achieved through so much hard work and personal success. After this, teaching became his mission and almost totally occupied his waking hours. It was a tragic irony that his terminal illness robbed him of his ability to speak and thus, his lifelong passion, teaching. He confronted his final illness with a stubbornness and apparent good cheer that should serve as a lesson to everyone.

1995–1997
A lifetime of incessant smoking leads to laryngeal cancer and inability to speak

1997
Miller's death

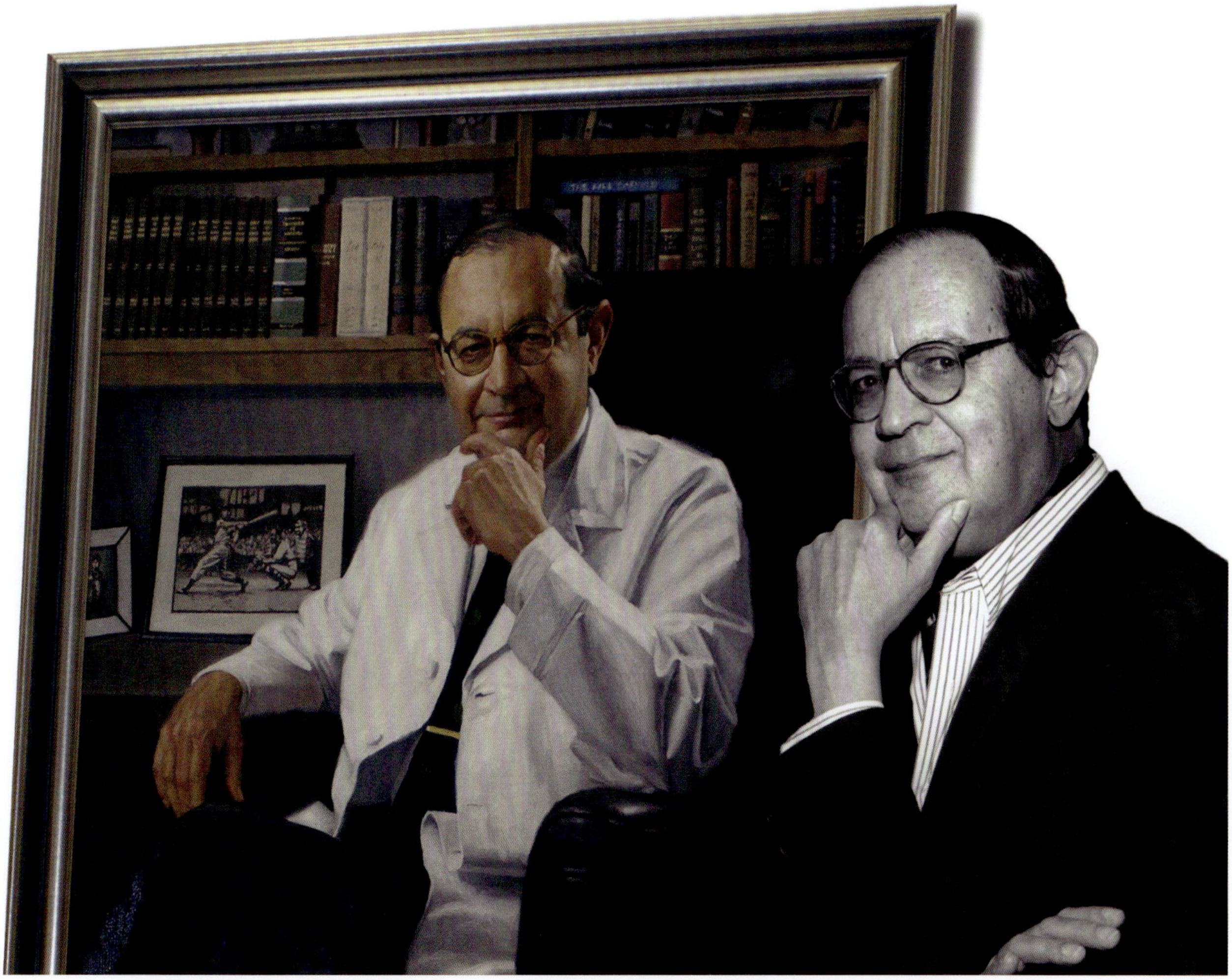

Leonard Miller at the presentation of his portrait. Note the baseball picture that he kept in his office. He was as obsessively knowledgable about the history of this sport as he was about surgery.

Notes

[1] Barker, Clyde. Dr. Leonard Miller, Teacher and Surgeon. *University of Pennsylvania Almanac*, Vol 44, No 1. https://almanac.upenn.edu/archive/v44/n01/deaths.html.

[2] Kastor, John A. *Governance of Teaching Hospitals, Turmoil at Penn and Hopkins* (Baltimore: The Johns Hopkins University Press: 2004) p. 17.

CHAPTER 24

A Period of Turbulence, 1968–2000

1968
Alfred Gellhorn becomes dean of Penn's medical school

Gellhorn proposes emphasis of social issues and is critical of Penn's "narrow focus on sciences"

Conservative faculty and Jonathan Rhoads disagree

At the University of Pennsylvania Medical Center, the last third of the twentieth century was a period of turmoil. For the medical school and the university hospital, this turmoil lasted from 1968, when Alfred Gellhorn was appointed dean, until the dismissal of Dean William Kelley in the year 2000.[1] For surgery, the period was shorter, but the turmoil spoiled the careers of two talented department chairs, and the instability in leadership delayed progress.

Dean Gellhorn, a medical oncologist, was recruited from New York. He agreed to take the job only if he was given control of HUP as well as the School of Medicine. He was determined to reform Penn Medicine into a full-time, salaried faculty system and to integrate the clinical practices so that money could be shared between the clinical and basic science departments, as well as between financially wealthy and impoverished clinical departments.[2] In addition, he planned to alter what he viewed as Penn's overly narrow focus on science and emphasize social and community issues and diversity. Jonathan Rhoads, chairman of surgery at the time, was very much opposed to Gellhorn's socialist plans, as were many powerful senior faculty members in other departments, especially those with lucrative private clinical practices. But in 1972, Rhoads completed his twelve-year term as chairman of surgery and could no longer effectively counter Gellhorn. Thereafter, for several years, uncertainty over who would succeed Jonathan Rhoads was a dominant issue. For the first time in the surgery department's long history, the chairmanship was not automatically passed on to the next most senior Penn faculty member, thus ensuring that an internal candidate would become the next chairman. This time, Gellhorn set up a national search for surgery's chairman. Senior members of the surgical faculty were determined that an internal candidate be selected

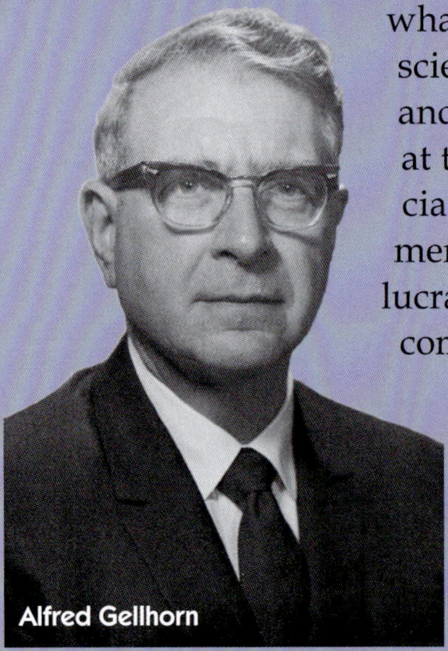
Alfred Gellhorn

to maintain the status quo of departmental independence. But many leaders of other departments favored Gellhorn's position and the appointment of an outsider. Prominent surgeons from around the country were interviewed, including James Maloney, Thomas Starzl, Sy Schwartz, and others. The signs of a pending showdown over restructuring the practice plan were pretty obvious. Further diminishing the interest of external candidates was that governance of the school, the teaching hospital (HUP), and the clinical practices all seemed shaky. Because of these uncertainties, no serious offers of the chair were sought or made, and the search went on.

The logical internal contender was fifty-five-year-old Brooke Roberts, longtime chief of vascular surgery. In 1972, Roberts heard from an unidentified source that he would soon be offered the chairmanship. He even called a meeting of his vascular division to inform its members (including me) that this was about to be announced. Possibly, this information was provided to him by his surgical colleague and friend, William Fitts, who was a member of the search committee. Whatever the source, the information was wrong. Maybe Roberts was too conservative for Gellhorn. Anyway, if there was a plan to appoint Roberts, it was dropped. Instead, within a few days it was announced that Bill Fitts would be the new chairman.

The selection of Fitts came as something of a surprise for several reasons. One, Fitts was a member of the search committee, even though it was unusual for a member of the department searching to be placed on the search committee. Second, Fitts had recently been ill, hospitalized, and absent from the faculty. In fact, it soon turned out that choosing him was unwise, despite his popularity and fine credentials as an academic surgeon. It has always been my feeling that if he had been appointed at a younger age while in good health, he would have been an ideal chairman. But in the troubled, highly charged atmosphere of 1972, the appointment of Fitts should have been recognized as risky.

As soon as he was installed as chairman, Fitts found himself pressured by his boss, Dean Gellhorn, and like-minded others to endorse Gellhorn's liberal philosophy and vision, including an integrated practice plan, with surgery as a member. Fitts may have had some liberal tendencies, but his senior surgical colleagues did not. They were fiercely independent and conservative. The idea of sharing the funds of strong departments or the hospital with the school, research programs, or less financially successful departments was to them anathema.

The ugly conflict that ensued and surrounded Fitts was too much for him. Within three years of his appointment, he gave up most of his activities as chairman, turning them over—at first, informally—to his young protégé, Leonard Miller. In 1975, he resigned. Until his death five years later, he continued to operate, teach, and participate actively in departmental and university activities. He was a beloved citizen of the

1972
Rhoads retires.
Fitts appointed chairman of department of surgery

Pressure for surgery to join integrated practice plan is too much for Fitts

1973
Demoralized by lack of support, Gellhorn resigns after five years as dean

1975
Fitts resigns after only three years as chairman. Ed Stemmler becomes acting dean, appoints Leonard Miller as acting chairman of surgery

1977
Failed attempt to appoint outsider as surgery chairman

1978
Internal candidate Leonard Miller is appointed John Rhea Barton Professor and Chairman of Surgery

surgery department, medical school, and the university, and his funeral was attended by almost a thousand individuals.

Even before Fitts resigned, Gellhorn was in trouble. From the start, he was playing against a stacked deck. Not for another thirty years would Penn be ready for the kind of changes Gellhorn wanted. Soon, a group of clinical department chairs went to University President Martin Myerson, insisting that Gellhorn's control of the hospital was a mistake and should be rescinded.[3] The trustees, also a conservative group, didn't trust Gellhorn, didn't like him or his philosophy, and couldn't understand why he had been appointed. Gellhorn concluded that virtually nobody at Penn wanted him to continue as dean. He resigned at the end of 1973, returning to New York as chairman of a new department at City College of New York, which would emphasize social issues.

After an extended period in an acting role, Ed Stemmler, who had been Gellhorn's assistant, was appointed dean in 1975. He soon chose Len Miller to lead surgery but only as an acting chair. Thus, for several years, the search resumed.

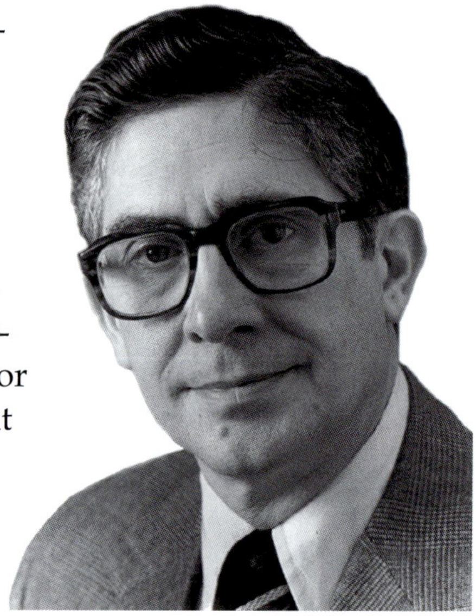
Edward J. Stemmler

The next step in this convoluted process was the appointment of, or rather, the attempt to appoint as surgery chair, an external candidate, Bill Drucker. Drucker was a surgeon, but at the time was dean at the University of Virginia. He was apparently offered or promised the offer to be surgery chairman at Penn. This offer seemed definite enough. It was leaked to the local Charlottesville newspapers and soon reached Philadelphia. The Penn surgical faculty members were outraged and responded by organizing a meeting with Dean Stemmler to abort this appointment. Drucker was criticized with some justification as a nonoperating surgeon and thus hardly fitting the image of the department's leader. Led at this uncomfortably contentious meeting by urologist John Murphy, surgery's opposition proved so powerful that Dean Stemmler, to his embarrassment, was forced to back down, reverse the appointment of Drucker, and give up on the plan for an external candidate. In 1978, Stemmler formally appointed Leonard Miller as JRB Professor and chairman of the department of surgery.

As a new chairman, Miller was well-liked by his surgical colleagues on a personal basis, and his research was highly respected. But detractors characterized him as a nonoperating surgeon and one that might not be strong enough to overcome the push for change in the practice plan and to preserve the independence of the department of surgery. Miller's appointment was only barely favored over potential outsiders by his surgical colleagues because they hoped he would try to avoid the department's joining CPUP, the integrated clinical practice group being organized by Stemmler. But the pressure for surgery to join this clinical practice group continued and built up steam. Other than surgery, most departments were now members. Actually, Miller secretly favored joining CPUP, recognizing the benefits integration might bring despite surgery's loss of independence. As it turned out, consolidation and integration of the practices were not only inevitable, but necessary for Penn Medicine to survive the difficult times ahead.[4] Miller quietly tried to recruit younger members of the surgery department (including myself) to this position. He now found himself uncomfortably trapped between two very powerful forces. This was surely a major factor in impairing his health, soon causing him to take a leave of absence for several months while Brooke Roberts acted for him, and then to resign as chairman in 1981, only three years after he had been appointed.

1978–1981
Pressure for surgery to join CPUP and Miller's illness impairs his performance as chairman

1981
Miller resigns

1981–1983
Brooke Roberts is appointed acting chairman of surgery

He negotiates compromise over Surgery joining CPUP

From 1981 to 1983, Brooke Roberts was acting chairman and proved to be quite skilled and effective as a leader. He smoothed the rough waters and negotiated a truce with the university. Surgery would need to join CPUP, the last department to do so, but senior faculty of the department would be exempt and could continue to practice independently. Junior members had to either join CPUP or leave the university and HUP. Amazingly, this compromise was accomplished without the defection of any surgery faculty members. Over the same issue, ophthalmologist Harold Scheie, a major figure in his field, pulled his department out of HUP and set up an independent institute at Presbyterian Hospital.

1984
Clyde Barker appointed chairman of surgery

But the national search for a surgery chairman resumed. Initially, the search committee had the strong feeling, and perhaps instructions from the dean, that an internal candidate was not acceptable. Hiram Polk, Tony Monaco, Mel Williams, Ernie Rosato, Alden Harken, and others were interviewed. The committee eventually decided that I was the best fit, and in 1983, I was appointed as the JRB Professor and chairman. This was a long and painful eleven years after Rhoads retired. Fortunately, the CPUP issue was now resolved, sparing me from the pressure that spoiled the academic careers of Fitts and Miller. For the department of surgery at least, the turbulent period seemed over. For other departments, the problems were just beginning.

In the mid-1980s, troubles resurfaced on another front. Surgery seemed to be okay financially, but both CPUP and HUP started to lose money. At least partly at fault, perhaps, was that the department chairmen, who were now in control of CPUP, had their own priorities. Lacking firm leadership, they squabbled over resources. HUP's losses of $6 to $8 million per year, at the time, were small compared with what was coming. But the university was concerned enough to consider divesting itself of its ownership of the hospital and clinical practices. During this period, in an attempt to place its strongest leader in charge, the university gave Dean

1989
After HUP begins to lose money, Bill Kelley is recruited as dean and CEO

1990–1998
Kelley's period of building: basic science, clinical, and financial success

Stemmler control of the hospital and CPUP.[5] The change in leadership failed to stem the losses. In addition to the shaky financial status of HUP and CPUP, several factors probably encouraged Stemmler to resign. He was under pressure to generate funds for a new building to provide badly needed research space. He would have preferred to be dean or CEO of the medical center, rather than both. Therefore, he first appointed Arthur Asbury as acting dean. Eventually, he resigned as CEO, leaving Asbury as acting in both jobs. After several more years of financial woes, Asbury was quietly replaced by Michigan's successful chair of medicine, William Kelley.

In 1989, Bill Kelley, another iconic figure, was given the combined position of dean and CEO of CPUP and HUP.[6] He arrived with a reputation as a brilliant and very tough leader. He was called by some "Neutron Bill," suggesting that in his wake, the people were all found dead, but the buildings were left standing.[7] He deserves to have a chapter to himself. He was a strong and interesting leader with a strange mix of personality traits: energetic, decisive, effective, and in turn, either supportive or ruthlessly critical of his staff and department leaders. And to many, he was totally intimidating. Most of the department chairs were afraid of him. They had reason to be, since he would eventually replace virtually all of them.

The Kelley years were the best of times and the worst of times. Kelley and his heavy-handed chief of operations, Bud Pittinger, quickly reversed the financial losses.[8] Business practices were skillfully applied and costs ruthlessly cut. Accounts receivable were sold and converted to cash. Half

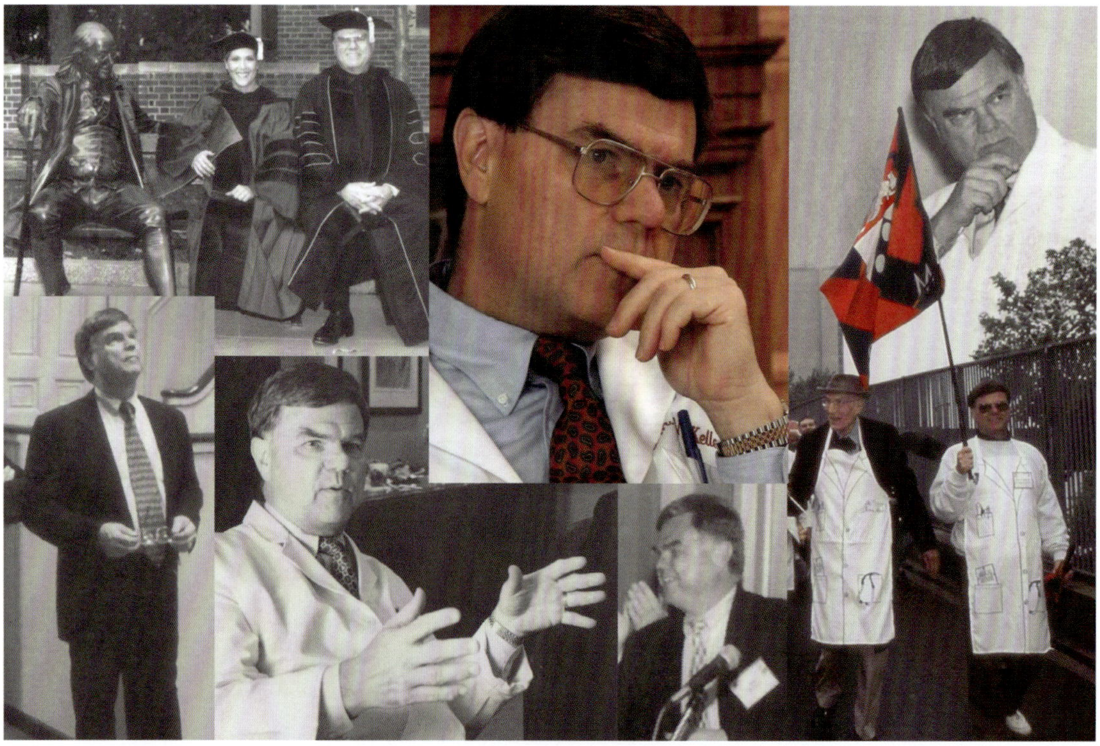

Bill Kelley: A man of many faces.

of the hospital's senior staff were replaced. Before long, annual surpluses of $70 to $97 million were generated. Kelley used the money to build strong academic and clinical programs. In his ten and a half years as everyone's boss, even his detractors admit that he transformed Penn Medicine from a parochial, rather stodgy institution into a modern medical center, one of the most vibrant and successful anywhere. He bought three hospitals and 270 primary care practices, and built two research buildings and one new hospital building. He renovated over a million square feet of space in the school and hospital. He recruited and supported dozens of bright young investigators whose research lifted Penn from tenth to second in NIH funding. Penn now trailed only Hopkins.

1998–2000
HUP loses money, $300 million over two years

2000
Bill Kelley is dismissed by Penn President Judith Rodin

In spite of these accomplishments, one issue should have made Kelley uneasy. It was apparent before long that Kelley and the new president of the university, Judith Rodin, could not get along.[9] Kelley's enthusiasm and aggressiveness led to spectacular success during his eight initial years of building, but also to ill-founded confidence and overreach. In 1998, financial losses resurfaced, this time to a greater extent than before. Over the next three years, the loss amounted to $300 million, $200 million of it in the year 2000 alone. If that wasn't enough trouble, also in the year 2000 came a well-publicized $30 million fine from Medicare for CPUP's overbilling.[10] In addition, Kelley's favorite research program of human gene therapy came apart and was closed by NIH when a patient, Jesse Gelsinger, died from the treatment for ornithine transcarbamylase deficiency.[11]

Kelley addressed the financial problem by dismissing 3,000 employees and through other austerity measures advised by the university's downsizing consultant specialists, the Hunter Group. These measures seemed to be working, and a small surplus was projected for 2001. But by now, Judith Rodin had gathered enough excuses and support for her to fire Kelley in 2000, which she had wanted to do anyway.[12] Since Kelley had made few friends, when he got into trouble, few tried to protect him. Yet many of his detractors and enemies would have agreed with former NIH director James Wyngarden that, "He made Penn the world-class institution it had every right to be."[13]

Because surgery never lost any money, and had strong clinical and research programs, Kelley had no reason to go after me, although he found reasons to replace virtually all of the other chairman, both basic science and clinical. I got along with him well, though always looking over my shoulder to be prepared for trouble. Perhaps because Kelley had a surgical personality, he provided strong support for me and the department of surgery. He even named a wing of HUP for a surgeon (Jonathan Rhoads). While he was in the process of firing most of the chairmen, he praised surgery for its research, nominated me for awards, and appointed me for an unprecedented third six-year term as chairman.

1983–2001
Department of surgery is productive and financially stable

2001
Surgery survives the period of turbulence

Kelley was satisfied to let me run my department with little interference. He pressured me only on a few issues. One was to replace academically accomplished Henry Edmonds as chief of cardiothoracic surgery because Kelley and Pittinger wanted CT surgery to focus exclusively on generating income for the institution, rather than on research. Another strong suggestion from Kelley was to turn the modest liver transplant program into a large institutional moneymaker by recruiting a proven clinical expert in the field. Kelley was correct in the suggestion, and his insight paid off.

In retrospect, it's hard to see why my support should have been strong in a department that hadn't bothered to defend two of its favorite members, Fitts and Miller, when, as chairmen, they were in trouble. Other than practice vascular surgery to make a living, my professional life to this point had been spent half doing immunology research in genetics, a basic science department, and half doing clinical research in transplantation, a new field which was generating no money for me, the department, the hospital, or the school of medicine. Perhaps I lasted because I was surrounded by friends, including the dean, and had no political agenda. I could have been happy inside or outside of CPUP. There was no particular reason to expect me to last longer than the three years Fitts and Miller averaged. There was no assurance that the turbulence for surgery would be over. But it was. While all of the basic science chairs and most of the clinical chairs were replaced by Kelley, I survived for eighteen years. Maybe it was by lying low, stepping on no toes, and making no unpopular changes, anticipating that after this period of chaos, Penn would be just the same as before. But no, in the next eighteen years, surgery, like the rest of the institution, would change substantially. It was an exciting time.

Notes

1 John A. Kastor. *Governance of Teaching Hospitals, Turmoil at Penn and Hopkins* (Baltimore and London: The Johns Hopkins University Press: 2004).

Kastor's 2004 book is based on his experience as a former faculty member at the Hospital of the University of Pennsylvania (HUP) and his interviews of 317 individuals involved with resolving the turmoil. The book is a review of William N. Kelley's experience as dean and CEO at Penn during his building phase, troubled phase, and dénouement. Kastor also touches on the ambitions and troubles of Penn's previous dean, Alfred Gellhorn, which impacted the careers of several surgical chairmen.

2 Ibid., p. 13.

3 Ibid., p. 16.

4 Quinn, Peter. CPUP at 40 *Penn Medicine News* (April 12, 2016).

Despite the organizational complexity necessary and resultant cultural and psychological impact, CPUP was necessary. Its integrated system allowed management of resources and cross-subsidization. The unified response was necessary to confront difficulties, such as virus epidemics.

5 Kastor. *Governance of Teaching Hospitals,* pp. 20–23.

6 Ibid., p. 31.

Although Penn later named a prominent research building for Stemmler, I thought its abrupt dismissal of him was inappropriate and shabby, considering all he had done to elevate the school's performance and reputation. In his fourteen years as dean, this gentleman-scholar always conducted himself with thoughtful intelligence, grace, and honor.

7 The Penn, The Summer Pennsylvanian and Khatib, Kate. Medical Dean Survives Review. *The Daily Pennsylvanian* May 30, 1996.

8 Kastor. *Governance of Teaching Hospitals,* p. 33.

9 Ibid., pp. 112–121.

10 Ibid., p. 58.

11 Jesse Gelsinger. (2021, August 5) In *Wikipedia.* https://en.wikipedia.org/wiki/Jesse_Gelsinger: "Gelsinger joined a clinical trial run by the University of Pennsylvania that aimed at developing a treatment for infants born with the severe form of the disease [ornithine transcarbamylase deficiency].

On September 13, 1999, Gelsinger was injected with an adenoviral vector carrying a corrected gene to test the safety of the procedure. He died four days later [. . .] apparently having suffered a massive immune response triggered by [. . .] the viral vector [. . .], leading to multiple organ failure and brain death."

12 Kastor. *Governance of Teaching Hospitals,* p. 121.

13 Ibid., p. 132.

CHAPTER 25

Engineer of the Department's Truce with the University

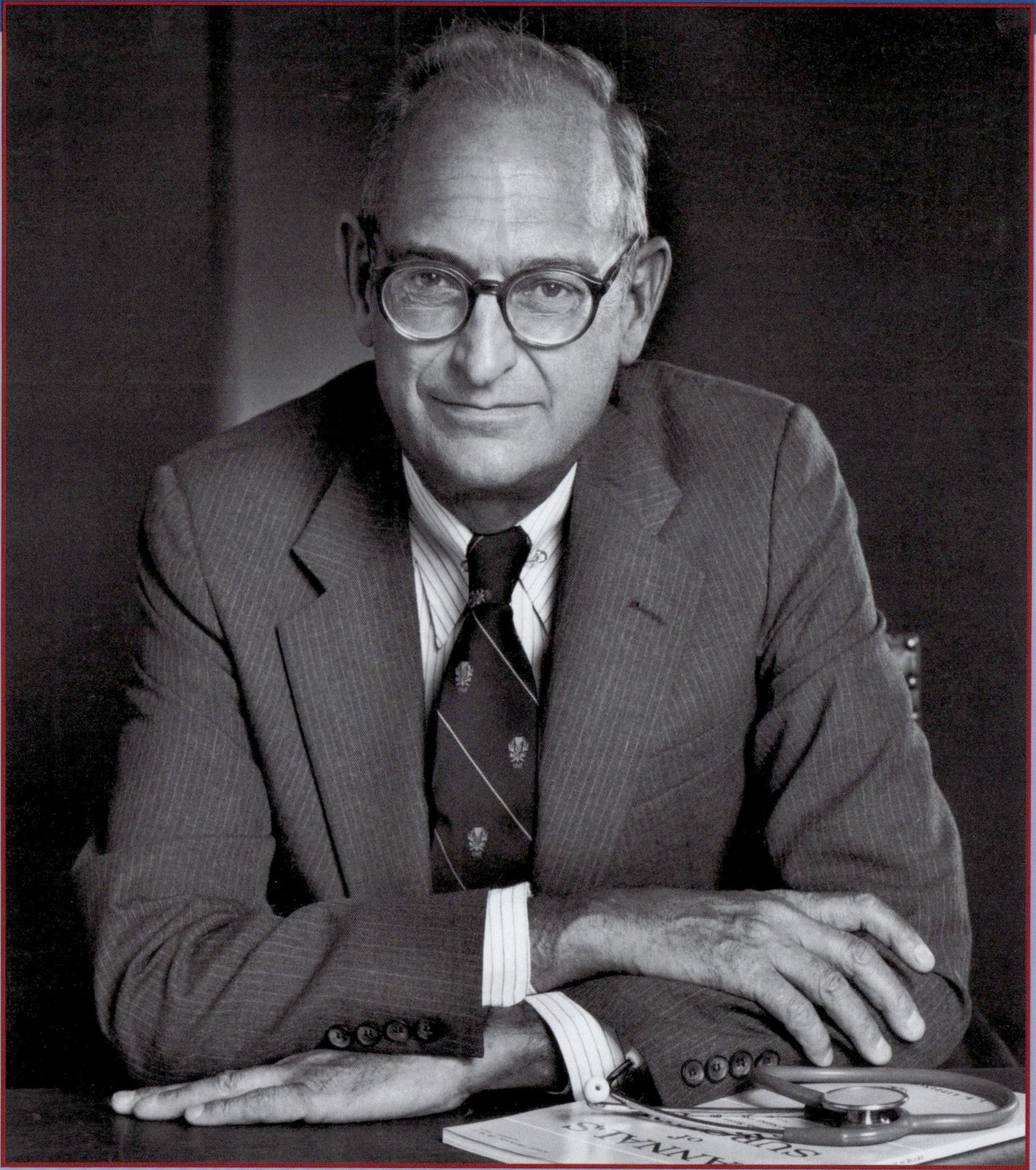

Brooke Roberts (1917–2003)

Acting Chairman of Surgery (1981–1983)

Brooke Roberts was born March 23, 1917, into one of Philadelphia's founding families.[1] He grew up at Pencoyd, the family estate that was granted to his forbearers by William Penn. He was educated at St. Paul's School and Princeton where he played hockey and rowed on the crew team, though he was not at the level of his son who became a member of the US Olympic crew team. At Penn's medical school, he distinguished himself, graduating in 1943 AOA and as winner of the Spencer Morris prize as the top student in medicine. After internship at HUP, he served for two years in the US Army at a military hospital in Germany, where he acquired enough experience in orthopedics to allow him to care for fracture patients and to pin broken hips throughout his later career.

Brooke returned to civilian life in 1947 as a surgical resident under I. S. Ravdin. He was appointed to the Penn faculty and for several years was Ravdin's understudy and assistant in management of his busy general surgery practice. In 1954, Ravdin appointed Brooke as chief of the new division of vascular surgery, just as this specialty was expanding beyond treatment of varicose veins to complex arterial surgery. Brooke's career charted the development of the field of vascular surgery. His more than 100 publications indicate that he was often an innovator. By 1956, he and his colleagues were able to report in the *JAMA* their treatment of 100 patients with aortic aneurysms and other arterial lesions with homografts preserved in their bank of cadaver arteries.[2] In a landmark *New England Journal of Medicine* paper of 1961, he and his colleagues defined the subclavian steal syndrome with careful hemodynamic studies.[3]

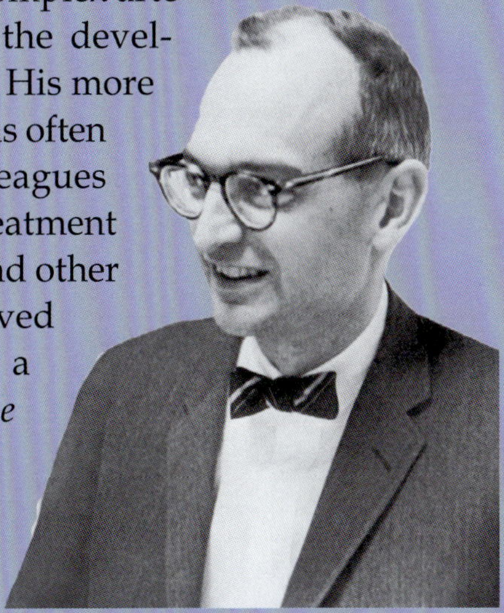

1917
Brooke Roberts is born into one of Philadelphia's first families

1943
MD at Penn

1944
HUP intern

1945–1946
Service in US Army hospital

1954
Appointed chief of vascular surgery at HUP

1956
Reports experience with 100 operations for aortic aneurysms

1961
New England Journal report of subclavian steal syndrome

1964
Report of heparin-induced emboli. Starts vascular fellowship

1964–1982
As chief of vascular division, Roberts trains a series of fellows. One, Peter McCombs, becomes chief of surgery at Pennsylvania and VA Hospitals

1981–1983
Acting chair of the department

1982
Strittmatter Award

1983
Negotiates with university to bring department of surgery into CPUP

Brooke's 1964 report was the first to describe heparin-induced arterial thromboses.[4] In the late 1970s and early 1980s, his series of reports with Ernie Ring and other radiology colleagues pioneered the era of transluminal balloon angioplasty for stenotic arteries.[5] Shortly thereafter, their use of streptokinase infusions to recanalize occluded arteries was similarly innovative.[6] In recognition of these and other research contributions, in 1983 the department dedicated its new research laboratories to Brooke.

Brooke was one of the most prominent and highly respected members of the entire Penn medical school faculty. He served as the chairman of the medical board of HUP and was frequently called upon by the dean to chair important interdepartmental committees. He served as vice chairman of the department of surgery under Leonard Miller and from 1981–1983 as the department's acting chairman. During this tempestuous political interval, he succeeded in converting surgery's private practice group to its status as a university-based practice plan. Remarkably, he accomplished this without any faculty defections. Following his tour as chairman and retirement from surgical practice, he remained active for a number of years in teaching anatomy to the medical students.

In 1964, Brooke started a vascular training program, the first and, for many years, the only accredited vascular fellowship in the Philadelphia area. In addition to being the region's most prominent vascular surgeon, Brooke had leadership roles in many other aspects of surgery and medicine. He served as President of the Philadelphia Academy of Surgery, the College of Physicians of Philadelphia, and the Philadelphia County Medical Society. In 1982, the County Medical Society recognized his contributions to Philadelphia medicine with the prestigious Strittmatter Award. He was also president of the Eastern

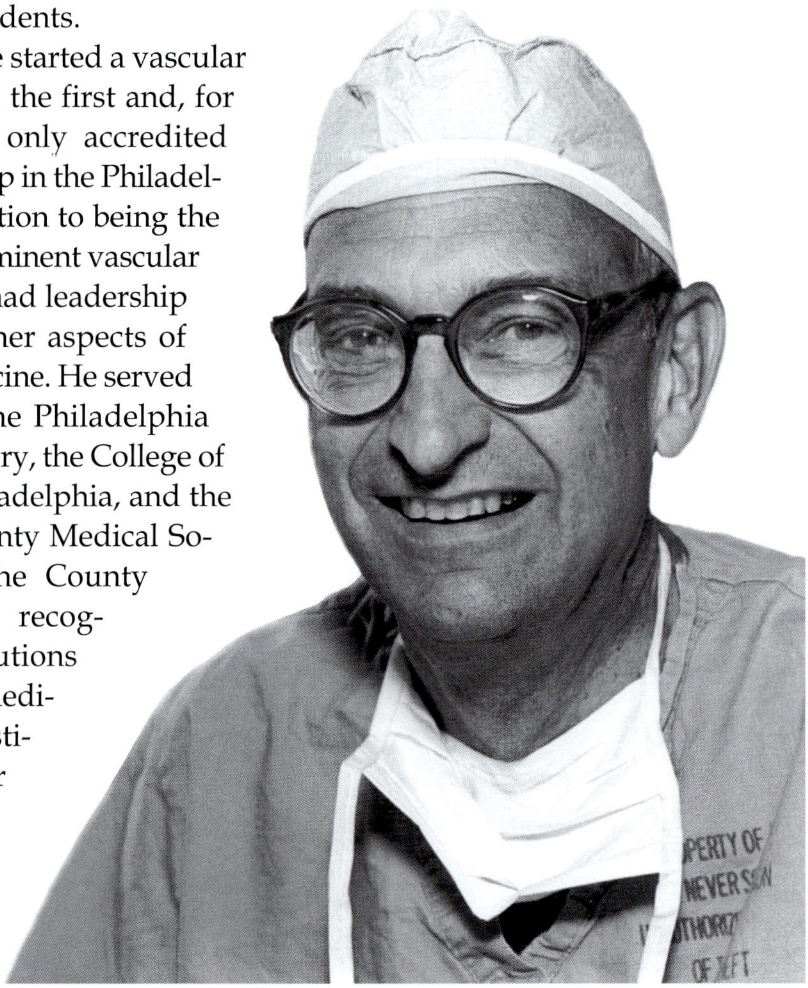

Brooke Roberts

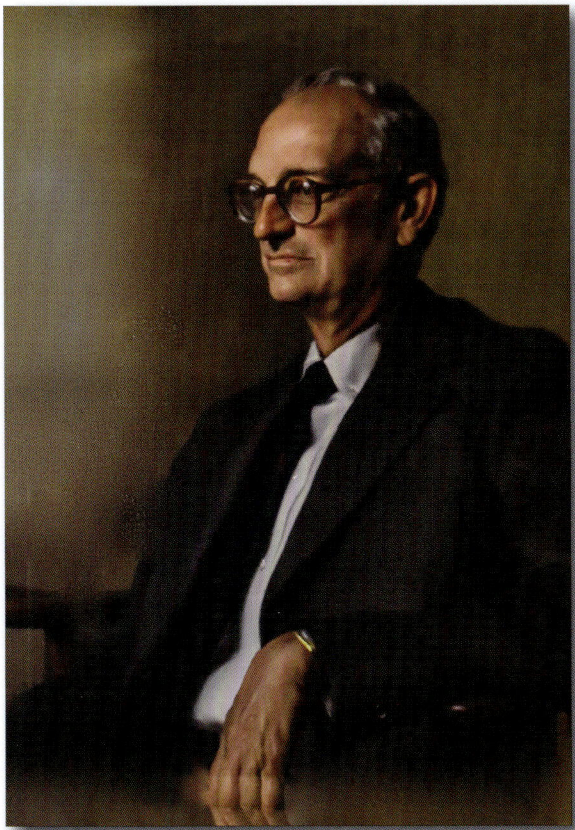

Portrait by Nelson Shanks on display in the Brooke Roberts Research Laboratories

Vascular Society. Other professional society memberships included the Society for Vascular Surgery, the Society of University Surgeons, the American Surgical Association, and the James IV Association of Surgeons. His influence extended beyond surgery and medicine to the trusteeship of St. Paul's School, Blue Cross of Philadelphia, and the William Measey Foundation, which he chaired. Despite the breadth of his important activities and research, teaching, and administration, Brooke considered himself first and foremost a practicing surgeon. His expertise in this regard was reinforced by his report more than four decades ago of 100 consecutive resections of aortic aneurysms without a death, during an era when the usual mortality of this operation was considerable.[7] His attention to detail, compassion, and conscientiousness in following each patient were unmatched. Even after he was the department's senior surgeon, he insisted on making careful daily rounds on every patient no matter how late he might have been detained by his operative schedule or administrative obligations. This was sometimes frustrating for residents and fellows who, in order to lighten his load, had seen the patients, reassured them that all was well, and predicted that Dr. Roberts would not have time to visit them until the next day. However, Brooke's inevitable visit later the same night was never a source of complaint by his grateful patients, even if they had to be awakened for it.

Brooke's death on February 23, 2003, came when, at age eighty-five, he was still vigorous and active in family, community, and professional affairs. Ironically, his terminal illness from hepatocellular carcinoma was undoubtedly the result of patient care, a needlestick during an operation many years before, which led to chronic hepatitis. Brooke was survived by his wife of fifty-nine years, Anna Ingersoll Roberts, and their sons Jared, Thomas, and Andrew, who became a vascular surgeon. His family, friends, colleagues, and patients expressed their love and respect for Brooke by endowing a surgical professorship in his name at the University of Pennsylvania.

1984–2003
Continues active role in department of surgery; e.g., recruits Tim Gardner, teaches students anatomy

2003
Death of Brooke Roberts

Notes

[1] Barker, Clyde. Brooke Roberts: 1917-2003. *Trans Meet Am Surg Assoc Am Surg Assoc.* (2003) 121:372–373.

[2] Blakemore WS, Lehr HB, Roberts B. Experience with Arterial Homograft Bank: Report of One Hundred Consecutive Arterial Homografts. *JAMA* (1956) 162(13):1220–1222.

[3] Reivich M, Holling HE, Roberts B, Toole JF. Reversal of blood flow through the vertebral artery and its effect on cerebral circulation. *N Engl J Med* (1961) Nov 2; 265:878–885.

[4] Roberts B, Rosato FE, Rosato EF. Heparin—a cause of arterial emboli? *Surgery* (1964) 55:803–8.

[5] Freiman DB, Ring EJ, Oleaga JA, Berkowitz H, Roberts B. Transluminal angioplasty of the iliac, femoral, and popliteal arteries. *Radiology* (1979) 132(2):285–288.

[6] Hargrove III, WC, Barker, CF, Berkowitz, HD, Perloff, LJ, McLean, GK, Freiman, D, Ring, EJ, and Roberts, B. Treatment of Acute Peripheral Arterial and Graft Thromboses with Low Dose Streptokinase. *Surgery* (1982) 92:981–993

[7] Volpetti G, Barker CF, Berkowitz H, Roberts B. A twenty-two year review of elective resection of abdominal aortic aneurysms. *Surg Gynecol Obstet* (1976) 142(3):321-324.

CHAPTER 26

HUP Chief Residents During Drs. Fitts, Miller, and Roberts's Chairmanships

Despite political turbulence that caused rapid turnover of chairmen, HUP's residency continued to produce leaders in academy surgery. Of the sixty-five graduates of the program during this eleven-year period, four became department chairs at US universities, and thirteen became heads of divisions in major teaching hospitals.

1973 **Butler, Charles J.** MD University of Pennsylvania; practice of general surgery in Voorhees, New Jersey.

Cayten, C. Gene. BA Cornell University; MD New York University 1967; MPH Yale University School of Medicine 1971; assistant professor of surgery and director of emergency health services 1974–83; chief of trauma division, University of Pennsylvania 1980–83; professor of surgery, New York Medical College, Valhalla, since 1983; director of surgery, Our Lady of Mercy Medical Center, Bronx, NY, since 1983; member of injury control steering committee, New York State Department of Health in 1989; Trauma Advisory Council since 1992.

Edynak, Eugene M. MD Johns Hopkins University; internship and residency at HUP; University of Miami Master's in health administration; from 1966 to 1968, director and chief surgeon III Corps, US Army, Special Forces, Hospital for Civilian Irregular Defense Group, Republic of Vietnam; military awards include Bronze Star and Vietnamese Medal of Honor; professor of surgery, SUNY Downstate College of Medicine; recent practice as surgeon and family physician treating patients in New York City; in the past, served as associate professor of surgery at Eastern Virginia School of Medicine and CEO of Healthcare Management Consultants of South Florida.

Mullen, James L., Jr. BA Harvard University; MD University of Pennsylvania; professor of surgery, University of Pennsylvania; see Chapter 33.

Ruberg, Robert L. BA Harvard University 1967; residency in general surgery at HUP 1967–73; residency in plastic surgery at HUP 1973–75; for many years, chief of plastic surgery at Ohio State; honors include an endowed chair and annual symposium in his name.

Samuels, Garth A. S. MD University of the West Indies; residency at HUP; practices general and vascular surgery in Baltimore, Maryland.

Steiger, Ezra. MD Ohio State; while a HUP resident, developed model for studying TPN in rats. After two years in Air Force, joined faculty of Ohio State where he has continued to be productive in research on nutrition. Now professor and head of IV nutrition program. Given 2022 Lifetime Achievement Award of American Society of Parenteral and Enteral Nutrition (ASPEN).

Sugarman, Harvey J. MD Jefferson University; general surgery residency at HUP; faculty for thirty years at Virginia Commonwealth University; David E. M. Hume Professor of Surgery and interim chairman; international acclaim for gastric bypass surgery and other contributions for metabolism and bariatric procedures. Died in 2020.

Mayer, Lawrence J. MD University of Pennsylvania; practice in the **1974**
Drexel Hill area and at Delaware County Memorial Hospital.

Mullis, William F. MD University of Pennsylvania; residency in general surgery and plastic surgery at HUP; practices general and plastic surgery in Charlotte, North Carolina; member of Southern Surgical Association.

Nowicki, Edward R. Practice in cardiothoracic and vascular surgery in Portland, Maine.

Reckard, Craig R. MD University of Pennsylvania; research in transplantation; with Barker and Ziegler, was the first to successfully transplant isolated pancreatic islets in an animal model; served as transplant surgeon at Walter Reed Army Hospital, the University of Chicago Hospital, and was chief of transplantation at Loyola Medical Center in Chicago and Lehigh Valley Medical Center in Allentown, Pennsylvania. Died at age eighty in 2021.

Thomas, James H. MD University of Kentucky; training in vascular surgery at the University of Kansas; chairman of the department of surgery at the University of Kansas for ten years; member of the Society for Vascular Surgery, the American College of Surgeons, the American Surgical Association, and the Society of University Surgeons.

White, IV, Raleigh R. MD University of Pennsylvania; resident in general and plastic surgery at HUP; practice of plastic surgery and chairman of surgery department at Texas A&M and Scott White Clinic.

Ziegler, Moritz M. MD University of Cincinnati; training in general and pediatric surgery at the University of Pennsylvania and CHOP; extensive research including joining Barker and Reckard in the first successful transplantation of pancreatic islets in an animal model. Assistant professor to full professor at the University of Pennsylvania; then chief of pediatric surgery at the University of Cincinnati, Boston Children's Hospital, and the University of Colorado; winner of the Ladd Medal.

1975 **Caplan, Howard, S.** Fellowship in plastic surgery at HUP; plastic surgery staff at CHOP.

Ellman, Barry R. MD University of Pennsylvania; practice of general surgery in Edison, New Jersey.

Frazier, Thomas G. MD University of Pennsylvania; senior attending surgeon and medical director of Bryn Mawr Hospital Comprehensive Breast Center; clinical professor of surgery at Thomas Jefferson University; program director for Bryn Mawr Hospital breast surgery fellowship program; has been principal investigator of the National Surgical Adjuvant Breast and Bowel Project and past president of both the Metropolitan Philadelphia Chapter of the American College of Surgeons and the Philadelphia Academy of Surgery.

Jacobs, William E. MD and AOA University of Pennsylvania; internship, general surgery residency, and fellowship in plastic surgery at HUP; practice of plastic surgery in Charlotte, North Carolina. Died in 2014.

Shesol, Barry F. BA University of Pennsylvania; MD Ohio State University College of Medicine; general surgery and plastic surgery residency at HUP; assistant chief of plastic surgery, Fitzsimmons Army Medical Center 1978–80; chief of plastic surgery, Denver VA Hospital in 1980–82; chief of surgery, Aurora Humana Hospital 1988–90; president of Society of Colorado Plastic and Reconstructive Surgeons 1990–91.

Shumate, George R. MD University of Pennsylvania; residency in general surgery and fellowship in vascular surgery at HUP.

Tomasello, Donald N. MD Jefferson University; residency in general and cardiothoracic surgery at Jefferson University; prominent cardiovascular surgeon practicing mainly at Lankenau Hospital.

Brown, Arthur S. MD, general surgery residency, and plastic surgery fellowship at the University of Pennsylvania and HUP; practice of plastic surgery in Moorestown, New Jersey. **1976**

Chu, Winston. MD Rangoon University; general surgery residency and plastic surgery fellowship at the University of Pennsylvania; successful career as a plastic surgeon in Erie, Pennsylvania; now retired; author of autobiography, *REBORN: Journeys from the Abyss* that tells the story of Win's father's World War II adventures and Win's own journey from government oppression in Burma to Philadelphia. See *Penn Surgery Society Newsletter*, Fall 2015.

Levin, John M. BA Harvard University; MD Georgetown University; general surgery residency at Albert Einstein Medical Center and HUP; practice in Media, Pennsylvania.

Melissinos, Emmanuel G. MD University of Athens; residency in general surgery and plastic surgery at HUP; clinical professor of surgery, division of plastic and reconstructive surgery and clinical professor, department of orthopedic surgery, University of Texas Health Science Center at Houston; experienced in microsurgical free tissue transfers; 300 publications; married to Adrian Starvetsky who was HUP's first transplantation nurse administrator.

Naji, Ali MD Shiraz University School of Medicine, Iran; general surgery residency at HUP; PhD in immunology, University of Pennsylvania; for many years, one of the nation's leading scientists in transplantation biology and specifically in pancreatic transplantation; J. William White Professor of Surgical Research; in 2017 and again in 2022 had the largest amount of NIH funding of any US surgeon; in 2023, appointed Jonathan E. Rhoads Professor of Surgery.

Roseman, James M. MD University of Pennsylvania; general surgery residency at HUP; associate professor of surgery at Eastern Virginia Medical School; practice of surgical oncology in Vero Beach, Florida. Died in 1998.

Rout, W. Robert. BA Centre College of Kentucky; MD University of Louisville; general surgery residency at HUP; fellowship in addiction medicine in the department of psychiatry at University of Florida, Gainesville; active duty in US Army, Walter Reed Institute of Research; chief of surgery of the 354th Combat Support Hospital and surgeon at Dwight D. Eisenhower Medical Center at Ft. Gordon, Georgia, during Operation Desert Shield/Storm; board certified in surgery and addiction medicine; has been member of the faculties of Johns Hopkins and University of Florida departments of surgery, psychiatry, and behavioral sciences; chief of surgery at the VA Medical Center, Gainesville, Florida;

for many years, a highly valued associate professor of surgery at the University of Florida, Gainesville; presently director of the addiction medicine fellowship program in the department of psychiatry of Tulane University School of Medicine.

1977 **Alpert, Jeffrey R.** MD University of Vermont College of Medicine; internship, residency, and vascular fellowship at HUP; practice of general and vascular surgery in New York City.

Goodwin, Cleon W., Jr. MD University of Pennsylvania; four-year fellowship in respiratory physiology with Robert Forster at Penn; many years' experience in burn therapy at the San Antonio Burn Center with Basil Pruitt and Doug Wilmore and as chief of the burn center at New York Hospital; past president of the American Burn Association and chief of the San Antonio Burn Center succeeding Basil Pruitt in this role; at present, head of Western States Burn Center in Greeley, Colorado.

Hill, Robert B. MD University of Texas Southwestern in Dallas; general surgical residency at HUP; lt. commander and surgeon on active duty in the US Navy on the *USS Nimitz* during the Iran crisis. Also, surgeon for the 7th Fleet aboard the *USS Midway;* served as trauma surgeon at Cooper Hospital in Camden, New Jersey, and also as assistant professor of surgery at Rutgers University of Medicine and Dentistry; later practiced in Haddenfield, New Jersey. Died in 2020.

Hoelzer, Dennis J. MD University of Rochester; general surgery residency at HUP; fellowship in pediatric surgery at CHOP; for many years, practice of pediatric surgery and director of pediatric residency program at Christiana Care Health Services; associate professor of surgery at UMDMJ–Robert Wood Johnson Medical School.

McCombs, Peter R. BA Yale University; MD Tufts University; residency in general surgery and fellowship in vascular surgery at HUP; practice in vascular surgery at Abington Hospital; chairman of surgery at Pennsylvania Hospital 2001–2006; chief of surgery at Philadelphia Veterans Affairs Medical Center 2006–2010; retired, living in Florida.

Oram-Smith, Jeffrey C. MD University of Pennsylvania; internship in surgical residency at HUP; practice of general surgery in Colorado Springs; now retired.

Wallack, Marc K. MD University of Pittsburgh; general surgery residency and three years research on tumor immunology at HUP; for many years, chief of surgery at the University of Miami; now chief of surgery at New York Metropolitan Hospital and professor of surgery at New York Medical College.

Zins, James E. MD University of Pennsylvania; internship, residency in general and plastic surgery, and fellowship in craniofacial surgery at HUP; fellowship in maxillofacial surgery at Great Ormond St. Hospital in London; honorary research fellowship at University College Hospital in London; chairman of the department of plastic and reconstructive surgery at Cleveland Clinic; founding member of the American Society of Craniofacial Surgeons; past president of the American Association of Plastic Surgeons and current director of the American Board of Plastic Surgery; professor of surgery at the Cleveland Clinic Lerner College of Medicine; serves on editorial boards of plastic surgery journals including *Annals of Plastic Surgery, Aesthetic Plastic Surgery,* and *Aesthetic Surgery.*

Belcastro, Vincent J. MD Loyola University Chicago Stritch School of Medicine; residency in general surgery at HUP; practices general surgery in Fort Myers, Florida. **1978**

Brownstein, Gary M. MD Thomas Jefferson University; BA in psychology from Temple University; resident in general surgery at HUP; chief resident in general surgery at Presbyterian Hospital; residency in plastic surgery at Case Western Reserve University; practice of plastic surgery, Case Western Reserve University; past president of the New Jersey Society of Plastic Surgeons; plastic surgery practice in Voorhees, New Jersey.

Frangipane, Leo G., Jr. MD Temple University; general surgery residency at HUP; HUP fellowship in vascular surgery; research in transplantation; practice of general surgery at Southern Regional Medical Center in Georgia; founded SEEK, a national support group to help terminally ill patients and their families deal with chronic illness and end-of-life issues; published books on wellness.

Kerr, Lawrence P. BA Hamilton College; MD SUNY Upstate Medical University; general surgery and plastic fellowship at HUP; practice of plastic surgery in Binghamton, New York.

Nakashima, Rolland K. MD University of Pennsylvania; general and plastic surgery residency at HUP; practices in Aiea, Hawaii.

Pollock, Thomas W. MD University of Pennsylvania; general surgery and research fellowship at HUP; very promising young assistant professor of surgery at SUNY Downstate; shot and killed in 1985 at Kings County Hospital by disgruntled patient who was searching for someone else.

Fakhraee, Michael S. MD University of Shiraz, Iran; intern at Jefferson University; resident in general and plastic surgery at HUP; practices plastic surgery and hand surgery at Jeanes Hospital. **1979**

Gertner, Marc H. MD Ohio State University; general surgery residency at HUP; practice of general surgery at Sinai Hospital in Baltimore.

Hargrove, III, W. Clark. MD Wake Forest University; residency and cardiothoracic fellowship at HUP; for many years, clinical professor of cardiothoracic surgery at the University of Pennsylvania; highly valued faculty surgeon who was considered to be one of the finest cardiac surgeons in the area; operated mainly at Presbyterian Hospital.

Lane, Michael F. MD SUNY Upstate Medical University; general surgery residency at HUP; practice of general surgery in Rockledge, Florida.

Reichman, Joseph H. MD Hahnemann University; general and plastic surgery residency at HUP and CHOP; practice of plastic surgery in Voorhees, New Jersey.

Sparenberg, C. Russell. MD University of Texas Medical Branch at Galveston; residency in general and plastic surgery at HUP; practice in Plano, Texas.

1980 **Hanno, Philip M.** MD Baylor University; associate professor at University of Pennsylvania and chief of Veterans Administration Hospital 1981–90; chairman of urology, Temple University 1990–1998; professor of urology, University of Pennsylvania 1999–2016; MPH University of Wisconsin 2005; clinical professor of urology, Stanford University 2016 to present.

Hobbs, Charles L. MD George Washington University; general surgery residency at HUP; practices general surgery at ChristinaCare Hospitals in Wilmington, Delaware.

Matthews, David C. MD University of Cincinnati; residency in general and plastic surgery at HUP; fellowship in pediatric plastic surgery at Royal Melbourne Hospital; practice of plastic surgery in Charlotte, North Carolina.

Rastegar, Hassan. MD Shiraz University of Medical Sciences; internship SUNY Downstate Medical Center; general surgery residency at HUP; fellowship in cardiothoracic surgery at Northwestern Memorial Hospital; professor of surgery, Tufts University School of Medicine.

Spence, Richard K. BA Rutgers University; MD Georgetown University; general surgery residency and vascular fellowship at HUP; research with Barker in transplantation; professor and chief of vascular division, Robert Wood Johnson School of Medicine and Dentistry, Camden, New Jersey; widely acclaimed for research and clinical aspects of bloodless surgery and transfusions in Jehovah's Witness patients; director of surgical education, Baptist Health Systems in Alabama.

Buzby, Gordon P. BA University of Pennsylvania; Phi Beta Kappa and for three years, All-American intercollegiate champion in sailing; MD University of Pennsylvania, AOA 1974; general surgery residency at HUP; with Jim Mullen, developed a prognostic nutrition index for pre- and postoperative nutritional support; associate professor of surgery, University of Pennsylvania; co-director of Nutrition Support Service, HUP; director of surgical metabolic unit at Philadelphia VA; board of directors, ASPEN; chairman of influential randomized trial of TPN in surgical patients; published in *New England Journal of Medicine*; with his wife, endowed prize for annual lecture at HUP on leadership; director of HUP general surgery residency 2001–2003. Died in 2003. **1981**

Cooper, Arthur. BA Harvard University; MD University of Pennsylvania; fellowships in pediatric surgery and critical care at CHOP; emeritus professor at Columbia College of Physicians and Surgeons; founding member and past chairman of American Board of Disaster Medicine; Medical Director of Pediatric Injury and Prevention Program for NYC Health Hospitals, Harlem.

Dafoe, Donald C. BA and MD University of Wisconsin; residency and fellowship in transplantation at HUP; associate professor of surgery, University of Michigan; professor and chief of transplantation division, HUP; chief of transplantation, Stanford University; chairman of department of surgery, Jefferson University; director of pancreas and kidney transplantation and director of surgical education and Eris M. Field Endowed chair in diabetes research, Cedars-Sinai; chief of transplantation surgery, University of California, Irvine.

Gadzik, James P. BA Yale University; MD University of Pennsylvania; general surgery residency at HUP; general surgery practice in Westport, Connecticut.

Smale, Brian F. MD Hahnemann University; general surgery residency at HUP; practice of general and colorectal surgery in Morrisville, Vermont.

Barot, Lenora R. MD University of Pennsylvania; general and plastic surgery residency at HUP; practice of plastic surgery in Voorhees, New Jersey. **1982**

Caldwell, Michael D. BS University of South Carolina 1964; PhD in physiology Vanderbilt University 1980; general surgery residency at HUP 1980–82; fellow ASPEN 2013; Gwen Sebold Award for outstanding research 2012; practice of general surgery in Marshfield, Wisconsin.

Chang, Alfred E. BA Dartmouth University; MD Harvard University; residency Duke University 1974–76; oncology fellow surgical branch National

Cancer Institute 1976–79; residency HUP 1979–82; senior investigator, National Cancer Institute 1982–87; Hugh Cabot Professor of Surgery, University of Michigan 1987 to present; director of breast center, director of GI oncology program, associate director of translational research and clinical affairs, University of Michigan; extramural funding of tumor immunology research for twenty-five years; director of T32 training grant in oncology.

Schwartz, Ira. MD Jefferson University; residency in general surgery and urology at HUP.

Boraas, Marcia C. MD University of Pennsylvania; general surgery res-
1983 idency at HUP; seven years faculty at University of Pennsylvania (clinical associate professor); practices at Jeanes Hospital specializing in breast surgery.

Fairman, Ronald M. BA Muhlenberg College; MD Thomas Jefferson University; general surgery residency and vascular surgery fellowship at HUP; chief of surgery, Jeanes Hospital; Clyde F. Barker—William Maul Measey Professor of Surgery, chief of division of vascular surgery and endovascular therapy, and vice chairman for clinical affairs in the department of surgery, HUP; performed the first endovascular abdominal aortic aneurysm repair (EVAR), endovascular thoracic aortic aneurysm repair (TEVAR), and carotid stent with distal protection to prevent stroke at the University of Pennsylvania; has performed well over seventy clinical trials since the mid-1990s and has served as PI for virtually all of them; in 2010, was awarded the University of Pennsylvania Health System Luigi Mastroianni Clinical Innovator Award; in 2015, received the University of Pennsylvania Health System Master Clinician Award; in his tenure as division chief at Penn, mentored ten fellows who became division chiefs or department chairman at major academic institutions; served as president of the Society for Vascular Surgery (SVS) and is a "Distinguished Fellow" of the Society; member of the Halsted Society, the American College of Surgeons, the Society for Clinical Vascular Surgery, and the American Surgical Association; has published over 250 peer-reviewed manuscripts and over 100 book chapters and reviews; on the editorial board of most major vascular surgical and endovascular journals; in 2016, was elected to membership in the American Philosophical Society, a unique honor for both a physician and surgeon.

Kusiak, Joseph F. General and plastic surgery residency at HUP; practice in Voorhees, New Jersey, and Ft. Myers, Florida.

Ruben, Garry D. BA Tufts University; MD University of Maryland; general surgery residency at HUP; vascular surgery fellowship, Albert Einstein Hospital, Philadelphia; practice of general and vascular surgery in Silver Springs, Maryland.

CHAPTER 27

For Surgery, the End of Turbulence

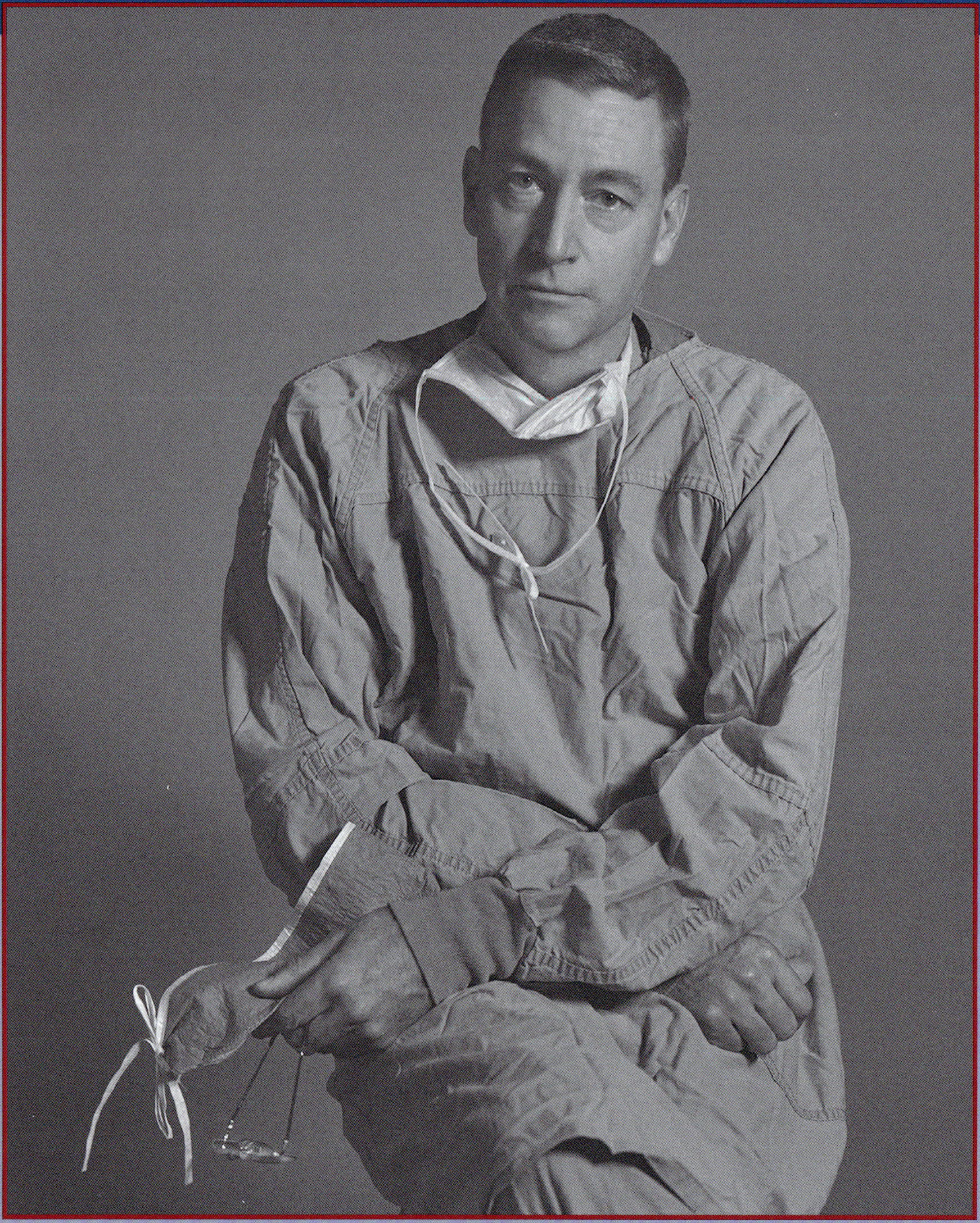

Clyde F. Barker (1932–)

JRB Professor and Chairman of Surgery (1983–2001)

Contributed by Ronald M. Fairman

Introduction

In writing this chapter, I came across some correspondence from Dr. Tom Starzl to the American College of Physicians regarding the *John Phillips Memorial Award for Outstanding Work in Clinical Medicine*, dated April 25, 2011. Starzl wrote, "Dr. Clyde Barker's contributions to clinical medicine over the last fifty years have been so consistently innovative (and sustained over time) that he has emerged as the prototypical physician-investigator envisioned by Claude Bernard, the nineteenth-century father of experimental medicine." Furthermore, "the immune tolerance of Barker and Billingham was the *de facto* cornerstone of all categories of transplantation and for that matter immunology generally. Barker created a new field, a branch of transplantation in which alloengraftment depends in large part on achieving and maintaining immune ignorance of allografts." Starzl concluded, "What Barker accomplished before, during, and after his eighteen-year tenure as Chairman of Surgery at the University of Pennsylvania required a unique dual personality: the able administrator who is also a working and inventive scientist. His career provides a model that deserves study of how to advance medicine and surgery against the grudging opposition posed by the unknown. Central to his effort was the attitude that research laboratories are to help people, and more specifically, sick patients; Barker created the profile of an extensive laboratory program interwoven into a world-class clinical endeavor. The result was

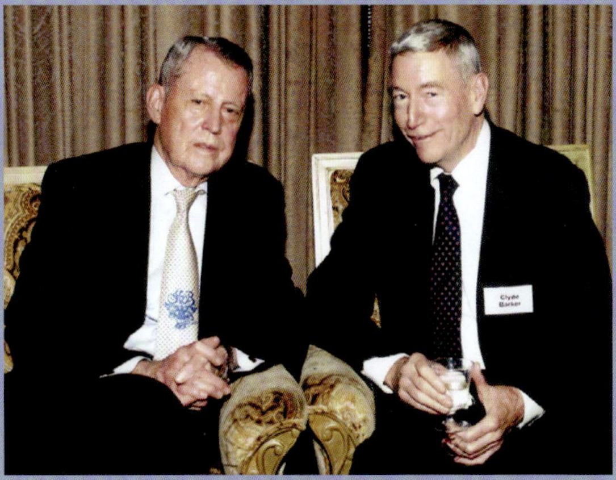

Tom Starzl and Clyde Barker

1849
Barker family reaches Utah

1943–1958
All four Barker brothers obtain doctorates. Which one is most academically accomplished can be debated.

Hal directed Columbia Presbyterian Hospital's metabolic unit and ICU. He was also director of medical affairs, in charge of new programs.

Roland's PhD thesis was based on nine papers he published on quantum theory with his mentor Henry Eyring, the founder of the field.

Earl directed Penn's third-year medical school class

complete dissolution of the artificial barrier between *basic* and *clinical* science."

When Barker finished his third six-year term as John Rhea Barton Professor and Chairman of Surgery in 2001, he marked the longest tenure of anyone in this leadership position in the oldest medical school and oldest university hospital in the United States. As I researched and composed this chapter, I came to the realization he was the most unique and transformative chairman in the history of Penn Surgery.

The Early Years

Clyde F. Barker (CFB) was born in Salt Lake City in 1932. His father, Fred G. Barker, was a professor of psychology at the University of Utah, and CFB added that he was an author and Shakespearean scholar.[1] The Barker family originally arrived in Salt Lake City in 1849, two years after the city was founded by Brigham Young. Tragically, his father died at fifty-five years of age from a coronary occlusion; CFB was thirteen years old. His mother, Jennetta, was from Ogden, north of Salt Lake City, was college educated, and to fund her children's education worked as a high school teacher. She died at ninety-four years of age. CFB was the youngest of four children. Hal was his oldest brother and was fifteen years older than CFB. Notably, he was captain of the tennis team at the University of Utah and spent his last two

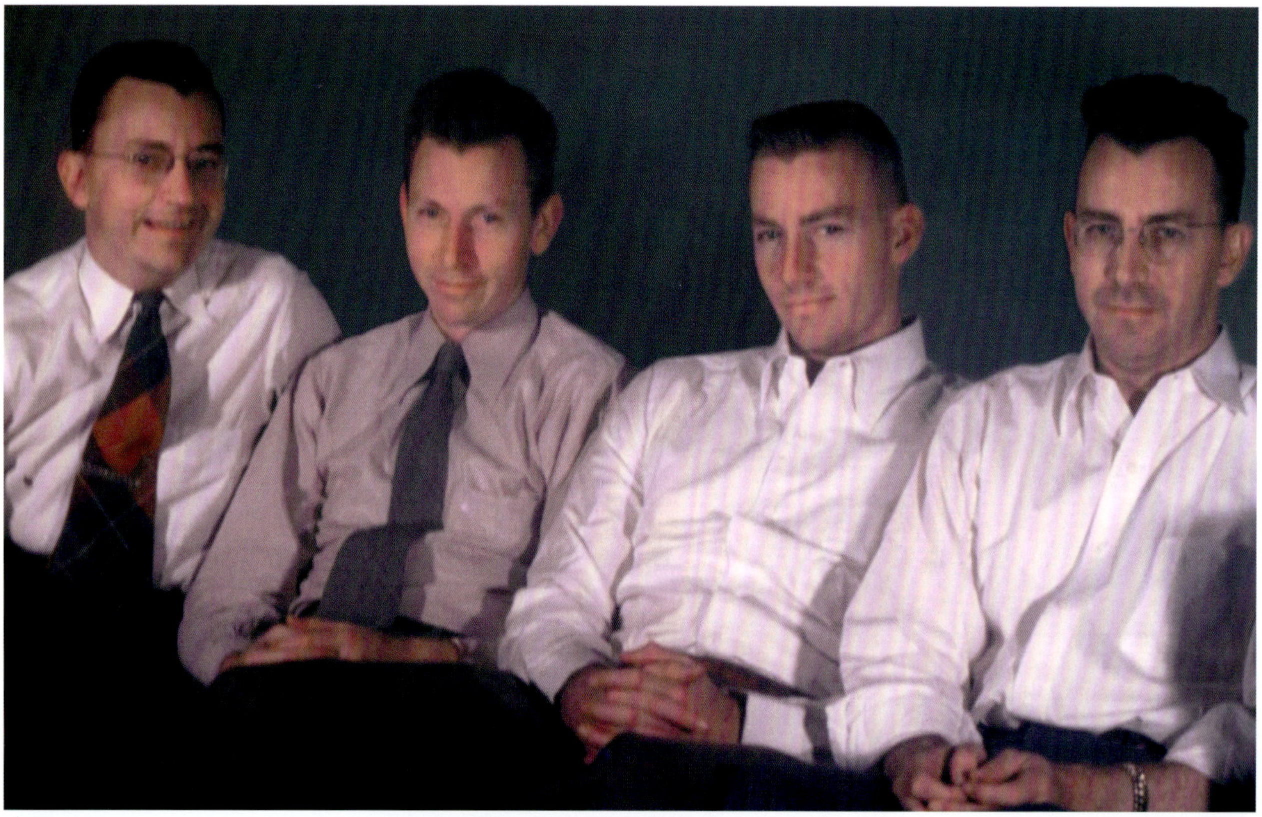

Barker brothers: (l to r) Earl, Roland, Clyde, and Hal

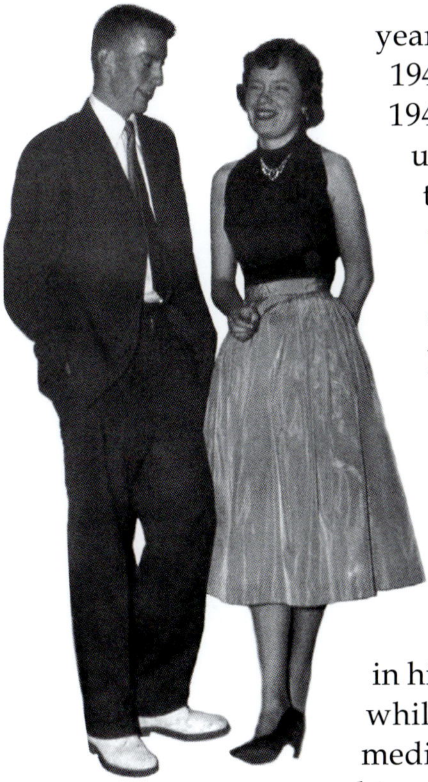

Clyde and Dode are classmates at Cornell. Meet on a blind date.

years of medical school at Penn, graduating in 1943. After serving in the wartime Army from 1943 to 1945, he did his surgical residency under I. S. Ravdin at Penn and then joined the faculty for one year. He was recruited to Columbia, promoted to full professor, had a huge clinical practice as a general surgeon, had twenty-two consecutive years of NIH research funding, and spent his entire career there.[2] His brother Roland, who was thirteen years older than CFB, received his PhD in chemistry from Princeton but died at age thirty-six of rheumatic heart disease. His other older brother Earl, who was twelve years older than CFB, graduated first in his class in college at the University of Utah, while also playing varsity tennis. He went to medical school at Penn and stayed at HUP for his residency in internal medicine. He became a nephrologist and spent his entire career at Penn.

Hal, as the oldest brother, had great impact on CFB following the death of their father. Hal encouraged CFB to be educated at Phillips Exeter Academy, and he enrolled there at fifteen years of age (1947) as a sophomore. Like Hal, CFB played competitive tennis and was captain of the tennis team at Exeter and their number one player. He was ranked first in both the intermountain and New England states and third nationally while at Exeter. Exeter served as an eye-opening educational and social experience for CFB, while he admitted he was not a dedicated student. He decided to attend Cornell University where he continued to develop his tennis prowess. As a junior and senior, he played number one singles and doubles for Cornell and was captain of the team as a senior. He met his future wife Dorothy (Dode was her nickname from childhood) in February of his junior

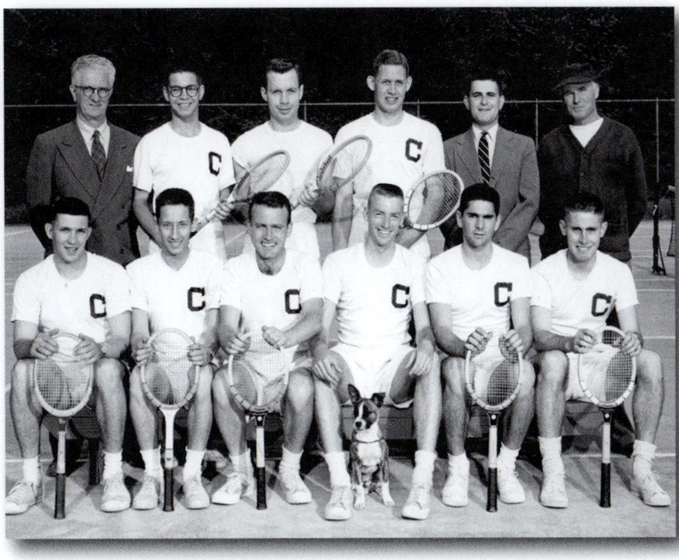

Cornell University tennis team with Oliver, captain CFB's dog

1947–1950
CFB at Phillips Exeter Academy

1950–1954
Clyde and Dode are classmates at Cornell

1953
Clyde and Dode meet on a blind date at Cornell

1953
Cornell's once-beaten tennis team holds Cornell's record for most wins

1954
CFB is number one player and team captain

1956
Clyde and Dode are married after his second year of medical school

1954
A summer of tournament tennis

1954–1958
Medical school at Cornell

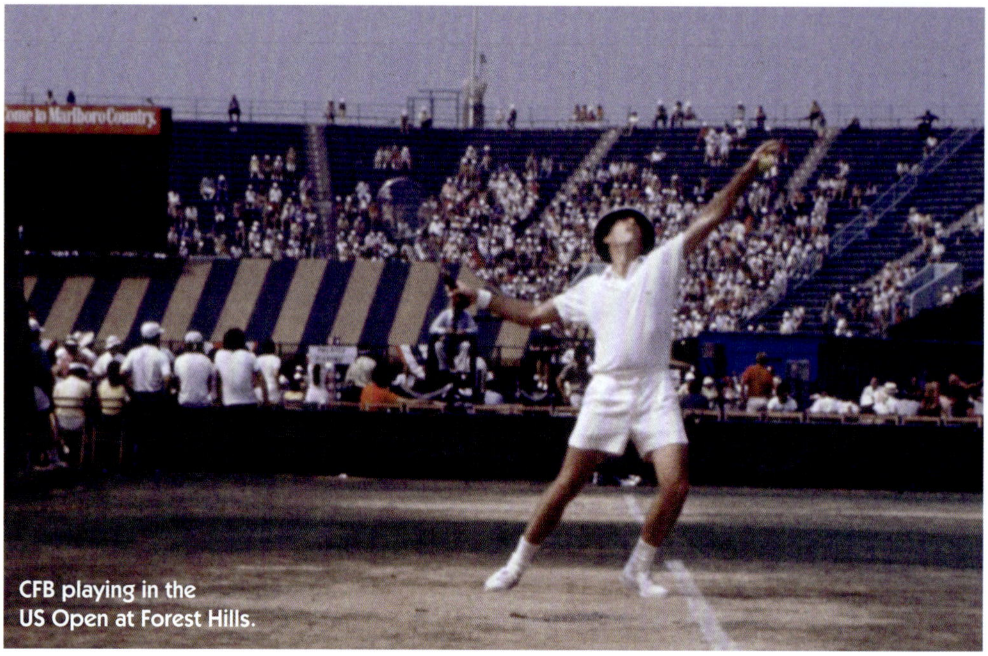

CFB playing in the US Open at Forest Hills.

year on a blind date. From then onward, they were a couple. Dorothy majored in French literature at Cornell and was from Chicago.

Tennis remained a huge focus, and the summer following graduation from college, he played in the eastern grass court tournaments and the US nationals, earning a national ranking in the men's division. CFB went on to Cornell Medical School, and Dorothy returned to Chicago after college graduation to pursue a work opportunity. While his brothers wanted CFB to postpone marriage, he and Dode disagreed, and they were married in Chicago after he completed his second year of medical school in 1956. Tennis took a back seat during medical school, and he became, perhaps for the first time (in his own view), a serious student. He thrived academically and personally in medical school.

Postgraduate Training

CFB followed his brothers' advice and came to HUP as a rotating intern in 1958. He clearly knew all about Penn from both Hal and Earl. He stayed on as a surgical resident while I. S. Ravdin was still chairman for the first six months of his residency. Jonathan Rhoads then became Chairman of Surgery in 1960. Notably influential Penn physicians during his residency included I. S. Ravdin, Bob Mayock (a former roommate of Hal's), Francis Wood,

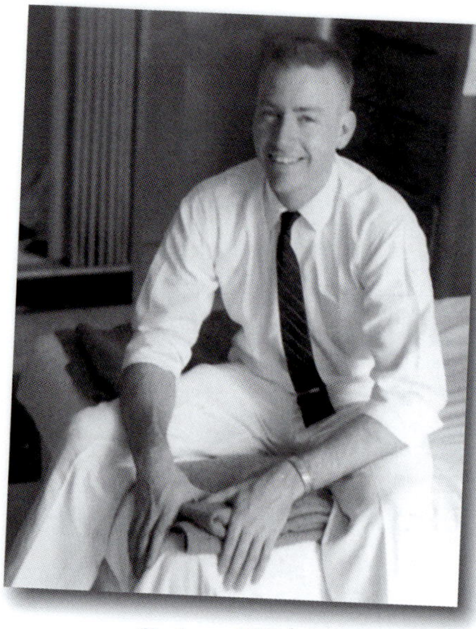

Clyde as HUP intern

Bill Hanson, Truman Schnabel, and Sylvan Eisman. He was a surgical resident from 1959 to 1964.

1958–1964
CFB's HUP internship and general surgery residency

Influential surgical faculty included Jerry Peskin, Jack Mackie, Julian Johnson ("J. J."), Jim Thompson, and Jonathan Rhoads. CFB performed research as a resident with Jerry Peskin on portacaval shunts[3] and introduced/managed a machine for gastric cooling in HUP patients to stop upper gastrointestinal bleeding.[4] While Julian Johnson was known as an intensely demanding cardiovascular surgeon who was feared by the house staff, CFB considered J. J. a favorite mentor and admired his technical prowess and dedication, more so than any other surgical faculty. The surgical residency program at Penn was very much aligned with the traditional, rigorous pyramidal training models of that period (Halsted/Ravdin residency). There were twelve residents in his first year, and only three completed surgical training at HUP.

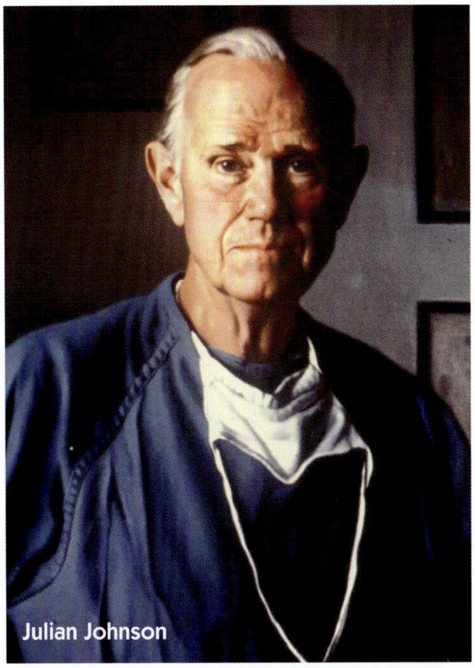
Julian Johnson

CFB's favorite mentor during his residency

1964
While a chief resident, CFB visits US transplant centers. He scrubs with Tom Starzl on a kidney transplant

1964–1965
CFB spends a year as vascular fellow under Brooke Roberts

While contemplating a career in transplantation, as a chief resident, he visited the handful of active US transplant centers that existed at the time, including scrubbing with Tom Starzl on a kidney transplant at the University of Colorado. This brief clinical experience of working with Starzl was transformative and cemented his desire to pursue a career as a transplant surgeon. He spent one month studying the basics of transplantation research in Paul Russell's laboratory at MGH. Passing up J. J.'s offer of a fellowship to train as a cardiac surgeon, he chose a vascular fellowship with Brooke Roberts at Penn from 1964–65. He was Roberts's second vascular fellow; Harry Nelson was the first. He viewed his vascular fellowship as a necessary pathway to transplantation.

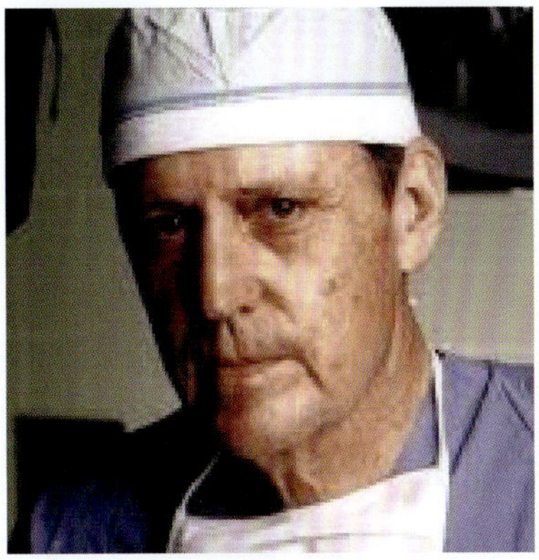
Tom Starzl

CFB and Dode began their family during his residency and went on to raise four children (Fred, John, Bill, and the youngest, Elizabeth) who all excelled academically and as adults have gone on to highly successful careers.

1965–1972
CFB is a junior member of HUP surgical faculty and also Billingham's postdoctoral fellow and a junior faculty member in the Department of Genetics

1967–1972
CFB is associate in Department of Genetics, sharing a bench with Billingham for their work on privileged sites. They define the principle of immunologic ignorance

1976–present
Vacations of Barker family at their Adirondack retreat

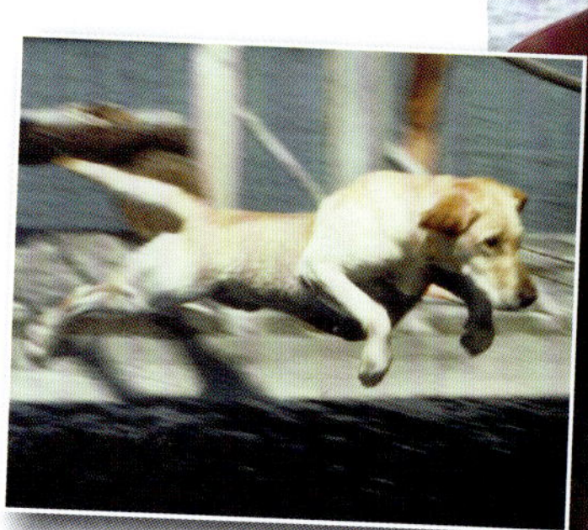
Max

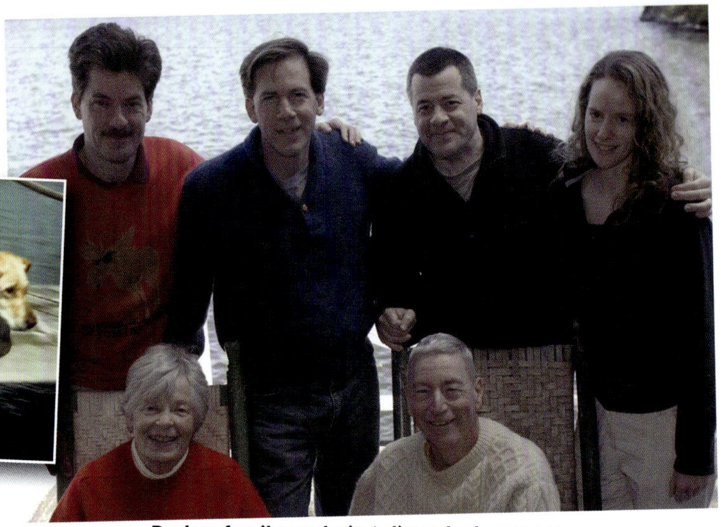
Barker family at their Adirondack retreat: (back row, l to r) John, Bill, Fred, and Elizabeth

Early Penn Faculty Career

Following his vascular fellowship, he joined the faculty and became Roberts's junior associate in the vascular division. While focused on advancing transplantation, CFB performed the first infrapopliteal vein bypasses at HUP,[5] many to the level of the foot. He also performed the first resection of a suprarenal aortic aneurysm at HUP. He collaborated with Roberts and Ernie Ring (interventional radiologist) and pioneered transluminal angioplasty[6] and thrombolysis of occluded arteries with streptokinase.[7]

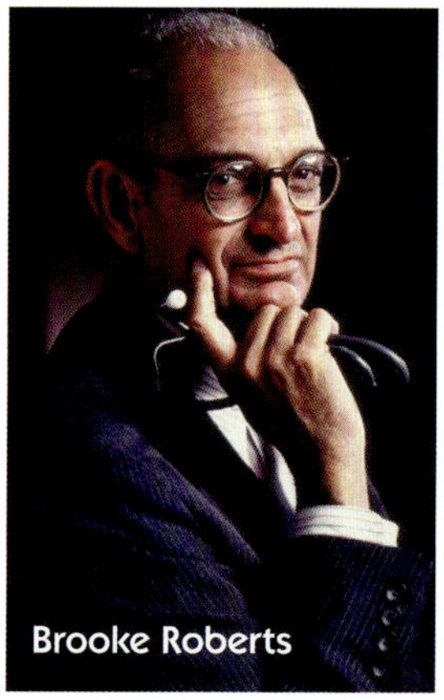
Brooke Roberts

In 1966, Rupert Billingham moved to Penn from England and became chair of the genetics department. Billingham was Peter Medawar's former graduate student and played a major role in the research responsible for Medawar receiving the Nobel Prize for transplantation tolerance in 1960.[8] CFB be-

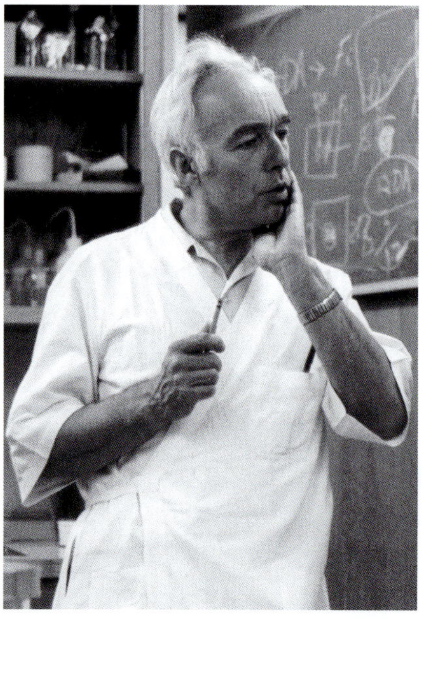

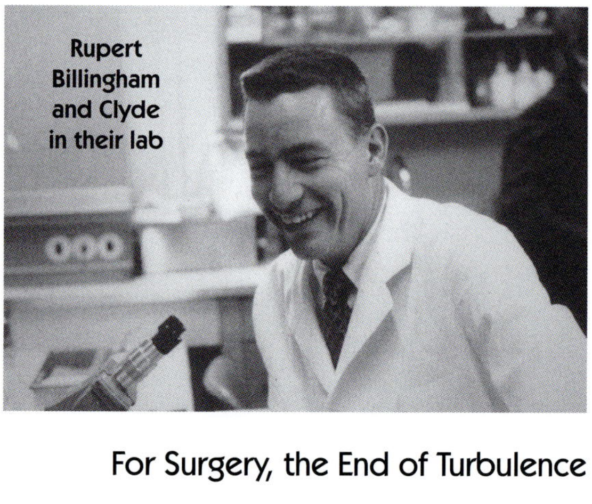
Rupert Billingham and Clyde in their lab

1966 (Feb.)
While a fellow in Billingham's genetics department, CFB performs HUP's first kidney transplant

came one of Billingham's first postdocs and was a junior faculty member of his Department of Genetics for six years. They shared a research laboratory where they worked together on the same research projects.

With Billingham, CFB published twelve highly regarded basic research publications. Their first paper was a classic. It established a fundamental law of transplantation—immunologic ignorance. This principle is that the immune system cannot recognize the presence of foreign antigen that fails to reach host lymphoid tissue.[9] The decisive experiment leading to this conclusion was their demonstration that skin allografts transplanted to a surgically constructed, vascularized pedicle lacking lymphatic drainage completely escaped rejection (see illustration).[10] Their dissection of this seemingly simple surgical model and of other privileged sites, such as the hamster cheek pouch, had profound impact.[11] The principal of immune ignorance remains a cornerstone of transplantation immunology and is one of the most important findings of the last half century.[12] Barker's presentation of this work at international meetings and publications of it in prestigious journals led to his recognition as one of the best-known researchers in the early years of transplantation biology. The enduring relationship with Billingham propelled CFB academically, and they remained lifelong, close friends.

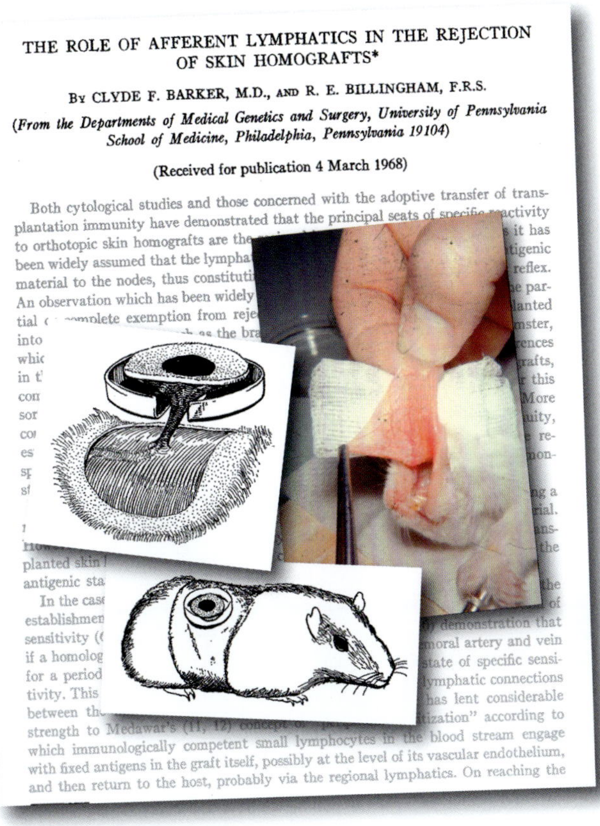
THE ROLE OF AFFERENT LYMPHATICS IN THE REJECTION OF SKIN HOMOGRAFTS*

By CLYDE F. BARKER, M.D., and R. E. BILLINGHAM, F.R.S.

(From the Departments of Medical Genetics and Surgery, University of Pennsylvania School of Medicine, Philadelphia, Pennsylvania 19104)

(Received for publication 4 March 1968)

Both cytological studies and those concerned with the adoptive transfer of transplantation immunity have demonstrated that the principal seats of specific reactivity ... which immunologically competent small lymphocytes in the blood stream engage with fixed antigens in the graft itself, possibly at the level of its vascular endothelium, and then return to the host, probably via the regional lymphatics. On reaching the

Fifty years later, the importance of immune ignorance was reinforced by Fadi Lakkis's demonstration that skin allografts cannot be rejected by mice genetically lacking lymph nodes.[13] As an accomplished microsur-

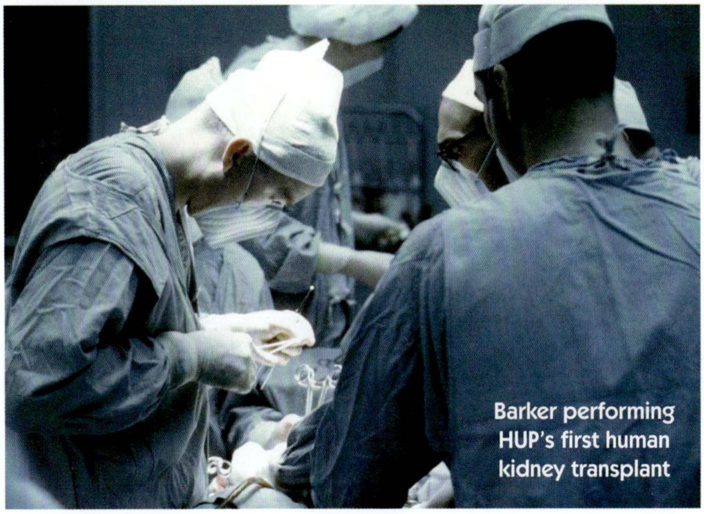
Barker performing HUP's first human kidney transplant

1969
Ex vivo microsurgery to resect renal artery aneurysms

geon, Barker used organ transplants in rodents to sort out basic differences in the rejection of skin and vascularized organ transplants.[14]

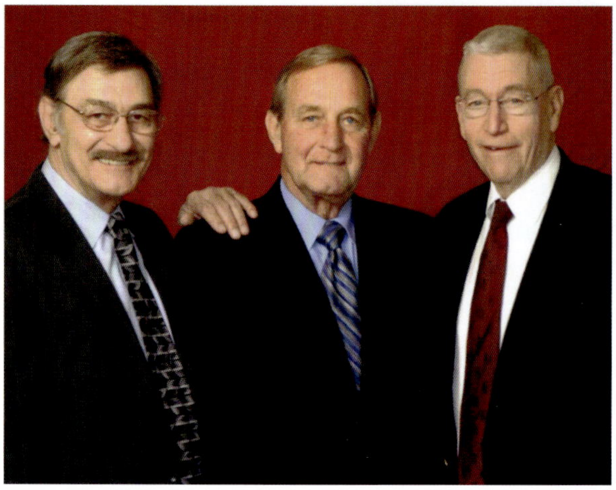

Five decades later: kidney donor, Joe; his brother the recipient, Howard; and the surgeon, Clyde Barker.

In February 1966, while still a postdoctoral fellow in Billingham's genetics department, CFB performed HUP's first human kidney transplant. The kidney functioned normally for forty-eight years until the otherwise healthy patient died of a coronary occlusion. This early transplant was one of only about ten in the world to survive that long. It was Billingham's support for CFB and his clout with the Penn nephrologists (who were skeptical of kidney transplantation) that led the young CFB to perform this first kidney transplant at Penn. Billingham moved to the University of Texas Southwestern Medical Center in 1971.

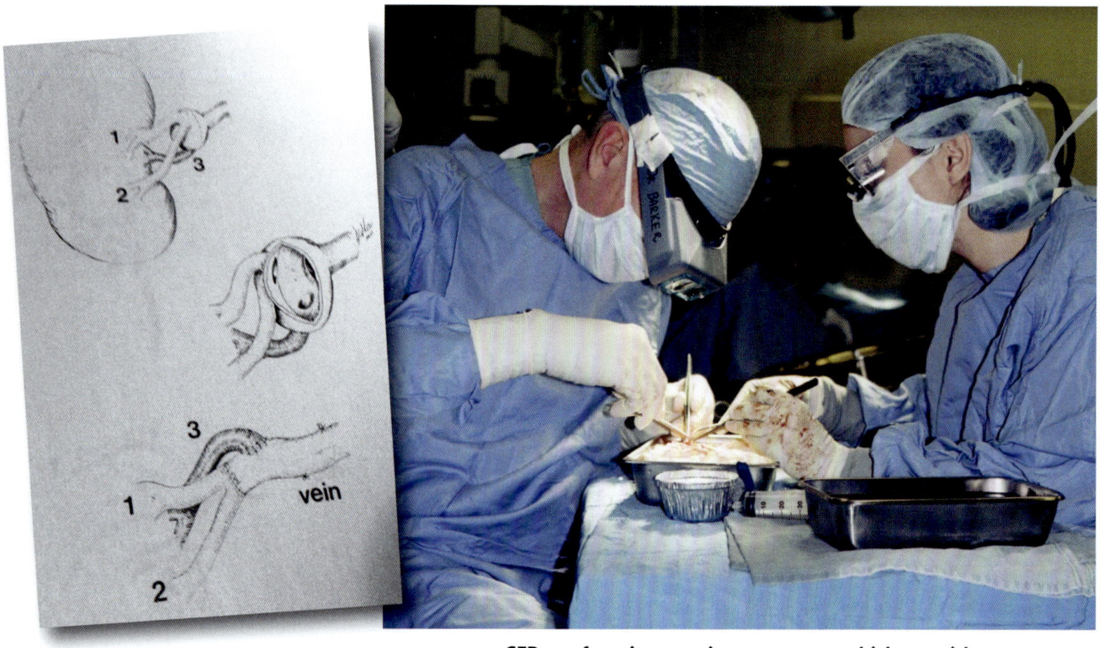

CFB performing ex-vivo surgery on kidney with his vascular fellow, Omaida Velazquez.

CFB became chief of the transplantation program at Penn in 1966 and held this position until 2001. Transplantation became a Penn surgery division in 1969. CFB employed his technical skills as a kidney transplant surgeon to pioneer ex vivo renal artery surgery focused on complicated renal artery aneurysms at Penn.[15] This involved removing a kidney with multiple renal artery aneurysms, cooling it, resecting the aneurysms, and reconstructing the renal arteries on a back table, following which he would re-implant the kidney into the pelvis of the patient. He was able to achieve both immediate and long-term successful results in this highly complicated group of patients who otherwise would have faced loss of the kidney and life-threatening complications. His results remain the gold-standard even today.

From 1968–1974, CFB was a Markle Scholar.[16] The Markle Foundation was founded in 1927 by a Pennsylvania coal magnate, John Markle. The now-extinct scholar program was intended to identify and support the country's most promising teachers and investigators in academic medicine early in the course of their careers. By a uniquely competitive process, it was awarded to individuals who were identified as the future leaders of academic medicine. This provided CFB financial support over five years and, because of the Markle Foundation's influence, was instrumental in his early academic success. Most of the Markle Scholars became department chairmen or deans.

In 1972, CFB began pancreatic islet transplant research and explored the idea—not widely accepted at the time—that Type 1 diabetes mellitus was an autoimmune disease. In 1972, CFB with surgical residents Craig Reckard and Mory Ziegler reported the first complete and lasting reversal of diabetes in an animal model by pancreatic islet transplantation.[17] His research studies were the first to systematically dissect the immunological barriers to islet allograft acceptance. While CFB had numerous research collaborations, his graduate students Ali Naji and Jim Markmann, both surgeons and PhDs, became his most enduring collaborators.

1968–1974
CFB is Markle Scholar

1972
CFB begins research in transplantation of isolated pancreatic islets

1972
CFB with research fellows Reckard and Ziegler reports the world's first complete and permanent reversal of diabetes by islet transplantation

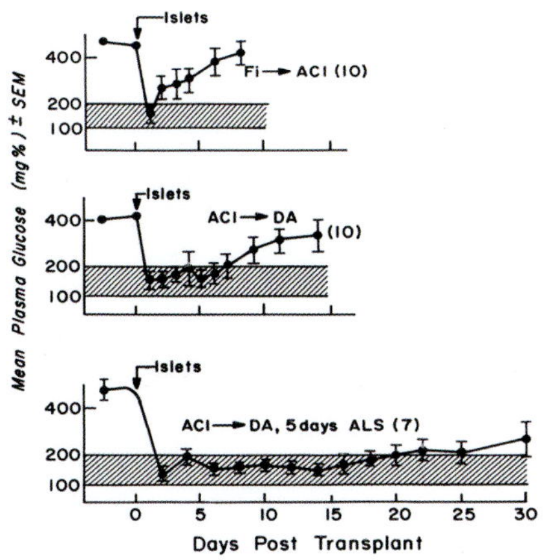

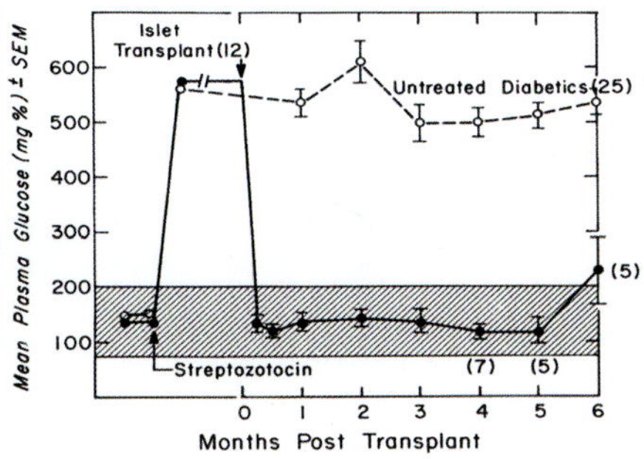

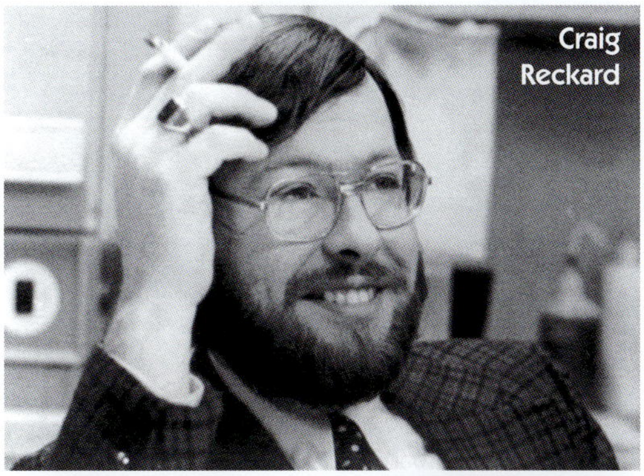
Craig Reckard

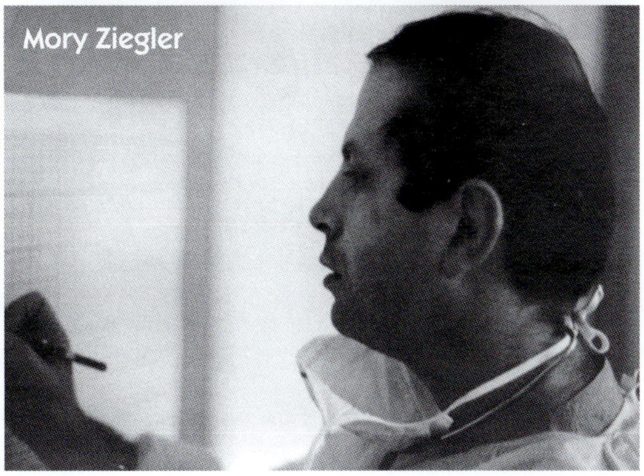
Mory Ziegler

1973
CFB appointed full professor

1974
CFB and other Philadelphia surgeons found organ-sharing program

1982–2001
CFB is chief of vascular division. One of his fellows, Marc Mitchell, was chief of surgery at Presbyterian and the VA Hospital before becoming chairman of surgery at the University of Mississippi. Two others also become surgery department chairs, Jeffrey Carpenter at Cooper Medical School of Rowan University and Omaida Velazquez at the University of Miami

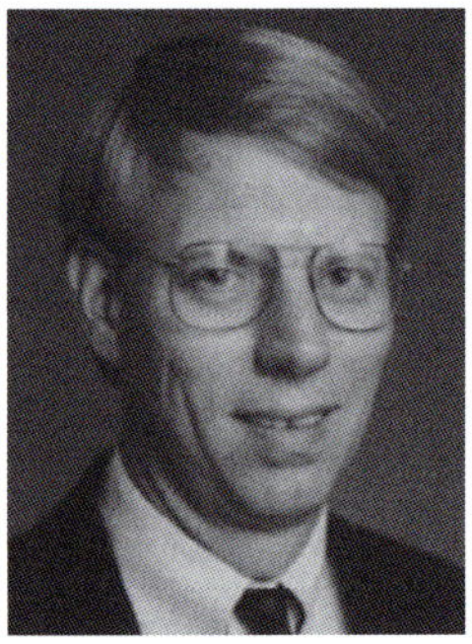

Marc Mitchell

1982
Reports with Naji in *Science* that autoimmunity alone can destroy transplanted islet allografts.

He was proud to acknowledge that they later became more accomplished in research than him. Objectively, the Penn pancreatic islet research program went on to become the best in the country. Also in 1972, CFB performed the first liver transplant at HUP. The patient survived only a few days, and CFB declared a moratorium on further liver transplants awaiting further resources and better immunosuppression.

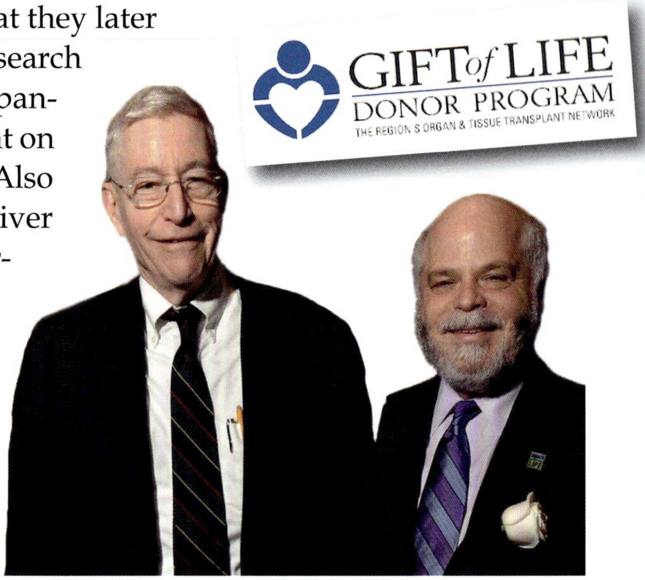

Clyde Barker and Howard Nathan

By the mid-1970s, the Penn kidney transplant program was performing large numbers of procedures with excellent outcomes, establishing it as one of the most respected clinical transplant centers in the country. In 1974, CFB with other Philadelphia transplant surgeons founded the Organ Procurement Organization (OPO), later named Gift of Life. After Barker and his colleagues appointed Howard Nathan as director, it became the largest OPO in the United States. As of the end of 2021 and for the fourteenth consecutive year, Gift of Life has coordinated the most organs for transplant achieving the highest number of organ donors (705) ever recorded for a US-based OPO. Those donations resulted in 1,732 transplants, the most in the US in 2021, and 1,007 kidney transplants, the most ever.

CFB was promoted to professor of surgery in 1973, the J. William White Professor of Surgical Research in 1978, and the Donald Guthrie Professor of Surgery in 1982. From 1974 until 1999, CFB had RO1 NIH funding of his research for twenty-five consecutive years, including a MERIT grant (1987–1996). From 1979 through 1981, he served on the NIH immunobiology study section. CFB became chief of the Penn Division of Vascular Surgery in 1982 and held this position until 2001. Gary Gross and Ron Fairman were his first vascular fellows in 1982. In this same year, Barker and Naji published in *Science* that in an animal model of spontaneous diabetes, transplanted islet allografts exempt from rejection because of neonatal-induced tolerance are destroyed instead by autoimmunity alone.[18] This sentinel finding was the best evidence at the time that diabetes is an autoim-

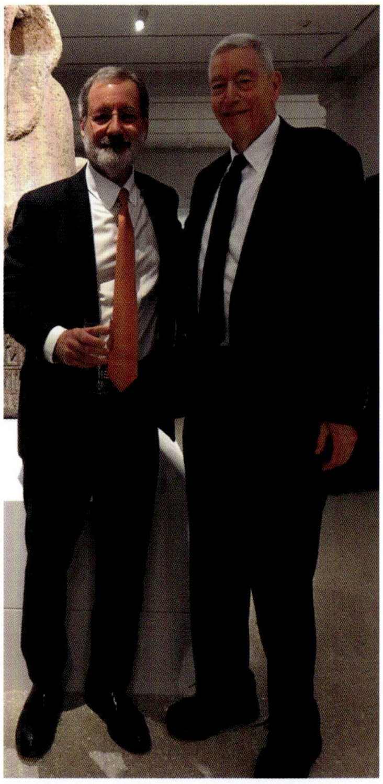

Ron Fairman and Clyde Barker

mune disease. These studies also provided the first description of immunotherapy for autoimmune diabetes and identified recurrent autoimmunity as a barrier to the success of clinical islet transplantation.

1983
Four chairmen celebrate CFB's appointment as JRB professor on the day his appointment is announced

Chairman Years

CFB was appointed the John Rhea Barton Professor and Chairman of the Department of Surgery at Penn and director of the Harrison Department of Surgical Research in 1983, following Brooke Roberts who was interim chairman for one year. He went on to serve as chairman for eighteen years until 2001.

Shortly after CFB became chairman, the rules governing the training of general surgical residents began to change. The Residency Review Committee (RRC) mandated that all residents have an identical clinical program, effectively ending the pyramidal model. In 1984, Barker began to provide all HUP surgery residents with an opportunity to be supported for two years of research. Vice chair Jim Mullen was responsible for the day-to-day operations of the general surgery residency. CFB had strong collaborations in the medical school and university; Mullen's close relationship with hospital administration created innovative programs within Penn Surgery and throughout HUP. The CFB–Mullen collaboration resulted in big dividends for the department. The William T. Fitts Library and Education Center opened on the fourth floor of the Maloney Building in 1994. Mullen was responsible for the concept and funding. Mullen's enduring contributions included the development of the hospital-wide Nutrition Support Service and its extension into the adjunct Home Total Parenteral Nutrition (TPN) program. For Mullen's numerous other accomplishments, see chapter 31.

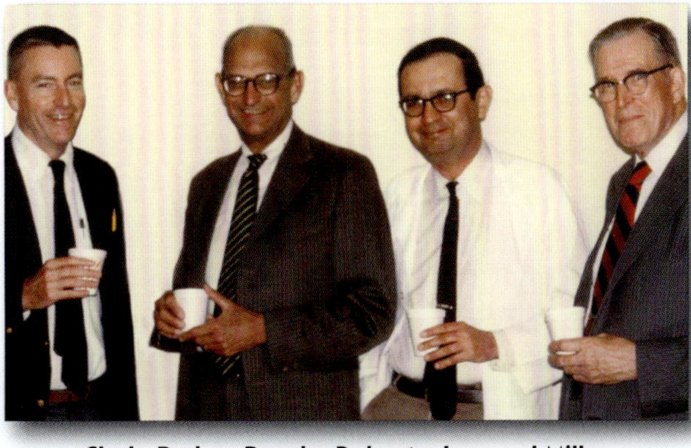

Clyde Barker, Brooke Roberts, Leonard Miller, and Jonathan Rhoads

While there were academic and clinical stars among the surgical faculty in 1983 when CFB became chairman, the department was relatively small with approximately twenty full-time faculty and only a few who were

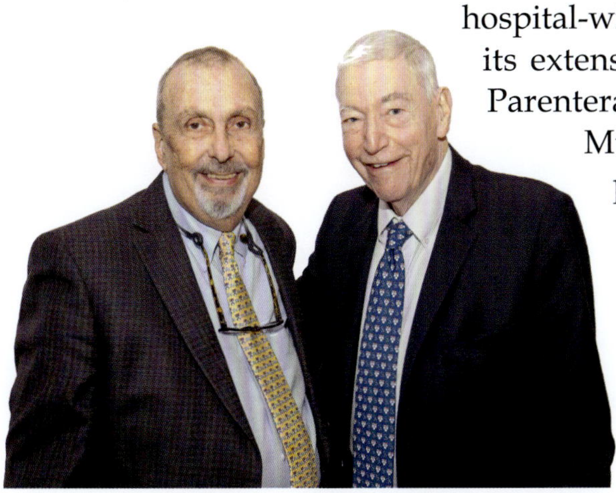

Jim Mullen and Clyde Barker

1985
John Daly recruited to head a new division, Surgical Oncology

1985
Liver transplant program begins

academically focused and productive. The general surgical residency training program was highly regarded, but not among the very best in the US. Barker's vision was to recreate Penn Surgery into a department comprised of highly productive, nationally recognized faculty who were both clinically and academically exceptional. He realized there needed to be significant programmatic changes in order to bring Penn Surgery to the forefront nationally. He felt it would be necessary to recruit outsiders rather than perpetuating Penn's usual pattern of inbreeding. What follows is a timeline that highlights CFB's successful transformation of Penn Surgery as chairman, yet while all these recruitments and events were occurring, remarkably CFB remained productive in clinical surgery, laboratory research, and teaching. He uniquely was a "triple threat" in the true sense.

- In 1984 as the new chairman, CFB and his department hosted the annual meeting for the Society of Clinical Surgery. This and other Penn-hosted meetings, such as the Halsted Society in 1989 and the International Surgical Group in 1996, garnered national exposure for Penn Surgery.
- In 1985, he recruited John Daly from Memorial Sloan Kettering as the first chief of a new Division of Surgical Oncology. Daly served until 1993 when he left to become chairman of surgery at Cornell. Doug Fraker was then recruited from NIH to succeed Daly as chief of the division, a position he continues to hold today.

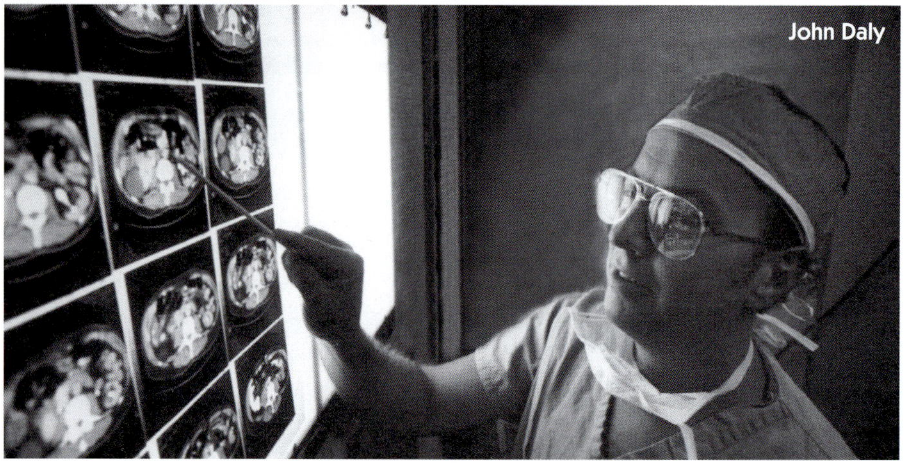
John Daly

- In 1985, Ira Fox was recruited from Pittsburgh to start the liver transplant program, and Mory Ziegler was sent to Pittsburgh to train with Tom Starzl. Fox, with Don Dafoe, Ali Naji, Ziegler, and CFB, spearheaded the program.
- CFB's other notable clinical events in the early 1980s included the first pancreas transplant and small bowel transplant (with Jim Mullen) at HUP.

- In 1986, CFB served as chairman of clinical practices of the University of Pennsylvania (CPUP) and held this position until 1989.

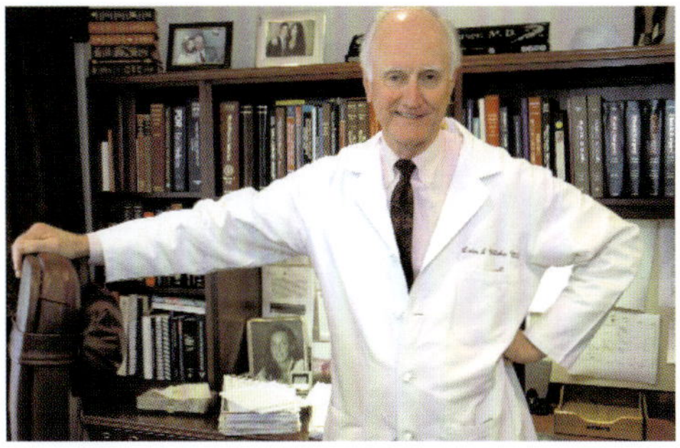

Linton Whitaker

- He appointed Linton Whitaker as chief of plastic surgery in 1987, and Linton founded the Center for Human Appearance and the craniofacial surgery program.

1986–1989
CFB is chairman of clinical practices of the University of Pennsylvania

1987
Linton Whitaker appointed chief of plastic surgery division

1987
Bill Schwab recruited to head new division, Trauma

1988
Ernie Rosato appointed head of new division, Gastrointestinal Surgery

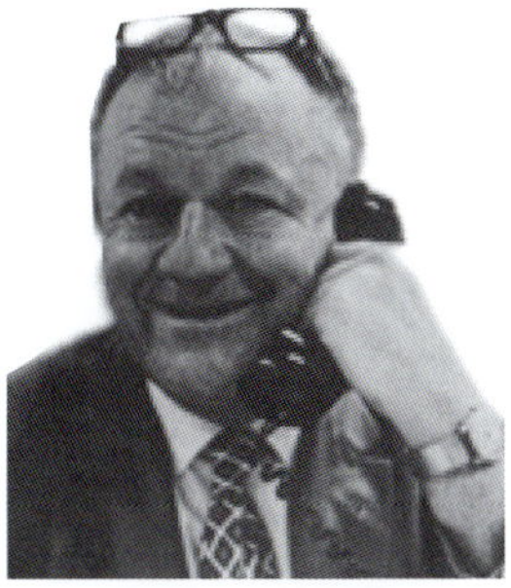

William T. Fitts

- While faculty member Bill Fitts was a nationally respected leader in trauma,[19] who was president of the American Association for the Surgery of Trauma and editor of its journal, his untimely death in 1980 left a hole in the residency training program. CFB recruited William Schwab from New Jersey in 1987, who went on to develop one of the most respected clinical and academic trauma centers in the world. Schwab also started the PennStar helicopter service. Mike Rotundo, Schwab, et al., introduced the concept of "damage control" for severe abdominal injuries.[20] This revolutionary paradigm, though initially rejected, was eventually adopted worldwide and expanded over time to include the delayed closure of abdominal incisions following some general surgery procedures.[21]

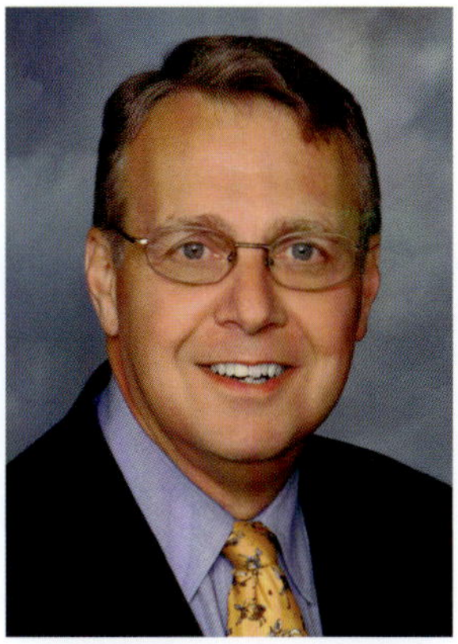

Bill Schwab

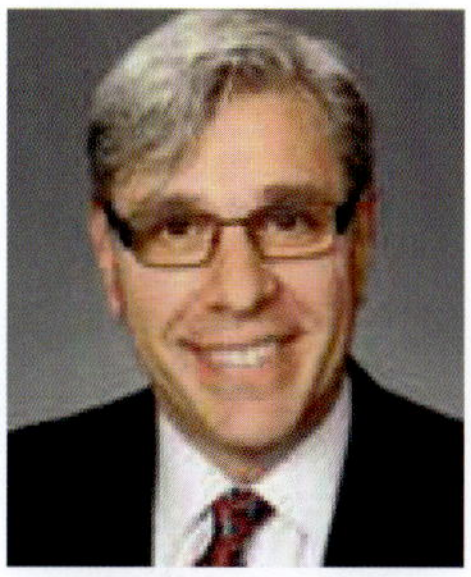

Mike Rotondo

- In 1988, CFB appointed Ernest Rosato as chief of a new Division of Gastrointestinal Surgery. Rosato compiled the record for the largest consecutive number of chief resident teaching awards; he was the busiest gastrointestinal surgeon in the region, technically exceptional, and beloved by all the Penn medical students and residents.

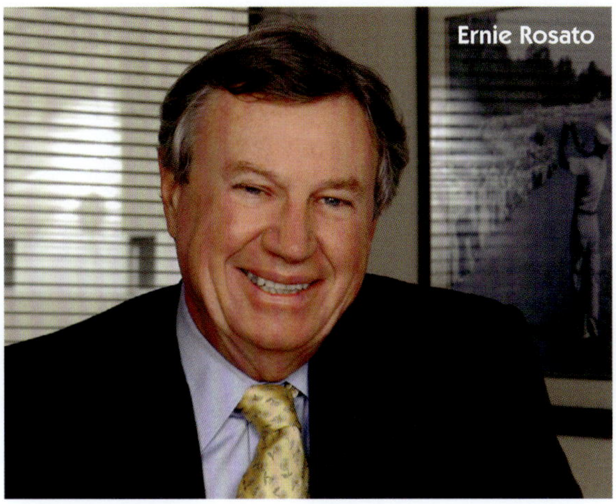

Ernie Rosato

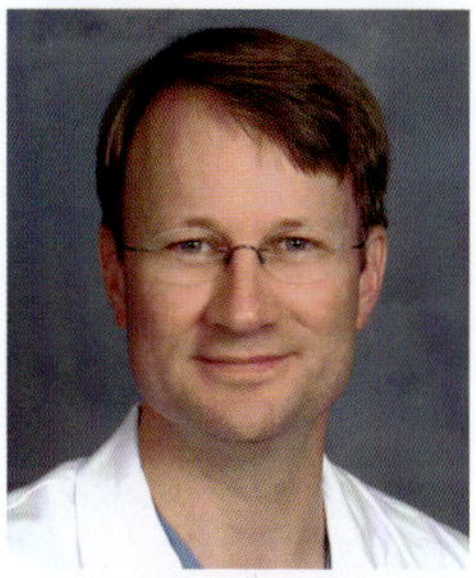

Mike Nance

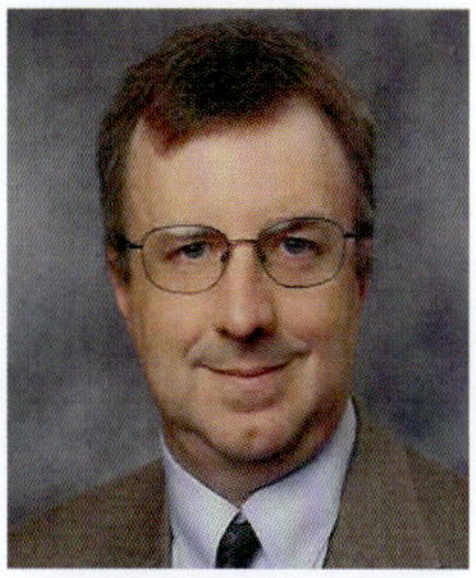

Pat Reilly

1989
Bill Kelley appointed dean and CEO

1989–2000
Chairman of Radiology Stan Baum kept track of chairmen's retirements, resignations, and dismissals. In his office he exhibited this collage of the chairs and marked with an X each chairman's demise. Eventually CFB was the only one left without an X

1990
CFB, et al., introduce the concept of intrathymic tolerance, illustrated on the cover of *Science*

1991
Larry Kaiser recruited to start lung transplantation.
New section: General Thoracic Surgery

- In 1989, Bill Kelley was appointed dean and CEO of HUP. A strong leader, he is credited with transforming Penn into a modern medical center, expanding research and faculty, and building three new buildings.[22] Kelley was supportive of CFB; in fact, CFB was the only chairman of a department who did not get dismissed, retire, or resign during the Kelley years.[23] Kelley served until 2000 when he was fired by University president Judith Rodin over the institution's financial setbacks (see chapter 24).[24]

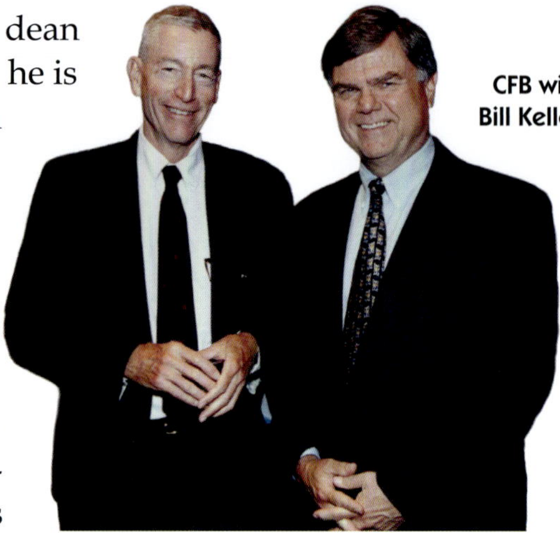

CFB with Bill Kelley

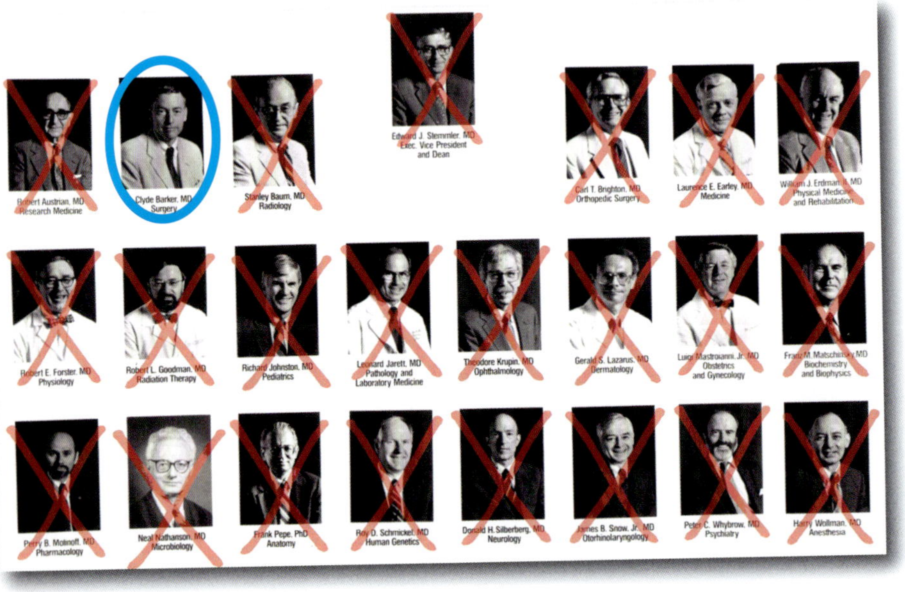

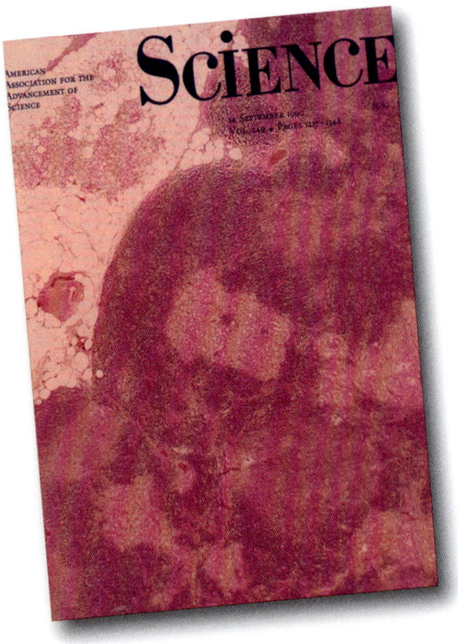

- In 1990, Andy Posselt, Ali Naji, CFB, Jim Markmann, and Mike Choti reported in *Science* that the thymus is a privileged site and that intrathymic islet allografts can induce tolerance.[25]

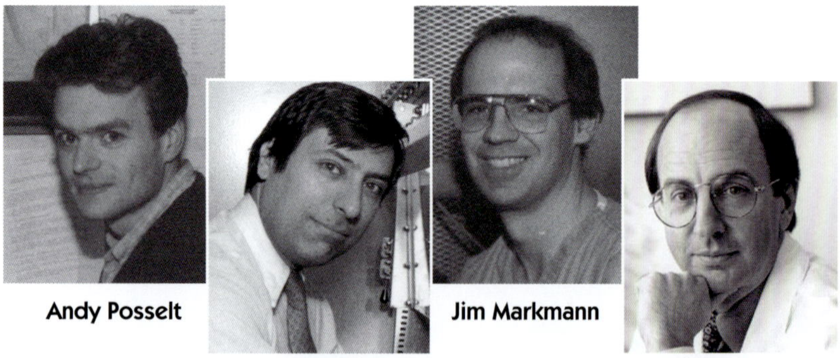

Andy Posselt Ali Naji Jim Markmann Michael Choti

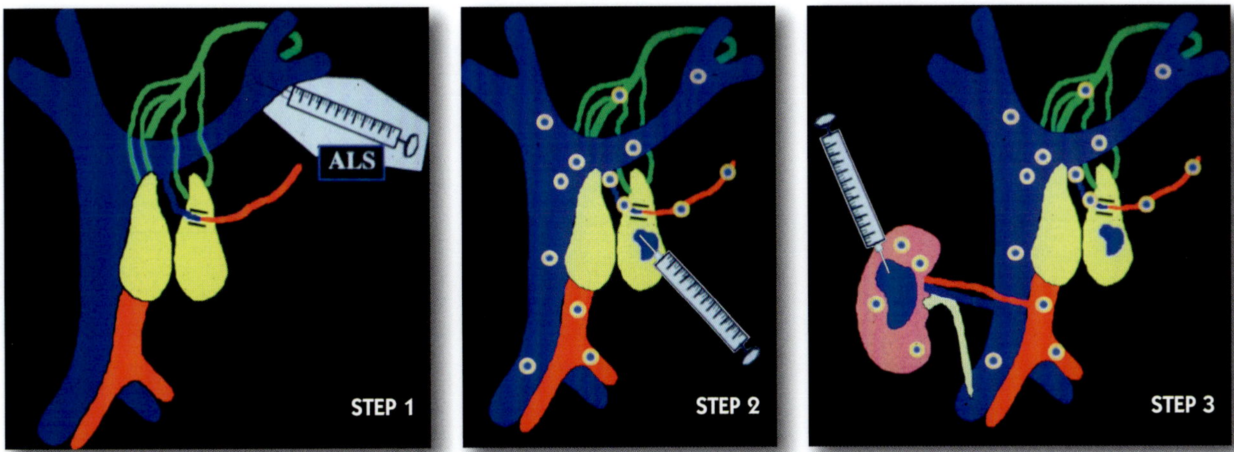

Induction of Intrathymic Tolerance—Induction of Donor Specific Unresponsiveness by Intrathymic Islet Transplantation. *Science* 249:1293-1295, 1990.

- In 1991, CFB recruited Larry Kaiser from Memorial Sloan Kettering to start a lung transplant program at Penn. Kaiser became chief of the new section of General Thoracic Surgery and later became the next John Rhea Barton Professor and Chairman following CFB.
- In 1992, with Andy Posselt and others, CFB reported that intrathymic implantation of a subtherapeutic number of islets in newborn BB rats could prevent the development of diabetes.[26]

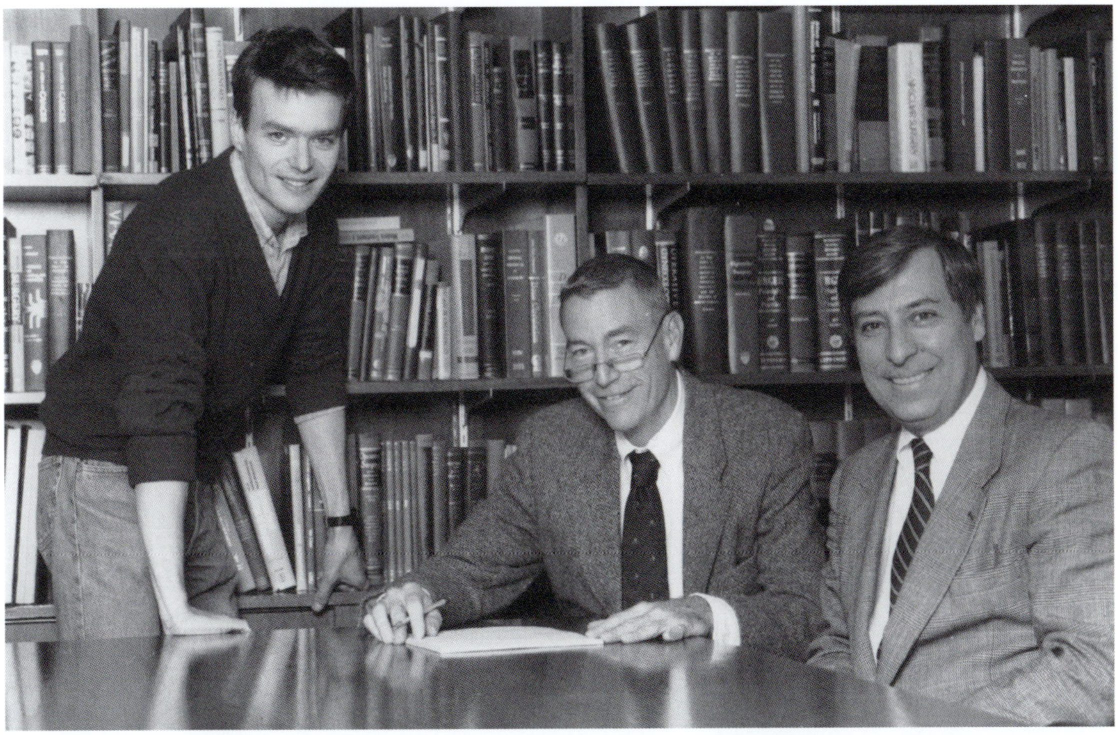

Andy Posselt, CFB, and Ali Naji at a press conference on intrathymic tolerance.

- In 1992, CFB was elected president of the American Society of Transplant Surgeons.

1993
Tim Gardner recruited to succeed Hank Edmunds as chief of CT division

1995
A new liver transplant team recruited

1995
Scott Adzick recruited as chief of pediatric surgery

1997
CFB elected president of American Surgical Association

1998
Jim Markmann recruited

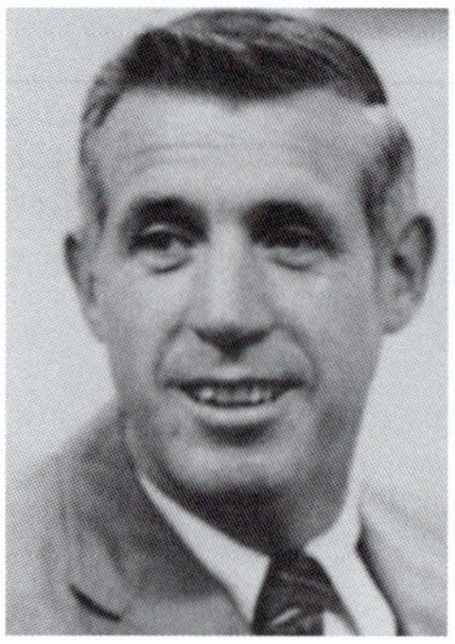
Henry Edmunds

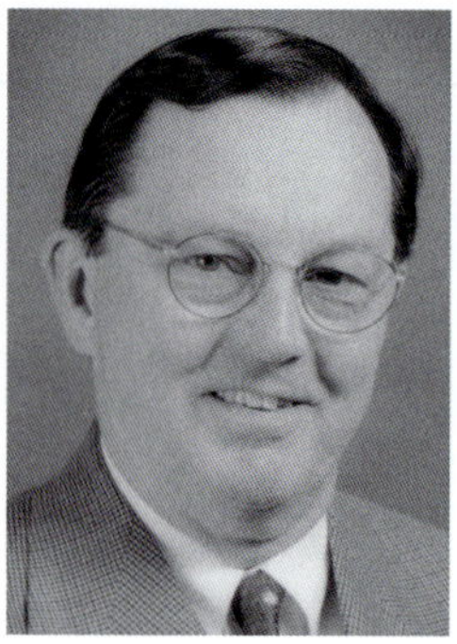
Tim Gardner

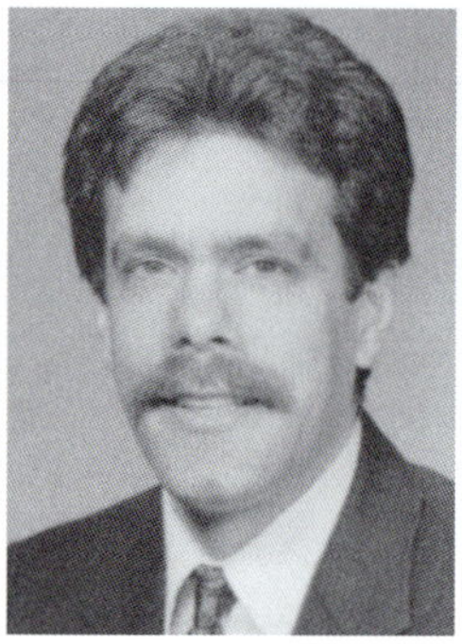
Mike Acker

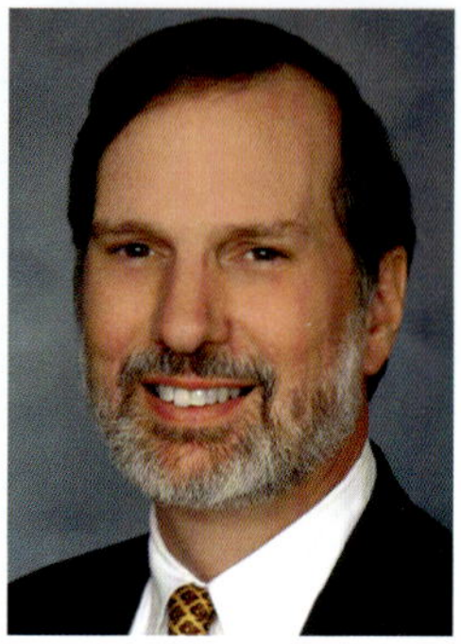
Joseph Bavaria

- In 1993, he recruited Tim Gardner from Johns Hopkins to succeed Henry Edmunds as chief of the Division of Cardiothoracic Surgery. Gardner held this position until he was succeeded by Barker's former resident Michael Acker in 2003, who had returned to HUP with Gardner in 1993.
- HUP resident Joseph Bavaria was appointed in the cardiac division in 1990. He developed an internationally-praised program to treat thoracic-aortic aneurisms.
- In 1995, CFB recruited Abraham Shaked and Kim Olhoff from UCLA. They transformed liver transplantation at HUP into one of the largest and most respected in the country.

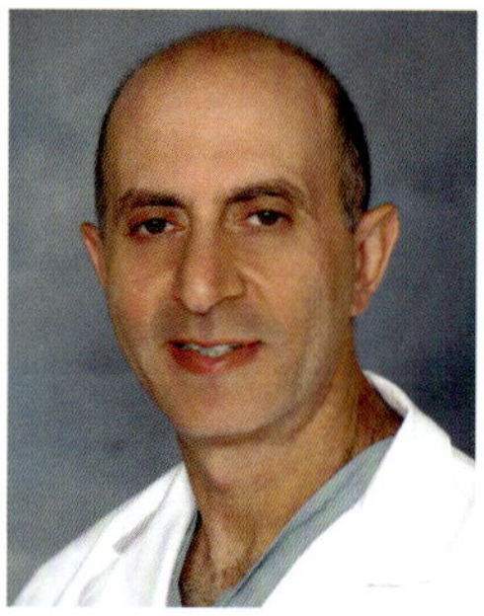
Avi Shaked

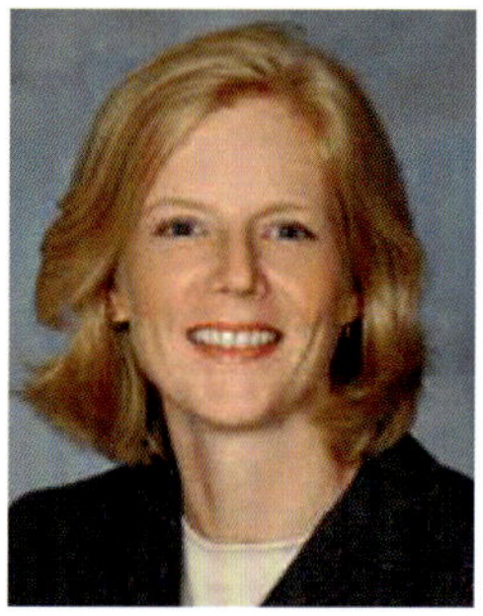
Kim Olthoff

- That same year, Scott Adzick was recruited as chief of surgery at Children's Hospital of Philadelphia (CHOP) and initiated the fetal surgery program, the largest in the world.
- In 1997, CFB was elected president of the American Surgical Association, once again propelling Penn Surgery to the forefront nationally and internationally.[27]
- In 1998, he recruited Jim Markmann to the transplant division. Markmann's research and clinical contributions to Penn Surgery were substantial. He left Penn in 2009 to become chief of the Division of Transplantation at Massachusetts General Hospital and surgical director of the liver, pancreas, and islet transplant programs.

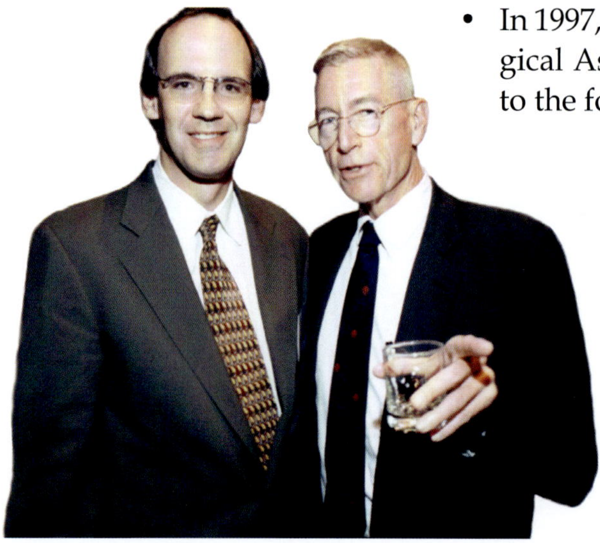
Jim Markmann and Clyde Barker

Between 1995 and 2000, Penn Medicine experienced several major setbacks and hurdles.[28] There were financial losses of roughly $200 million dollars, a substantial Medicare fine of $30 million dollars for inadequate billing documentation, and the gene therapy patient Jesse Gelsinger tragically died, leading to the closure of the Penn gene therapy program by the NIH. During these tumultuous years, CFB as surgery chairman maintained the department's professional and financial stability, as well as forward thinking and optimism.

1995–2000
Penn Medicine loses money, Bill Kelley is fired

From the start, CFB made it clear his goal was to train residents who would become national leaders in academic surgery. As chairman, CFB kept hanging in his office a framed picture of all his research, transplant, and vascular fellows. He also initiated hanging photographs of the graduating general surgery residents outside the Fitts Library on the fourth floor of the Maloney building (see illustration below). During his eighteen years as chairman, he trained sixteen chief residents and fellows who have become chairs at university medical schools, and well over thirty who became chiefs of academic divisions. Remarkably, forty-six trainees of his were ultimately promoted to the rank of full professor in university departments as of 2021. During CFB's years as chairman, the general surgery residency and fellowship training programs grew in numbers and stature, and Penn Surgery became one of the most coveted places to train in the United States.

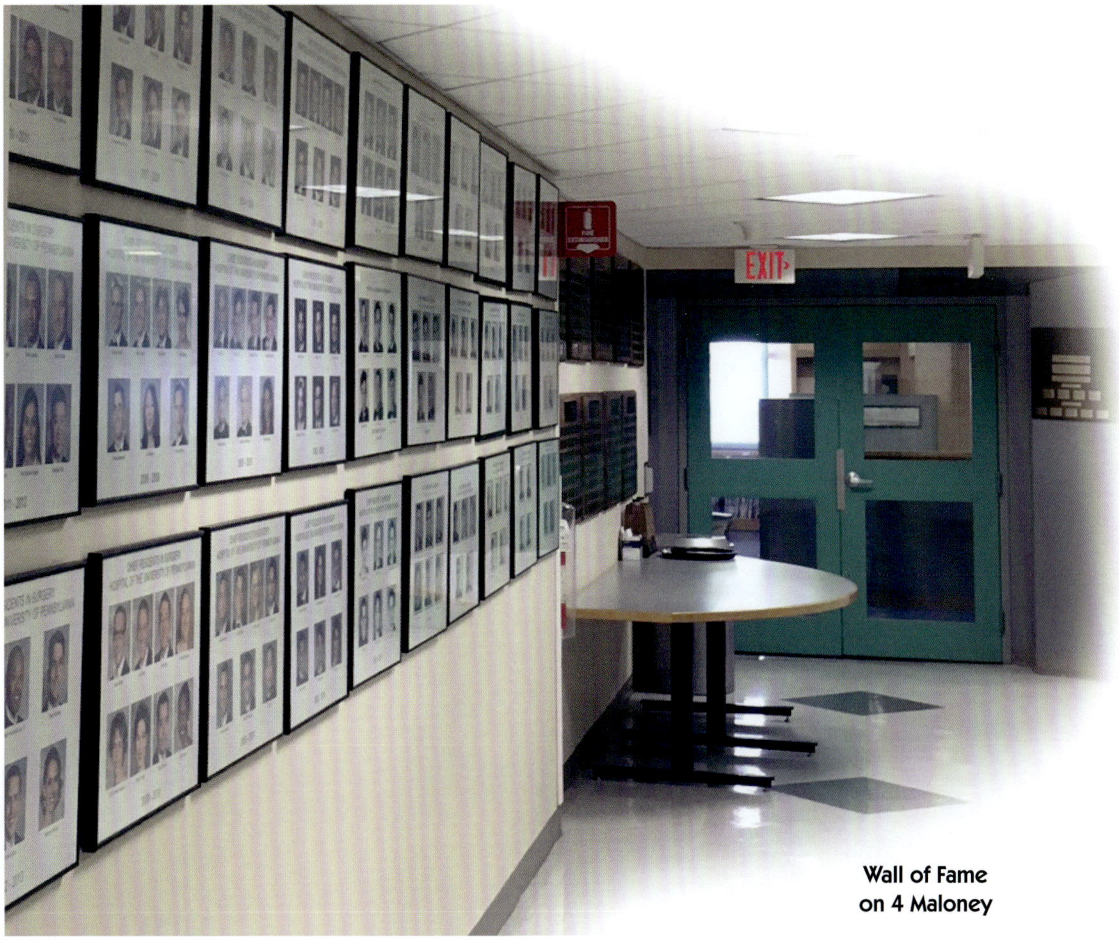

Wall of Fame on 4 Maloney

While many chairs of large academic departments cease to practice clinically or to maintain an independent lab with NIH funding, CFB continued all of his professional activities. He remained chief of transplantation, as well as vascular surgery, while he was chairman. As a clinical surgeon, he was unflappable in the operating room and highly capable. On a personal level, he was a pleasure to operate with, had a good sense of humor, never seemed to fatigue, and his clinical skills were exceptional. It is utterly remarkable how he successfully navigated the day-to-day administrative imperatives while also advancing his academic and clinical goals during his eighteen years as chairman. Many of us recall finding Clyde, Ali Naji, and Fran Ramirez (his administrative assistant) in his office, working late into the night on a grant or abstract deadline.

In 2001, he finished his third six-year term as John Rhea Barton Professor and Chairman of Surgery. It is worth repeating, this was the longest tenure of anyone in this leadership position in the oldest medical school and oldest university hospital in the United States. This same year, a successful human pancreatic islet transplant program was initiated at HUP.[29] The degree to which he was respected throughout the university clearly enhanced the programmatic development he supported within Surgery. I was recruited back to Penn in 1996, and when our Division of Vascular Surgery embarked on "first in man" endovascular clinical trials for abdominal aortic aneurysms, CFB had the standing to successfully deal with the aggressive pushback we were subjected to from some sectors.[30] He understood the importance of clinical research in advancing the care of surgical patients, and his steadfast support was integral to our clinical research successes at the divisional level. I learned from CFB the importance of "leading from behind." As chairman and throughout his career, he was a role model for multiple generations of surgical trainees and faculty members at Penn. Beyond the obvious as an incredibly successful academic and clinical surgeon who, as chairman, promoted internationally recognized faculty, clinical divisions, and research programs, he was a committed husband, father, and avid tennis player. I recall CFB and Dode would travel to Kauai, Hawaii, every January just so they could watch the Australian Open *live.* He continued to play competitive tennis well into his eighties.

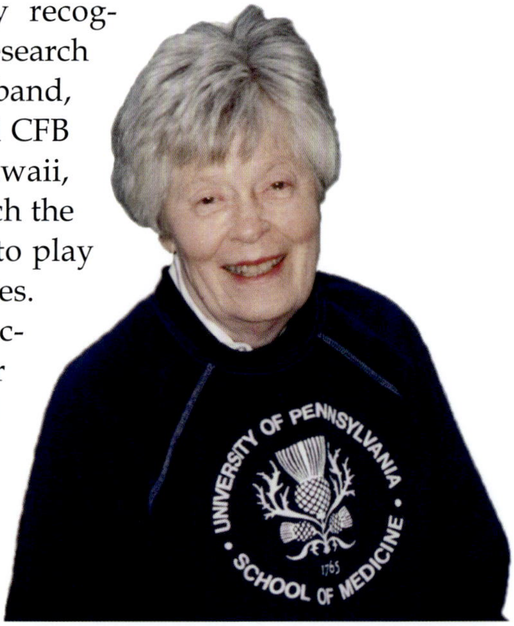

I would be remiss if I did not acknowledge Clyde's wife Dode in her own right. She opened her home and regularly welcomed faculty, residents, and students; she was a devoted wife/partner, mother, and huge supporter of Penn. From 1995 to 2001, Dode organized and di-

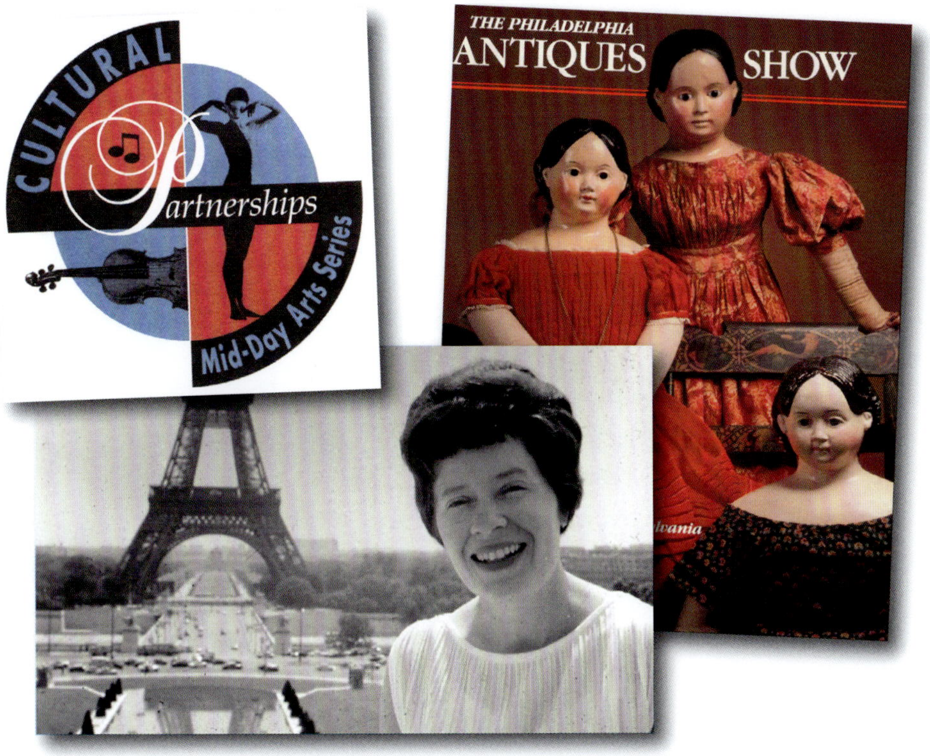

rected a weekly lunchtime arts and performance program for residents, faculty, patients, staff, and students. It was frequently attended by as many as 250 guests. During the years CFB was chairman, Dode hosted a Christmas party each year in her home for over 200 house staff, faculty, and other members of the hospital community, as well as a summer picnic for interns, residents, and faculty. She also started the surgical residents' library and was chair of the annual Philadelphia Antiques Show, the proceeds of which supported HUP. Dode was well known and admired by everyone at Penn, and we were all blessed to have her active involvement for so many years in our professional and personal lives. Sadly, Dode passed away in 2019 at the age of eighty-seven.

Post-Chairman Years

Following his chairmanship, CFB has remained a huge force in Penn Medicine, and his contributions in support of Penn Surgery have continued uninterrupted. Both during his chairman years and since then, he successfully expanded the number of endowed chairs within Penn Surgery made possible by his chairmanship of the Benjamin and Mary Siddons Measey Foundation. Other Penn Surgery Measey Board members included Jonathan Rhoads, Brooke Roberts, and currently Ron Fairman. While a detailed discussion of Measey Foundation support for Penn Surgery is beyond the scope of this chapter, our faculty and surgical trainees have been the recipients of its career-transforming academic and educational support.

Notably, Jonathan Rhoads died in 2002. Clearly, Rhoads significantly influenced CFB over the course of their careers; they developed a close

2011–2017
CFB is president of American Philosophical Society.

W.W. Keen, Jonathan Rhoads, and CFB are the only three surgeons that have held this office in the APS, which Benjamin Franklin founded in 1743

relationship that became even more strongly cemented over time. In the same year, CFB was elected president of the United Network for Organ Sharing in the United States (UNOS) and the following year was awarded the Medallion for Scientific Achievement by the American Surgical Association. He continued to accumulate awards; in 2009, he was named the Society of University Surgeons Lifetime Achievement Awardee, was awarded the Thomas Starzl Prize in Transplantation and Immunology, and the following year, 2010, received the Medawar Prize, the highest award of the International Transplantation Society.[31] Starzl provided the Medawar Prize nomination, demonstrating his admiration for CFB's career achievements. Other notable awards include the Roche Pioneer Award of the American Society of Transplant Surgeons, the Sheen Award of the American College of Surgeons, the Jonathan Rhoads Gold Medal of the American Philo-

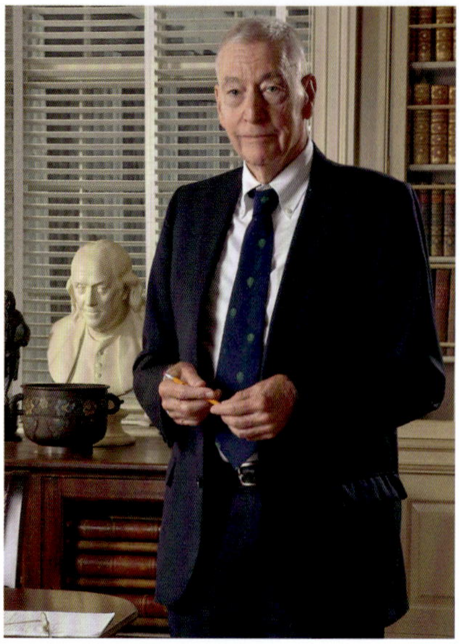

CFB as president of the American Philosophical Society

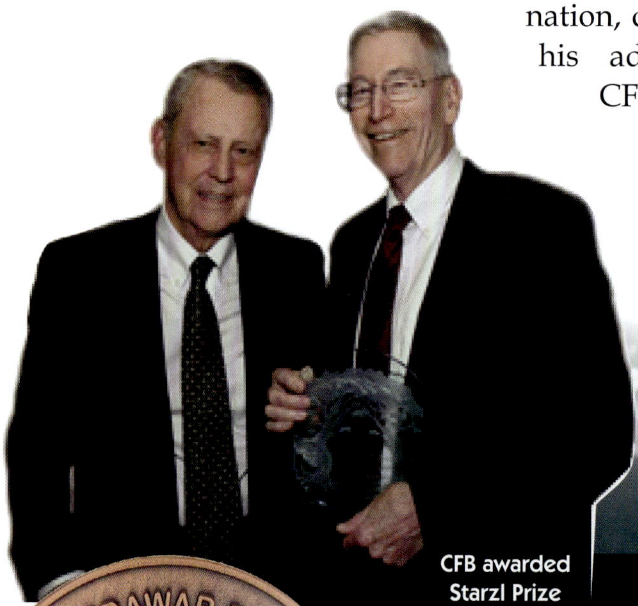

CFB awarded Starzl Prize

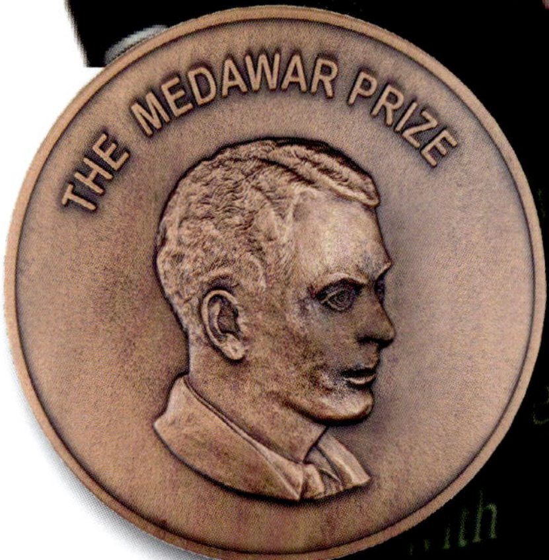

Medawar Prize

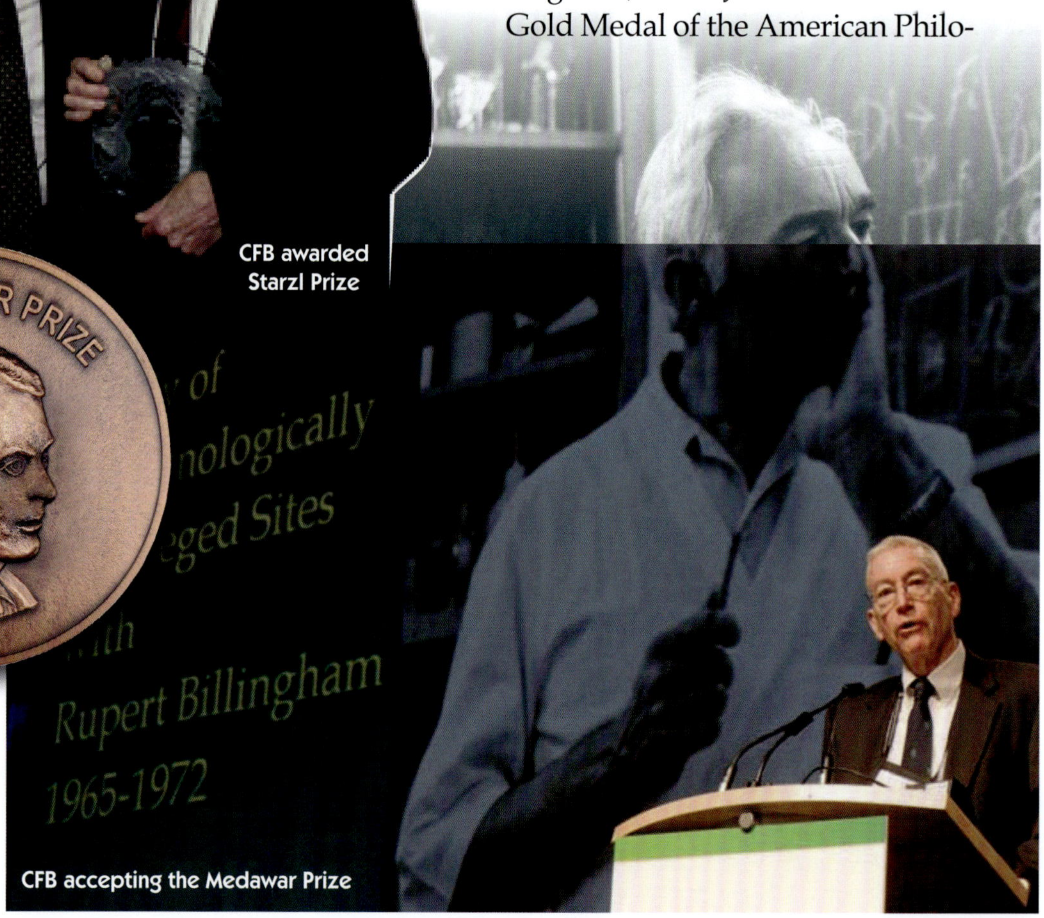

CFB accepting the Medawar Prize

2012
Transplant House is named for CFB

sophical Society, the Distinguished Graduate Award of the School of Medicine at the University of Pennsylvania, and the American Philosophical Society's Henry Allen Moe Prize in the Humanities (2010).[32]

Clearly one of the most prestigious and unique accomplishments for a physician and surgeon came in 2011 when CFB was elected president of the American Philosophical Society (APS) for a six-year term.[33] The following year in 2012, the Clyde F. Barker Transplant House was opened. This is not a medical facility, but a guest house at 3940 Spruce Street designed to meet the unique needs of transplant patients and their families and caregivers. It was designed by Rafael Vinoly and built entirely through the generosity of private donors.

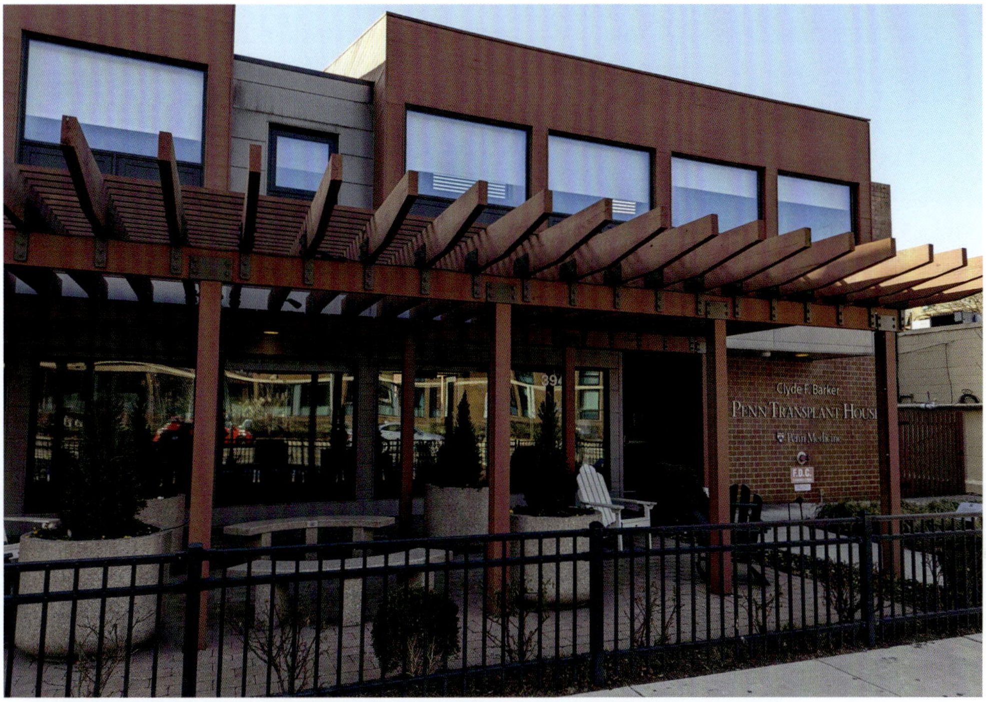

During the course of his career, he published well over 450 scientific papers and served on twelve editorial boards, including *Diabetes, Transplantation, Journal of Surgical Research, Archives of Surgery, Surgery, Journal of the American College of Surgeons,* and *Annals of Surgery.* His scientific memberships not already mentioned include the American College of Surgeons, the National Academy of Medicine, the Association of American Physicians, the American Association for the Advancement of Science, and the American Academy of Arts and Sciences. He has also been president of the Halsted Society and the US chapter of the International Society of Surgery. He has served as a visiting professor at more than ninety different universities in the United States and abroad and is an honorary fellow of the Royal College of Surgeons of England and of the Royal College of Surgeons in Ireland.

As this book indicates, Barker's knowledge of the history of Penn Surgery is an ongoing passion that has served to strengthen and reconnect former graduates of Penn Surgery training programs. He is the editor-in-chief of the *Penn Surgery Society Newsletter* that is published quarterly and broadly distributed. It spotlights the accomplishments of our current and former trainees as well as faculty, introduces new faculty members, and typically includes a historical component. Candidly, I look forward to reading every issue. Along the same theme, Barker has remained closely engaged with the achievements of his former trainees. Two recent examples include his presence in San Diego when I delivered my presidential address to the Society for Vascular Surgery in 2018, and when he and Dode were present as Dan Dempsey received the Philadelphia County Medical Society's Strittmatter Award in 2019 (Clyde had also received the Strittmatter Award in 2001).

In preparing this chapter, I was again reminded of how uniquely fortunate we have all been to know and work alongside a "living legend" for so many years. As he approaches his ninety-first birthday, he may no longer effortlessly spring over a tennis net following a win, but his intellect, enthusiasm, and ongoing desire to increase pride in everything related to Penn Surgery remain robust.

—Ron Fairman, MD

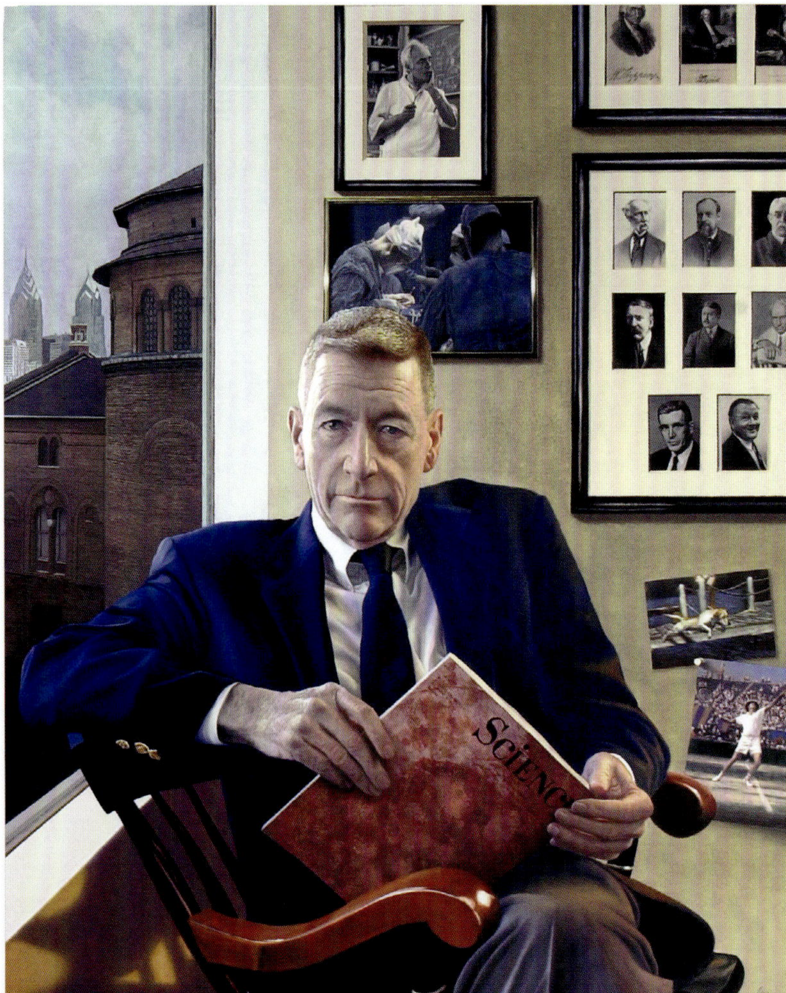

CFB portrait by artist Jon R. Friedman

Notes

[1] Barker, FG. *Forty-Minute Plays from Shakespeare* (New York: MacMillan, 1936). Fred G. Barker's grandson (Fred G. Barker II) is professor of neurosurgery at Harvard and Massachusetts General Hospital.

[2] Hardy, Mark A. Memoir of Harold G. Barker. *Transactions of the American Surgical Association*, Vol 129 (2011) p. 264.

[3] Peskin GW, Miller LD, Barker CF and Evans GW. Comparative Effects of Portosystemic Shunting on Liver Function: Use of New Technique: Half and Half Shunt. *Surgery* 54:67–77 (1963).

[4] Barker CF, Nance FC and Peskin GW. Regional Hypothermia for Massive Bleeding. *Surgery* 56:624–627 (1964).

[5] Nicholas GG, Barker CF, Berkowitz HD and Roberts B. The Effect of Reconstructive Surgery Distal to the Popliteal Trifurcation on the Natural History of Arterial Occlusive Disease. *Arch. Of Surg.* 107:652–656 (1973).

[6] Berkowitz HD, Spence RK, Freiman DB, Barker CF, Roberts B, McLean G and Ring EJ. Long Term Results of Transluminal Angioplasty of the Femoral Arteries. CT Dotter, A Gruntzig, W Schoop, E Zietler, eds. In: *Percutaneous Transluminal Angioplasty*. New York: Springer-Verlag, 207–214 (1983).

[7] Hargrove, III, WC, Barker CF, Berkowitz HD, Perloff LJ, McLean GK, Freiman D, Ring EJ and Roberts B. Treatment of Acute Peripheral Arterial and Graft Thromboses with Low Dose Streptokinase. *Surgery* 92:981–993 (1982).

[8] Billingham RE, Brent L, Medawar PB. Actively acquired tolerance of foreign cells. *Nature* (1953) 172(4379):603–606.

[9] Starzl, Thomas E and Barker, Clyde F. The origin of clinical organ transplantation revisited. *JAMA* 301 19 (2009): 2041–3.

[10] Barker CF and Billingham RE. The Role of Afferent Lymphatics in the Rejection of Skin Homografts. *J. Exp. Med.* 128:197–221 (1968).

[11] Barker CF and Billingham RE. The Lymphatic Status of Hamster Cheek Pouch Tissue in Relation to its Properties as a Graft and as a Graft Site. *J. Exp. Med.* 133:620–639 (1971). Barker CF and Billingham RE. Immunologically Privileged Sites. HG Kunkel and Frank J. Dixon, eds. In: *Advances in Immunology*. New York: Academic Press, 25:1–54 (1977).

[12] Starzl TE. Acquired immunologic tolerance: with particular reference to transplantation. *Immunol Res.* (2007) 38(1–3):6–41.

[13] Lakkis FG, Arakelov A, Konieczny BT, Inoue Y. Immunologic 'ignorance' of vascularized organ transplants in the absence of secondary lymphoid tissue. *Nature Medicine.* (2000 June) 6(6):686–688.

[14] Barker CF and Billingham RE. Histocompatability Requirements of Heart and Skin Grafts in Rats. *Transplant.* Proc.3:172–175 (1971).

[15] Foley, Paul, Wang, Grace, Jackson, Benjamin, Naji, Ali, Carpenter, Jeffrey, Barker, Clyde, Fairman, Ronald, Woo, Edward. PS70. A Contemporary Experience of Open Surgical Treatment of Renal Artery Aneurysms. *J Vas Surg.* 53 (2011).

[16] Each year, North American medical schools were allowed to nominate one young faculty member from any of its departments. The nominees lived with and were evaluated in a two-and-a-half day interview-retreat by a panel of business executives, college presidents, and their spouses. Twenty per year were selected.

[17] Reckard CR and Barker CF. Transplantation of Isolated Pancreatic Islets across Strong and Weak Histocompatibility Barriers. *Transplant*. Proc. 5:761–763 (1973). Reckard CR, Ziegler MM and Barker CF. Physiological and Immunological Consequences of Transplanting Pancreatic Islets. *Surgery*, 74:91–99 (1973). Ballinger WF, Lacy PE. Transplantation of intact pancreatic islets in rats. *Surgery* (1972) 72(2):175–186.

Ballinger and Lacy are often identified as the first to succeed with islet transplantation. Their work, simultaneous with Barker's, was published a few months earlier, but their correction of hyperglycemia was partial and of brief duration.

[18] Naji A, Silvers WK, Bellgrau D and Barker CF. Spontaneous Diabetes in Rats: Destruction of Islets is [not] prevented by Immunological Tolerance. *Science* 213:1390–1392 (1982).

Subsequently, David Sutherland confirmed this in humans by finding that autoimmunity destroyed islets transplanted from an identical twin donor (Sutherland DE, Sibley R, Xu XZ, et al. Twin-to-twin pancreas transplantation: reversal and reenactment of the pathogenesis of type I diabetes. *Trans Assoc Am Physicians* (1984) 97:80–87.)

[19] Kim PK, Nance FC, Nance ML, Schwab CW. William T. "Billy" Fitts Jr, MD: an AAST visionary. *J Trauma* (2007) 63(1):221–227.

[20] Rotondo MF, Schwab CW, McGonigal MD, et al. "Damage control": an approach for improved survival in exsanguinating penetrating abdominal injury. *J Trauma* (1993) 35(3):375–383.

[21] Stawicki SP, Brooks A, Bilski T, et al. The concept of damage control: extending the paradigm to emergency general surgery. *Injury* (2008) 39(1):93–101.

[22] John A. Kastor. *Governance of Teaching Hospitals, Turmoil at Penn and Hopkins* (Baltimore: The Johns Hopkins University Press: 2004) p. 7

[23] Ibid., p. 7

[24] Ibid., p. 118

[25] Posselt A, Barker CF, Tomaszewski JE, Markmann JF, Choti MA and Naji A. Induction of Donor Specific Unresponsiveness by Intrathymic Islet Transplantation. *Science* 249:1293–1295 (1990).

[26] Posselt AM, Barker CF, Friedman AL and Naji A. Prevention of Autoimmune Diabetes in the BB Rat by Intrathymic Islet Transplantation at Birth. *Science* 256:1321–1324 (1992).

[27] Barker CF. Science, Specialization and the American Surgical Association. *Annals of Surgery* 226: 211–228 (1997).

[28] Kastor, John A. *Governance of Teaching Hospitals, Turmoil at Penn and Hopkins* (Baltimore: The Johns Hopkins University Press: 2004) pp. 89–98.

[29] Markmann JF, Deng S, Huang X, Desai NM, Velidedeoglu EH, Lui C, Frank A, Markmann E, Palanjian M, Brayman K, Wolf B, Bell E, Vitamaniuk M, Doliba N, Matschinsky F, Barker CF, and Naji A. Insulin independence following isolated islet transplantation and single islet infusions. *Annals of Surgery, 237*(6), 741–750 (2003).

[30] Fairman, Ronald M. Measuring the worth of a vascular surgeon: Making it personal through a career of service, *Journal of Vascular Surgery,* Vol 67, No 5 (2018) pp. 1321–1327.

[31] Barker CF. Medawar Prize, Acceptance Speech, *Transplantation,* Vol 90, No 12 (December 27, 2010) pp. 1253–1259.

[32] Barker, Clyde F. The Jayne Lecture: Thomas Eakins and His Medical Clinics. *Proceedings of the American Philosophical Society* 153, No 1, 1–47 (2009).

[33] In the 275-year history of the American Philosophical Society, only two other surgeons have been president—W. W. Keen and Jonathan Rhoads.

CHAPTER 28

HUP Chief Residents During Dr. Barker's Chairmanship

This was a remarkable group of ninety-one HUP surgical residents. Fully two thirds of them pursued an academic career. Thirty-six of them have become full professors, and thirteen of them chairs of departments of surgery in US university medical schools.

1983–1984

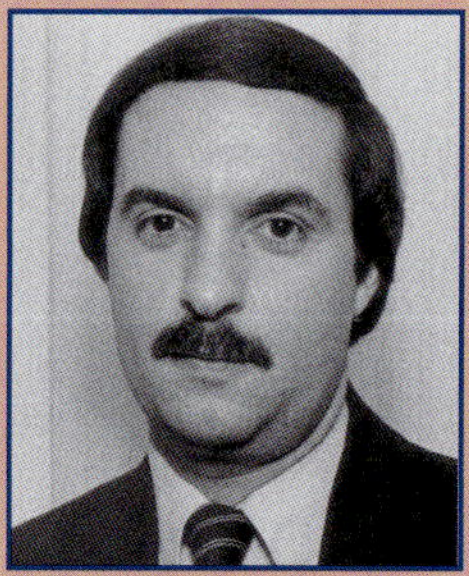

Frederick R. Armenti. MD Rutgers University; fellow in CT, HUP; practices thoracic surgery at Hurley Medical Center, Flint, Michigan.

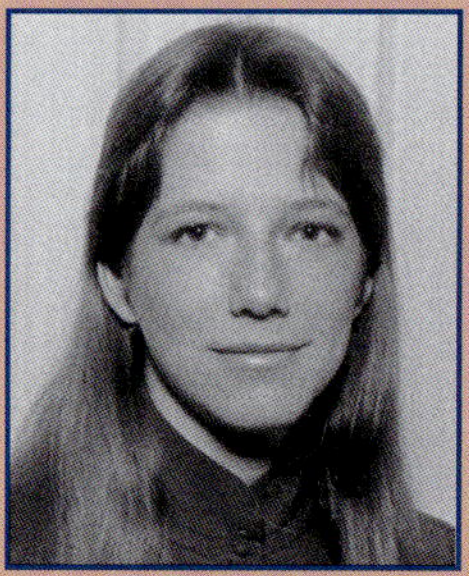

Donna Barbot. SUNY Nursing School (1972); MD SUNY Downstate (1978); research fellow with Ernest Rosato (1985); instructor of surgery, Jefferson (1985–full professor 2001); Drexel Medical College (2004–2005); University of Pennsylvania Chestnut Hill (2006–2015); chief of surgery, Jeanes Hospital and professor and chief of general and minimally invasive surgery, Temple (2015–2018); president of Philadelphia Chapter of the American College of Surgeons (2000–2001); president of Philadelphia Academy of Surgery (2001).

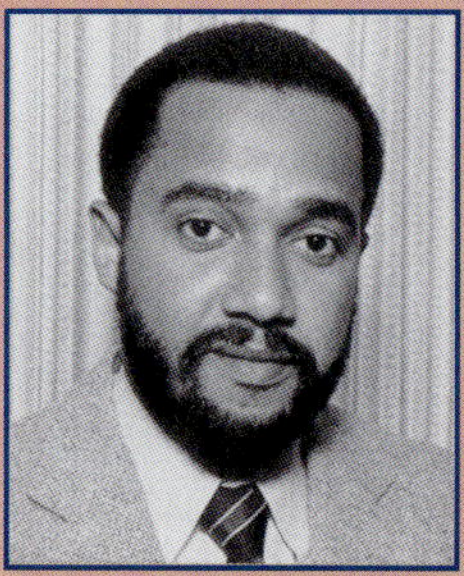

Paul J. Creary. MD Cornell University; practices general surgery at Harrisburg Hospital and has served as Lou Patterson's assistant in supervising HUP residents rotating there.

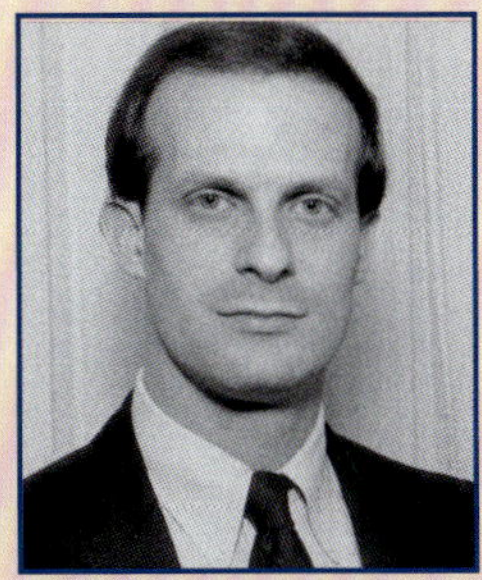

John E. Gatti. BA St. Joseph's University; MD Georgetown University; plastic surgery fellowship, HUP; chief of plastic surgery, Our Lady of Lourdes Hospital; volunteers for cleft surgery in Guatemala.

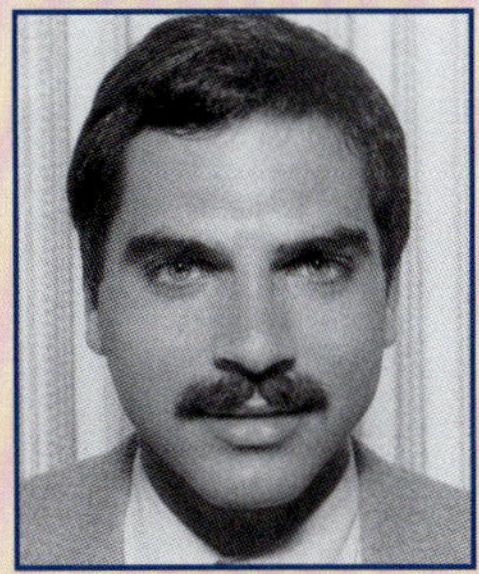

Burt M. Greenberg. BA Cornell University; MD SUNY Downstate (Brooklyn); plastic surgery fellowship, University of Pennsylvania; hand fellowship, MGH; practice in Great Neck, New York; adjunct assistant professor of surgery, NYU Long Island School of Medicine, Northshore University Hospital.

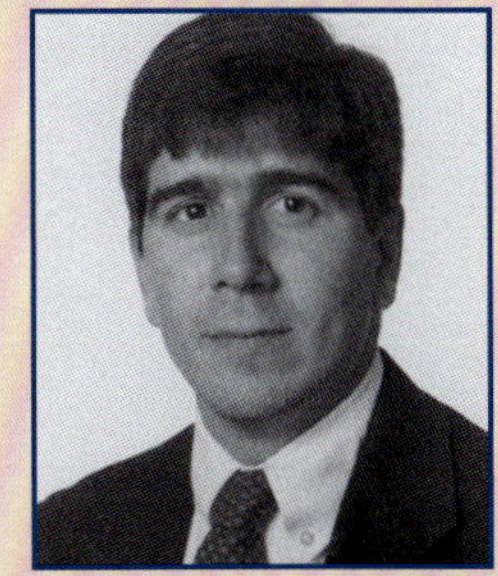

Stephen Bartlett. MD University of Chicago; transplantation research with Barker and Willys Silvers; vascular fellowship, Northwestern; chief of transplantation, University of California, Davis; chief of transplantation, University of Maryland; chairman of Department of Surgery, University of Maryland (2004–2018); University of Pennsylvania Department of Surgery Distinguished Graduate Award (2009). **1984–1985**

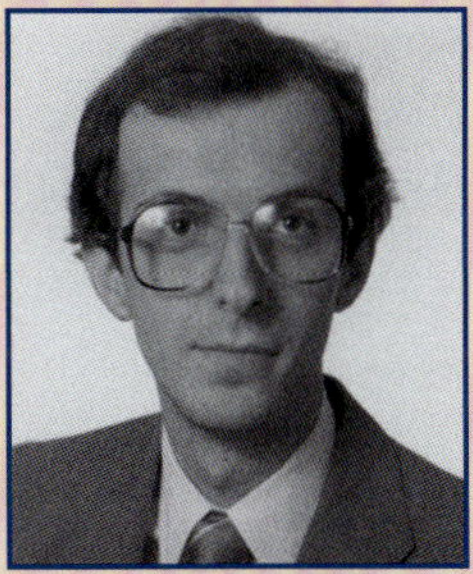

John Ricci. MD NYU; surgical oncology fellow, Memorial SKCC 1985–1987; practice in Lake Success, New York; assistant professor of surgery, Hofstra Northshore; chief of surgical oncology, Northshore University Hospital.

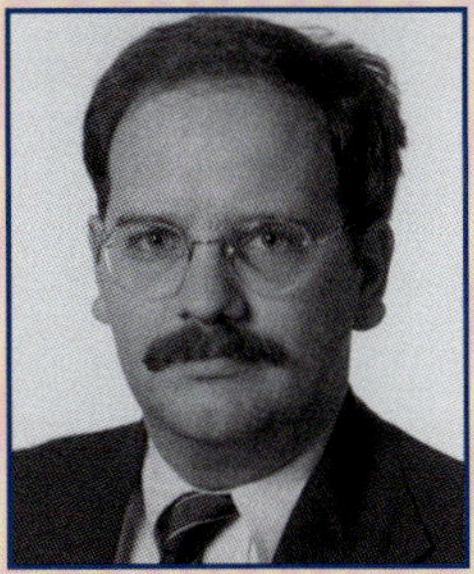

Nicholas Tepe. BA Harvard University; MD Jefferson University; fellow in cardiothoracic surgery, HUP; practice of cardiac surgery, Southeastern Michigan Cardiovascular Surgeons (2002–2010); assistant professor, Oakland University William-Beaumont School of Medicine (2010–present).

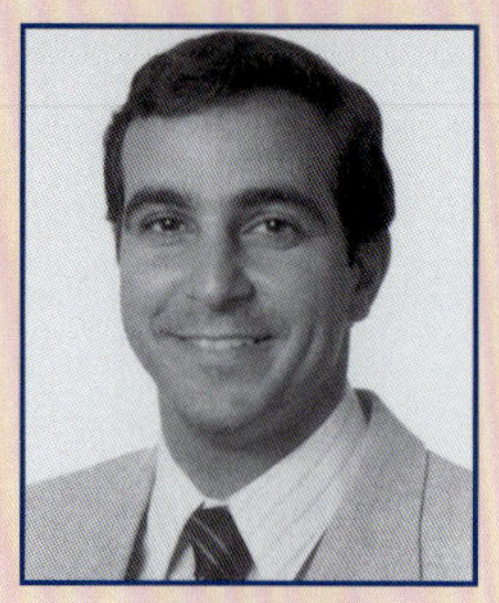

Michael Torosian. BA Princeton University; MD University of Pennsylvania; surgical oncology fellowship, Memorial SKCC; surgical faculty to associate professor at HUP (1993); family practice in Wayne, Pennsylvania.

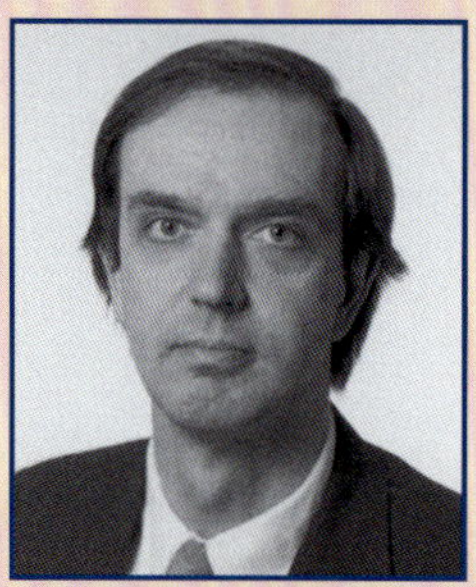

J. Frederick Villars. BA in classics, Harvard University; BA in biology, MIT; MD Harvard Medical School; fellow in cardiovascular surgery, CHOP and HUP (1985–1988); CT practice in Philadelphia; resident in psychiatry, University of Pennsylvania (1998–2001); practice of psychiatry.

1985–1986

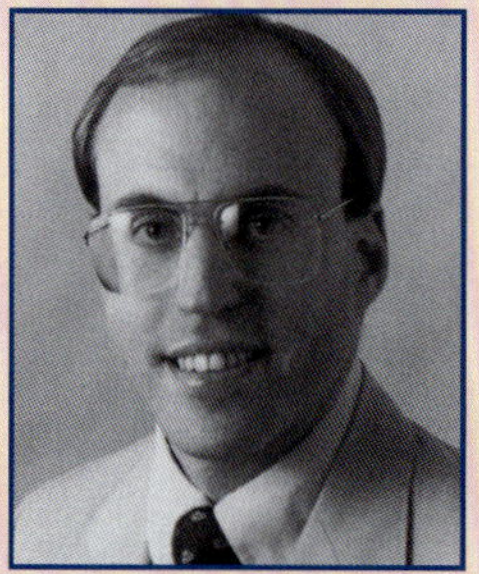

James Balshi. MD Jefferson University; vascular fellow, HUP; endovascular fellowship, Cleveland Clinic; practice of vascular surgery, Bethlehem, PA, St. Luke's Hospital; director of Vascular Center, St. Luke's Hospital.

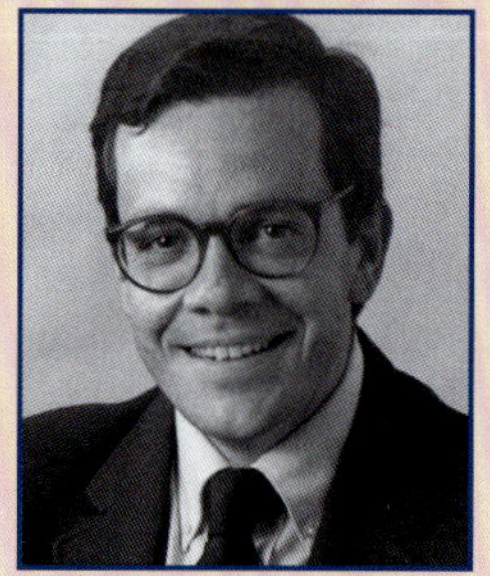

Dan Dempsey. BA in classics, Princeton University; MD University of Pennsylvania; assistant professor of surgery, Temple University; professor and chief of surgery, Pennsylvania Hospital; chairman of surgery, Temple University (2000–2010); chief of GI surgery, University of Pennsylvania (2011–2021); president of Philadelphia County Medical Society (2016); Strittmatter Award (2019).

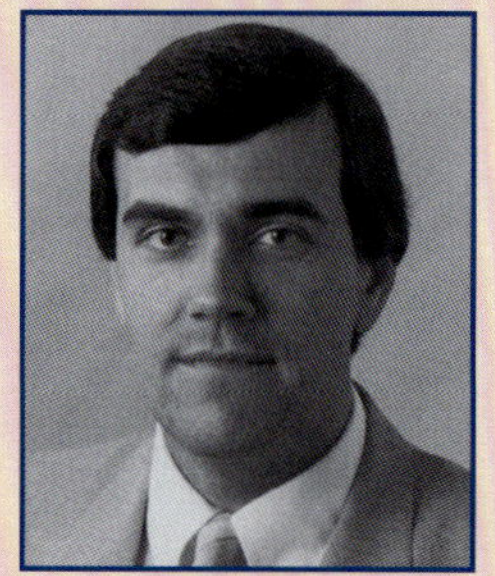

John Francfort. MD Rutgers University; transplantation research fellow with Barker and Naji; vascular fellowship, Northwestern University; assistant professor of surgery, Jefferson University; clinical assistant professor of surgery, SUNY Stonybrook; chairman of surgery, Good Samaritan Hospital; past president, Eastern Long Island Chapter of American College of Surgeons.

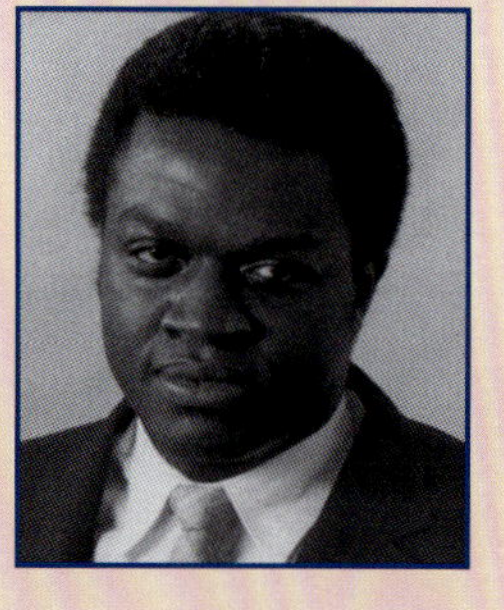

Danny O. Jacobs. Philips Exeter Academy; BA Harvard University; MD Washington University; research fellow and MPH to associate professor at Harvard (1986–2000); associate director, Brigham's Clinical Research Center; professor and chairman Department of Surgery, Creighton University (2000–2003); David Sabiston Professor and Chairman of Surgery, Duke University

(2003–2012); executive vice president, provost, and dean, University of Texas Medical Branch (2012–2018); president of Oregon Health Services University (2018–present); research on critical illness and malnutrition effect on metabolism; twelve editorial boards; 300 manuscripts; member of National Academy of Medicine; University of Pennsylvania Department of Surgery Distinguished Graduate Award (2010).

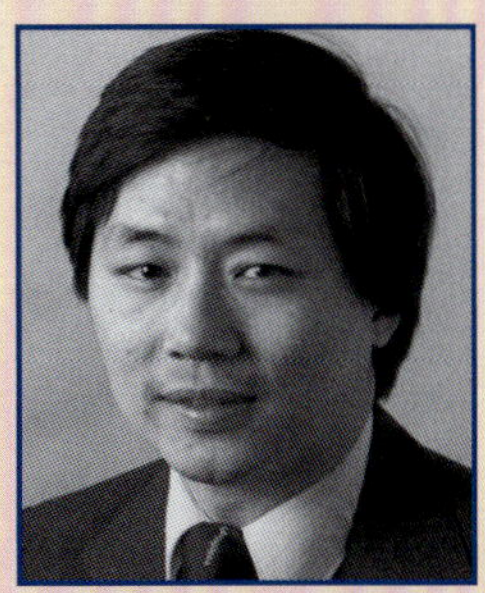

David Low. BA Harvard University; MD Harvard University; fellowship in plastic surgery HUP; assistant professor to professor at University of Pennsylvania and CHOP (1989–present); seven major teaching awards; extraordinary artist and medical illustrator; ninety peer-reviewed publications and illustrations of 156 others and seven books; free care provided to underserved patients in Venezuela and Guatemala.

1986–1987

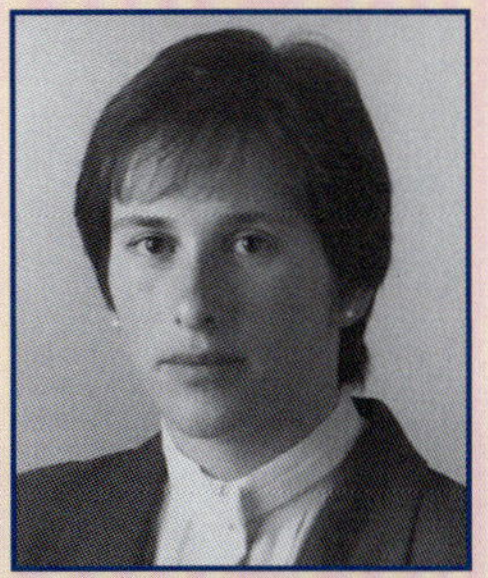

Patricia Bailey. BA Clark University; MD University of Massachusetts; research with Drs. Mullen and Buzby; practice of general surgery, Chestnut Hill Hospital; faculty appointments at Temple (1987–1990); Jefferson (1990–1996); Penn at Chestnut Hill.

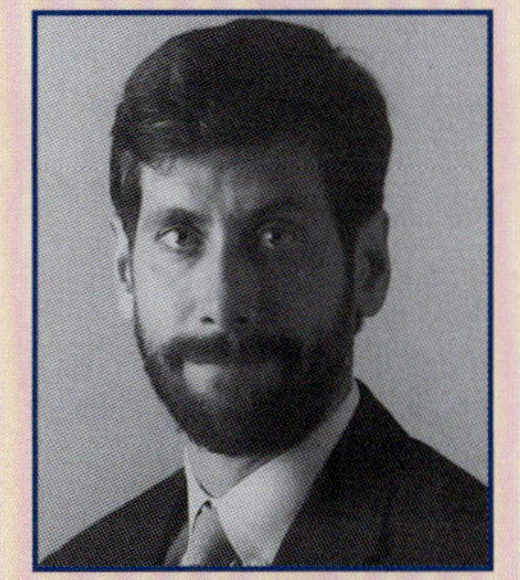

Robert Hinks. MD Jefferson University; practice of surgery in Jacksonville, North Carolina; Naval Medical Center, Camp Lejeune.

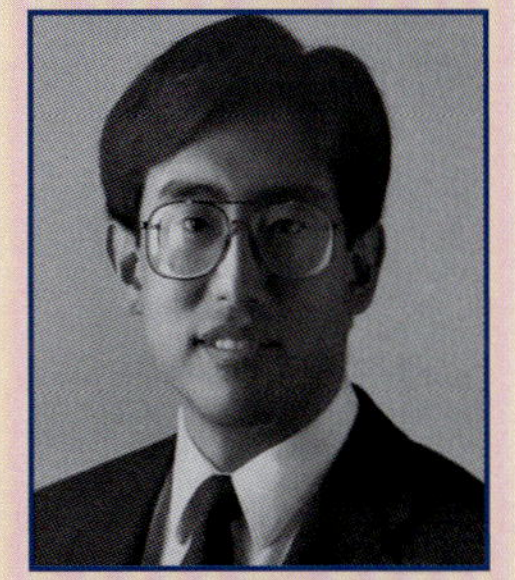

Norman Kato. BA Swarthmore College; MD University of Pennsylvania; fellow in physiology at Penn (1987–1989); CT fellowship, NYU (1989–1991); assistant professor, UCLA (1991–1997); practice of CT surgery, Encino, California; CEO, Alvarda.

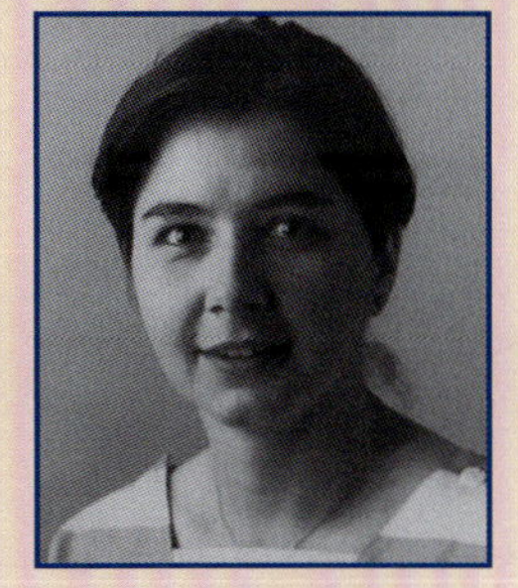

Jane Kugaczewski. MD SUNY Brooklyn; fellowship in pediatric surgery, University of Pennsylvania (Presbyterian campus 1985–1986); practice of pediatric surgery, Mt. Sinai; practice of pediatric surgery, SUNY Stonybrook.

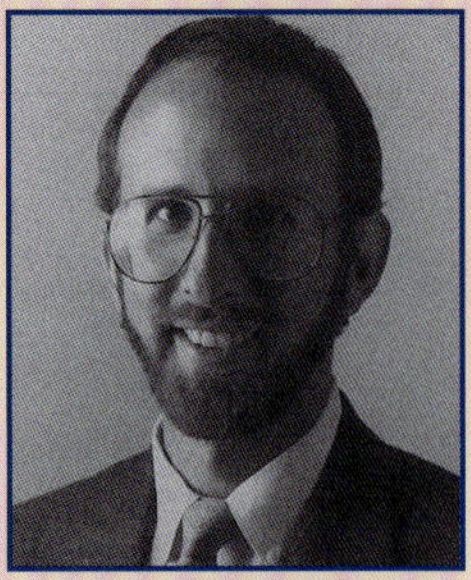

Robert Fried. BA Washington University; MD Washington University; practice of surgery, Paoli Hospital; chief of surgery and vice president of medical affairs, Paoli Hospital; past president of medical staff and chief of staff of Main Line Health System.

1987–1988

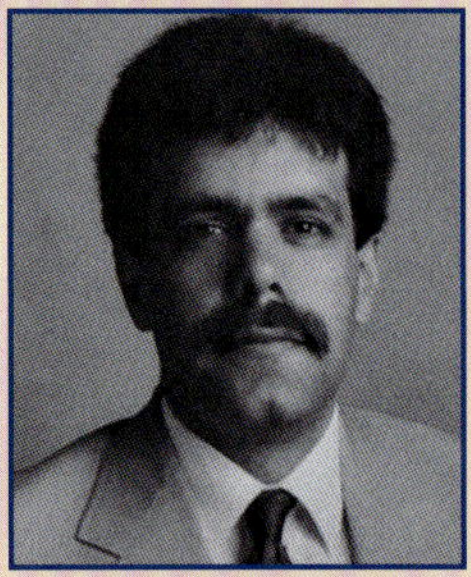

Michael Acker. BS Brown University; MD Brown University 1981; CT residency, Johns Hopkins; Julian Johnson Professor and chief of division of CV Surgery, HUP; director of Heart and Vascular Center, HUP; Alfred Stengel Health System Award; Gordon Buzby Leadership Award; classical guitarist.

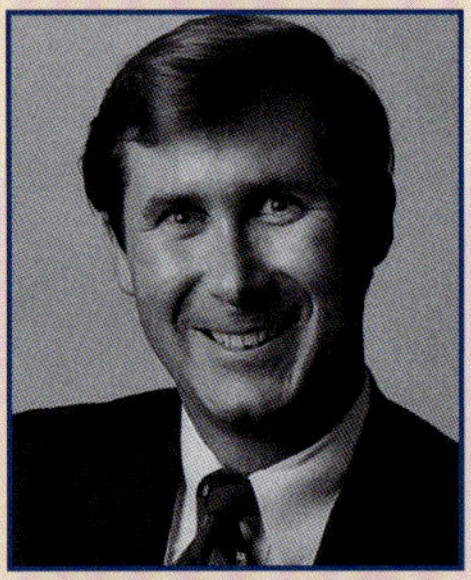

Robert Donoway. MD University of Pennsylvania; surgical oncology fellow, Memorial SKCC; medical director and chief of surgery of Memorial Regional Hospital, Hollywood, Florida.

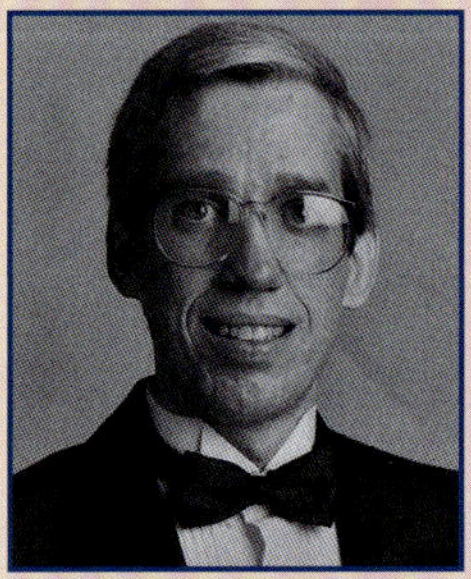

Jeffrey Kappa. MD Duke University; vascular fellowship at HUP; practice of general and vascular surgery in Johnson City, Tennessee.

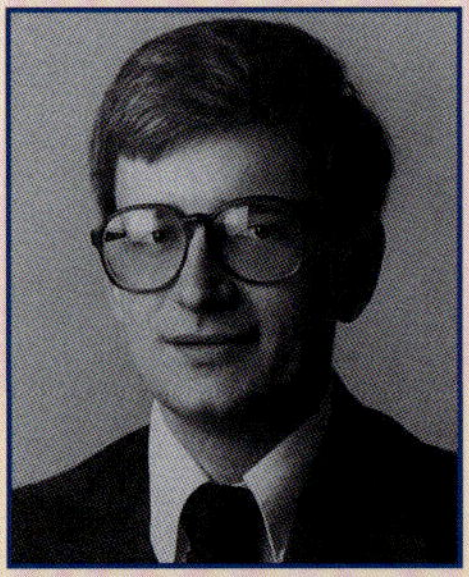

Mark Koruda. MD Yale University; professor of surgery and chief of GI division, University of North Carolina; 1989 Stanley Dudrick Award in Nutrition from American Society for Parenteral and Enteral Nutrition.

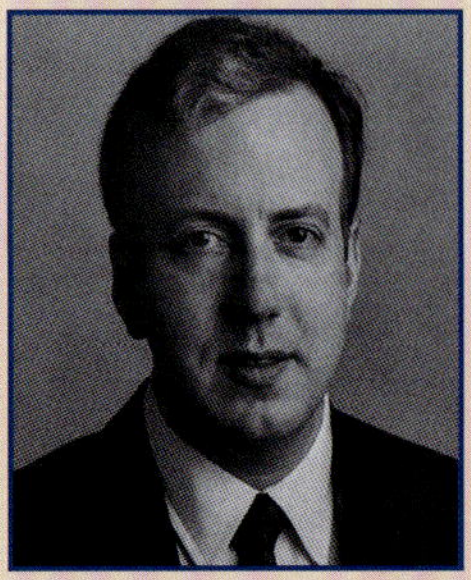

Mark Ratcliffe. BA Denison University; MD Case Western Reserve University; intern and junior resident, Johns Hopkins University; senior resident, HUP; CT fellowship HUP; faculty University of Pennsylvania; since 1993, San Francisco General and VA Hospitals; director, Cardiac Biomechanical Laboratory; professor-in-residence and chief of surgery at San Francisco VA Hospital; vice chairman, UCSF.

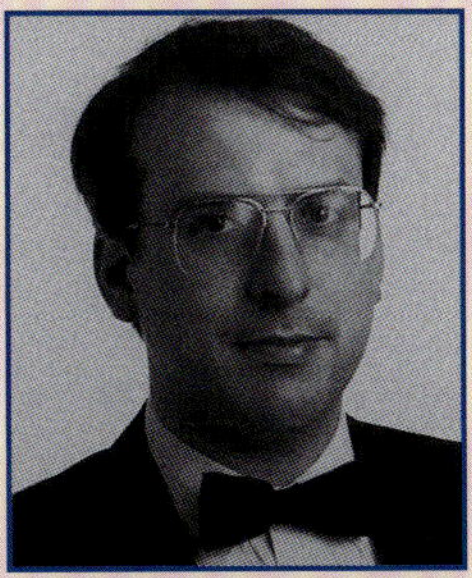

James Andersen. MD Jefferson University; fellowship in plastic surgery, University of Pennsylvania; further plastic training, University of Southern California; twenty-six years on faculty at Keck University of Southern California; professor and director of plastic surgery, City of Hope Medical Group, Duarte, California. 1988–1989

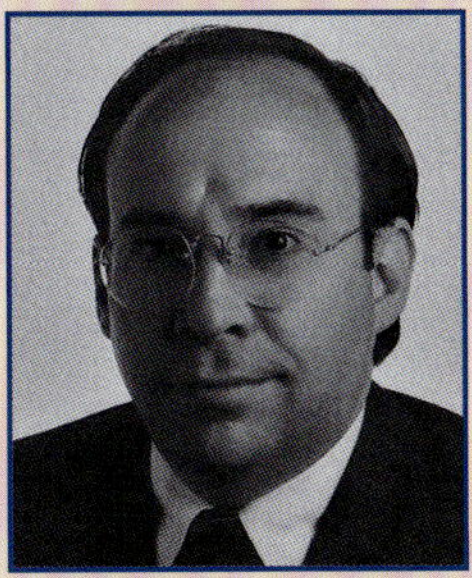

Ken Brayman. BS University of Massachusetts; MD University of Pennsylvania; postdoctoral fellowship in transplantation with Clyde Barker and Ali Naji, HUP; fellowship in transplantation, University of Minnesota (1989–1992); assistant to associate professor of surgery, University of Pennsylvania (1992–2002); director of pancreas transplantation, HUP and kidney transplantation, CHOP; 2002 director of renal, pancreas, and islet transplantation, University of Virginia; 2009 division chief of transplantation, University of Virginia; chief of islet transplantation, University of Virginia; Nabi Professor of Transplantation, University of Virginia; University of Pennsylvania Department of Surgery Distinguished Graduate Award (2017).

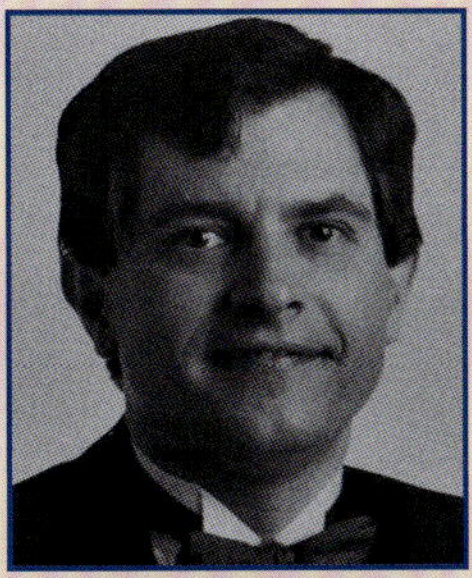

Earl Cottrell. BA University of Utah; intern Penn State University, Hershey; vascular fellow at University of Arizona (1989–1991); assistant clinical professor, University of Nevada; practice at University of Southern Nevada (Las Vegas).

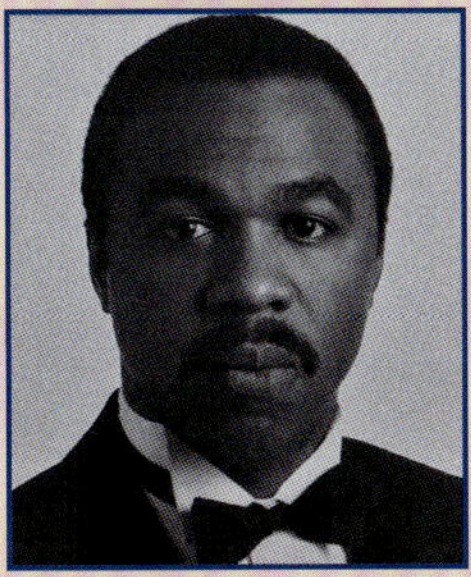

Martin Karpeh. BA University of Pennsylvania; MD Penn State University; surgical oncology fellowship, Memorial SKCC; ten years on faculty at Memorial SKCC; chief of surgical oncology, SUNY Stonybrook (2003–2007); chief of surgery, Beth Israel Hospital (2007–2014); founding chairman of surgery, Hackensack-Meridian School of Medicine at Seton Hall University; president of Society of Black Academic Surgeons; Chairperson Department of Surgery, Northwell Health Eastern Region at Huntington, Long Island.

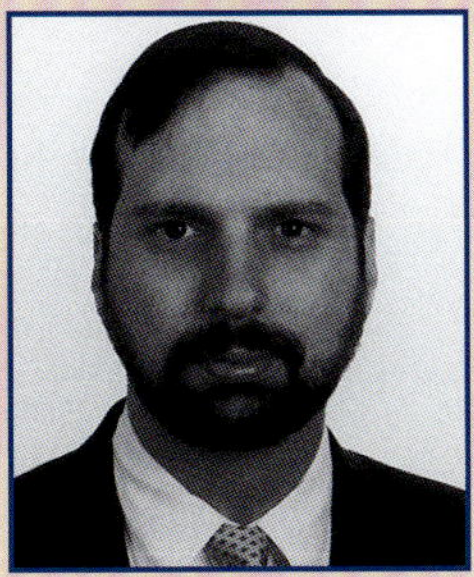

Joseph Bavaria. American High School (Paris); Indiana High School (Cincinnati); University of Edinburgh; MD Tulane University; CHE Tulane University School of Engineering; fellowship in CT surgery, HUP and CHOP; research in CT fellowship with Hank Edmunds, HUP; Brooke Roberts/Measey Professor of Surgery, HUP; vice chief of division of CV surgery, HUP; director of 1989–1990 thoracic-aortic surgery program, HUP; president of Society of Thoracic Surgery (2018); Sheen Award of American College of Surgeons; honorary fellow, Royal College of Surgeons of Edinburgh.

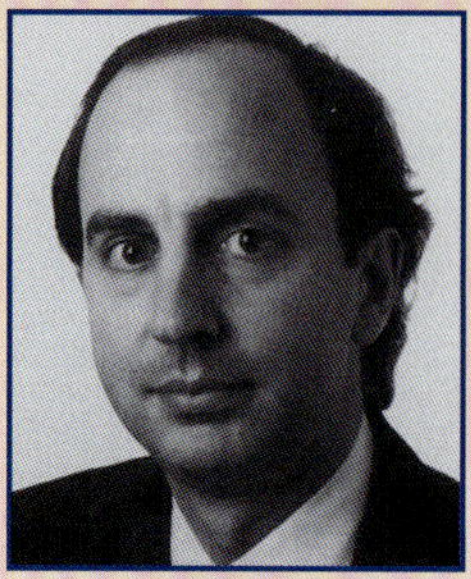

Michael Choti. MD Yale University; fellowship in surgical oncology, Memorial SKCC; assistant professor to professor, Johns Hopkins (1992–2013); vice chair and chief of Division of Surgical Oncology, Johns Hopkins; chairman of Department of Surgery, Southwestern Medical School; University of Pennsylvania Department of Surgery Distinguished Graduate Award (2013).

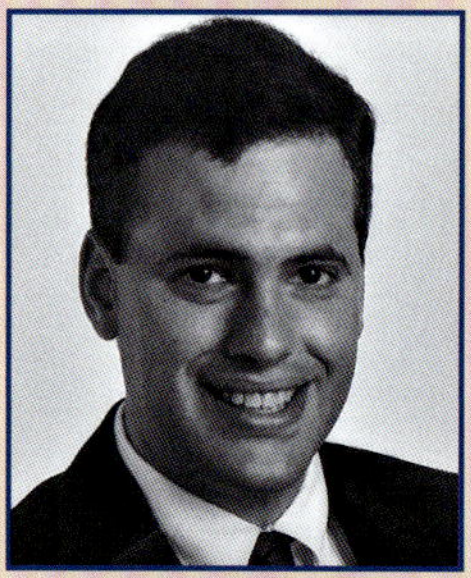

Andrew Fox. MD Yale University; vascular fellow at University of Massachusetts (1999–2003); MBA at MIT (2004–2006); president and CEO of Wadsworth Medical Technologies (2005–present); Venture Mentoring Services at MIT (2010–present).

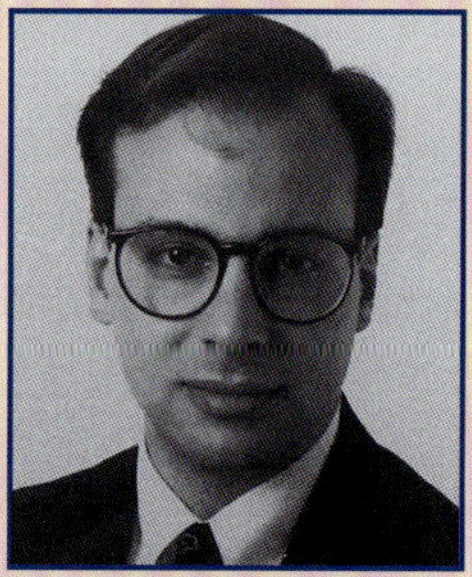

Scott Kripke. BA Harvard University; MD University of Pennsylvania; two years research on nutrition and metabolism at HUP; surgical oncology fellowship at Memorial SKCC; surgical practice at Paoli Hospital; President of Surgical Specialists of Main Line.

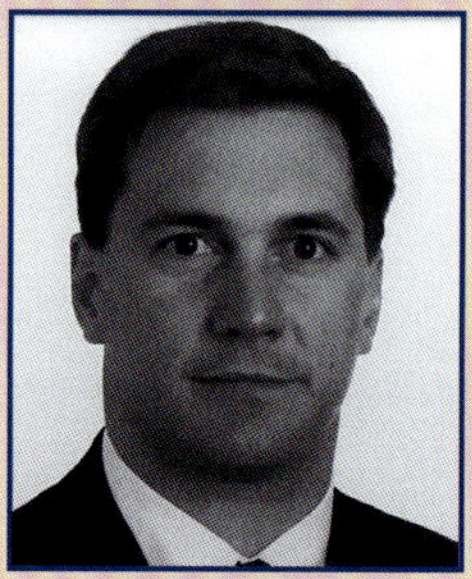

Russell Stahl. BA Cornell University; MD New York University; cardiothoracic resident, HUP (1990–1992); assistant professor of surgery, University of Massachusetts (1992–1997); cardiac surgery associate, NEPA (1997–2000); Premcare Surgical (2000–2013); Geissinger Clinic (2013–2016); chief of County Medical Center, Scranton, Pennsylvania; Grand Strand Heart and Vascular (2016–present), Myrtle Beach, South Carolina.

1990–1991

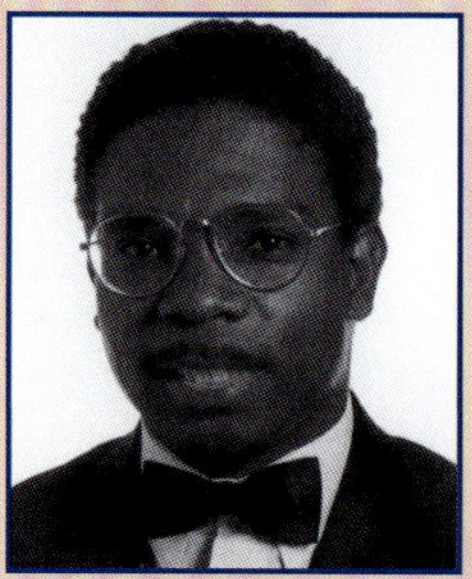

Charles Bridges. MD Harvard University; professor of surgery, University of Pennsylvania; chief of cardiac surgery, Pennsylvania Hospital; global chief technology officer, Pulmonary Hypertension Therapeutic Area; Jannsen Pharmaceuticals Research and Development, Johnson & Johnson; professor and chairman of cardiovascular, thoracic, and vascular surgery at Carolina Healthcare System, University of North Carolina.

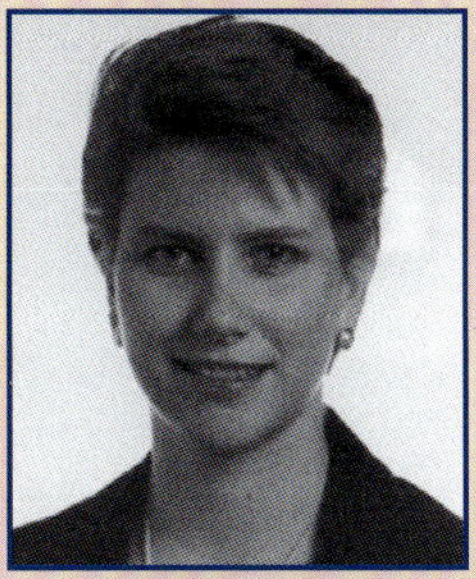

Linda Callans. MD Johns Hopkins University; practice of surgical oncology, specialty of breast surgery, Ardmore, Pennsylvania.

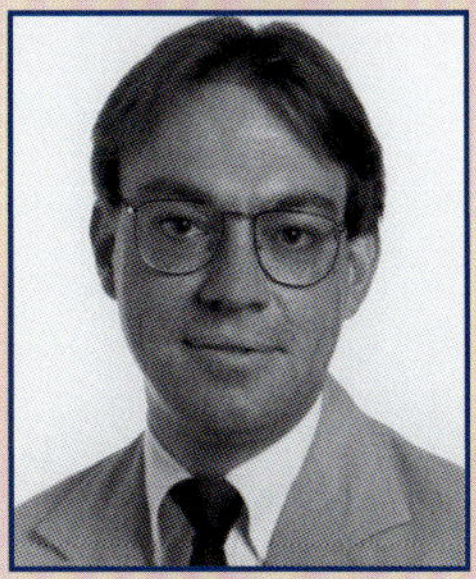

Jeffrey Carpenter. BA Amherst College; MD and MDiv Yale University; vascular fellowship, HUP; assistant professor to professor, HUP (1992–2008); chairman, Department of Surgery, Robert Wood Johnson School of Medicine (2008–2013); chairman, Department of Surgery, Cooper University Healthcare of Rowan University (2013–present); pioneered early devices for endovascular surgery; president of Philadelphia Academy of Surgery (2012).

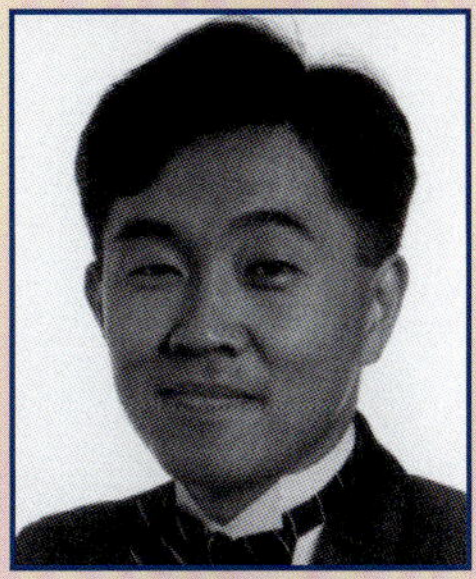

Satoshi Furukawa. MD University of Pennsylvania; cardiothoracic fellowship, HUP; professor of CT surgery at Temple (1993–2013); chief of CT surgery, Reading Health System (2013–2014); professor of clinical surgery and chief of CV surgery, Pennsylvania Hospital (2014–present).

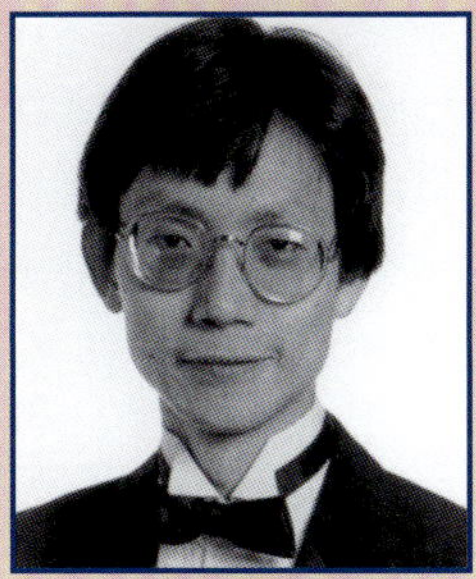

Jack Yu. MS University of Pennsylvania; MD University of Pennsylvania; fellowship in plastic surgery, University of Pennsylvania; Hatcher Professor and chief of section of plastic surgery, Medical College of Georgia; director of Cranial-Facial Center; research on stimulation to prevent age-related muscle and bone loss.

1991–1992

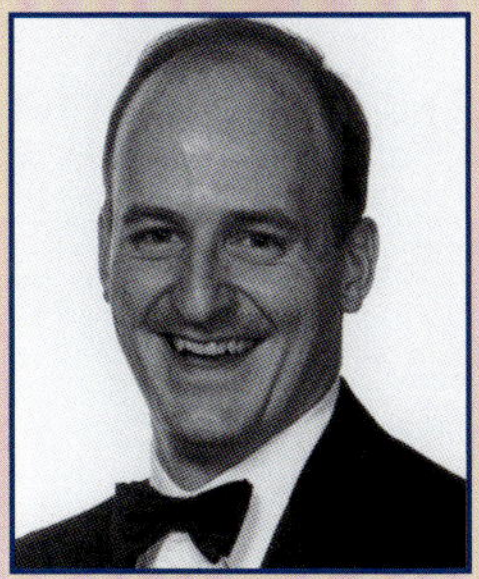

David Deaton. BA Haverford College; MD Duke University; vascular fellowship, UCLA; former chief of vascular and endovascular surgery, MedStar-Georgetown University Hospital; also affiliated with University of Maryland and North Carolina; pioneer of endograft devices.

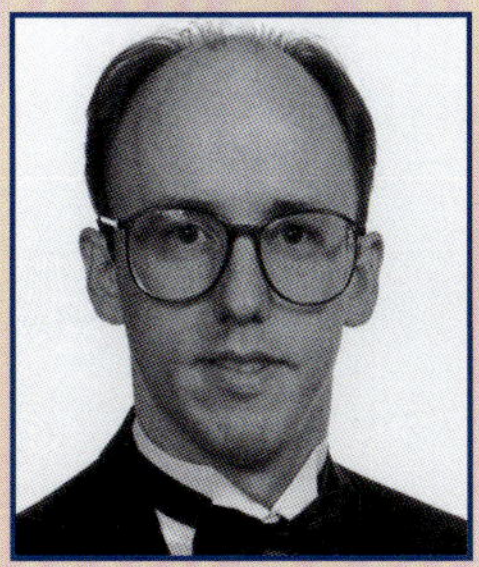

Steven Fishman. BS Northwestern University; MD Northwestern University; pediatric surgery fellowship, Boston Children's Hospital; faculty—assistant professor to professor, Boston Children's Hospital; director of vascular anomalies, Boston Children's Hospital; professor and chief of surgery, Boston Children's Hospital (2019–present).

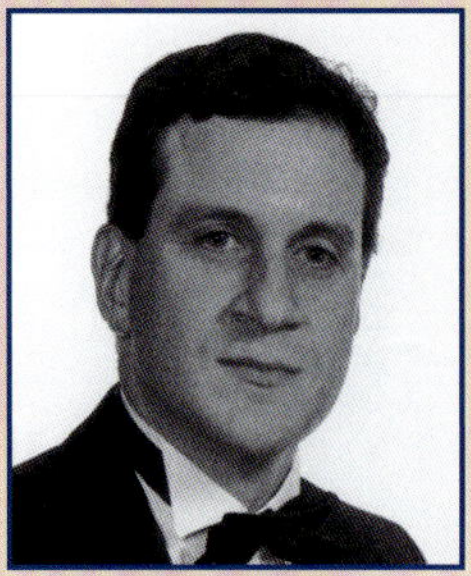

Michael Lieberman. MD University of Pennsylvania; fellow in surgical oncology, Memorial SKCC; director of Surgical Oncology and Pancreas Center, New York Hospital, Weill-Cornell; associate professor of clinical surgery, Cornell.

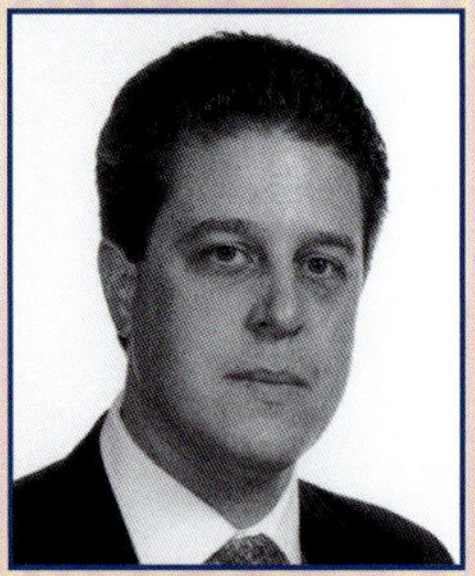

Edward Savage. MD Yale University; cardiothoracic fellowship, Brigham and Womens Hospital; chief of CT at Cook County and associate professor at Rush Medical School; chair of Department of CT Surgery, Cleveland Clinic in Florida (2009–2018); since 2018, clinical professor and director of CV services at Cleveland Clinic Lerner College of Medicine.

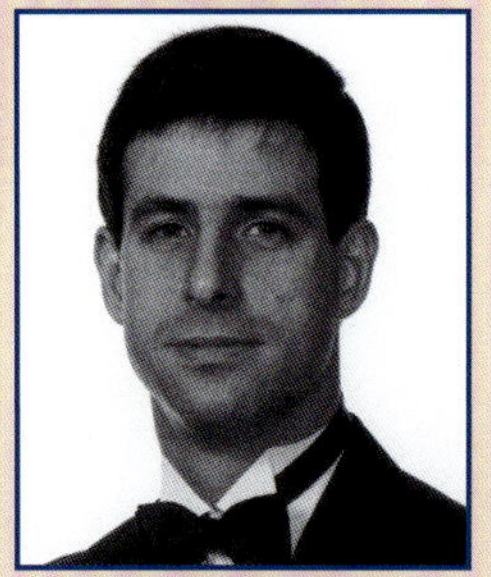

Mark Shachner. MD Yale University; research fellow in immunology and transplantation, University of Pennsylvania; president of South Florida Surgical Specialists; clinical associate professor at NOVA Southeastern University.

1992–1993

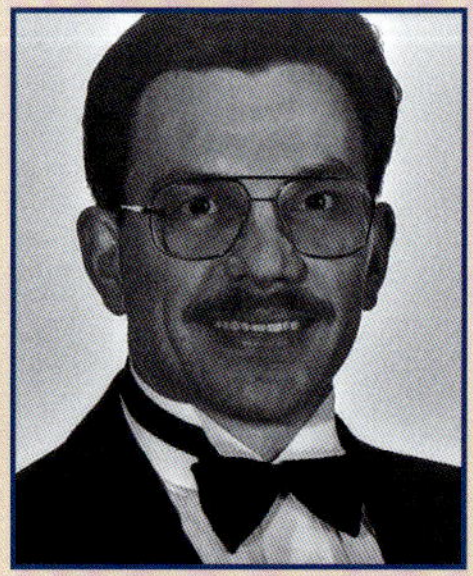

James Luketich. BA Old Dominion University; MA Vanderbilt; MD Medical College of Pennsylvania; postdoctoral research in nutrition with Jim Mullen; fellowships in thoracic and CT at Cleveland Clinic and Cornell; fellowship in surgical oncology at Memorial SKCC; faculty at University of Pittsburgh CT Division; Henry T. Bahnson Professor and Chairman of CT Division, University of Pittsburgh; 2010 Inaugural Chair of Department of CT Surgery, University of Pittsburgh; University of Pennsylvania Department of Surgery Distinguished Graduate Award (2012).

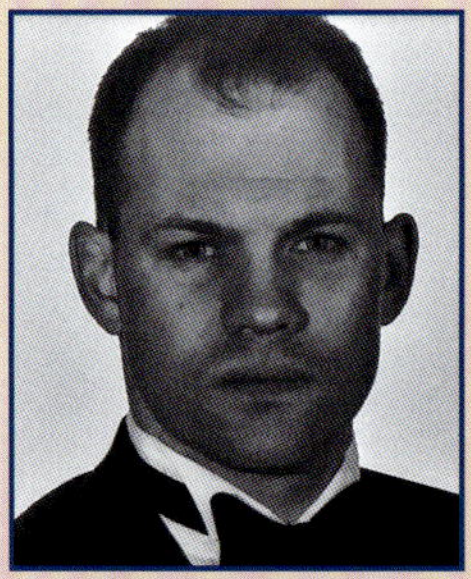

Stephen Downing. MD Georgetown University; cardiothoracic fellowship, Washington University; Inouye and Rhoads awards as resident; chairman of surgery at Mercy Hospital, clinical assistant professor of Surgery, SUNY Buffalo.

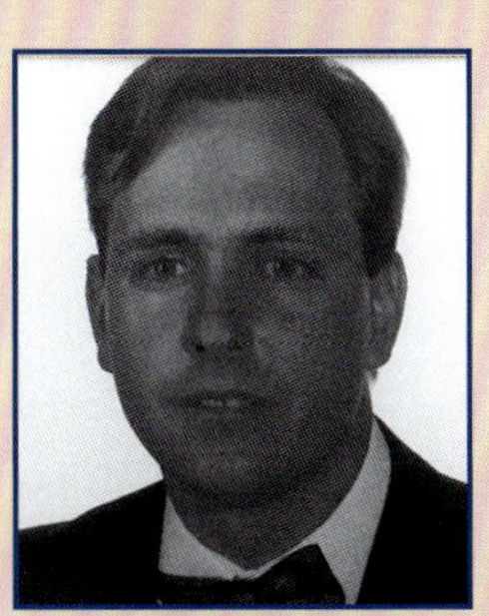

David Bartlett. MD University of Pennsylvania; fellowship in surgical oncology, Memorial SKCC; Bernard Fisher Professor of Surgery, University of Pittsburgh; after two decades at Pitt, since 2020, chairman of surgery, Alleghany Health Network Cancer Institute; president of Society of Surgical Oncology (2019).

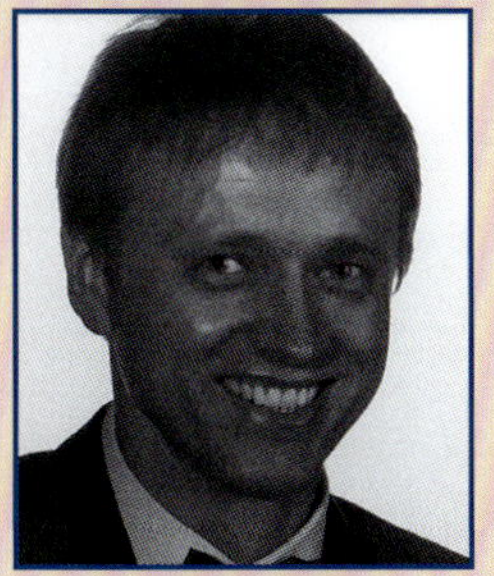

Christian Schunn. MD Ludwig Maximilian University of Munich; practice of vascular surgery in Richmond and Midlothian, Virginia.

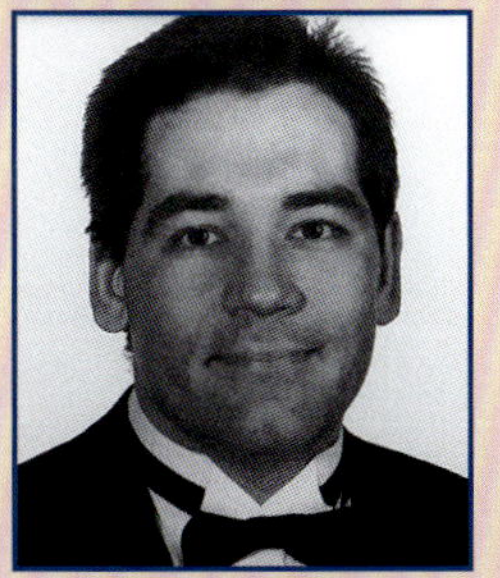

James McCaughan. MD Wright State University; practice of thoracic surgery in Toms River, New Jersey; father was one of Ravdin and Rhoads's residents.

1993–1994

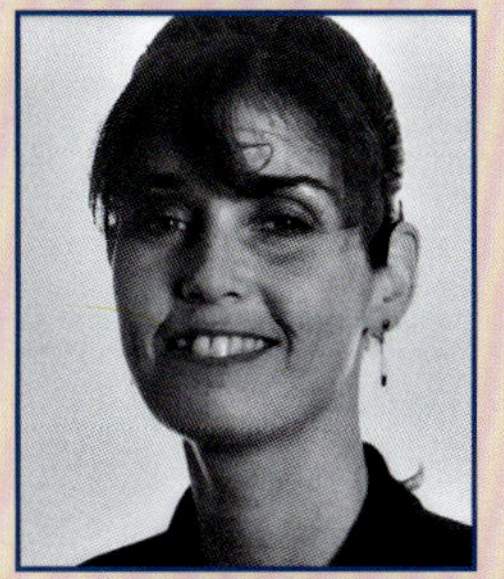

Abigail Hanna. MD Cornell University; practice of general surgery in West Hartford, Connecticut; research at Yale.

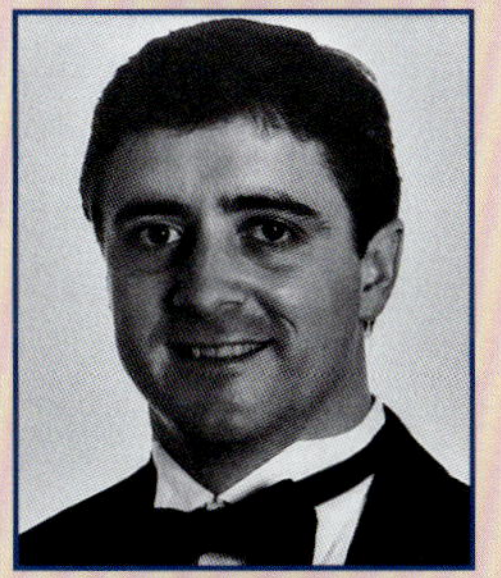

Steven Hendrickson. MD Duke University; fellowship in CT surgery, Duke University; practice of CT surgery, Moses Cone Hospital, Greensboro, North Carolina.

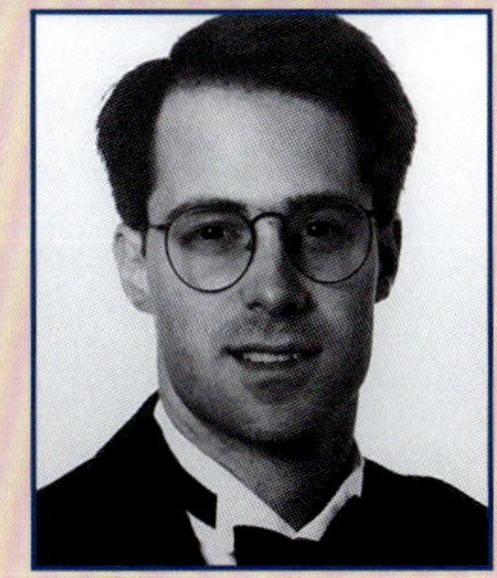

Jon Odorico. BS Duke University; MD New York University; postdoctoral fellowship at HUP in islet transplantation and thymic tolerance; transplantation fellowship, University of Wisconsin, Madison; professor, University of Wisconsin; director of pancreas and islet cell program; active NIH-supported research on stem cell tolerance; past president of International Pancreas and Islet Cell Transplantation Association.

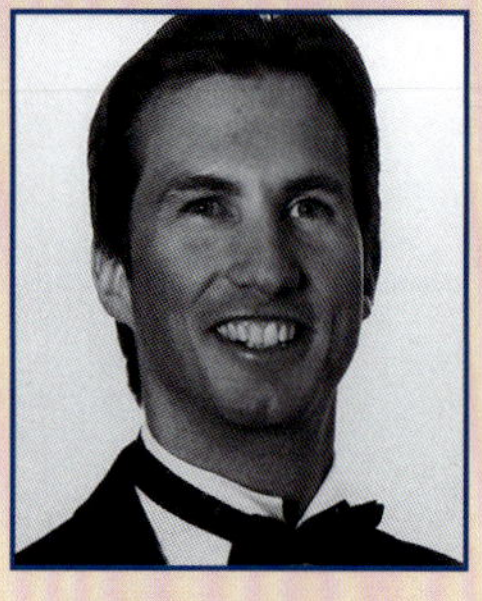

Hansell Stedman. BS MIT; MD Harvard University; associate professor at Penn, active surgeon at VA Hospital; research focus on molecular aspects of muscular dystrophy; Department of Surgery's most active NIH-supported investigator; recent paper in *Nature* is important progress in his lifelong research on muscular dystrophy. He showed that mUtro is a highly functional, non-immunogenic substitute for dystrophin; it can prevent the deleterious histological and physiological aspects of muscular dystrophy in small and large animal models. These findings constitute a model in which utrophin-derived therapies might be used to treat clinical dystophin deficiency (muscular dystrophy).

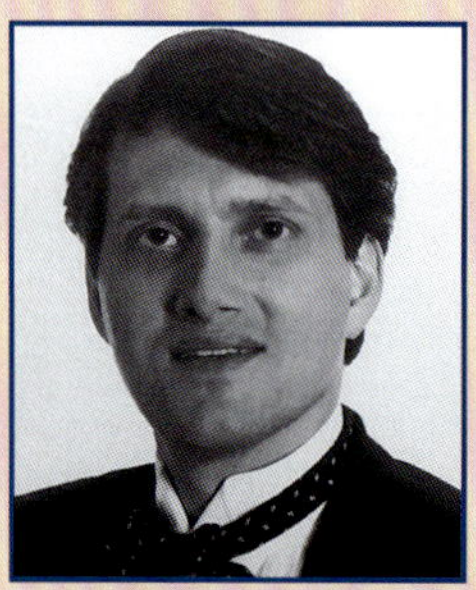

David Theodoro. MD Washington University; fellow in cardiothoracic surgery, Mayo Clinic; practice of thoracic surgery, Hazelwood, Missouri; chairman of SSM Health Heart and Vascular Institute and Gateway Quality Physician Alliance, St. Louis, Missouri.

1994–1995

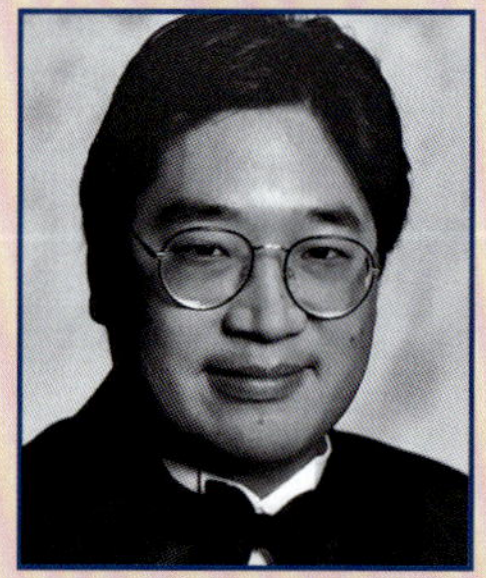

Donald Liu. BA Johns Hopkins University; MD and PhD in immunology, Jefferson University; fellow in pediatric surgery, University of Michigan; professor and chief of pediatric surgery and surgery-in-chief at University of Chicago Children's Hospital; internationally recognized for introducing minimally invasive techniques in children; NIH-supported research in the microbiome; died in 2012 during rescue of drowning child in Lake Michigan.

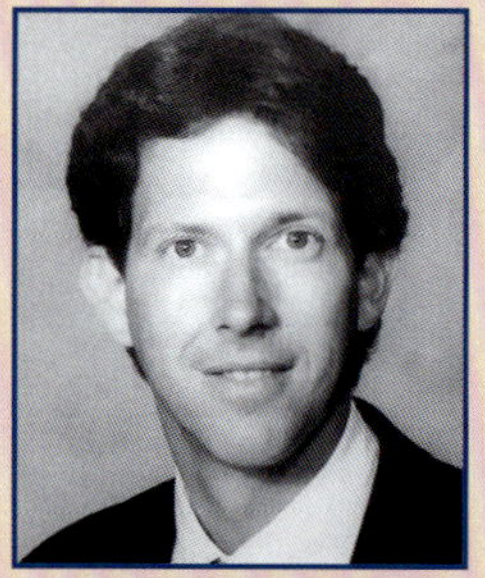

Mark Mantell. MD University of Pennsylvania; vascular fellowship, HUP; clinical associate professor and director of vascular access at Penn-Presbyterian Hospital.

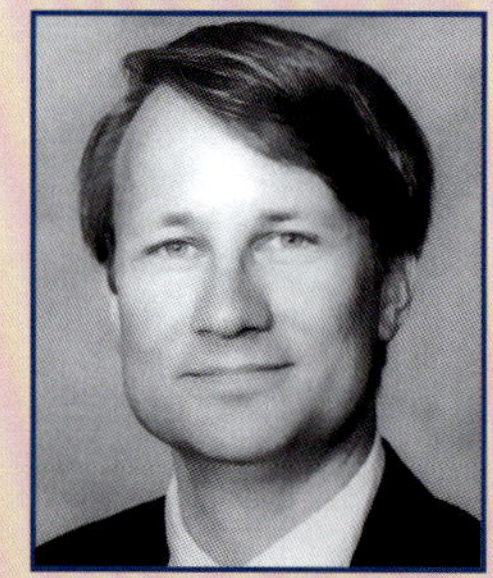

Michael Nance. MD Louisiana State University, Shreveport; fellowship in critical care medicine at HUP; fellowship in pediatric surgery, CHOP; director of pediatric trauma program, CHOP; Josephine J. and John M. Templeton Professor of Surgery, CHOP; chief of Division of Pediatric Surgery, CHOP; chief of Division of Trauma Surgery, CHOP; father was Rhoads's resident and well-known trauma surgeon at LSU.

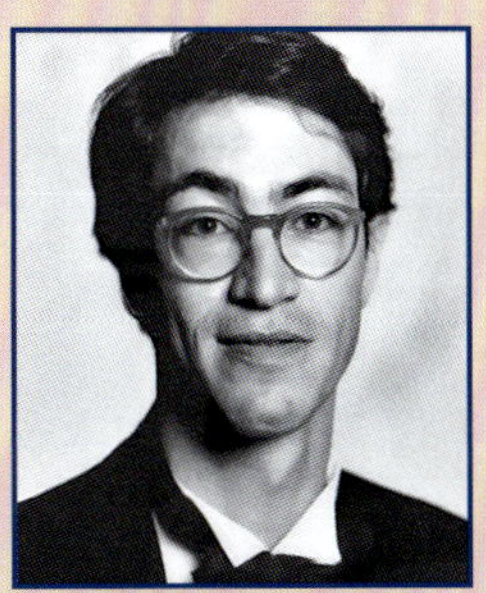

Joseph Shrager. BA Amherst College; MD Harvard University; thoracic surgery fellowship, MGH; chief of general thoracic division, HUP (2003–2007); professor and chief of Division of Thoracic Surgery, Stanford University; member of editorial board of *Annals of Thoracic Surgery.*

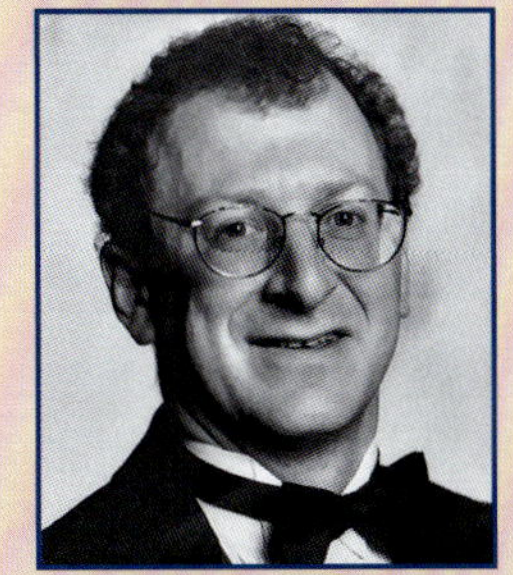

Scott Steinmetz. MD Johns Hopkins University; practice of general surgery, Bel Air, Maryland; affiliated with University of Maryland Upper Chesapeake Medical Center.

1995–1996

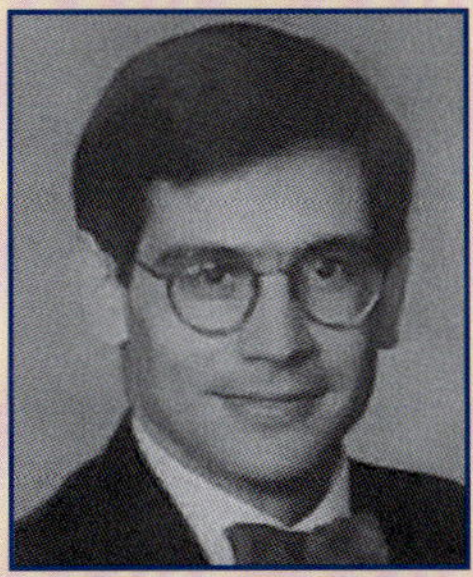

Alex Cech. BS/MS Yale University; MD Duke University; research with John Daly; plastic surgery fellowship, HUP; fellowship in surgical oncology, HUP; fellowship in microsurgery and cancer, Memorial SKCC; fellowship in craniofacial surgery, Chang Gung Memorial Hospital; assistant clinical professor, University of Connecticut.

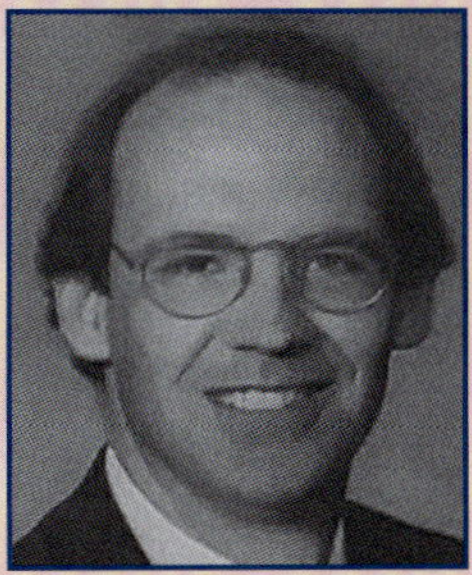

James Markmann. BA LaSalle University; MD University of Pennsylvania; PhD University of Pennsylvania (1983–1989); fellowship in transplantation, UCLA; assistant to associate professor, University of Pennsylvania (1998–2007); chief of transplantation, MGH; pioneer of islet transplantation research; with Naji, initiated HUP's human islet transplant program; Claude Welch Professor of Surgery at Harvard University; University of Pennsylvania Department of Surgery Distinguished Graduate Award (2016).

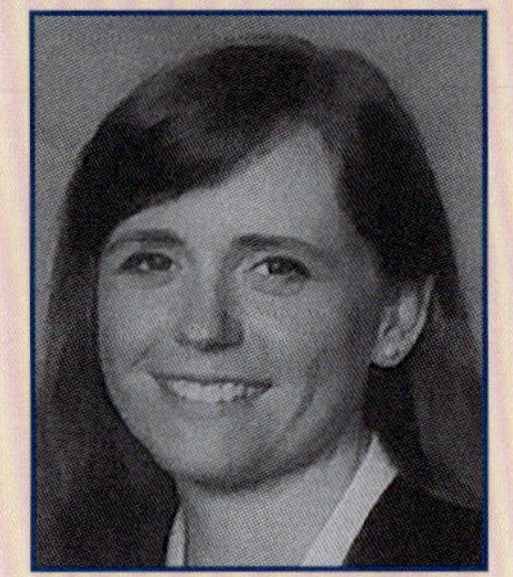

Kathleen Reilly. BA University of Pennsylvania; MD University of Pennsylvania; professor of surgery, Lewis Katz School of Medicine, Temple University; pianist and pilot; two years nutrition research with John Rombeau.

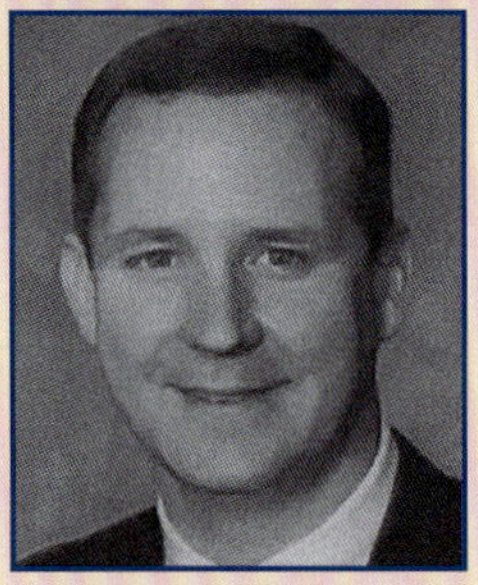

Roy Smythe. BS Baylor University; MD Texas A&M; CT fellowship, HUP; research with Larry Kaiser and Steve Albelda on gene transfer, oncology, mesothelioma; faculty at MD Anderson; professor and chairman of Department of Surgery, Texas A&M (2004); later switched to industrial activities, CEO of Somalogic; global leader in health information; University of Pennsylvania Department of Surgery Distinguished Graduate Award (2011).

1996–1997

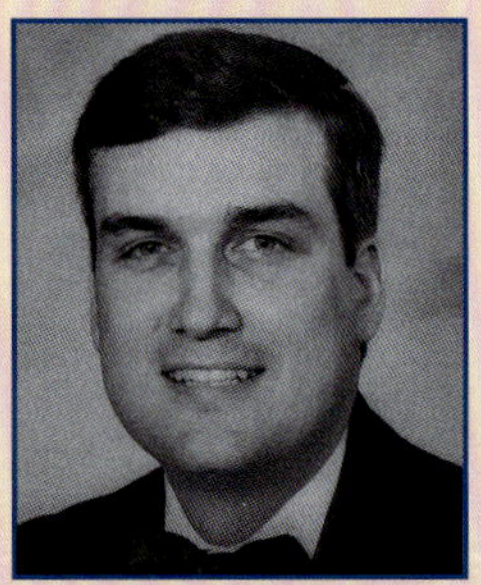

William Adamson. MD Duke University; fellowship in pediatric surgery, CHOP; chief of pediatric surgery, University of North Carolina Medical School (2004–2018); division chief of pediatric surgery, Nemouns Children's Health System, Orlando, Florida.

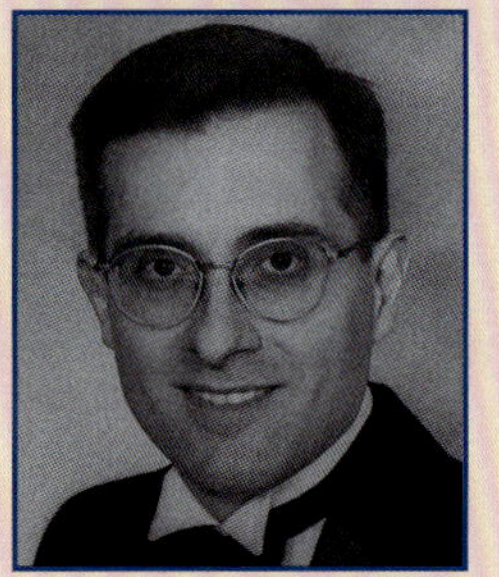

Ron DeMatteo. MD Cornell University Medical College; four-year research fellowship with Jim Wilson and Steve Raper; surgical oncology fellowship at Memorial SKCC; faculty at Memorial SKCC (1999–2017); head of Division of General Surgery and vice chair of the Department of Surgery at Memorial SKCC (2006–2017); John Rhea Barton Professor and Chairman, Department of Surgery, University of Pennsylvania (2017–present); member of American Society of Clinical Investigation, Association of American Physicians, and National Academy of Medicine. University of Pennsylvania Department of Surgery Distinguished Graduate Award (2007).

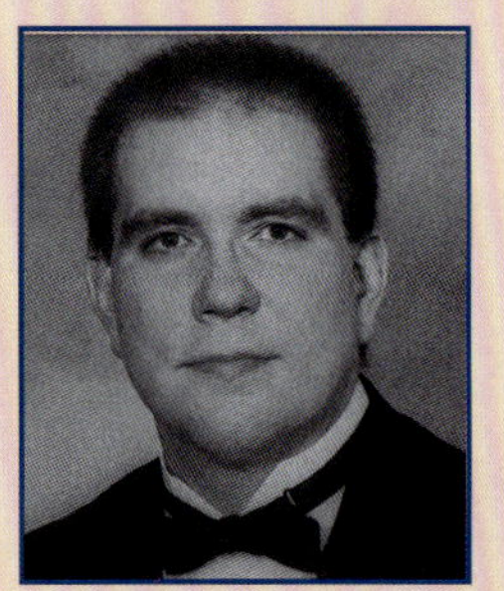

Frank DiPierro. MD University of Chicago; fellow in cardiothoracic surgery, Cleveland Clinic (1997–2000); CT surgery staff, Eastern Maine Medical Center (2000–2012); surgical staff, Cleveland Clinic (2012–2015); fellow in critical care anesthesiology (2016–2017); cardiothoracic intensivist and assistant professor of anesthesia (2017–present).

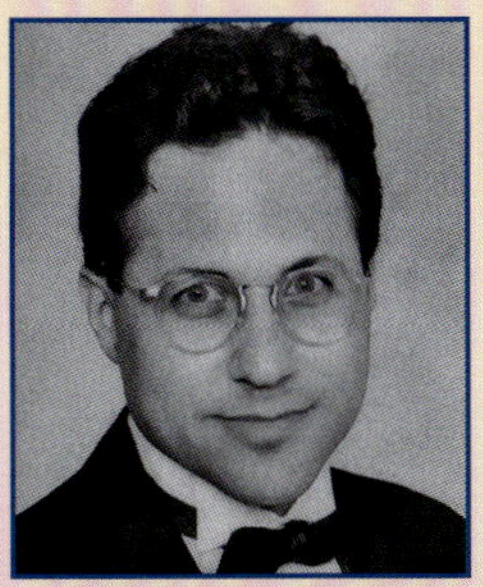

Mark Levy. MD University of Pennsylvania; transplantation research with Ken Brayman on intrathymic islet transplantation in dogs; Inouye Award; president of Agnew Society; fellow in vascular surgery, HUP (1997–1998); H. M. Lee Professor in vascular surgery, Virginia Commonwealth University; chief of Division of Vascular Surgery, Virginia Commonwealth University; vascular fellowship program director, Virginia Commonwealth University; founder of Richmond's first endovascular program.

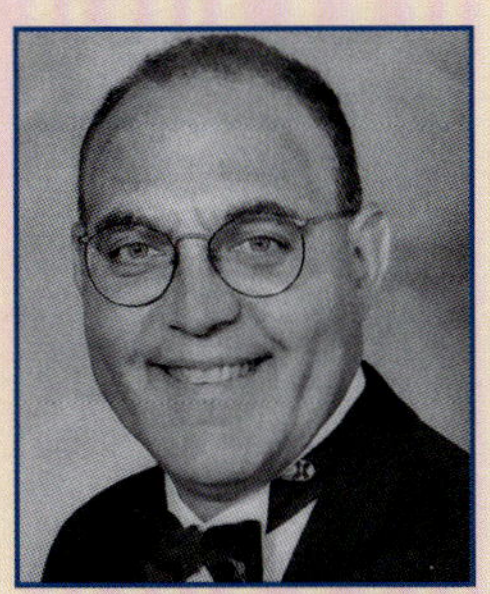

Noel Williams. MD Royal College of Surgeons, Ireland; Rhoads/Harrington professor of clinical surgery, University of Pennsylvania; director of Penn Metabolic and Bariatric Surgery Program; director of William Fitts Surgery Education Center; honorary fellow, Royal Society of Surgeons in Ireland, 2023.

1997–1998

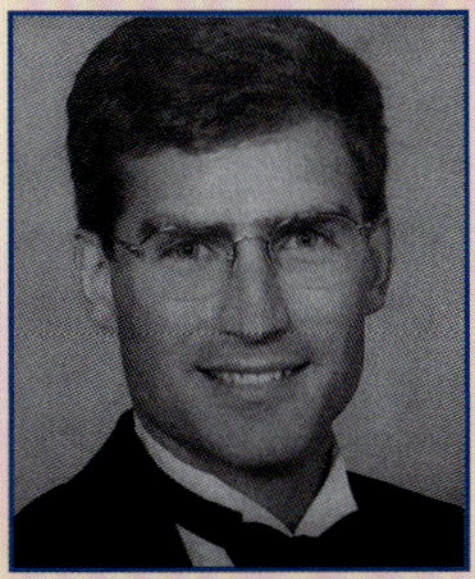

Thomas Hamilton. MD Cornell University, pediatric surgery fellowship, Boston Children's Hospital; assistant professor, Harvard Medical School; assistant program director, pediatric surgery fellowship, Boston Children's Hospital; associate professor of surgery, CHOP.

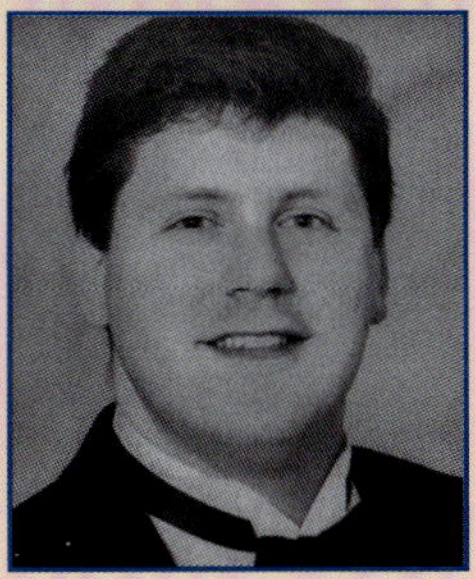

Robert Larson. MD University of Pennsylvania; vascular fellowship, HUP (2000–2001); surgical staff, Guthrie Clinic; associate professor of surgery, Virginia Commonwealth University.

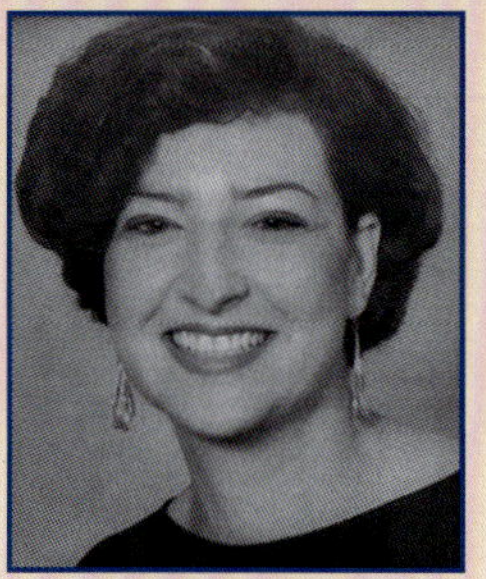

Susan Lerner. MD University of Pennsylvania; transplantation fellowship, UCLA; director of liver transplantation program, Penn State University, Hershey; associate professor of surgery and medical education, Mt. Sinai Medical School.

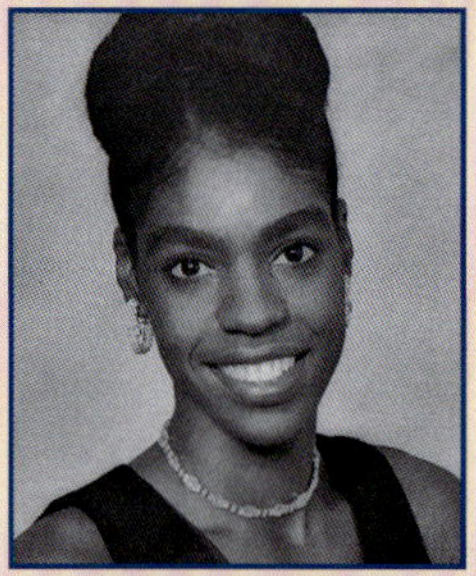

Wendy Olivier. MD Duke University; fellowship in plastic surgery, New York University; practice of plastic and reconstructive surgery, Brooklyn, New York; clinical assistant professor, Cornell University.

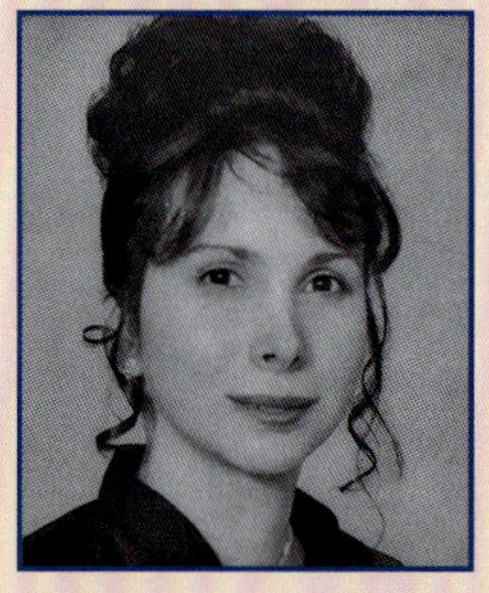

Omaida Velasquez. BS Stevens Institute of Technology; MD UMDNJ; fellow in vascular surgery, HUP; assistant professor to associate professor, HUP (2000–2007); research in nutrition with Jonathan Rombeau; research in endothelial biology with Meenhard Herlyn at Wistar Institute; 2007 professor and chief of Division of Vascular Surgery and executive dean for research, University of Miami; 2015 chair of Department of Surgery, University of Miami; member of American Society for Clinical Investigation; member of National Academy of Medicine; University of Pennsylvania Department of Surgery Distinguished Graduate Award (2015).

1998–1999

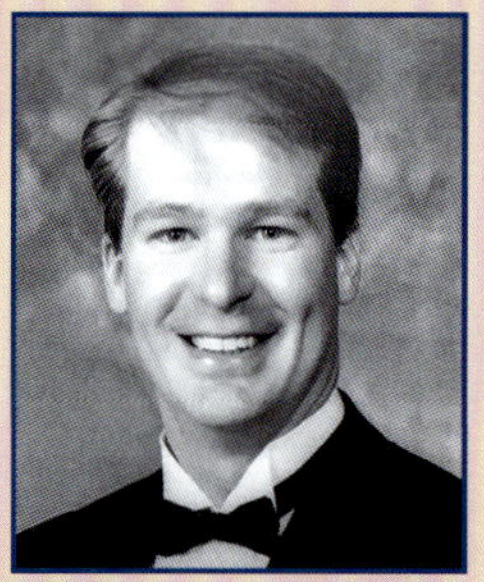

James Greelish. MD Wake Forest University; cardiothoracic fellowship, Brigham and Women's Hospital (1999–2000); associate professor, Vanderbilt University (2000–2010); director of cardiac surgery, Caremont Regional Medical Center, Gastonia, North Carolina; medical director cardiac physician administrator, Caremont Regional Medical Center, Gastonia, North Carolina (2010–present).

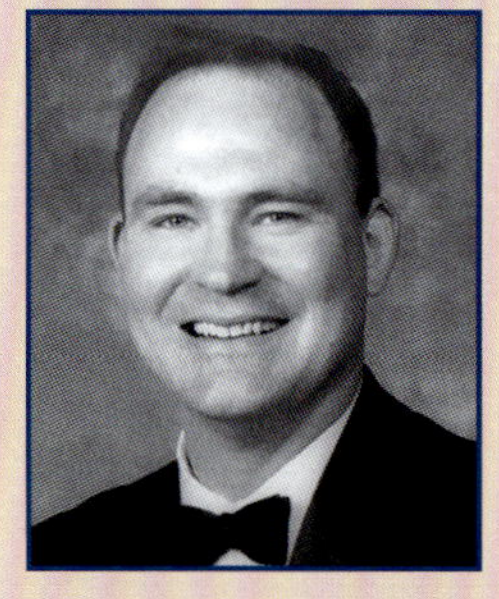

John Kucharczuk. BCE Villanova University; MD University of Pennsylvania; fellowship in thoracic surgery, HUP; associate professor and chief of Division of Thoracic Surgery, University of Pennsylvania.

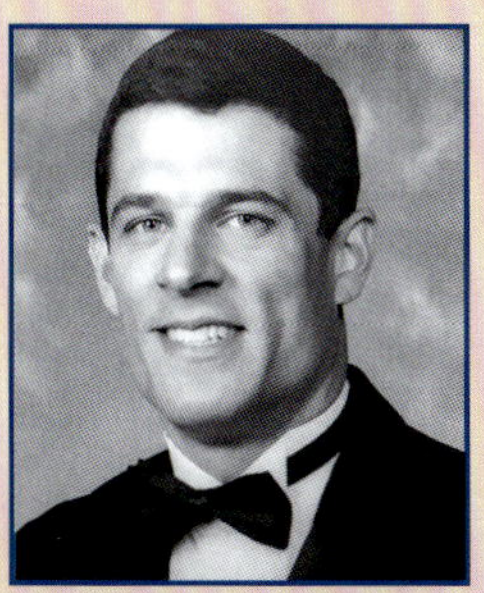

Steven McClane. BA Princeton University; MD Cornell University; colorectal fellow, Cleveland Clinic; chief of Division of Colorectal Surgery, MD Anderson Cancer Center at Cooper University, New Jersey.

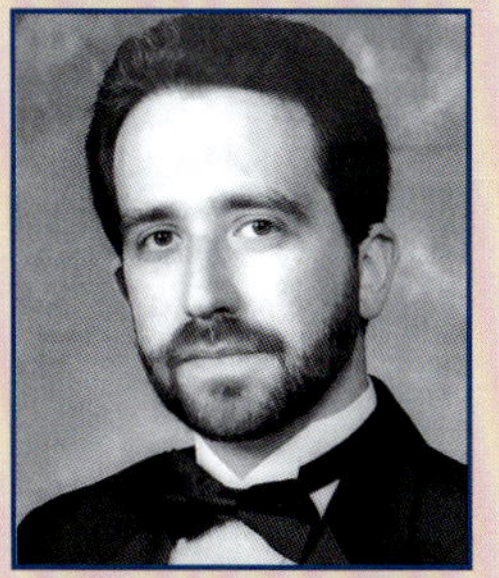

David Neschis. MD Rochester University; vascular fellowship, HUP; clinical associate professor, University of Maryland.

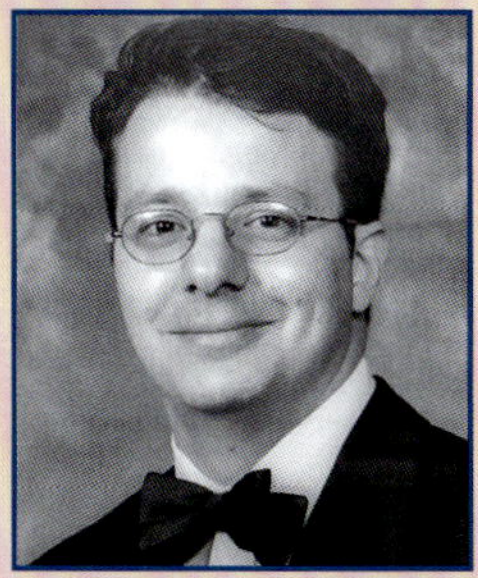

Nabil Rizk. MD Yale University; cardiothoracic fellowship, Brigham and Women's Hospital (2000); surgical oncology fellowship, Memorial SKCC (2001); cardiothoracic fellowship, Cornell University (2002–2004); chairman of thoracic surgery, Hackensack University Medical Center (2015–present); EMPH from Columbia University in Hospital Management; MS in Research Design, Columbia University; associate professor, Cornell University.

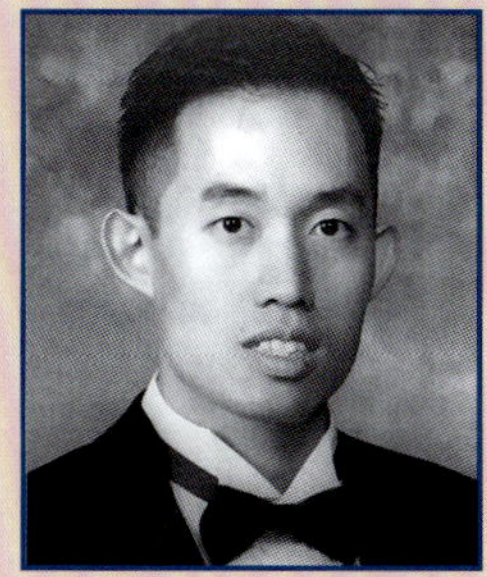

Joe Woo. BS MIT; MD University of Pennsylvania; fellowship in CT surgery, HUP; NIH-supported research in molecular studies of cardiac ischemia; faculty at University of Pennsylvania—assistant professor to professor (2002–2013); Norman Shumway Professor and Chairman of Stanford Department of Cardiothoracic Surgery (2013–present); University of Pennsylvania Department of Surgery Distinguished Graduate Award (2021).

1999–2000

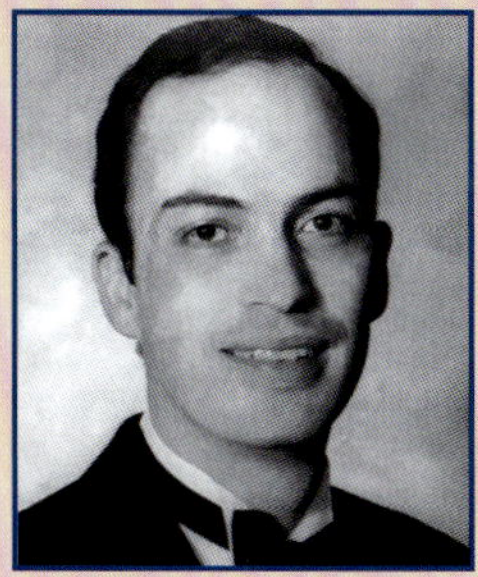

Luis Campos. MD LaSalle University, Mexico City; transplant fellowship, HUP (2000–2003); assistant professor, University of Maryland (2003–2008); associate professor and director of kidney transplantation, Methodist Hospital, University of Tennessee (2008–2020); liver transplantation and hepatobiliary director, Cleveland Clinic, Abu Dhabi.

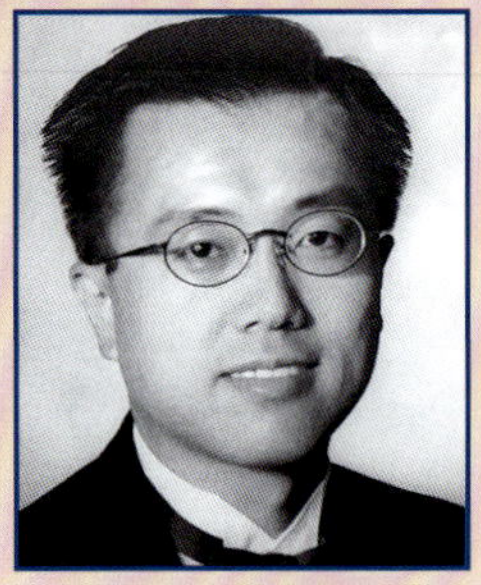

Michael Chang. MD University of Michigan; cardiothoracic fellow, Brigham and Women's Hospital; faculty at Brigham and Women's Hospital (2002–2006); thoracic surgeon, Kaiser-Permanente, Los Angeles.

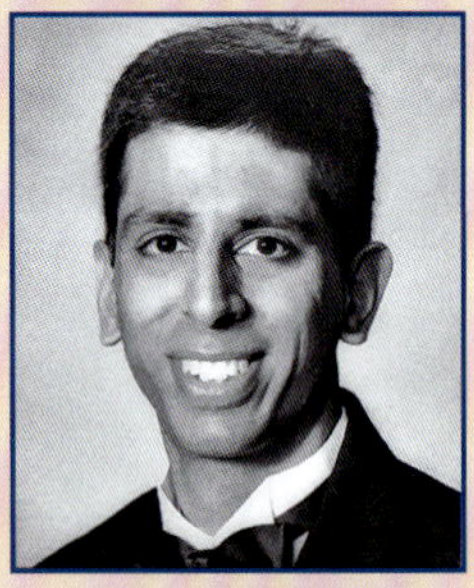

Niraj Desai. MD Washington University; transplantation fellow, HUP; assistant professor and director of kidney, pancreas and islet transplantation, Johns Hopkins University.

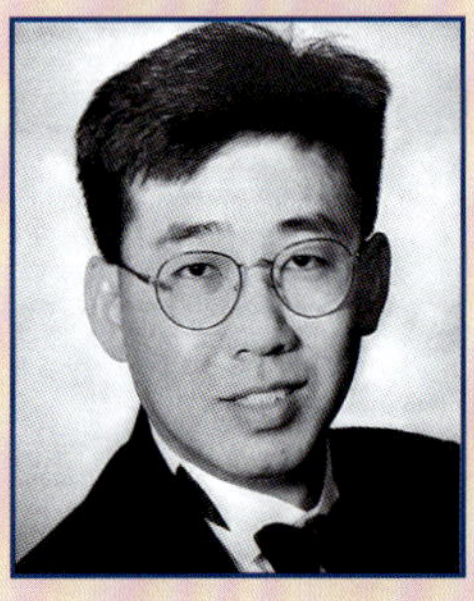

Heung Bae Kim. Yale University; MD Albert Einstein; fellowship in pediatric surgery, Boston Children's Hospital; fellowship in liver transplantation, Lehey Clinic; research with David Sachs on transplantation tolerance and with Alan Flake on in-utero tolerance; research on bowel lengthening (STEP) and expansion of arteries to avoid use of prostheses; started only intestinal transplant program in New England; professor of surgery, Harvard University; Weitzman Family Chair in Surgical Innovation, Boston Children's Hospital; vice chair of surgery for clinical operations, Boston Children's Hospital; director of Pediatric Transplant Center and co-director Mid-Aortic and Renal-Vascular Hypertension Center, Boston Children's Hospital. University of Pennsylvania Department of Surgery Distinguished Graduate Award (2023).

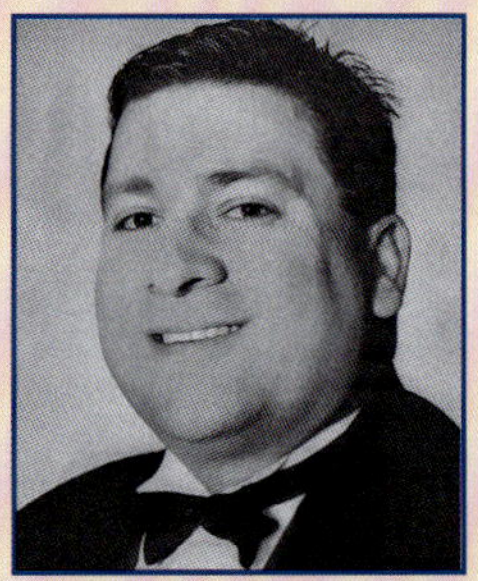

Scott Kelly. MD Columbia University; fellowship in CT oncology research, HUP; fellowship in surgical oncology, Lee Mofitt Cancer Center, Tampa; associate professor of surgery, University of South Florida, Lakeland Regional Health Medical Center.

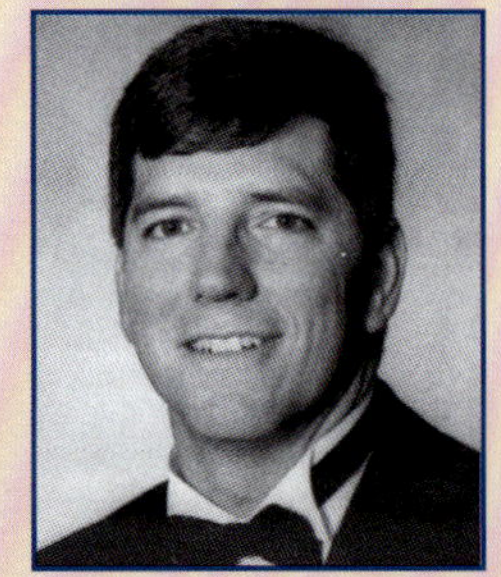

Harold N. Lovvorn III (Bo). Groton School; BA Duke University; MD University of Tennessee, Memphis; research fellowship, CHOP; pediatric surgery fellowship, LeBonheurand St. Jude Children's Research Hospital of the University of Tennessee, Memphis; assistant professor to professor of pediatric surgery, Vanderbilt University (2002–2020); vice chair of research and education, Vanderbilt University; chief of trauma and residency program director, Vanderbilt; chief of Division of Pediatric Surgery, Vanderbilt.

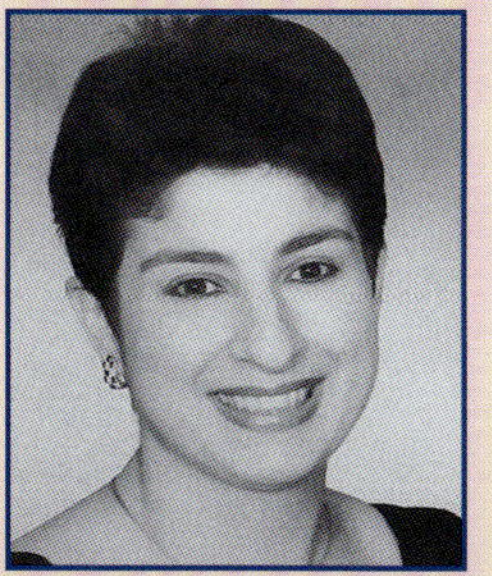

Isabelle Bedrosian. MD Northwestern University; surgical oncology fellowship, MD Anderson Cancer Center; professor Department of Breast Surgery Oncology, Division of Surgery, University of Texas MD Anderson Cancer Center; active NIH research-supported molecular biology study of breast cancer; University of Pennsylvania Department of Surgery Distinguished Graduate Award (2022).

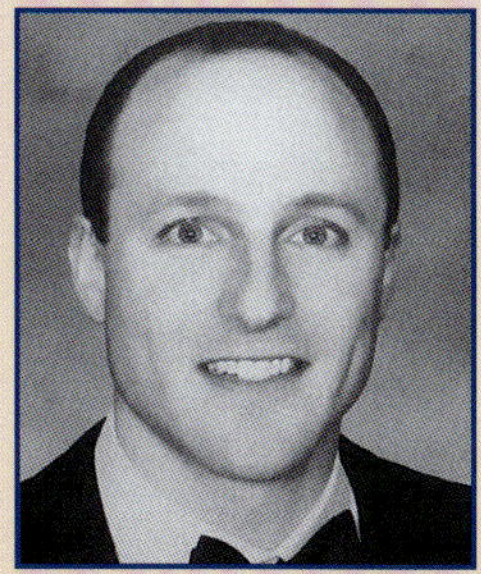

Seth Force. BA Davidson College; MD Tulane University; cardiothoracic fellow, Washington University and Barnes Hospital with Alec Patterson and Joel Cooper; Kamal Mansour Professor of Thoracic Surgery, Emory University; chief of general thoracic surgery, Emory University; as director of lung transplantation, tripled volume of lung transplants when appointed at Emory in 2003.

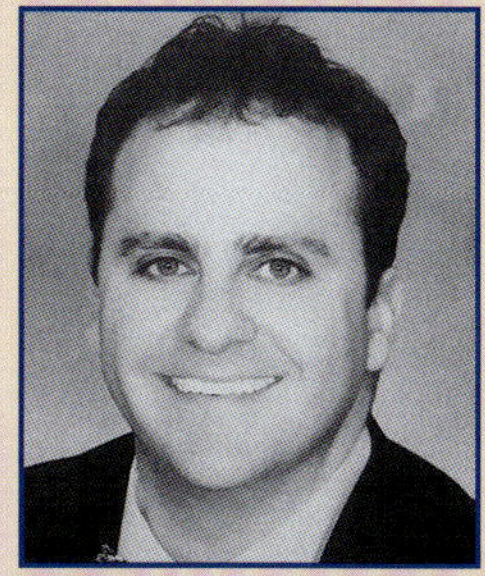

Michael Lanuti. MD University of Pennsylvania, cardiothoracic fellowship, MGH; associate professor of surgery, Harvard Medical School; director of thoracic oncology, MGH.

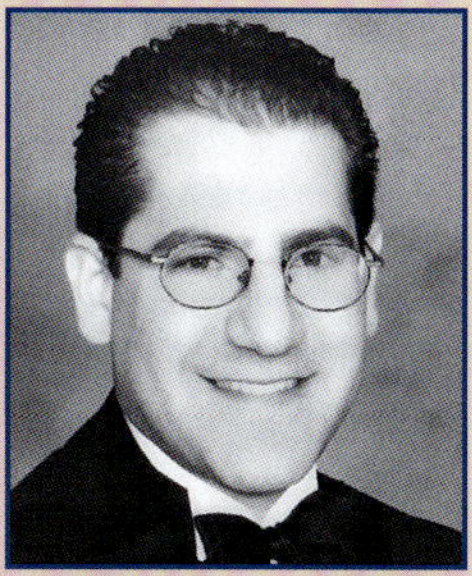

Ross Milner. MD University of Pennsylvania; vascular fellowship, HUP; Marco Polo Fellow of Society for Vascular Surgery; research fellowship, Utrecht, Netherlands; Emory University director of vascular fellowship; chief of vascular surgery, Loyola University, Chicago; professor of vascular surgery, University of Chicago and director of Center for Aortic Diseases (2009–present); chief of Division of Vascular and Endovascular Surgery, University of Chicago.

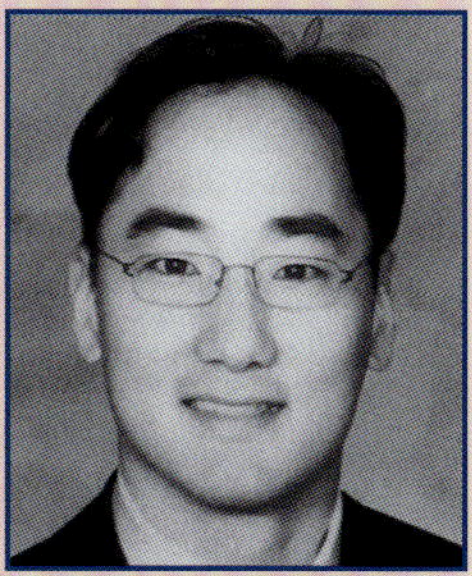

Howard Song. Yale University; MD Stanford University; cardiothoracic fellow, Emory University; PhD in immunology, University of Pennsylvania; professor of surgery and chief of cardiothoracic division and director of heart failure and transplantation, University of Oregon.

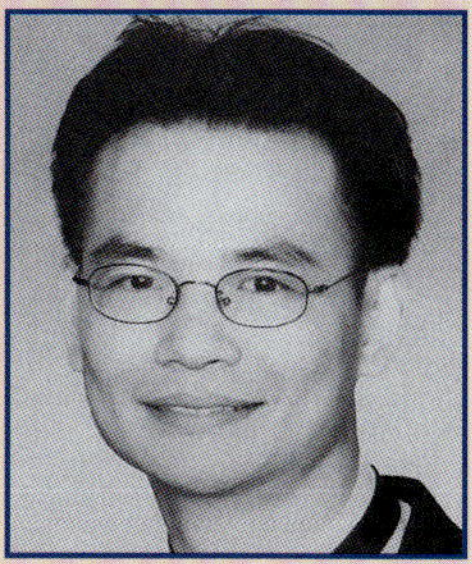

Henry Zhu. Harvard University; MD Harvard University; cardiothoracic fellow, HUP; practices at Sacramento Medical Center Kaiser-Permanente.

CHAPTER 29

A New Approach, A New Division

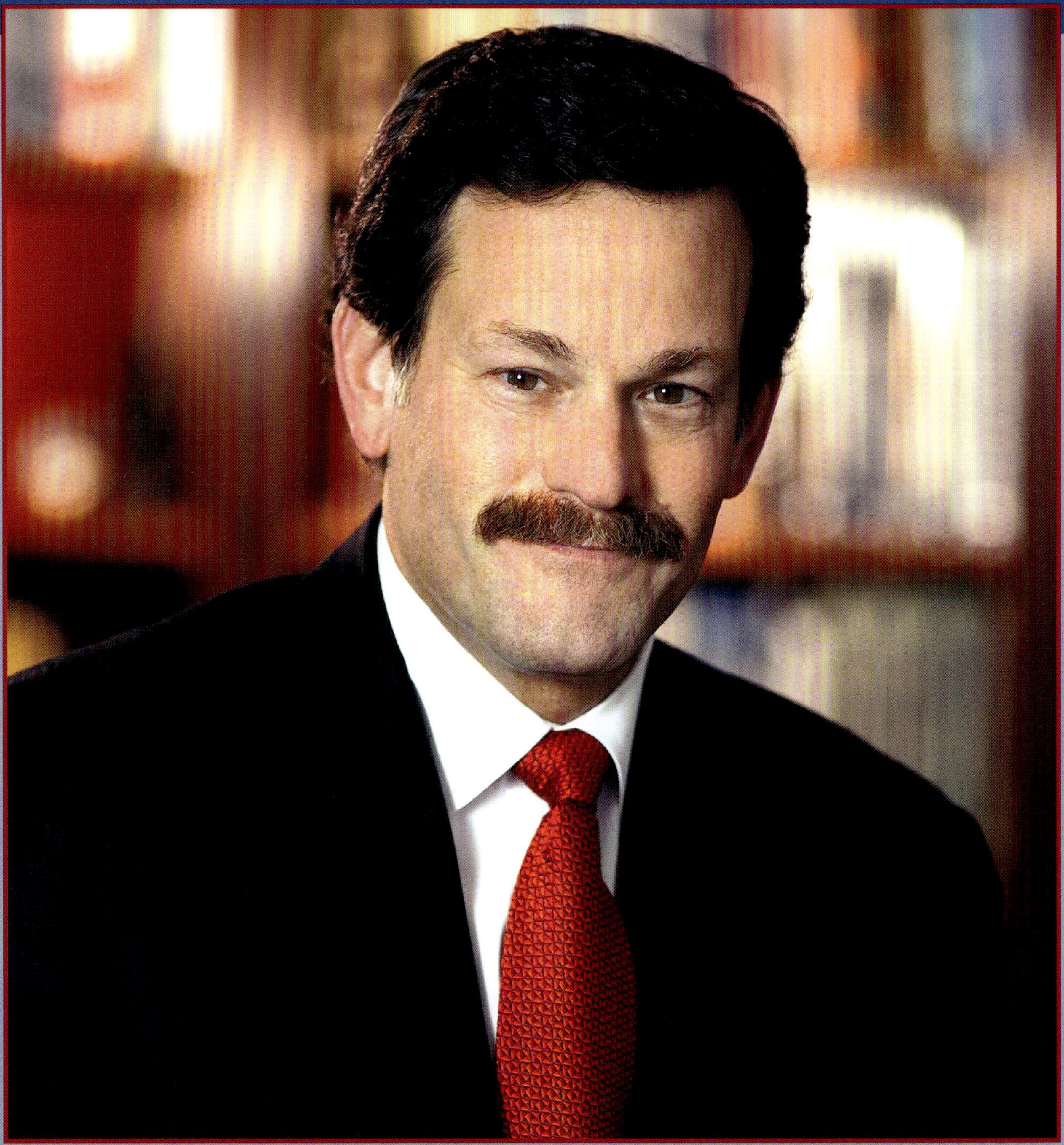

Larry R. Kaiser (1952–)

JRB Professor and Chairman of Surgery (2001–2008)

In 1991, it seemed important for the department to begin a program in lung transplantation which, though not yet a particularly common procedure, already existed at another Philadelphia institution (Temple). To lead it, Hank Edmunds recommended Larry Kaiser, who had experience with lung transplantation at the pioneering lung transplant institutions: the University of Toronto[1] and Washington University in St. Louis.[2]

Kaiser earned a BS in chemistry and his MD AOA from Tulane University. He completed a residency in general surgery and a fellowship in surgical oncology at the University of California, Los Angeles. He had additional training in cardiovascular and thoracic surgery at the University of Toronto and Memorial Sloan Kettering. He was then for three years a faculty member at Washington University in St. Louis before coming to Penn in 1991.

1973
BS Tulane Phi Beta Kappa

1977
MD Tulane AOA

1977–1983
Intern and general surgery resident, UCLA

1979–1981
Oncology research fellow, UCLA

1983–1985
Cardiac and thoracic surgery resident, University of Toronto

1985–1988
Memorial Sloan Kettering and Cornell Faculty

1988–1990
Faculty Washington University

Soon after he was recruited to Penn, Kaiser started a successful lung transplant program. But before long, he became more involved with general thoracic surgery than transplantation. The leadership in HUP's lung transplantation was delegated to others, and Larry concentrated very successfully on general thoracic surgery which soon morphed into a division. His broad experience and expertise in this field promptly allowed him to dominate it in the Philadelphia region and to achieve national recognition. To enlarge his division, several young surgeons were appointed to the faculty. These included Joe Schrager, a

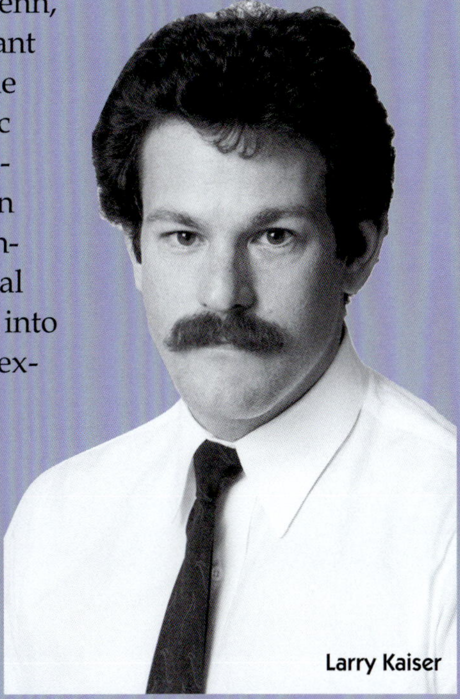

Larry Kaiser

1991–2001
Kaiser moves to Penn and founds lung transplant program, heads the Division of General Thoracic Surgery

1997
Kaiser appointed Eldridge Eliason Professor of Surgery

HUP resident and MGH fellow, who after several faculty years at Penn, moved to Stanford, where he became and remains chief of thoracic surgery. Another was Joe Friedberg, an MGH resident, who after thoracic fellowship at Brigham and Women's Hospital and several faculty years at Penn has led thoracic surgery programs at the University of Maryland and now at Temple. Jo Buyske, an MGH-trained surgeon, was also recruited. She rapidly became an important member of the faculty and chief of surgery at Presbyterian Hospital. She is now executive director of the American Board of Surgery.

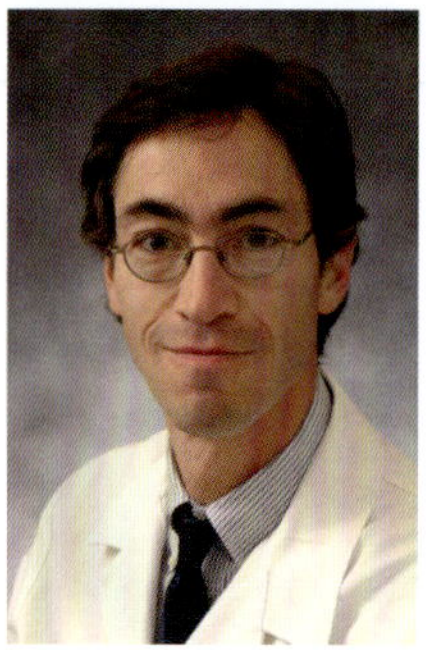

Joe Shrager

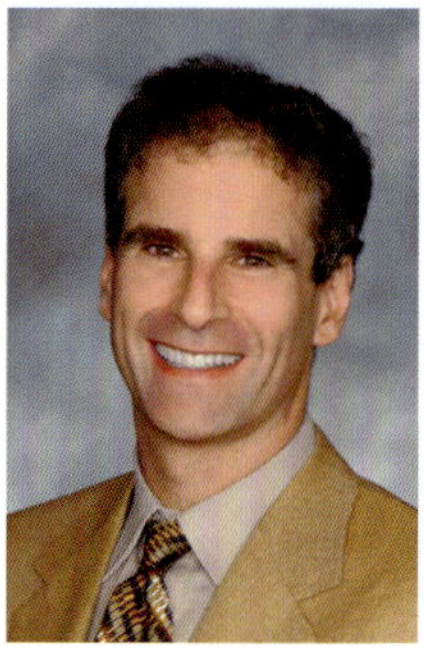

Joe Friedberg

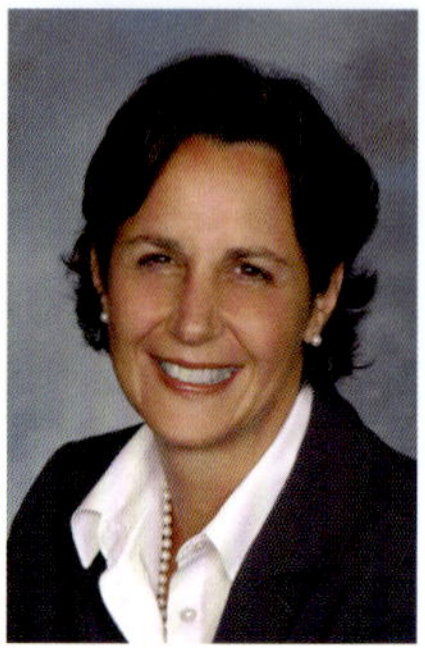

Jo Buyske

Larry's practice grew rapidly, and he became a force in the department. His enthusiasm and clinical expertise allowed him to attract and mentor as fellows a series of HUP residents, including Roy Smythe, Seth Force, Dan Kreisel, John Kucharczuk, and Sunil Singhal. They proved to be leaders nationally, and the last two eventually became his successors as chief of HUP's thoracic division.

Kaiser was primarily a clinical surgeon and an exceptionally good one. He won the department's admiration when he skillfully managed Brooke Roberts's serious illness, an abscess in his chest complicating an upper respiratory infection. Because of his large practice, HUP administrators and Dean Kelley were concerned that Larry might accept one of the multiple recruitment offers coming to him from other institutions, especially the one from HUP's crosstown competition, Jefferson. I was encouraged to find a way to keep him at Penn. Appointing him to an endowed chair probably helped, and he stayed.

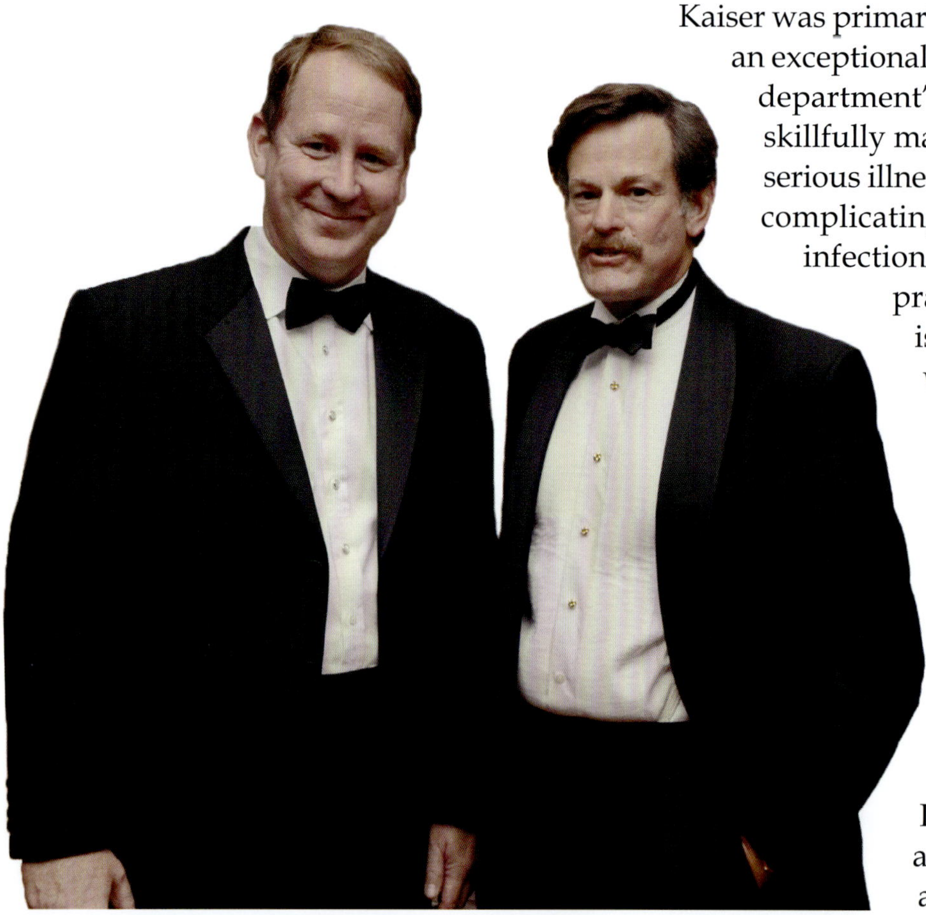

Roy Smythe and Larry Kaiser

Larry was hardly one-dimensional. His background in oncology and molecular biology, along with his abundant ambition and energy, also allowed him to become effective in research. He developed a collaborative relationship with Steve Albelda of the Department of Medicine. They conducted pioneering gene therapy research on animal models of mesothelioma. Larry and Steve Albelda, with their exceptionally talented and hard-working surgical fellow, Roy Smythe, were the first to evaluate adenoviral vectors in transfer of genes for the treatment of cancer.[3] They presented an important paper on this novel approach at the American Surgical Association meeting.[4] This animal experiment became the basis for a clinical trial at HUP, which was one of the world's first human gene therapy trials for cancer and the world's first for mesothelioma.[5] In a series of high-impact publications, they further explored thymidine kinase, followed by ganciclovir as suicide gene therapy for cancer.[6]

When my term as chairman finished in 2001, Larry competed effectively for the chair against a panel of worthy external candidates and became John Rhea Barton Professor and Chairman. Some faculty members were critical of Larry's aggressive ambition, but I admired his direct approach. I thought he was off to a good start as chairman. He started a new Division of Colon and Rectal Surgery and recruited Bob Fry as its chief. He revised and improved the teaching schedule and the morbidity and mortality conference. With financial support from his father-in-law, he enlarged the department's conference room and modernized its audio-visual system. He collaborated well with Gordon Buzby, the residency program director, and after Gordon's illness and premature death, Larry got along famously with his friend, Jon Morris,

1994–1998
Kaiser's pioneering gene therapy research for cancer. A series of publications examined the promise of suicide gene therapy strategy

2001
Kaiser appointed John Rhea Barton Professor and Chairman of Surgery

2002
Kaiser starts new Division of Colon and Rectal Surgery, recruits Bob Fry as its chief

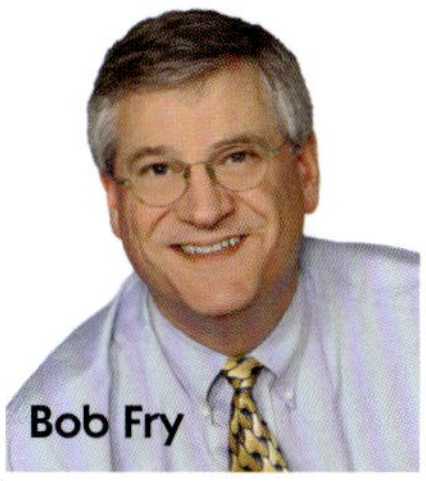
Bob Fry

2004
Kaiser wins I. S. Ravdin Master Clinician Award of Excellence, University of Pennsylvania

2005
Kaiser is elected to National Academy of Medicine.

Kaiser recruits Joel Cooper as chief of General Thoracic Division.

Kaiser marries Lindy Snider

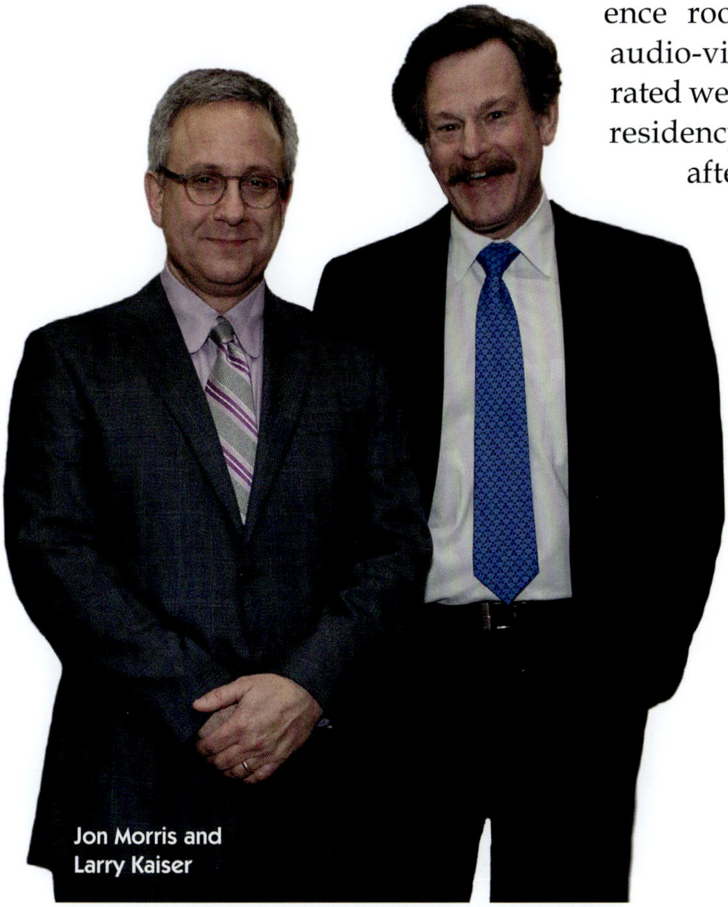
Jon Morris and Larry Kaiser

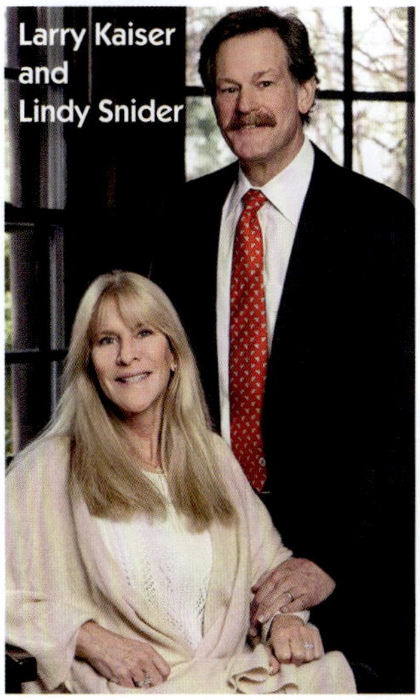
Larry Kaiser and Lindy Snider

2007
Kaiser finishes first six-year term as chairman and is reappointed

2008
President of Halsted Society

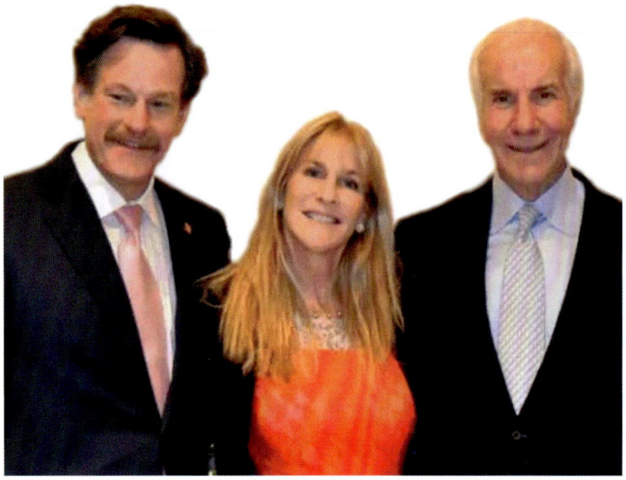

Larry Kaiser with wife Lindy Snider and her father Ed Snider, owner of the Philadelphia 76ers and Flyers.

who became director of the residency program. Together they improved student and residency education.

While Larry was obviously in favor of change, he also maintained respect for the history and traditions of the department. He further enhanced the reputation and effectiveness of the thoracic division in 2005 by recruiting from Washington University his own former mentor, Joel Cooper, the surgeon who performed the world's first successful lung transplants. It was clear that Larry aspired to advance the perception of Surgery as the leading department at Penn and also nationally. He became widely known for several procedures and surgical advances that had been started by Cooper, including: (1) improving pulmonary function by reducing the volume of emphysematous lungs[7]; and (2) minimally invasive thoracoscopic procedures.[8]

By the time Kaiser finished his first six-year term as chairman, he was not only a major figure in his field of thoracic surgery but broadly respected in American academic surgery. He was elected to memberships in all of the prestigious societies of thoracic and general surgery, including the Society of Clinical Surgery, the American Surgical Association, the National Academy of Medicine, and the Halsted Society of which he was elected president. He authored all or part of seventeen books and more than 300 peer-reviewed publications, many in basic oncology and molecular biology.

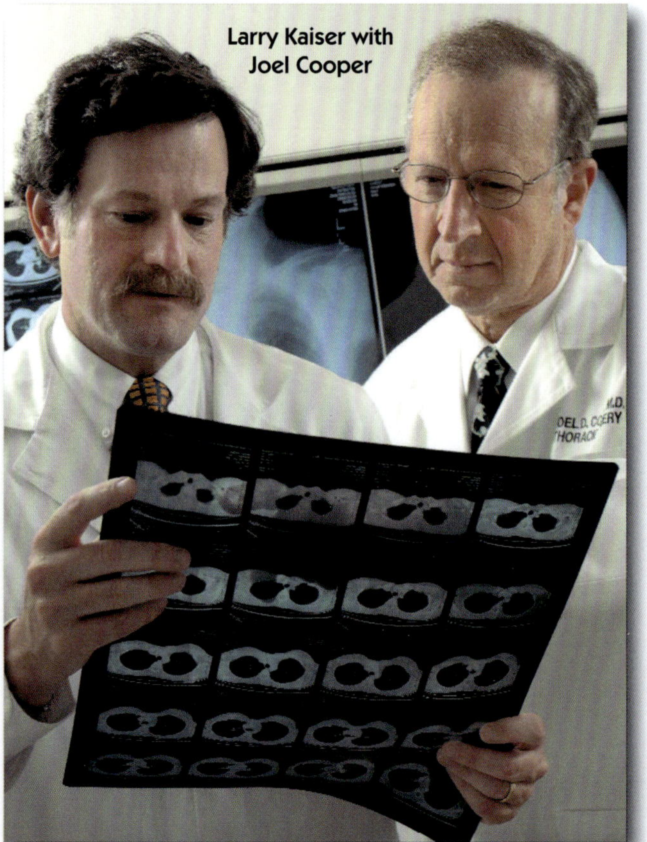

Larry Kaiser with Joel Cooper

Larry was very supportive of me as the former chairman. I thought he was doing very well as the department's leader. Shortly after Larry was appointed to a second six-year term as chair, during an awkward departmental meeting with the dean, it seemed likely that he and Larry were not in tune. The reasons were obscure and never explained, but in 2008 they may have influenced Larry's acceptance of an offer to become president of the University of Texas Health Science Center at Houston, the largest of six health-related campuses of the University of Texas. After three years there, he made another change, returning to Philadelphia to become president and CEO of the $2.2 billion Temple University Health System and dean of Temple University's Lewis Katz School of Medicine. He deserves praise for his accomplishments at Temple over the next eight years, including the acquisition of Fox Chase, an NCI-designated Comprehensive Cancer Center. Despite limited resources, he successfully developed a number of programs, including lung transplantation, cardiovascular surgery, thoracic surgery, neurosurgery, and orthopedic surgery. In 2017, *Modern Healthcare* named Kaiser as one of the 50 Most Influential Leaders and Executives in the entire healthcare industry. I think Temple made a mistake in not recruiting him as the university's president.

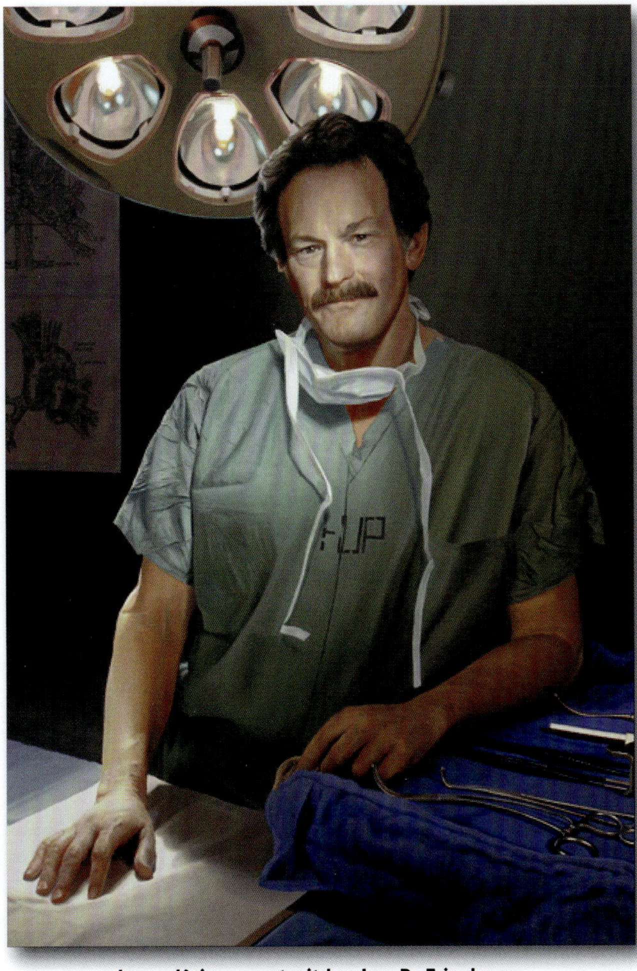

Larry Kaiser portrait by Jon R. Friedman

In 2019, after eight years as chief executive of Temple University Health System, Larry stepped down. He is now a managing director with Alvarez & Marsal's Health Care Industry Group in New York.

2008
Kasier leaves Penn, becomes president of University of Texas Health System at Houston

2011
Kaiser returns to Philadelphia as president, CEO, and dean at Temple University

2019
Kaiser leaves Temple for other position in health care

Notes

[1] Kaiser LR, Cooper JD, Trulock EP, Pasque MK, Triantafillou A, Haydock D. The evolution of single lung transplantation for emphysema. *Journal of Thoracic & Cardiovascular Surgery* 102(3): 333–341 (Sept. 1991). Kaiser LR, Pasque MK, Trulock EP, Dresler CM, Low DE, Cooper JD. Bilateral sequential lung transplantation: The procedure of choice for double-lung replacement. *Annals of Thoracic Surgery* 52(3): 438–446 (Sept. 1991).

[2] Trulock EP, Cooper JD, Kaiser LR, Pasque MK, Ettinger NA, Dresler CM. The Washington University-Barnes Hospital experience with lung transplantation. Washington University Lung Transplantation Group, *Journal of the American Medical Association* 266(14): 1943–1946 (Oct. 9, 1991).

[3] Smythe WR, Hwang HC, Amin KM, Eck SL, Davidson BL, Wilson JM, Kaiser LR, and Albelda SM. Use of recombinant adenovirus to transfer the herpes simplex virus thymidine kinase (HSVtk) gene to thoracic neoplasms: an effective in vitro drug sensitization system. *Cancer research, 54*(8), 2055–2059 (1994). Smythe WR, Kaiser LR, Hwang HC, Amin KM, Pilewski JM, Eck SL, Wilson, JM, and Albelda, SM. Successful adenovirus-mediated gene transfer in an in vivo model of human malignant mesothelioma. *The Annals of thoracic surgery, 57*(6), 1395–1401 (1994). https://doi.org/10.1016/0003-4975(94)90090-6.

[4] Smythe, WR, Hwang, HC, Elshami AA, Amin KM, Eck SL, Davidson BL, Wilson JM, Kaiser, LR, and Albelda SM. Treatment of experimental human mesothelioma using adenovirus transfer of the herpes simplex thymidine kinase gene. *Annals of surgery, 222*(1), 78–86 (1995). https://doi.org/10.1097/00000658-199507000-00013.

[5] Sterman DH, Treat J, Litzky LA, Amin KM, Molnar-Kimber K, Albelda SM, Amin KM, Wilson JM, Kaiser LR. Adenovirus-mediated herpes simplex virus thymidine kinase gene delivery in patients with localized malignancy: Results of a Phase I clinical trial in malignant mesothelioma. *Human Gene Therapy* 9(7): 1083–1092 (May 1, 1998).

[6] Kucharczuk JC, Raper ST, Elshami AA, Amin KM, Sterman DH, Wheeldon EB, Wilson JM, Litzky LA, Kaiser LR, Albelda SM. Safety of intrapleurally administered recombinant adenovirus carrying herpes simplex thymidine kinase cDNA followed by ganciclovir therapy in non-human primates. *Human Gene Therapy* 7(18): 2225–2233 (Dec. 1, 1996). Lanuti M, Gao GP G, Force SD, Chang MY, Kouri C, Amin K, Hughes JV, Wilson JM, Kaiser LR, Albelda SM. Evaluation of an E1E4-deleted adenovirus expressing the herpes simplex thymidine kinase (HSVtk) suicide gene in cancer gene therapy. *Human Gene Therapy* 10(3): 463–475 (Feb. 10, 1999). Lambright ES, Force SD, Lanuti M, Wasfi DS, Amin K, Albelda SM, Kaiser LR. Efficacy of repeated adenoviral suicide gene therapy in a localized murine tumor model. *Annals of Thoracic Surgery* 70(6): 1865–1870 (Dec. 2000). Sterman Daniel H, Recio Adriana, Vachani Anil, Sun Jing, Cheung Lumei, DeLong Peter, Amin Kunjlata M, Litzky Leslie A, Wilson James M, Kaiser Larry R, Albelda Steven M. Long-term follow-up of patients with malignant pleural mesothelioma receiving high-dose adenovirus herpes simplex thymidine kinase/ganciclovir suicide gene therapy. *Clinical Cancer Research* 11(20): 7444–7453 (Oct. 15, 2005). Sterman DH, Kaiser LR, Albelda SM. Gene therapy for malignant pleural mesothelioma. *Hematol Oncol Clin North Am.* (1998 June) 12(3):553–68. doi: 10.1016/s0889-8588(05)70008-3. PMID: 9684098. Singhal S, Kaiser LR. Cancer chemotherapy using suicide genes. *Surg Oncol Clin N Am.* (1998 July) 7(3):505–36. PMID: 9624215.

[7] Bavaria JE, Pochettino A, Kotloff RM, Rosengard BR, Wahl PM, Palevsky HI, Kaiser LR. Effect of volume reduction on lung transplant timing and selection for COPD. *Journal of Thoracic & Cardiovascular Surgery* 115(1): 9–18 (Jan. 1998). Keenan RJ, Landreneau RJ, Hazelrigg SR, Bavaria JE, Kaiser LR. Comparison of clinical results for unilateral and bilateral thoracoscopic lung volume reduction. *Annals of Thoracic Surgery* 69(6): 1670–1674 (June 2000).

[8] Smythe WR, Kaiser LR. History of thoracoscopic surgery. *Thoracoscopic Surgery*. Kaiser LR, Daniel TM (eds.). Boston: Little Brown & Co. pp. 1–16 (1993).

CHAPTER 30

Science and Surgical Leadership

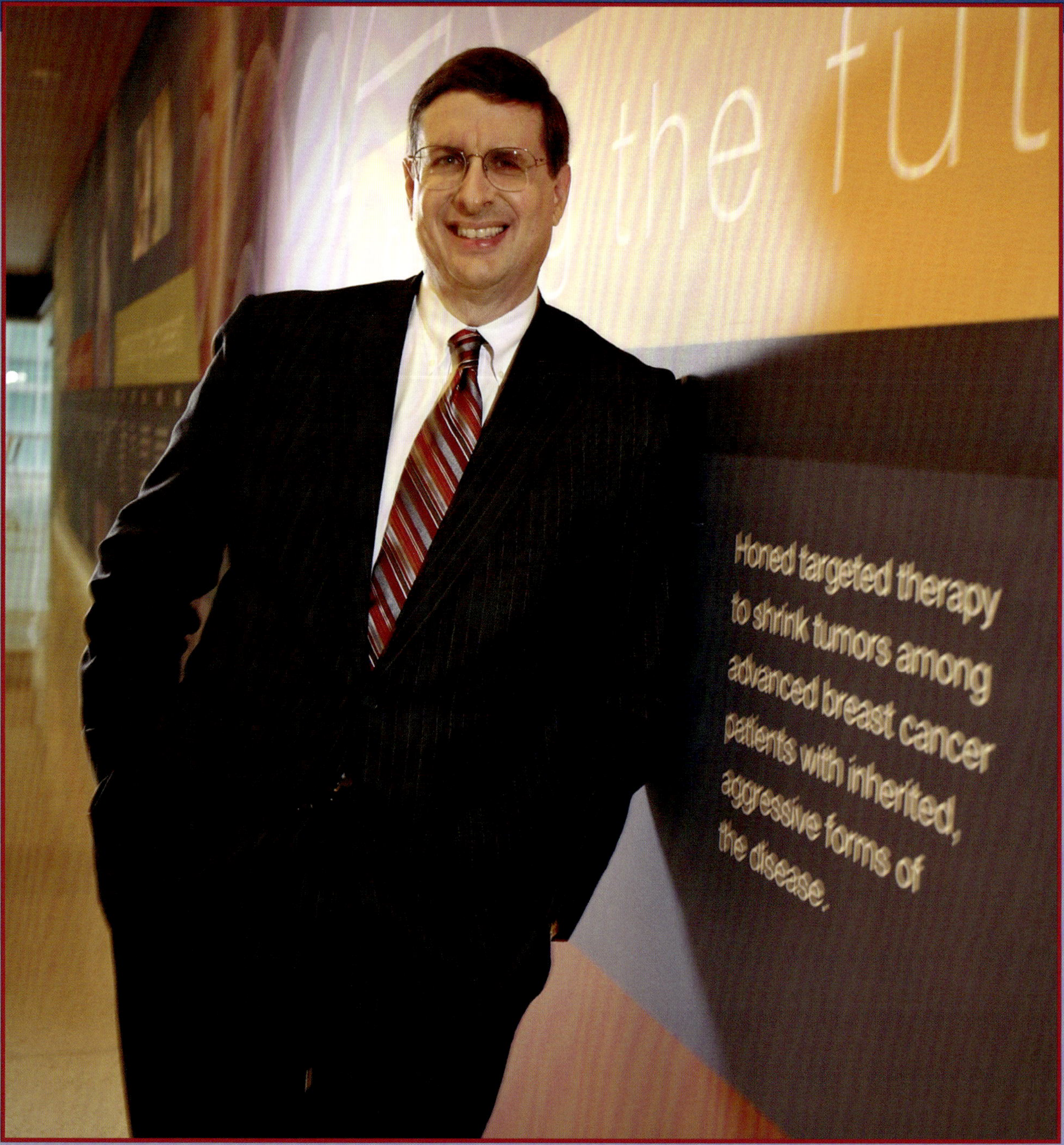

Jeffrey A. Drebin (1957–)

JRB Professor and Chairman of Surgery (2009–2017)

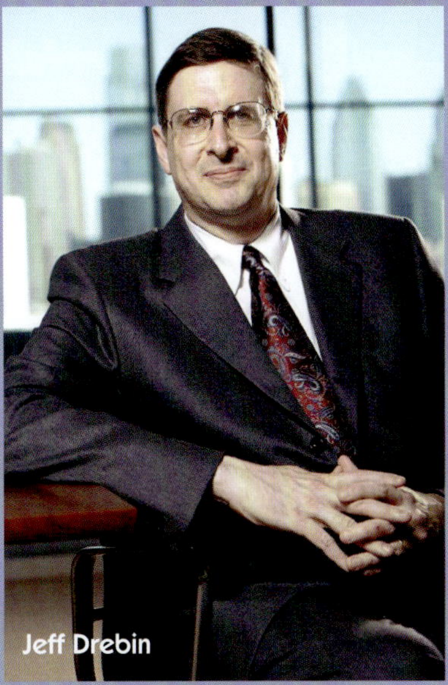

Jeff Drebin

Jeff Drebin obtained his MD and PhD at Harvard and his surgical training at Johns Hopkins. He was a member of the faculty at Washington University, rising to the rank of professor in 2002. In 2004, he was recruited to Penn as Chief of the Division of GI Surgery and vice chairman for research. In 2009, he was appointed John Rhea Barton Professor and Chairman of the Department of Surgery. After thirteen years of great accomplishments at Penn, in 2017 he was offered and accepted the position as chairman of surgery at Memorial Sloan Kettering Cancer Center.

On February 6, 2017, there was a reception in honor of Jeff Drebin as he departed Penn for Memorial. Speaking were CEO Ralph Muller, Dean Larry Jameson, and Dr. Drebin's scientific mentor, Mark Greene. I had the honor of speaking for the Department of Surgery. Below are some of my remarks.

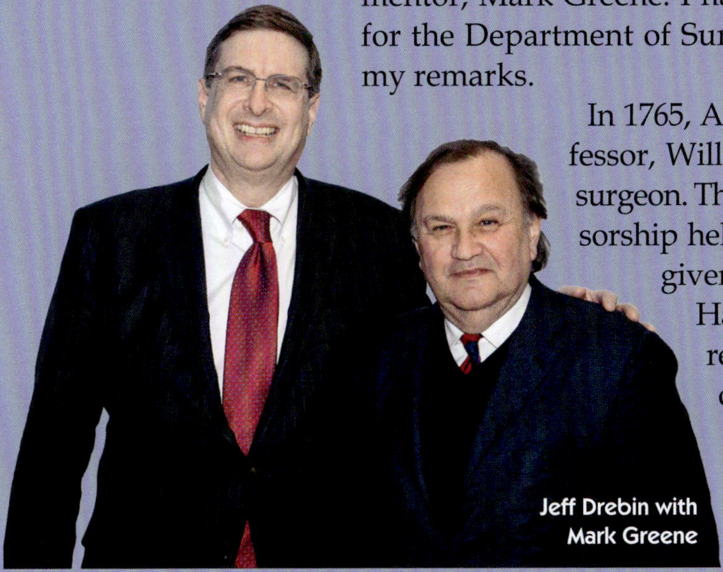

Jeff Drebin with Mark Greene

In 1765, America's first surgery professor, William Shippen, was a Penn surgeon. The John Rhea Barton professorship held by Jeff Drebin was first given to our school's icon, D. Hayes Agnew. Therefore, in reviewing the performance of a surgical chairman, we need to use historical perspective. So how does Jeff Drebin measure up as

1979
BA Oberlin,
Phi Beta Kappa

1987
MD/PhD Harvard.
Magna cum laude.
Conducts gene therapy research

1987–1994
Intern and resident at Johns Hopkins

1994–1995
Fellow in surgical oncology at Johns Hopkins

1995–2004
Assistant professor to professor of surgery, Washington University, St. Louis

1999
Member of NIH Study Section

2001
Member of Kettering Prize Selection Committee

2005–2009
Measey Professor and chief of Division Gastrointestinal Surgery, University of Pennsylvania

2009
Louis Duhring Outstanding Clinical Specialist Award of Penn School of Medicine

2009–2017
John Rhea Barton Professor and Chairman of Surgery, University of Pennsylvania

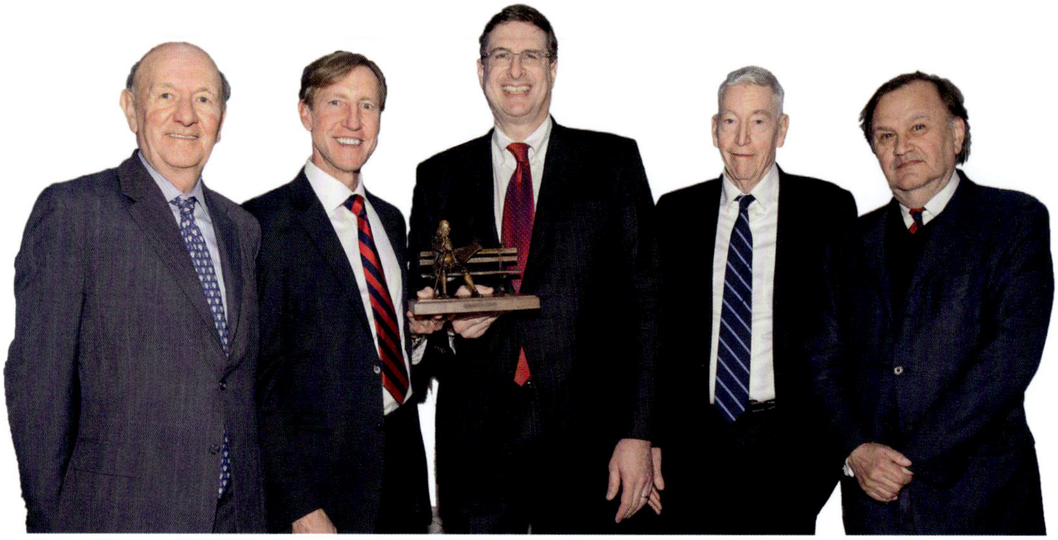

Reception Speakers: Ralph Muller, Larry Jameson, Jeff Drebin, Clyde Barker, and Mark Greene

compared to his professional forebears? My experience at Penn goes back far enough that I can compare him with six former department chairmen including I. S. Ravdin and Jonathan Rhoads. So what are the benchmarks? How should we measure the performance of a surgical chairman?

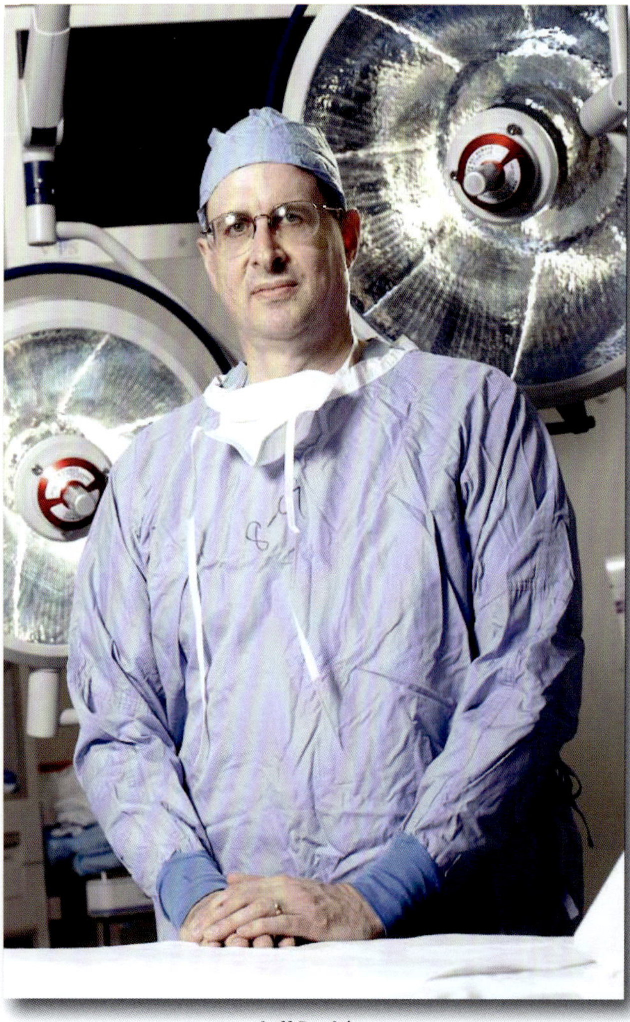

Jeff Drebin

For starters, how good is he as a surgeon? Perhaps only in surgery is the reputation of someone who has reached the administrative level of department chairman still rated and sometimes largely remembered for the level of their clinical skill in the performance of their specialty. In this case, some would disparage the specialty as a craft. Others might call it an art. Anyway, just how good was Jeff in the operating room? I'm not about to dredge up stories of how Ravdin and Rhoads were ranked as technical surgeons and are still remembered in this way by their surviving trainees. But I can tell you that on this scale, Jeff Drebin measures up very well. He is a master surgeon. At Penn, he developed a reputation for special expertise in pancreatic and other upper abdominal cancer operations.

A second criterion is how does he rate as a researcher and as a physician scientist? Sadly, and perhaps especially true of surgeons, this may be a dying breed. In fact, some say it is already extinct. Too bad! Yet for the rare surgical chairs with real scientific credentials, it is this more than anything else that in faculty meetings or over cocktails makes them comfortable as a true peer of their fellow chairs of more research-intensive departments. Jeff Drebin is one who can stand that test. He has the credentials of a surgeon scientist. In fact, he has them in spades. He even has a PhD, a distinction held by only one other Penn surgical chairman, and this was 146 years ago.

Helping to form his PhD thesis were the findings of ten high-impact papers by Drebin and his mentor, Mark Greene, that originated targeted gene therapy for cancer.[1] An unfortunate patent dispute between two drug companies obscures what would otherwise be accepted as their exclusive place in this story and the development of the widely used anticancer drug, Herceptin.

Further endorsement of Jeff as a scientist was provided by his election in 2013 to the Institute of Medicine of the National Academy of Sciences (subsequently renamed National Academy of Medicine). This is one of the nation's highest honors in medicine and one that very few surgeons achieve. Election to this academy is based mainly on research accomplishments. Excerpted here is part of the announcement of this honor by the IOM.

> Dr. Drebin's research has contributed significantly to the understanding of the genetic origins of cancer. His classic work with Mark Greene on monoclonal antibodies directed against the HER2/neu protein provided the scientific foundation for the evolution of targeted therapeutics for cancer and led to the development of the first generation of targeted monoclonal antibody drugs for the treatment of breast cancer [including Herceptin]. His research has been supported by the National Institutes of Health, the Department of Defense, and the Burroughs-Welcome Fund. He is currently the coprincipal investigator on a $22 million dollar clinical and translational "dream team" award from the Stand Up to Cancer Foundation for innovative studies in pancreas cancer. His

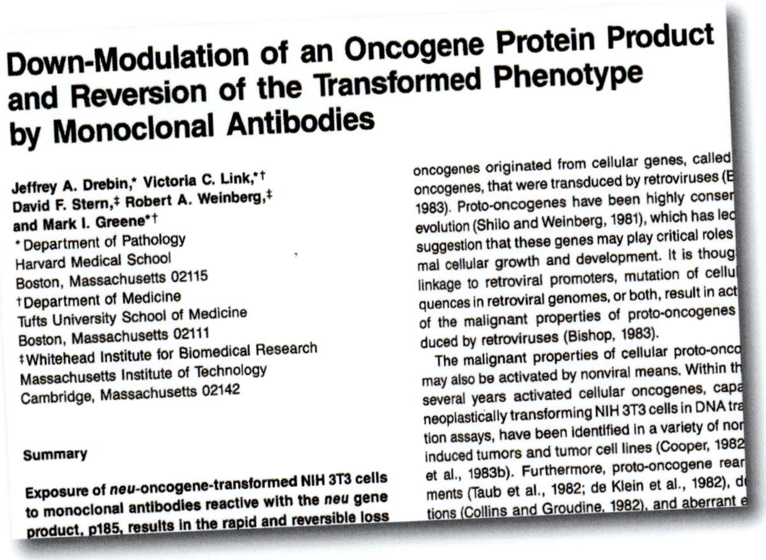

Down-Modulation of an Oncogene Protein Product and Reversion of the Transformed Phenotype by Monoclonal Antibodies

Jeffrey A. Drebin,* Victoria C. Link,*† David F. Stern,‡ Robert A. Weinberg,‡ and Mark I. Greene*†
*Department of Pathology
Harvard Medical School
Boston, Massachusetts 02115
†Department of Medicine
Tufts University School of Medicine
Boston, Massachusetts 02111
‡Whitehead Institute for Biomedical Research
Massachusetts Institute of Technology
Cambridge, Massachusetts 02142

Summary

Exposure of *neu*-oncogene-transformed NIH 3T3 cells to monoclonal antibodies reactive with the *neu* gene product, p185, results in the rapid and reversible loss

oncogenes originated from cellular genes, called oncogenes, that were transduced by retroviruses (B 1983). Proto-oncogenes have been highly conser evolution (Shilo and Weinberg, 1981), which has led suggestion that these genes may play critical roles mal cellular growth and development. It is thoug linkage to retroviral promoters, mutation of cellu quences in retroviral genomes, or both, result in act of the malignant properties of proto-oncogenes duced by retroviruses (Bishop, 1983).

The malignant properties of cellular proto-onco may also be activated by nonviral means. Within th several years activated cellular oncogenes, capa neoplastically transforming NIH 3T3 cells in DNA tra tion assays, have been identified in a variety of nor induced tumors and tumor cell lines (Cooper, 1982 et al., 1983b). Furthermore, proto-oncogene rear ments (Taub et al., 1982; de Klein et al., 1982), d tions (Collins and Groudine, 1982), and aberrant e

2010–2012
President, Society of Clinical Surgery

2013
Drebin elected to Institute of Medicine (now Academy of Medicine)

Gordon Buzby Leadership Award

2014
President, Philadelphia Academy of Surgery

2015
President of Society of Surgical Oncology

2016
American Association of Cancer Research Award

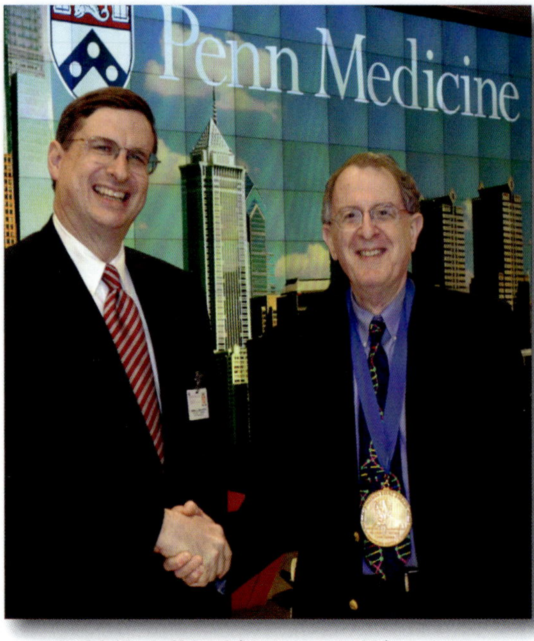

In 2015, Jeff Drebin presented his mentor Jeffrey I. Gordon, MD, with the 15th Annual Jonathan E. Rhoads Prize.

many clinical interests include pancreatic cancer, acute and chronic pancreatitis, and the use of new technologies to manage liver tumors, disorders of the bile ducts, and gallbladder disease. Dr. Drebin has published more than 100 peer-reviewed research papers, book chapters, and reviews and is co-inventor on two patents related to the treatment of cancer with monoclonal antibodies. He has served on the Board of Scientific Advisors of the National Cancer Institute.

A third factor is how the surgical chairman ranks on the national scene. The reputation of a surgical department, or at least its image, rests to a considerable degree on the chairman's recognition nationally and internationally. Again, Jeff has done us proud. He has been a director of the American Board of Surgery and president of the Philadelphia

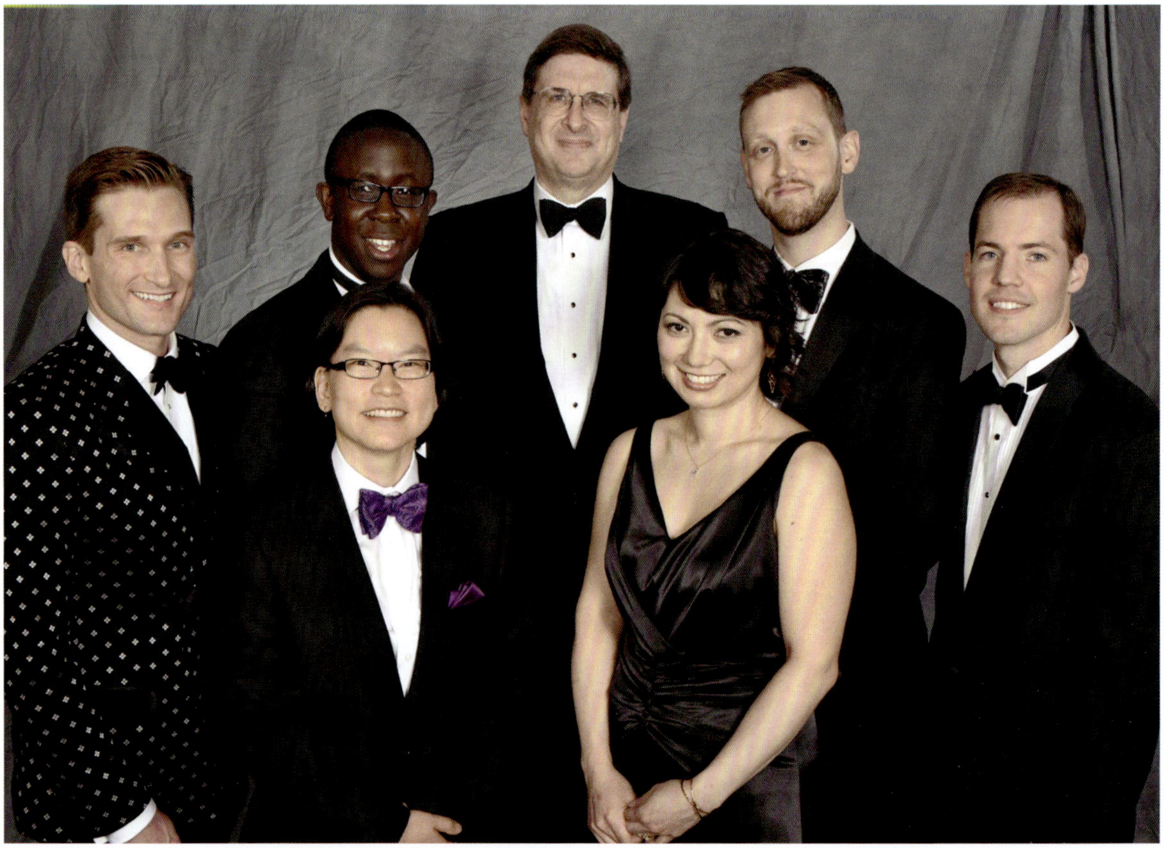

Dr. Drebin with the 2016 Chief Residents: (l to r) JW MacArthur, Kay Lee, Gbenga Okusanya, Heather Wachtel, Robert Caskey, and Ned Bartlett.

Academy of Surgery, the Society of Clinical Surgery, and the Society of Surgical Oncology. He is also an officer (recorder) of surgery's most prestigious senior society, the American Surgical Association.

Perhaps the criterion with most lasting importance, the only one by which the surgical chair can hope to impact the future, is as a teacher, educator, mentor, and role model. Unlike the other criteria, this one can actually be measured. Its metrics are the accomplishments of his residents and fellows. Do they pursue an academic life? How many are themselves teachers or physician scientists? To assess this, I looked up the career paths of Jeff's residents and compared them with those of the legendary I. S. Ravdin and Jonathan Rhoads.

Somewhat to my surprise, I found that less than half of Dr. Ravdin's and Dr. Rhoads's residents chose an academic career or achieved university appointments. Compared with this, almost 75 percent of Dr. Drebin's trainees appear headed for university careers.

Finally, how is Jeff viewed by his colleagues and in what kind of shape does he leave his department? Unlike some surgical geheimrats of the past, Jeff is never intimidating or ruthless. Instead, the effectiveness of his leadership style depends on his even temper, his approachability, and his consistently warm support of faculty and residents. He and his wife, Linda, have even restored a tradition employed by

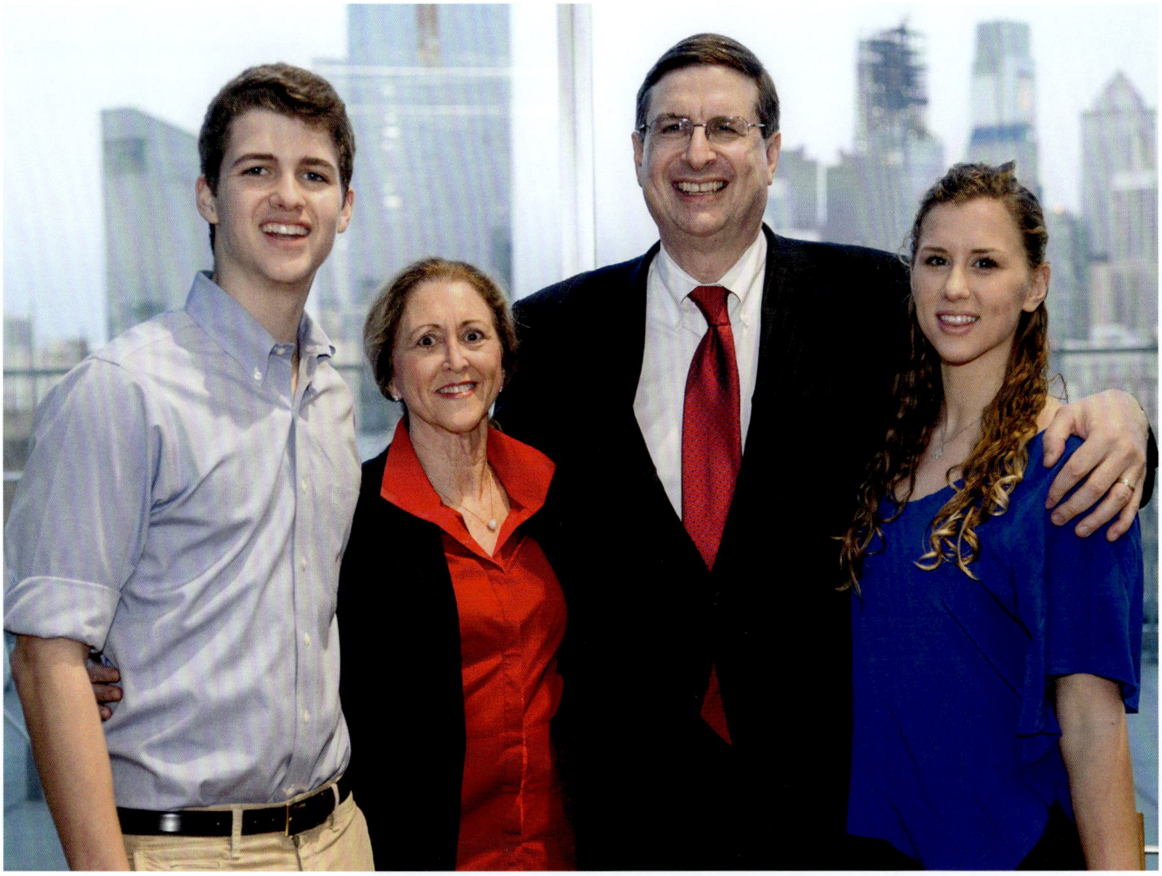

Drebin Family: Harrison, Linda, Jeff, and Lizzie

2017–present
Chair of Department of Surgery, Memorial Sloan Kettering Cancer Center, New York

2024
President-elect of American Surgical Association

I. S. Ravdin and others of welcoming faculty and residents into their home on holidays and special occasions.

Jeff Drebin leaves a department that is happy, academically and financially strong, and confident of its future. In every respect, he measures up very well with the best of his professional forebears. Small wonder that we are going to miss him. This will be a very hard act to follow.

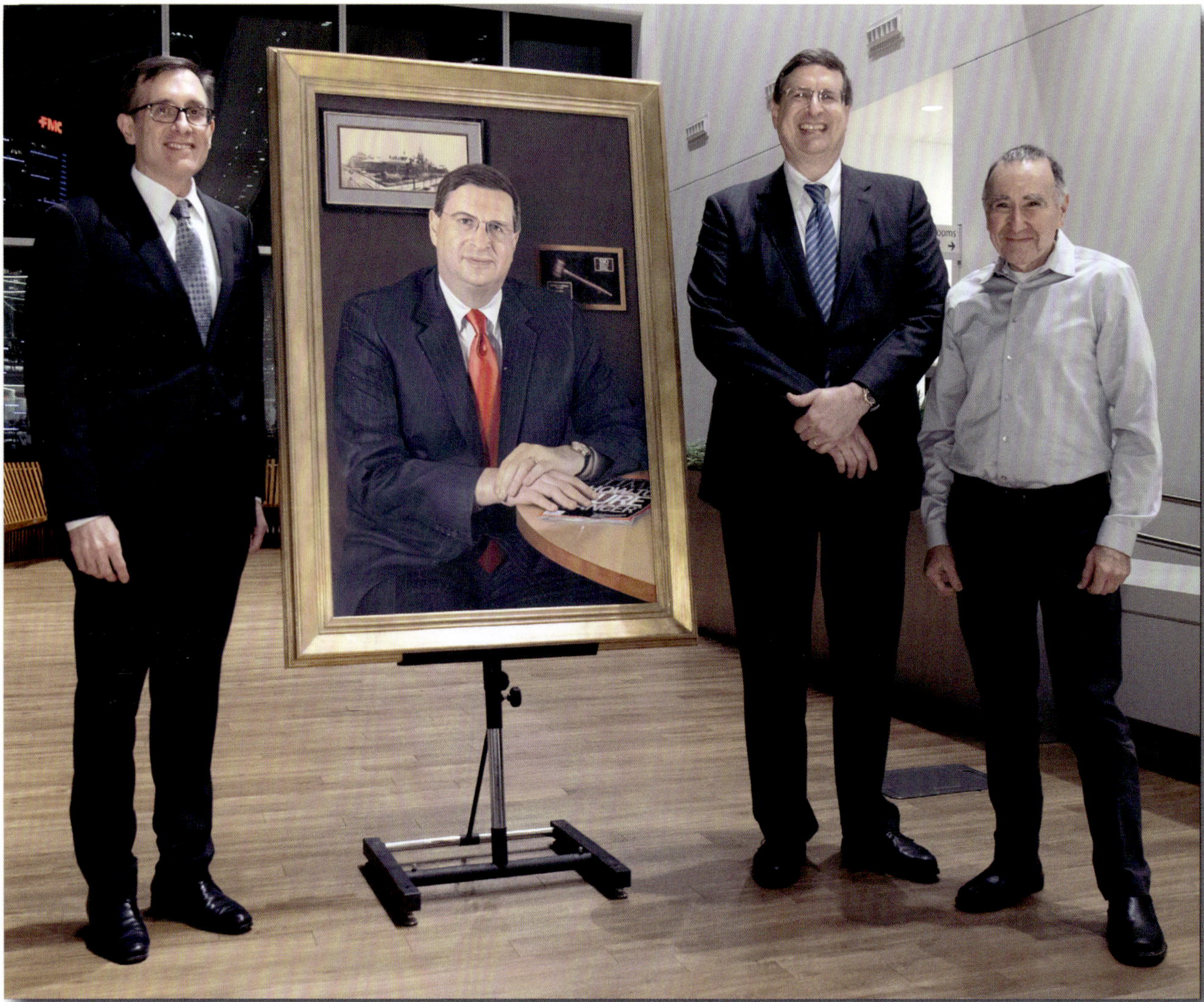

Ron DeMatteo and Jeff Drebin with the artist, Jon Friedman.

Notes

[1] Lowy A, Tominaga A, Drebin JA, Takeoki M, Benacerraf B, Greene MI. Identification of an I-J + antigen presenting cell required for third-order suppressor T cell activation. *Journal of Experimental Medicine* 157(1): 353–358 (Jan. 1983).

Schechter AL, Stern DF, Vaidyanathan L, Decker SJ, Drebin JA, Greene MI, Weinberg RA. The neu oncogene: An erbB related oncogene that encodes a 185,000 Mr tumor antigen. *Nature* 312(5994): 513–516 (Dec. 6–12 1984).

Drebin JA, Stern DF, Link VC, Weinberg RA, Greene MI. Monoclonal antibodies identify a cell surface antigen associated with an activated cellular oncogene. *Nature* 312(5994): 545–548 (Dec. 6–12, 1984).

Drebin JA, Link VC, Stern DF, Weinberg RA, Greene MI. Down-modulation of an oncogene protein product and reversion of the transformed phenotype by monoclonal antibodies. *Cell* 41(3): 695–706 (July 1985).

Kokai Y, Cohen JA, Drebin JA, Greene MI. Stage and tissue-specific expression of the neu oncogene in rat development. *Proceedings of the National Academy of Sciences (USA)* 84(23): 8498–8501 (Dec. 1987).

Drebin JA, Link VC, Greene MI. Monoclonal antibodies reactive with distinct domains of the neu oncogene-encoded p185 molecule exert synergistic anti-tumor effects in vivo. *Oncogene* 2(3): 273–277 (Mar. 1988).

Drebin JA, Link VC, Greene MI. Monoclonal antibodies specific for the neu oncogene product directly mediate anti-tumor effects in vivo. *Oncogene* 2(4): 387–394 (Apr. 1988).

Myers JN, Drebin JA, Greene MI. Biological effects of monoclonal anti-receptor antibodies reactive with the neu oncogene product, p185neu. *Methods in Enzymology* 198: 277–290 (1991).

Qian X, O'Roarke DM, Drebin JA, Zhao H, Wang Q, Greene MI. Identification of p185neu sequences required for monoclonal antibody- or ligand-mediated receptor signal attenuation. *DNA and Cell Biology* 16(12): 1395–1405 (Dec. 1997).

Roh H, Pippin J, Boswell CB, Drebin JA. Antisense oligonucleotides specific for the HER2/neu oncogene inhibit the growth of human breast carcinoma cells that overexpress HER2/neu. *Journal of Surgical Research* 77(1): 85–90 (June 1998).

CHAPTER 31

Does the World's Largest Explosion Inspire a New Field: Children's Surgery?

The Pioneering Roles of William Ladd, Robert Gross, and C. Everett Koop

Additional Contributions of Penn Surgeons, James O'Neill, Moritz Ziegler, Scott Adzick, and Steve Fishman

1946
I. S. Ravdin appoints C. Everett Koop as chief of surgery at CHOP.

Steven Fishman (HUP chief resident, 1992) is chairman of surgery at Boston Children's Hospital. This position is usually considered the top one in pediatric surgery, a view based in part on *US News & World Report*'s ranking of Boston Children's as the country's best pediatric hospital. This is arguable because CHOP has sometimes been ranked first and Boston Children's second, but in either case, Penn Surgery has played a major role in the development of this field. An interesting story is how the surgeons who led these two hospitals have interacted and determined the history and evolution of pediatric and cardiovascular surgery. Six of these surgeons have a strong Penn connection.

In 1946, when I. S. Ravdin returned to HUP from commanding World War II's 20th General Hospital, one of his first actions as department chairman was to appoint one of his residents, C. Everett Koop, as chief of surgery at CHOP. Koop was just finishing his HUP residency but had virtually no training or experience in children's surgery. To compensate for this inconvenience, Ravdin sent him to Boston Children's Hospital for a short course in pediatric surgery with the founders of the field, William Ladd and Robert Gross.

C. Everett Koop

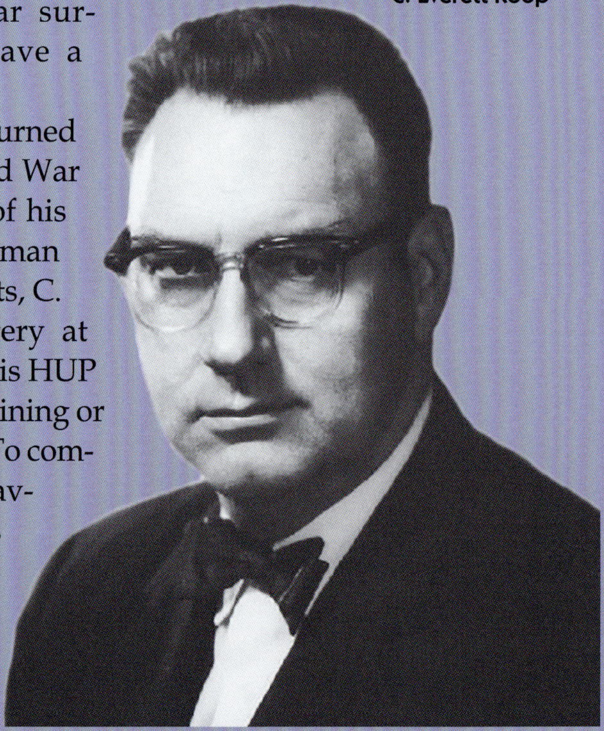

At the time, pediatric surgery as a specialty was quite new—in the United States only twenty years old. Legend has it that in this country, it began as the result of a tragic explosion. On December 6, 1917, a French munitions ship full of wartime explosives collided with a Swedish ship in Canada's Halifax harbor. This set off an explosion that was said to be the world's most powerful one prior to the first atom bomb in 1945.[1] Two thousand people were killed and 9,000 others injured. Thousands more were left homeless.

A Red Cross relief train came from Boston carrying enough equipment to set up a 500-bed hospital.[2] It was led by a young Harvard-trained surgeon, William Ladd. The experience of caring for 500 injured and burned children was claimed to be the reason he decided to become a pediatric surgeon. This is an exaggeration as he was already focused on children's surgery. But after his experience in Halifax, he decided to devote himself full-time to the field.[3] Moving his practice to Boston Children's Hospital as a junior attending, he studied, acquired clinical experience, chronicled, and wrote about surgical maladies of children, such as malrotation, pyloric stenosis, cleft palate, biliary atresia, and so forth. He became such an authority in the field that in 1927, he was appointed as chief of surgery at Boston Children's Hospital, and since then, he has been considered the father of pediatric surgery.

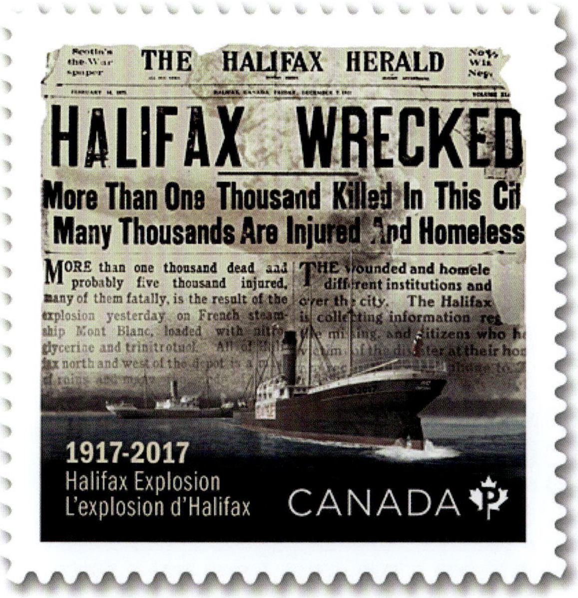
THE HALIFAX HERALD
HALIFAX WRECKED
More Than One Thousand Killed In This Cit
Many Thousands Are Injured And Homeless
MORE than one thousand dead and probably five thousand injured, many of them fatally, is the result of the explosion yesterday on French steamship Mont Blanc, loaded with nitroglycerine and trinitrotuol.
1917-2017
Halifax Explosion
L'explosion d'Halifax
CANADA

He also started the country's first formal training program in pediatric surgery. One of his residents, Robert Gross, was particularly accomplished and seemed to be Ladd's obvious heir apparent. Gross's interests were not limited to the general pediatric surgery he learned from Ladd. In fact, he was more interested in congenital cardiac abnormalities, which he studied in the department of pathology for two years. With animal experiments and dissection of human cadavers, he developed a plan for a new operation, ligation of the patent ductus arteriosus. In 1938, he told Ladd that he believed he

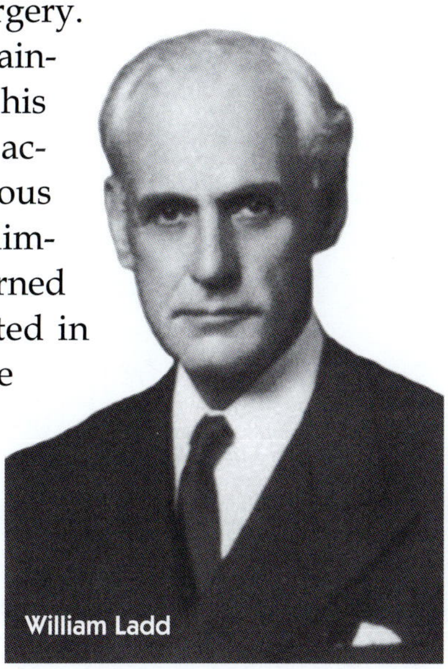
William Ladd

1917
Explosion in Halifax Harbor.

William Ladd leads Red Cross relief train

1927
Ladd appointed chief of surgery, Boston Childrens Hospital

1938
Ladd's resident Robert Gross plans to ligate a child's patent ductus arteriosus. Ladd forbids him.

While Ladd is away, Gross successfully performs the operation

1945
Ladd retires.
Koop serves as fellow at Boston Children's Hospital

1947
Robert Gross appointed chief of surgery, Boston Children's Hospital

1967
Gross retires as chief at Boston Children's Hospital, is succeeded by Judah Folkman

was prepared to do this operation, the first in a human patient. However, Ladd was convinced that this was too dangerous and explicitly forbade Gross to attempt it.

Disregarding his chief, Gross chose the opportunity of Ladd's absence on a European vacation and scheduled the operation. He then performed it successfully on a seven-year-old girl. When Ladd returned, he was furious that Gross had defied his order. According to Alden Harken (later a Gross resident), Ladd fired Gross, banishing him from Boston Children's Hospital for six weeks. Ladd never forgave Gross for this transgression, even though the operation Gross had done opened an entirely new field—heart surgery.[4] Nor did Ladd relent in 1945 when Gross was further acclaimed for performing the first successful operation for coarctation of the aorta.

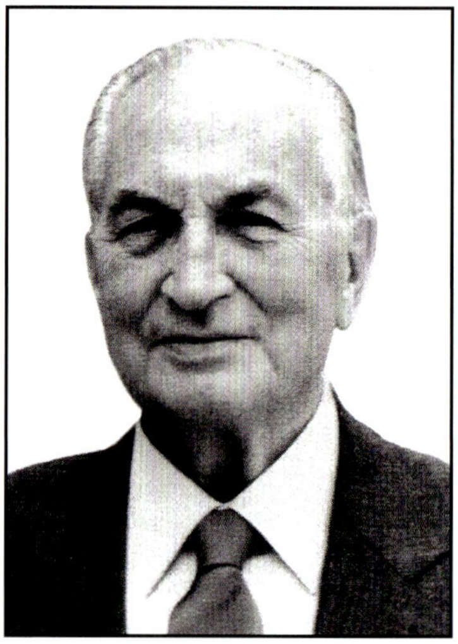
Robert Gross

As a result of their antagonism, when Ladd retired in 1945, he did his best to block Gross's appointment as his successor. According to Koop, as quoted in Ziegler's oral history of him, Ladd bitterly criticized Gross as an incompetent surgeon, a dishonest researcher, and even on moral and religious grounds.[5]

The antagonism between Ladd and Gross was at its height in 1946 when Koop showed up at Boston Children's for his fellowship. Ladd's criticism had delayed Gross's appointment as chief of surgery and poisoned the atmosphere. This unpleasantness resulted in Gross's frequent absence from the hospital and caused Koop to shorten his fellowship there from the planned twelve months to only eight. Nevertheless, in 1947, the widely-acclaimed Gross was appointed chief of surgery at Boston Children's. Recognized as the founder of cardiovascular surgery, he became one of the world's most praised and honored surgeons.

During his brief fellowship in Boston, Koop watched Gross operate, but he attached even more importance to his discussions with the recently retired Ladd on the complex art of caring for children and their families. Koop then returned to Philadelphia where at CHOP, he soon became a major figure in pediatric surgery.

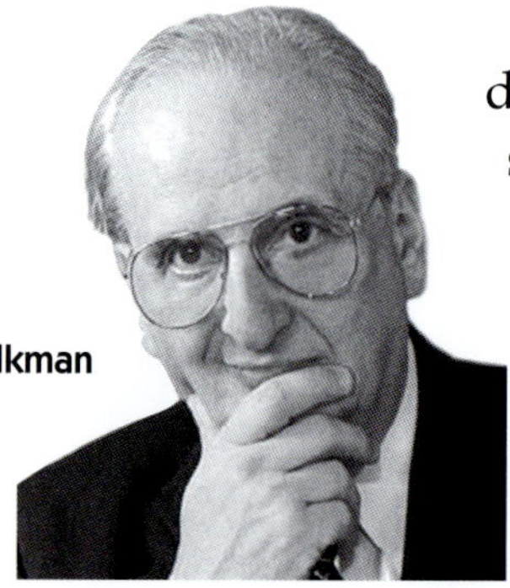
Judah Folkman

In 1967, when Robert Gross retired as Boston Children's chief surgeon, Harvard appointed as his successor Judah Folkman, then only thirty-four years old, brilliant but known mainly for his research on angiogenesis. During Folkman's surgical training at MGH, he had little exposure to the surgery of children. To prepare him for his new position, he came to Philadelphia for a six-month fellowship at CHOP with C. Everett Koop, who by then was considered the country's leading pediatric surgeon. Fourteen years later, Folkman retired from a successful career in children's surgery to devote himself to research full-time. He was succeeded by Hardy Hendren (no Penn connection). When Hendren retired in 1998, he was succeeded by Mory Ziegler, who was trained in general surgery at HUP and by Koop at CHOP. Ziegler's spectacular career was capped in 2016 by his winning the prestigious Ladd Medal. He was followed by Robert C. Shamberger (no Penn connection), who was chief from 2004–2019. Completing the circle, Steve Fishman, another HUP-trained surgeon, became chief of surgery at Boston Children's in 2019.

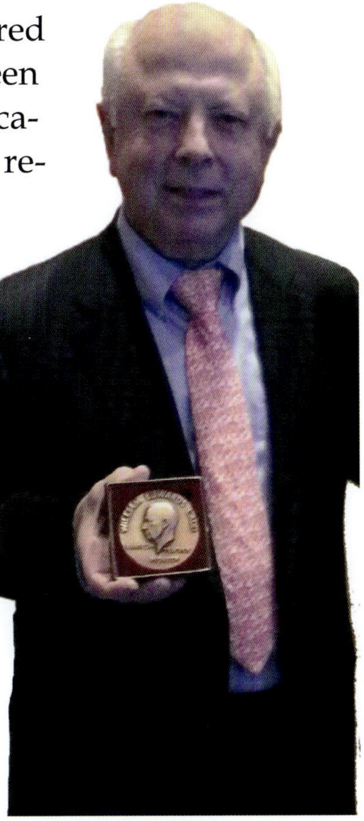

Mory Ziegler with Ladd Medal.

1968
Folkman serves as fellow to Koop at CHOP

1998
HUP and CHOP-trained Moritz Ziegler becomes chief at Boston Children's Hospital

2019
HUP-trained Steven Fishman becomes chief at Boston Children's Hospital

Steven J. Fishman is professor of surgery at Harvard Medical School and the Stuart and Jane Weitzman Family Chair in Surgery at Boston Children's Hospital where he is also vice-chair of surgery for clinical operations. He obtained BS and MD degrees at Northwestern University. As a HUP general surgery resident, Steve was president of the housestaff and won the Inouye Teaching Award, the Rhoads Research Award, and the Resident Scholar Award. After residency, he completed his pediatric surgery fellowship at Boston Children's Hospital in 1994. He has remained at Boston Children's for his entire career. Although always active in the practice and teaching of the broad spectrum of pediatric surgery, he has a particular clinical and research focus on vascular malformations.[6] In 1999, he became codirector of the Vascular Anomalies Center at Boston Children's Hospital. Annually this center's multidisciplinary group evaluates about 1,700 patients with hemangiomas, rare vascular tumors, and vascular malformations of all types. Steve originated and continues to maintain an international registry of hepatic hemangiomas. He is past president of the International Society for the Study of Vascular Anomalies.

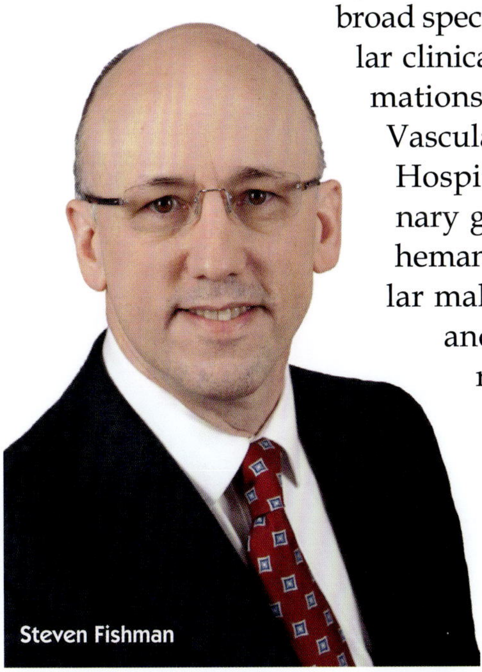

Steven Fishman

Dr. Fishman has authored over 200 scientific publications and chapters, as well as two books, including a comprehensive reference work on vascular

1916
Koop is born in Brooklyn

1937
BA Dartmouth

1941
MD Cornell

1941–1946
Intern at Pennsylvania Hospital. Surgical resident at HUP

anomalies. He has a particular interest in vascular abnormalities of the viscera. These anomalies are extremely rare, but Steve's international referral practice allows him to recognize patterns in their clinical presentation and opportunities for treatment. Dr. Fishman has extensive experience with resecting, debulking, and reconstructing vascular malformations and associated overgrown tissues of the torso, genitalia, neck, and extremities. He has also studied the role of dynamic contrast lymphangiography of the thoracic duct, which has led to the use of novel treatments and reconstruction of thoracic duct anomalies. He was the recipient of the Penn Department of Surgery's Distinguished Graduate Award in 2018.

C. Everett Koop, MD, DSc (1916–2013)

(Contributed by Moritz M. Ziegler, MD)

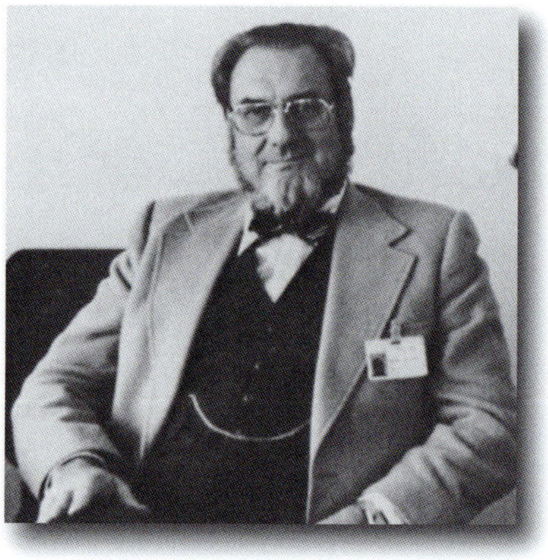

C. Everett Koop was born in Brooklyn as the only child of parents of Dutch and German heritage. He envisioned a career in surgery at a young age and attempted to satisfy that curiosity by observing operative procedures on Saturdays as a high school student.

Dr. Koop attended Dartmouth College, where he played football under Coach Earl Blaik until an injury terminated his career. It was at Dartmouth that friends for the first time called him "Chick." It was also there that he met visiting Vassar student, Elizabeth "Betty" Flanagan, whom he subsequently married. Betty Koop was an exceptional woman and a critical element—"the woman behind the man"—to Dr. Koop's success.

After graduating from Dartmouth in 1937, Koop attended Cornell University School of Medicine, graduating in 1941. His internship at Philadelphia's Pennsylvania Hospital was followed by a residency in surgery at HUP. He was also appointed as a fellow in the Harrison Department of Surgical Research where he studied the role of protein gels as a nutritional supplement and volume expander. This work, published in the *American Journal of Medical Science, Journal of Clinical Investigation,* and *Annals of Surgery,* was part of the foundation of the Harrison Department's nutrition program later led by Drs. Ravdin, Rhoads, Vars, Dudrick, and Wilmore that culminated in total parenteral nutrition.

With the advent of World War II, most of the Penn surgeons followed I. S. Ravdin to India, leaving Jonathan Rhoads and resident surgeons Harold Zintel and Koop in charge of Ravdin's HUP service. After the war, Ravdin appointed selected members of the returning faculty to new positions as surgical specialty leaders. Koop wanted to head the department's cancer program, but Ravdin instead offered him a position as surgeon-in-chief at the Children's Hospital of Philadelphia. Since during his HUP residency Koop had little experience in children's surgery, he needed a short course in pediatric surgery by Dr. William Ladd and Dr. Robert Gross at Boston Children's Hospital. During a few months, Ladd taught Koop the nuances of pediatric surgery, its philosophy, and how to evaluate and treat children and their families. He learned operative technique from pioneering vascular surgeon, Robert Gross.

1946
Appointed chief of surgery at CHOP. For eight months, Koop serves as fellow at Boston Children's Hospital with Ladd and Gross

Dr. Koop returned from Boston and began his pediatric surgical career at CHOP in 1946. Koop at once informed the CHOP pediatricians that they would no longer need to provide perioperative care since the surgical service would now assume that responsibility. This bold assertion was not welcomed, but it paved the way for a surgical service that eventually earned trust and respect from his medical peers. In 1948 at the age of thirty-two as an assistant professor of surgery, he was officially appointed surgeon-in-chief of CHOP. He was appointed professor of pediatric surgery in 1959. He eventually recruited to CHOP and University of Pennsylvania's faculty a number of associates in pediatric surgery: William Kiesewetter, Harry Bishop, Arie Verhagen, Charles Minor, Paul Mellish, Dale Johnson, Louise Schnaufer, Maurice Srouji, John Templeton, and Moritz Ziegler.

1956
At CHOP, Koop develops first ICU for babies

1959
Koop is promoted to full professor

Dr. Koop's innovations were numerous. The 1956 development of the nation's first neonatal intensive care unit for babies with surgical conditions was groundbreaking and undoubtedly contributed significantly to his many unprecedented accomplishments in newborn surgery. His support of his anesthesia colleagues, Drs. Deming, Bachman, and Downes, led to the development of a world-class Department of Pediatric Anesthesiology, another crucial element in favorable outcomes.

Koop's surgical trainees often spoke of the "Koopian Method"—an operative approach that emphasized, "Do what you do best; simplify

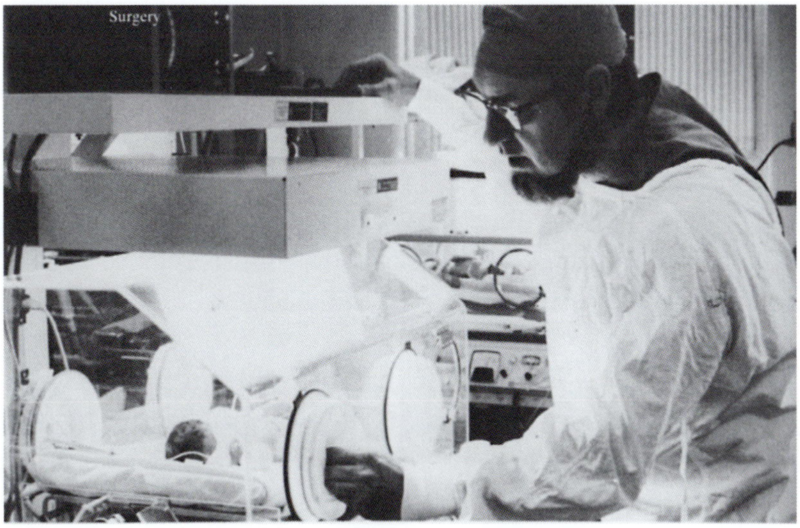

Dr. Koop in CHOP's first pediatric ICU.

1959
Koop separates conjoined twins

1964-1976
Koop is first editor of *Journal of Pediatric Surgery*

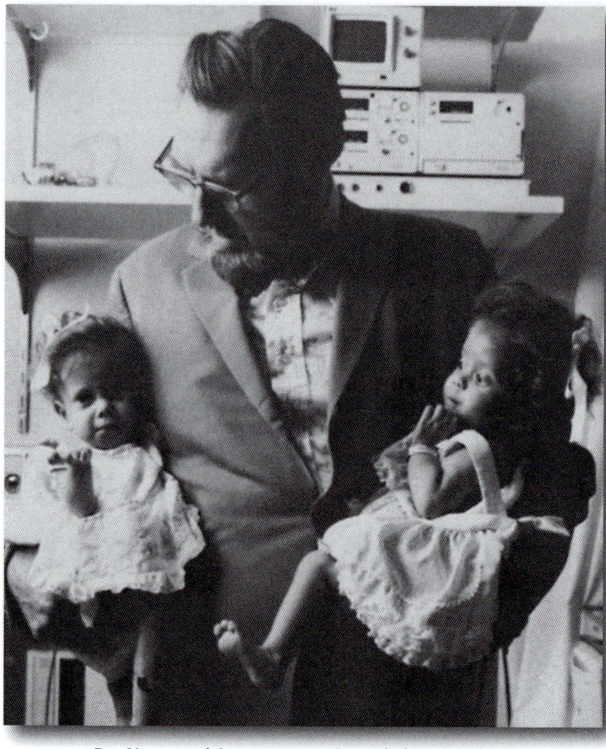
Dr. Koop with separated conjoined twins.

rather than complicate diagnostic and operative procedures; do an even better operation for the handicapped child, who deserves and needs it; maintain a sensitive respect for patients and their families; and enter difficult and complicated procedures with both physical and mental preparation for the job at hand." Dr. Koop's impact on pediatric operations ranged from simple, "routine" cases to the most complex. Hernia repair, orchidopexy, and pyloromyotomy were done quickly and precisely with a conservation of motion. For a complex neuroblastoma, perhaps his greatest clinical contribution in collaboration with pediatric colleagues Audrey Evans and Dan D'Angio, treatment ranged from observation alone to radical resection, to debulking, sometimes using as an instrument a kitchen "spoon" with which to scoop out tumor burden. Another example was the "no forceps, no touch" technique for infant intestinal anastomoses and esophageal atresia repair. Also in his list of technical accomplishments was the separation of multiple sets of complex conjoined twins for which he and his multidisciplinary team received considerable international recognition.

A goal emphasized by Koop was coordination of his surgical accomplishments with the evolution of his deep Christian faith. His colleagues recalled a deepening of this faith following the untimely death of his son David in 1968. The result was a pediatric surgical service that embodied a strong pro-life behavior. This encouraged the CHOP team to challenge prevailing attitudes of that time in pediatric surgery of "letting the poor baby die." Consequently, newborn babies stricken with such entities as cloacal exstrophy, conjoined twins, trisomy syndromes, and a variety of short bowel syndromes were all to become amenable to operative intervention.

Koop's pediatric residency nurtured more than thirty-five national and international trainees, many of whom became future leaders in the field. These men and women remained markedly loyal to him, and the support, mentoring, and friendship was always reciprocated. Another legacy was his vision of a multispecialty surgical faculty able to provide expertise in urology, cardiac surgery, neurosurgery, otolaryngology, plastic surgery, ophthalmology, and orthopedic surgery.

1975
Koop negotiates with American Board of Surgery to create a certificate of competence in Pediatric Surgery

1976
Awarded Ladd medal

Koop's influence on the development of pediatric surgery as a specialty became national and international. He was an important figure in the British Association of Pediatric Surgery, serving on its council and recognized by its highest honor, the Denis Browne Medal, in 1970. In France, he received the Legion of Honor, that nation's highest award. In the United States, he was a founding member and later chairperson of the first organization of pediatric surgeons, the Surgical Section of the American Academy of Pediatrics (AAP). In 1976, the AAP awarded him its highest recognition, the William E. Ladd Medal. Dr. Koop was also among several pediatric surgeons who negotiated with the American Board of Surgery a specialty board in pediatric surgery, culminating in a special certificate of competence exam in 1975. Dr. Koop was also a founding member of the American Pediatric Surgical Association, serving as its second president. Perhaps his most visible and lasting impact was his service from 1964 to 1976 as the first editor of the new *Journal of Pediatric Surgery.* The journal had a substantially positive impact on the new field, and today it remains the voice for APSA, the Surgical Section AAP, BAPS, the Canadian Association of Pediatric Surgery, and the Pacific Association of Pediatric Surgery. Dr. Koop was also a fellow of the American College of Surgeons, the American Academy of Pediatrics, a member of the American Surgical Association, and the American Philosophical Society. He held honorary fellowships in the Royal College of Surgeons of England, the Royal College of Surgeons of Edinburgh, and the Royal College of Physicians and Surgeons of Glasgow. He also held multiple university honorary degrees.

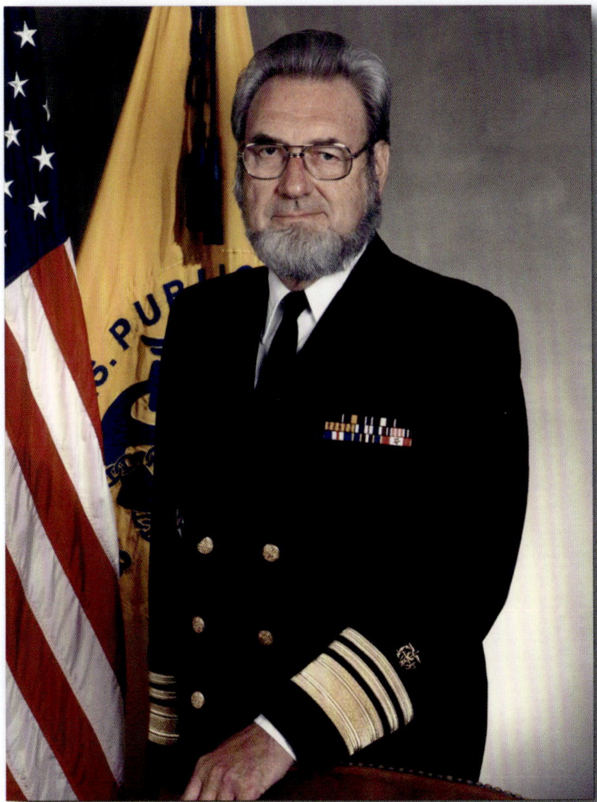

Another chapter of Dr. Koop's life took place during the final years of his tenure at CHOP when he became closely associated with theologian, Dr. Francis Schaeffer. They shared the philosophy of support for and sanctity of human life. As theologian and pediatric surgeon, they toured together on a traveling lecture series, supplemented with film and a book entitled *Whatever Happened to the Human Race?*

In 1981, soon after the election of Ronald Reagan as president, Dr. Koop was contacted about his potential interest in

1982
Appointed surgeon general of Public Health Service

the position of surgeon general of the Public Health Service (PHS). Because a long confirmation process was anticipated, the president first appointed Koop to the position of deputy assistant secretary of health. Not until November 16, 1981, was the confirmation realized. Appointment to the surgeon general position occurred on January 21, 1982.

Dr. Koop's many contributions as surgeon general were unprecedented. He brought his name and personal recognition to the position of surgeon general and unlike any predecessor or successor, he was deemed "America's doctor." The bond between the PHS and Dr. Koop was intense, and this deep respect continued even after Dr. Koop left Washington.

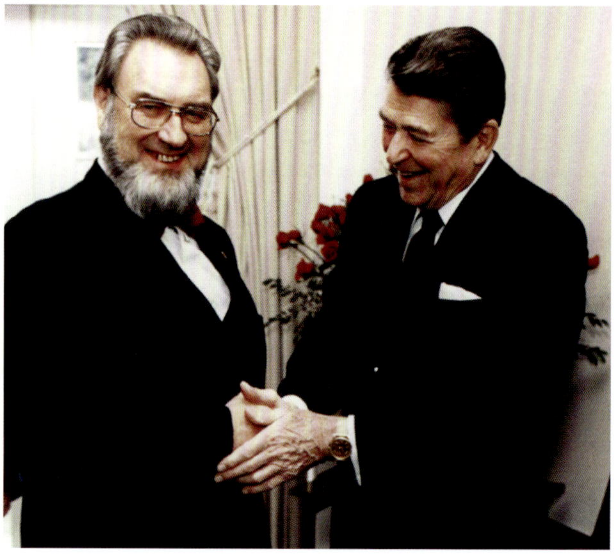

C. Everett Koop with President Ronald Reagan.

Koop's policies as surgeon general could be divided into several important components. The first was an antitobacco position in which he confronted the tobacco manufacturing and marketing industry with a formidable educational assault on the hazards of smoking, including the adverse effects of second-hand smoke. This effort is generally credited with the substantial decrease in the number of smoking Americans and the emergence of smoke-free environments.

Second was his early response to a new infectious epidemic that we know today as HIV/AIDS. This was a timely and brave program for public awareness and education. He focused on the fight against and protection from a transmissible disease instead of accentuating the most susceptible population. Mailing an educational brochure to every American household was controversial—it touted protection during sexual activity, including the use of condoms, and sex education of children. It was the largest public health educational initiative in American history.

Third was the national controversy over the death of a baby born with Downs Syndrome complicated by esophageal atresia and tracheoesophageal fistula following the withholding of operative therapy. Dr. Koop's position as prolife advocate and pediatric surgeon prompted him to weigh in. The legislated Baby Doe Amendment was a product of this intervention.

Also notable was Dr. Koop's position on abortion. In a report to the Reagan administration that expected a contrary view, Koop stated that he had found no evidence of harm to the psyche and well-being of a woman undergoing abortion in a safe and creditable environment. This was surprising since his confirmation was almost blocked by prochoice activists. Dr. Koop also conveyed his forward thinking on the obesity epidemic and on violence and safety in America, including firearm violence.

1982
Koop advocates Baby Doe Ammendment

1989
Koop resigns as surgeon general

1995
Koop is awarded Presidential Medal of Freedom

Dr. Koop finished his term as surgeon general in 1989, returning to private life and a position as senior scholar at the C. Everett Koop Institute at Dartmouth where he continued his advocacy for a healthier America. He was awarded the Public Welfare Medal from the National Academy of Sciences in 1990 and the Presidential Medal of Freedom from President Clinton in 1995.

In one of his last contributions to the literature (*Am Public Health* 2006; 98: 2090–2092), Dr. Koop defined the "core principles" that he felt would restore the credibility of American healthcare. They were:

1. Affirm a fundamental moral right to health by both preventions of disease and access to diagnostic and treatment regimens;
2. Disparities in healthcare, no matter what their description, are counter to this moral right;
3. The highest priority of health-care providers, whether public, private, or governmental agency, must be the improvement of the health of all people.

To characterize C. Everett Koop simply as a complex man would hardly do him justice. The first thirty-five years of his professional life in pediatric surgery are reflected in half of his more than 300 publications while the second thirty-one years as public health servant account for the rest. However, only by examining his personal value system can we begin to understand him. This value system encompassed integrity, ethics, generosity, compassion, truth, and friendship. In the long history of medicine, few physicians have achieved worldwide recognition for their importance in multiple careers. Among them is the towering figure of Charles Everett Koop, a pioneering pediatric surgeon, an extraordinarily effective public servant, and a thoughtful educator, with an impact ranging from the survival of

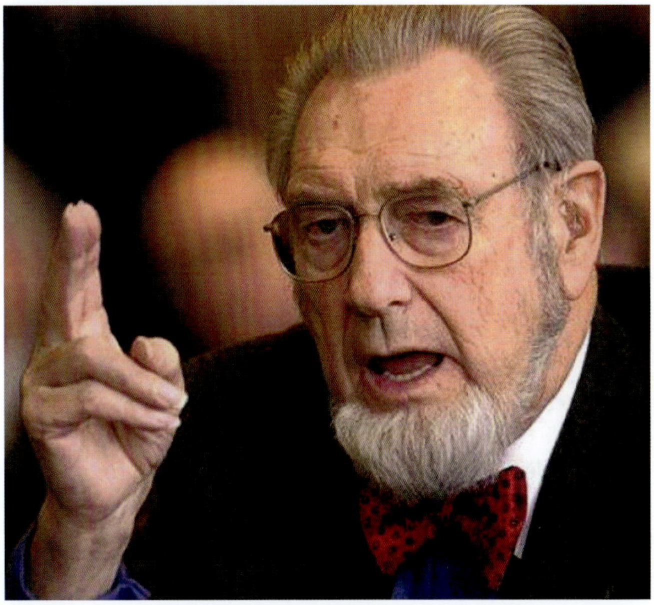

2013
Death of Koop

a single newborn with a congenital anomaly to the health of an entire nation.

In 2013, Charles Everett "Chick" Koop died at age ninety-six, peacefully in his home in Hanover, New Hampshire. In the church of his son, the Reverend Norman Koop, his multifaceted life was remembered, first, as father to Norman, Allen, David, and Betsy, and as husband to his wife Betty of more than sixty-nine years who died in 2007. He remarried in 2010 to long-standing family friend Cora Hogue who provided amazing support in his final days. From 1946 to 1981 as surgeon-in-chief at CHOP, he was a master clinician, teacher, administrator, and advocate for his patients and their families; friend and mentor to his trainees and faculty; and formative leader for the field of pediatric surgery. Finally, his contributions as surgeon general from 1981 to 1989 were characterized by his fight against smoking, his educational program that addressed the emerging AIDS epidemic, public awareness of traumatic injury and obesity, and his aggressive support for the handicapped child. Included was his life as a conservative Christian strongly committed to the sanctity of human life and dedicated to a continuous effort to strengthen the health of the nation. To be sure, this was a life lived to the fullest and a life whose contributions touched a broad swath of Americans.

James A. O'Neill

1959
O'Neill obtains MD from Yale

1959–1964
O'Neill's surgical residency at Vanderbilt

1965–1967
O'Neill serves in burn unit of Brooke Army Hospital in San Antonio

1967–1969
O'Neill is resident in pediatric surgery at Ohio State

1969–1971
O'Neill serves on faculty at Louisiana State University

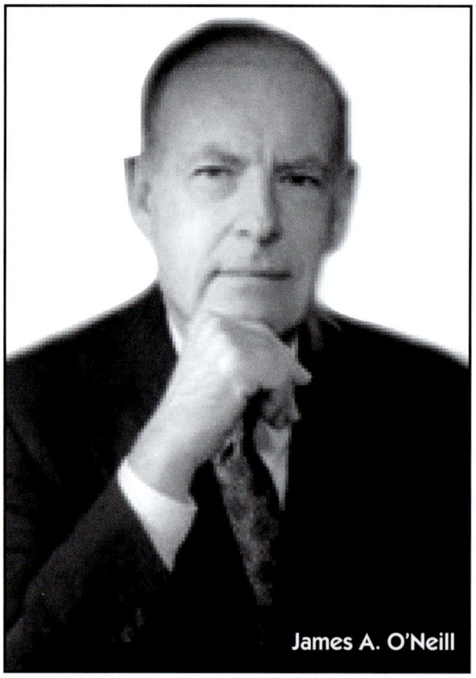
James A. O'Neill

Jim O'Neill succeeded C. Everett Koop as chief of surgery at CHOP in 1981 and served in this role until 1994. Dr. O'Neill was born in New York. His family had limited means, but he attended Georgetown University on scholarship, being the first one in his family to attend college. He obtained his MD at Yale and completed residency in general and thoracic surgery under H. William Scott at Vanderbilt. His two years in the Army were served under John Moncrief at the burn unit of Brooke Army Hospital in San Antonio. He decided on a career as a pediatric surgeon. There were few pediatric surgery training programs at this time of the early 1960s, but he was fortunate to be accepted at one of the best with Bill Clatworthy at Ohio State University in Columbus. Following this, for several years he served on the faculty of Louisiana

State University at Charity Hospital in New Orleans, where he was mentored by Isidore Cohn, a former Ravdin resident. He then founded a small pediatric surgery program at Vanderbilt, serving as chief of pediatric surgery there from 1971 to 1981. After considering several offers to be chief of pediatric surgery at larger programs, he accepted one at CHOP, where Dr. Koop had just retired and was departing to become US surgeon general.

1971–1981
O'Neill is Chief of Pediatric Surgery, Vanderbilt University

1981–1994
O'Neill is Chief of Surgery at CHOP

O'Neill initiated a research program at CHOP. Because he was so broadly trained in general and thoracic surgery as well as pediatric surgery, he was able to initiate or improve a number of CHOP's programs, including vascular surgery (especially congenital anomalies), cancer, burns, trauma, metabolism, and the separation of conjoined twins, which had begun under Dr. Koop. By his own assessment, he elevated the ranking of the hospital's pediatric surgery program during his years at CHOP from about fifteenth in the United States to first or second.

1994
O'Neill is appointed chairman, Department of Surgery at Vanderbilt University

2007
O'Neill awarded the Ladd Medal

In 1994, O'Neill was invited to return to Vanderbilt as the chairman of the Department of Surgery where he spent the remainder of his career. Especially during this phase, he devoted a considerable amount of his time to volunteering in services for the underprivileged in Guatemala, Kenya, and China. He also became deeply involved with administrative aspects of pediatric surgery, such as accreditation, development of societies, journals, and so forth. He published 300 peer-reviewed papers and seven books. The story of Jim O'Neill's life is told in great detail in an oral interview of the American Academy of Pediatrics.[7]

O'Neill won a number of awards, such as the American College of Surgeons/Pfizer International Volunteerism Award and the American Pediatric Surgery Association's Humanitarian Award. In 2007, he was awarded the Ladd Medal, the most prestigious award in pediatric surgery.

Moritz Ziegler

1964
Ziegler obtains BA from Capital University.

1968
Ziegler obtains MD from University of Michigan Medical School.

1968–1974
Ziegler does general surgery residency and transplant fellowship at HUP.

Moritz (Mory) Ziegler was HUP chief resident in 1974 and CHOP resident from 1975 to 1977. Although he passed up a chance to become chief of pediatric surgery at CHOP, he served in that role at three other university centers and as one of the most distinguished figures in the field.

Mory is a graduate of Capital University in Ohio where, as a varsity baseball player and member of the glee club, he was an example of "Altemeier's Rule"—that athletes and musicians make the best residents. After medical school at Michigan, he came to HUP as an intern. During residency, Mory was one of HUP's first research and clinical transplantation fellows. With Craig Reckard, he performed and reported the first successful pancreatic islet transplant experiments. After residency and a year of research at Fox Chase with immunologist Richard Prehn, he

1988
Zeigler promoted to professor of surgery at HUP and CHOP

1989
Zeigler appointed chief of surgery at Cincinnati Children's Hospital

1998–2004
Zeigler is chief of surgery at Boston Children's Hospital

2004–2009
Zeigler is chief of pediatric surgery at University of Colorado

2017
Zeigler receives the Ladd Medal

trained in pediatric surgery under C. Everett Koop at CHOP. For the next twelve years, he remained a faculty member at Penn, becoming full professor of surgery in 1988. As a mainstay of pediatric surgery under Dr. Koop and then Dr. O'Neill, he founded CHOP's laboratory of surgical research, the nutrition support service, and the transplant program. He also played an important role in the development of transplantation at HUP. After training with Tom Starzl in Pittsburgh, Mory helped start HUP's liver transplantation program and performed the first liver transplants at CHOP. In addition, for several years he directed HUP's adult kidney transplant program.

In 1989, Mory moved to the University of Cincinnati as chief of pediatric surgery. In 1998, he was recruited to Boston Children's Hospital as surgeon-in-chief. He was also the Robert E. Gross Professor at Harvard and chairman of Harvard Medical School's surgical executive committee.

After expanding the faculty size and the research program at Boston Children's, he became chief of pediatric surgery at the University of Colorado (2004–2009). Since then in retirement, Mory and his wife Barbara, a former HUP nurse, have lived in Cincinnati.

In 2017, Mory was awarded the William E. Ladd Medal of the Section on Surgery of the American Academy of Pediatrics. Named for the founder of the field, this is the highest award in pediatric surgery. In addition to the Ladd award, Mory has received many honors. He has been president of the American Pediatric Surgery Association and of the Section on Surgery of the American Academy of Pediatrics. He was secretary and then chairman of the surgical executive committee of the American Academy of Pediatrics. In 1997, he was selected as our own department's distinguished graduate awardee. In 2022, the University of Cincinnati named an endowed professorship for Mory. He is a member of the Society of University Surgeons and the American Surgical Association. In addition to 300 peer-reviewed publications, he is the author of the textbook recognized as the standard on operative pediatric surgery.[8]

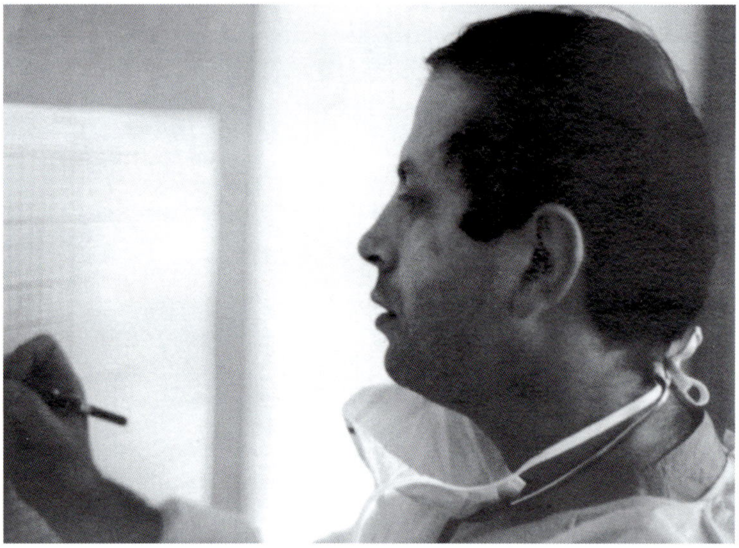

Mory Ziegler as a HUP Transplant Fellow.

During Mory's Festschrift in 2018, nineteen distinguished pediatric surgeons spoke on topics including gastroenterology, neuroblastoma, reform of pediatric surgery training, and quality in pediatric surgery. Most of the speakers were chiefs of pediatric surgery at university centers. Seven of them were Mory's trainees.

During his active career, Mory trained sixty-nine individuals, twenty-four as pediatric surgery residents. Seven of them have become chiefs of pediatric surgery at university centers: Brad Warner (Washington University), Edward Barksdale (Case Western Reserve), Daniel Von Altman (Cincinnati), Dai Chung (Vanderbilt), Franz Frazier (King's Daughters), David Whaoff (Minneapolis), and D. Dean Potter (Mayo Clinic).

Of forty-five others trained by Mory as fellows in laboratory research, seven became department or division chiefs (Irwin Krasra, Charles Howell, H. Naito, Martin Carpah, John Reynolds, Todasha Iwanaka, and Christopher Muratore). Thus of Mory's sixty-nine trainees, fourteen became department or division chiefs of pediatric surgery, 20.3 percent. I doubt that others can equal this record.

1975
Adzick obtains AB from Harvard

1979
Adzick obtains MD from Harvard

1980–1986
Adzick is resident in surgery at MGH

1983–1985
Adzick does research in fetal surgery at UCSF

1995
Adzick is appointed chief of surgery at CHOP

Scott Adzick

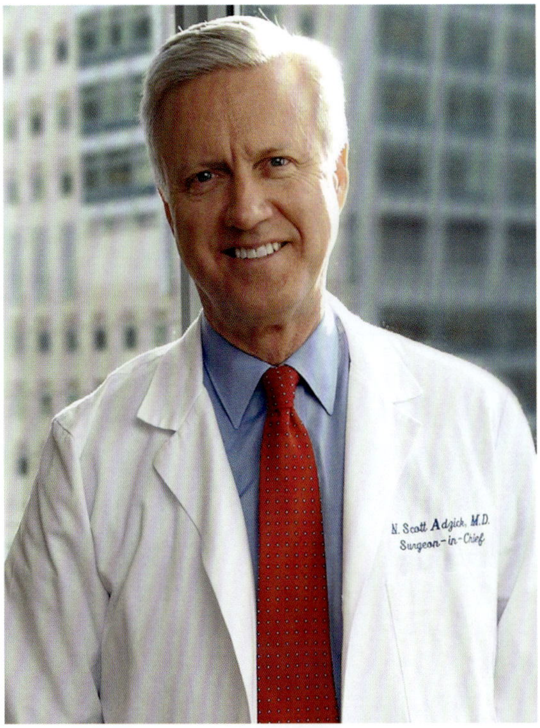

In 1994, Dr. Scott Adzick succeeded Jim O'Neill as surgeon-in-chief at Children's Hospital of Philadelphia (CHOP). He also became director of CHOP's Center for Fetal Diagnosis and Treatment, which he founded in 1995, and the C. Everett Koop Professor of Pediatric Surgery.

Dr. Adzick graduated from Harvard College where he played varsity baseball. He obtained his MD from Harvard Medical School in 1979. He completed his general surgical training at Massachusetts General Hospital in 1986. From 1983 to 1985, he was a postdoctoral scholar in the Department of Surgery of the University of California, San Francisco, where he worked with Michael Harrison in developing the first fetal surgical program, initially with animal models and then progressing to clinical application.

Dr. Adzick has dedicated his career to the pursuit of groundbreaking prenatal treatment for life-threatening and debilitating defects. He was the leader of a breakthrough randomized trial that demonstrated that performing fetal surgery for spina bifida results in significantly improved outcomes compared to the paralysis usually occurring despite conventional postnatal repair.[9] He is the most experienced and respected surgeon involved with this outstanding new treatment. Other fetal abnormalities that he has successfully treated by this approach include urinary tract obstruction that would fatally damage the kidneys, resection of lung lesions, and other life-threatening chest masses.[10] Although straightforward and bold in concept, the success of fetal surgery has required development of intricate methods of protecting the normal physiology and life of both the baby and mother. Dr. Adzick's productive research toward these goals has been supported by the NIH for more than thirty years. He has authored more than 600 peer-reviewed publications and has an H index of 103.

In addition to performing a full spectrum of standard pediatric surgical operations, Dr. Adzick has also performed more than 500 pancreatectomies for cure of hyperinsulinism, the most of any surgeon in the world. Dr. Adzick's many awards include the 1999 Presidential Class Contributions to the Republic of Poland, the 2012 Clinical Trial of the Year Award of the Society for Clinical Trials, the 2013 John Scott Award of the City Trusts of Philadelphia, and the Samuel D. Gross Prize of the College of Physicians of Philadelphia.

Dr. Adzick's memberships include the American Pediatric Surgical Association, the National Academy of Medicine, the Society of University Surgeons, and the American Surgical Association. He is an honorary member of the British Association of Pediatric Surgery, the Canadian Association of Pediatric Surgery, and the Chilean Society of Obstetrics and Gynecology. In 2021, he was given the Strittmatter Award of the Philadelphia County Medical Society.

As director of the CHOP pediatric surgery fellowship, he has trained more than thirty pediatric surgeons, many of whom serve in leadership positions in this field in the United States and around the world. In his research laboratory, he has trained more than fifty investigators, a number of whom have become professors at other university medical schools.

In 2021, Dr. Adzick stepped down as chief of the Division of Pediatric Surgery while remaining chief of surgery at CHOP.

Michael Nance

After a national search, Michael Nance was appointed Adzick's successor as chief of the Division of Pediatric General, Thoracic and Fetal Surgery as well as director of the Pediatric Trauma Program at CHOP.

Dr. Nance is recognized as one of the country's top pediatric surgeons. He earned his bachelor's degree in biology from Rhodes College, Memphis, Tennessee, his medical degree from Louisiana State University

School of Medicine, New Orleans, Louisiana, and completed his surgical residency at HUP. He also completed fellowships in pediatric surgery research and surgical critical care at the University of Pennsylvania. In 1997, Dr. Nance was the Louise Schnaufer Senior Fellow and chief resident at CHOP. As a faculty surgeon at CHOP for more than fifteen years, his major interest has been trauma.[11,12] He is a leading investigator in CHOP's Center for Injury Research and Prevention and a professor of surgery at the Pearlman School of Medicine where he holds the Josephine J. and John M. Templeton Jr. Chair in Pediatric Trauma. He has served as a member of the editorial board and guest editor and reviewer for more than a dozen medical journals.

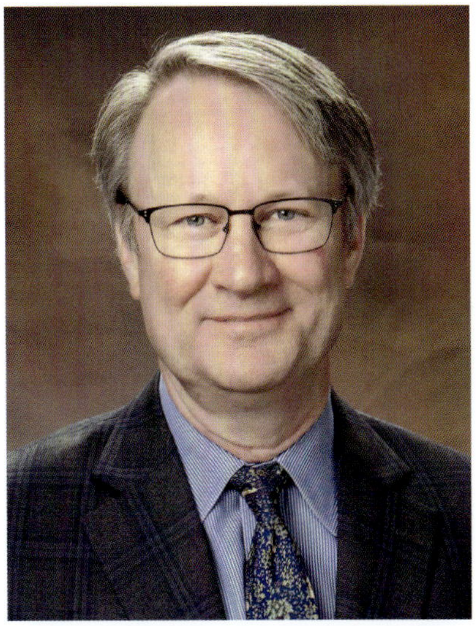

The large pediatric surgery faculty at CHOP is beyond the scope of this summary, but several members deserve special mention.

Holly Hedrick

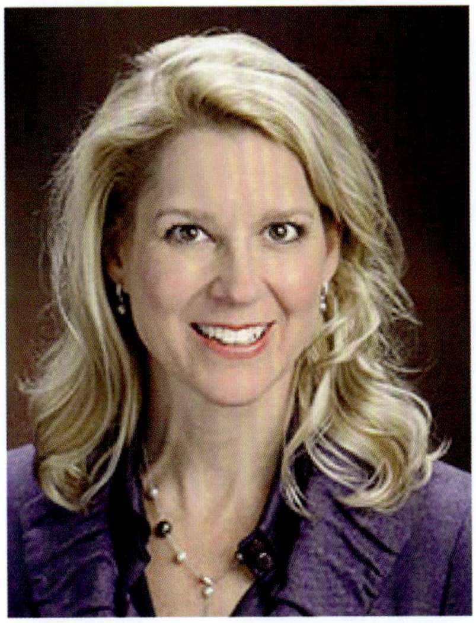

Holly Hedrick is the 2023 Strittmatter Awardee. She is professor of surgery in the Division of Pediatric General, Thoracic and Fetal Surgery, the Louise Schnaufer Endowed Chair in Pediatric Surgery, surgical director of the Extracorporeal Membrane Oxygenation Center, codirector of the Neonatal Surgical Team, director of the Pulmonary Hypoplasia Program, and investigator in the Center for Fetal Research.

Dr. Hedrick earned her bachelor's degree from Indiana University and her medical degree from Duke University School of Medicine. She completed her general surgery residency at Brigham & Women's Hospital/Harvard Medical School and her residency and fellowship in pediatric surgery at CHOP. Dr. Hedrick also completed research fellowships at Duke University and Harvard. She joined the CHOP staff as an attending surgeon in 1999. Her clinical specialty is treating children with congenital diaphragmatic hernia, especially those with resultant compromise in pulmonary function.[13]

Alan Flake

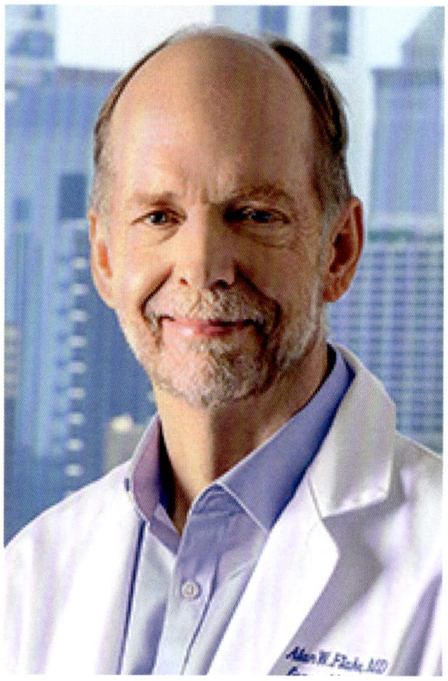

Alan Flake deserves special mention for his research in study of in utero transplantation and tolerance. His development of an artificial uterus is also promising as a method to sustain preterm infants.[14] Because his research is so intriguing, many HUP residents have chosen to spend their research time in his laboratory.

Other attending surgeons at CHOP are Myron Allukian, Thane Blinman, Joy Collins, Edward Doolin, Alexander Fairman, Thomas Hamilton, Pablo Laje, Peter Mattei, Gary Nace, Emily Partridge, and William Peranteau.

Notes

[1] Carter PL. The Halifax Explosion a century later: Lessons for our time. *Am J Surg.* (2018) 215(5):772–774.

[2] Nance ML. The Halifax disaster of 1917 and the birth of North American pediatric surgery. *J Pediatr Surg.* (2001) 36(3):405–408.

[3] Nakayama, Don K. The Halifax Explosion and the unofficial birth of pediatric surgery. *Bulletin of the American College of Surgeons* (May 1, 2017).

Ladd himself said that he had decided to be a pediatric surgeon ten years before the explosion.

[4] Wyckoff, Alyson Sulaski. Did you know? Surgical pioneer defied authority to conduct landmark operation. *American Academy of Pediatrics AAP News* (December 17, 2015).

[5] *Oral History of C. Everett Koop,* Interviewed by Moritz Ziegler, Pediatric History Center, American Academy of Pediatrics (May 8, 2006) p. 24.

[6] Fishman, Steven J. *Vascular Anomalies in Operative Pediatric Surgery* 7th edition CRC Press p. 6

[7] O'Neill, James. Interview. Conducted by George W. Holcomb III, MD (May 1, 2008). https://www.aap.org/en/about-the-aap/gartner-pediatric-history-center/oral-histories/?facets=%5B%5D&k=o%27neill&page=1

[8] Ziegler MM, Azizkhan RG, Allmen D, Weber TR, eds. *Operative Pediatric Surgery, 2e.* McGraw Hill (2014).

[9] Adzick NS, Thom EA, Spong CY, et al. A randomized trial of prenatal versus postnatal repair of myelomeningocele. *N Engl J Med* (2011) 364(11):993–1004. doi:10.1056/NEJMoa1014379. Adzick NS. Fetal surgery for spina bifida: past, present, future. *Semin Pediatr Surg* (2013) 22(1):10–17. doi:10.1053/j.sempedsurg.2012.10.003.

[10] Adzick NS. The IFMSS Tower Lecture: Fetal Surgery Past, Fetal Surgery Present, and Fetal Surgery Yet to Come! *Fetal Diagn Ther* (2020) 47(12):859–864. doi:10.1159/000507349.

[11] Sims CA, Wiebe DJ, Nance ML. Blunt solid organ injury: do adult and pediatric surgeons treat children differently? *J Trauma* (2008) 65(3):698–703. doi:10.1097/TA.0b013e3181574945.

[12] Nance ML, Carr BG, Branas CC. Access to Pediatric Trauma Care in the United States. *Arch Pediatr Adolesc Med* (2009) 163(6):512–518. doi:10.1001/archpediatrics.2009.65.

[13] De Bie FR, Avitabile CM, Joyeux L, et al. Neonatal and fetal therapy of congenital diaphragmatic hernia-related pulmonary hypertension. *Arch Dis Child Fetal Neonatal Ed* (2022) 107(5):458–466. doi:10.1136/archdischild-2021-322617.

[14] De Bie FR, Davey MG, Larson AC, Deprest J, Flake AW. Artificial placenta and womb technology: Past, current, and future challenges towards clinical translation. *Prenat Diagn* (2021) 41(1):145–158. doi:10.1002/pd.5821.

CHAPTER 32

Penn Trauma Surgeons in War and Peace

North American colonies of the British Empire fight against those of the French

John Jones is a cofounder of America's second-oldest medical school, Kings College (Columbia) (1767)

New Yorkers argue that Jones rather than Physick should be considered the Father of American Surgery

Benjamin Rush says John Jones is unmatched as an American surgeon

The French and Indian War (1754–1763)

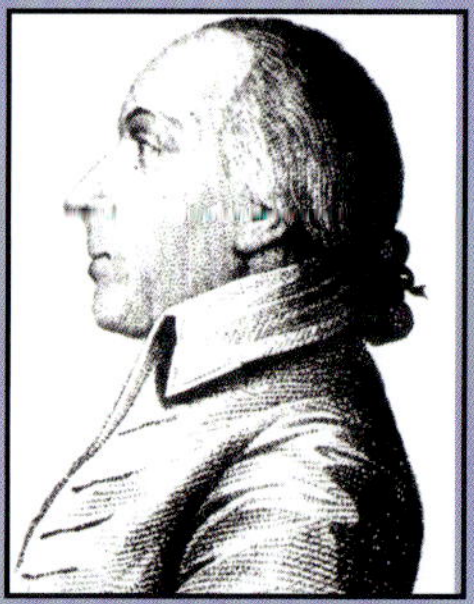

John Jones

Penn surgeons have served in all of America's wars, usually with distinction, sometimes with shame. In the French and Indian War, Penn Medicine's founder, John Morgan, served as an Army surgeon on the Western frontier shortly after graduating from college. Perhaps surprisingly, this future professor of medicine proved to be a talented operating surgeon.

In the same war, John Jones, a future Philadelphia surgeon, because of his wide reputation, was asked by the enemy to treat the wounds of captured French general Baron Dieskau (see Chapter 2).

The Revolutionary War (1775–1783)

Washington's First Surgeons General—All Failures

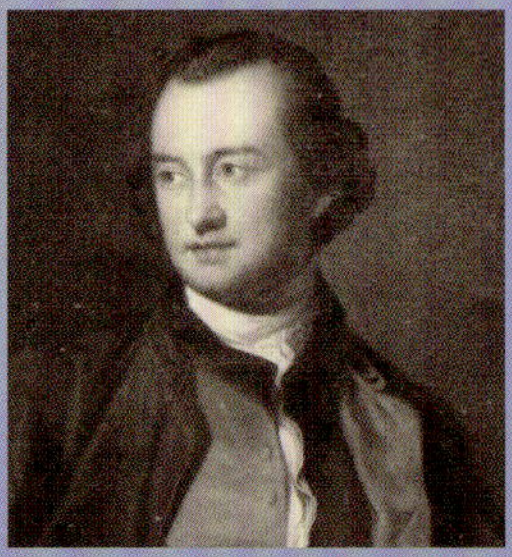

John Morgan
Oct. 1775–Jan. 1777

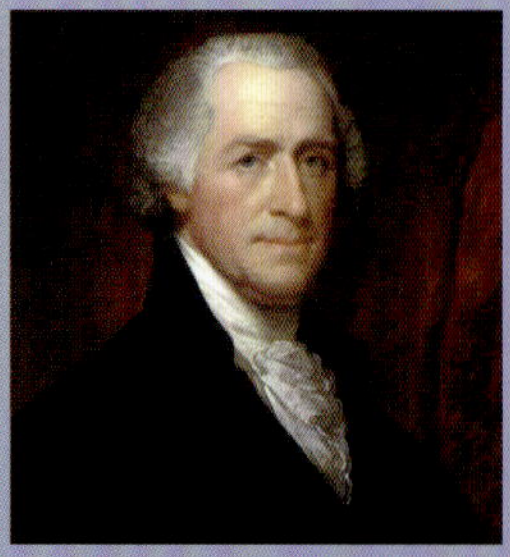

William Shippen Jr.
Apr. 1777–Jan. 1781

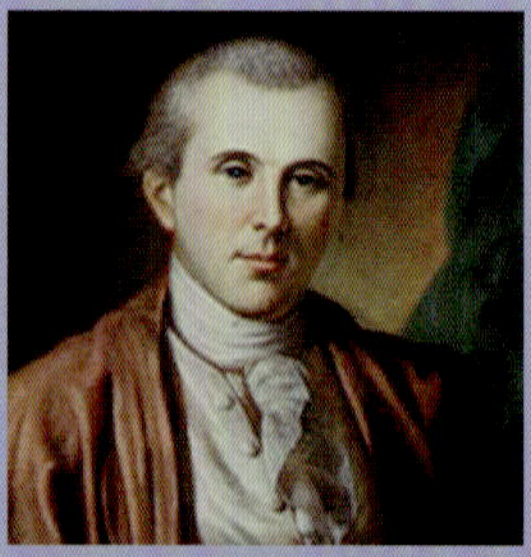

Benjamin Rush
Apr. 1777–Jan. 1778

At the beginning of the Revolutionary War, John Jones published a manual for military surgeons titled *Plain Concise Practical Remarks on the Treatment of Wounds and Fractures.* Although it was not a comprehensive surgical text, it was the first medical book of any kind to be printed in America.

As Washington's surgeon general, John Morgan, William Shippen Jr., and Benjamin Rush served in sequence. All of them made a mess of the job and were fired, forced to resign, or court-martialed (see Chapter 1).

On the positive side, Caspar Wistar, because he was a Quaker, declined to fight but volunteered as a nurse during the Battle of Germantown. That experience inspired him to be a doctor. Although he is usually categorized as a medical man, his longest university appointment by far was in the Department of Surgery. He was adjunct professor and Shippen's assistant for seventeen years. As Shippen's career declined and he became less active, Wistar probably gave more of the surgery lectures than the Chairman did (see chapter 2).

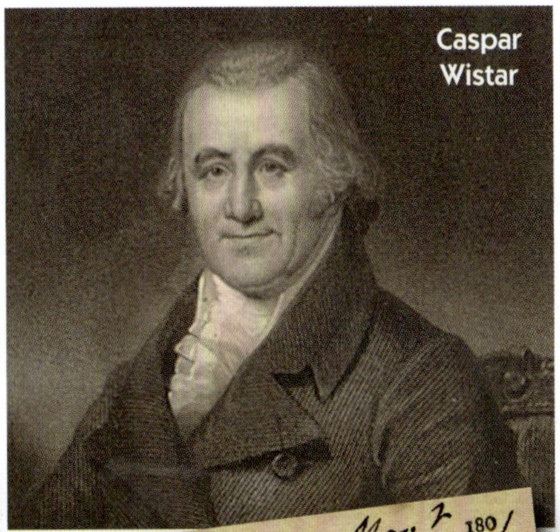
Caspar Wistar

Bones of giant sloth

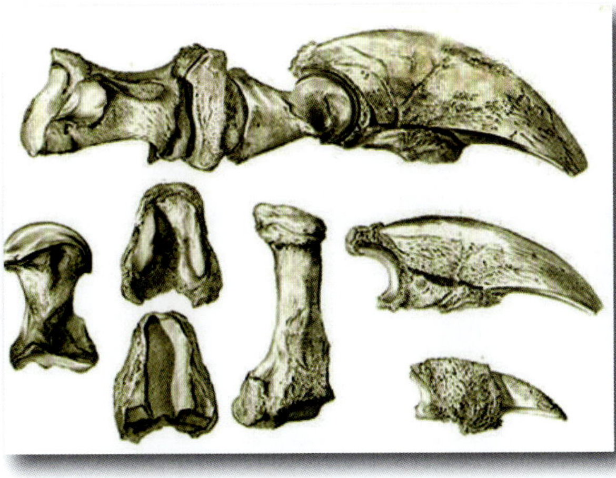

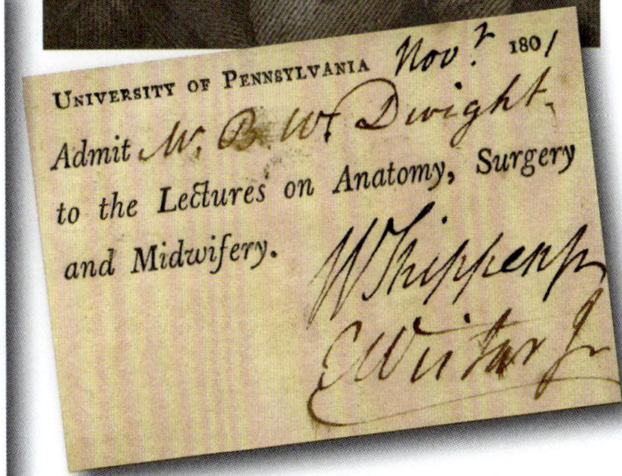
University of Pennsylvania Nov 2 1801
Admit Mr. B. Wt Dwight,
to the Lectures on Anatomy, Surgery
and Midwifery.
W Shippen Jr
C Wistar Jr

Admission ticket to student lectures on anatomy, surgery, and midwifery by William Shippen and Caspar Wistar.

At Pennsylvania Hospital, John Jones coaches Wistar in surgery, but Wistar never becomes confident in the OR

Wistar is an expert anatomist and writes the first US textbook on anatomy, *A System of Anatomy*

Wistar is probably best at anthropology. The bones shown here were sent to him by his friend Thomas Jefferson who thought they might be from a giant lion. Wistar figures out that they are instead from an extinct giant sloth

Although several novels and a recent television series portray Peggy Shippen and John Andre as lovers, there is no evidence that they are more than friends and conspirators

Although he betrayed America to their cause, the British never respect or trust Benedict Arnold

British Occupation of Philadelphia (1777–1778)

During the British occupation of Philadelphia, the complicated relationships between supporters of the revolution and British loyalists led to confusion and changing sides. This came to a climax that involved medical school faculty members and their families. William Shippen's seventeen-year-old cousin, Peggy, whose father and family were confirmed British loyalists, established a close friendship

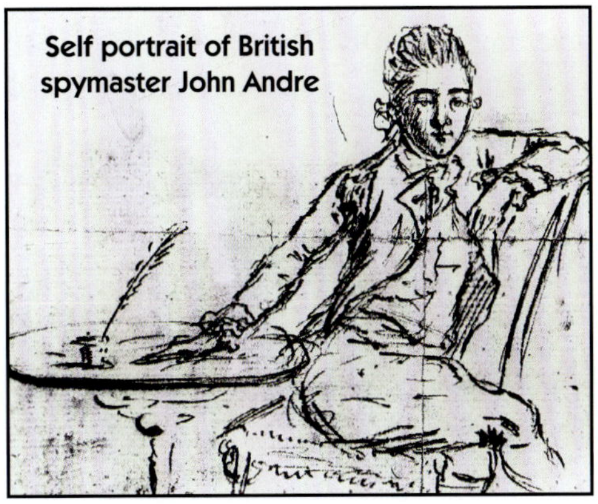
Self portrait of British spymaster John Andre

1780 (July)
Washington places Benedict Arnold in charge of the American fort at West Point

(September)
Arnold's plot discovered. He escapes

(October)
John Andre hanged

1781
Arnold as Brigadier General commands British troops in several battles

1782
After his treachery, Arnold is not trusted by the British in America; he soon moves to England

(and perhaps something more) with the handsome British spymaster, John Andre. When the British abandoned Philadelphia in June 1778, Peggy Shippen stayed in touch with Andre, although she married Benedict Arnold in April 1779. Soon after this, Benedict Arnold and John Andre began planning to turn over the American fort and garrison at West Point to the British.[1] Peggy Shippen was the conduit for their communications. In September 1780, the plot was discovered when Andre was caught with papers exposing their plans. Andre was hanged as a spy, but Benedict Arnold avoided capture, escaping to British-held New York and then to Canada where he was given a commission in the British army as a brigadier general. He successfully led several battles for the British before going to England in 1782.

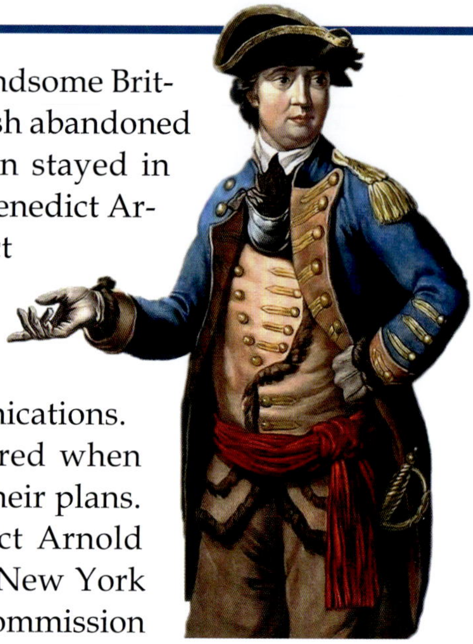

Benedict Arnold

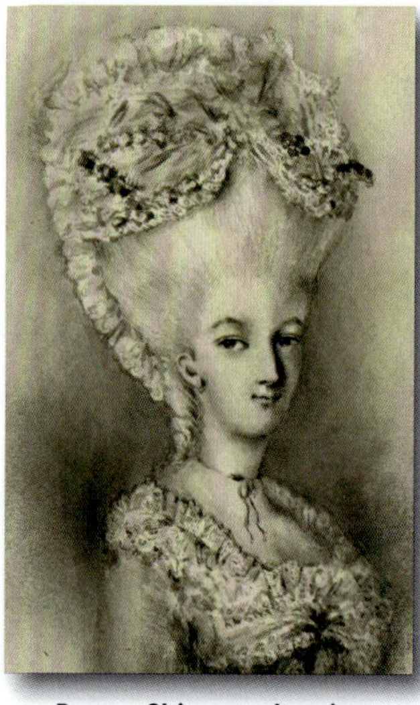

Peggy Shippen drawing by John Andre

Peggy Shippen avoided blame for her husband's treachery by feigning hysteria and claiming innocence during her interrogation. She was allowed to join her husband. Her important role in the plot remained hidden for 150 years until papers of British General Henry Clinton revealed it.

A number of the medical school's faculty were Loyalists. This was patently true of the provost William Smith. It was also true of Adam Kuhn, professor of materia medica, who refused to sign the oath of allegiance to the revolution and therefore was forced to spend the next several years in the West Indies. John Morgan also had Loyalist tendencies. He wrote an essay outlining the advantages of America remaining a British colony. During the city's occupation, he got along very well with the British and was observed walking arm-in-arm with British officers. When the occupation ended and the British prepared to leave Philadelphia, he acknowledged that he was tempted to go with them and at one point had decided to do it.[2] Instead, he eventually decided to stay in Philadelphia and continue battling with Congress to reverse the charges that led to his dismissal as Washington's surgeon general. Although it's doubtful that he aspired to regain his position as surgeon general, he was committed to continue his barrage of charges against his enemy, William Shippen.

Fortunately, for his reputation, there is no suggestion that William Shippen participated in or even knew about Benedict Arnold's plot. His branch of the Shippen family was known to be in firm support of the revolution.[3]

War of 1812 (1812–1815)

During the War of 1812, William Edmonds Horner, later a Penn anatomist, surgeon, and dean, interrupted his studies at Penn medical school to volunteer as an Army surgeon in battles near the Canadian border.

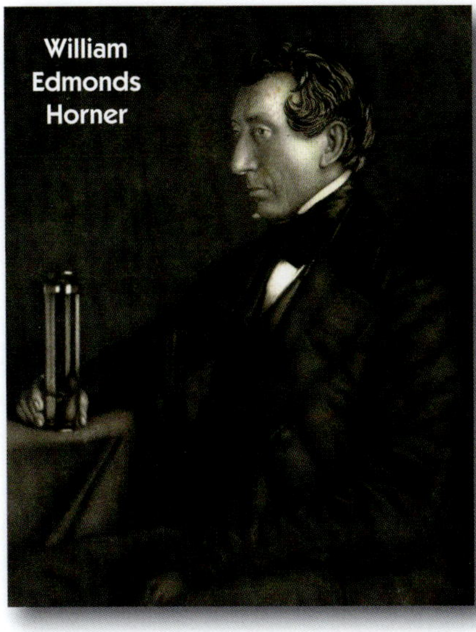

William Gibson, chairman of surgery at the University of Maryland, and soon to move to Penn as Physick's successor, was called to care for the wounded American hero of the war, Winfield Scott. During the war and a riot in Baltimore, Gibson treated a patient who had a gunshot wound of the groin. To stop the bleeding, he ligated the common iliac artery. Collateral circulation allowed the leg to remain viable. This was one of the first vascular procedures done in America (see Chapter 4).

1838
Joseph Barnes obtains MD at Penn and trains for a year at Blockley. Later becomes US surgeon general

1846
Barnes is head of medicine in US Cavalry when Mexico City is captured

1847
Elisha Kent Kane, graduate of Penn medical school, joins the Army to fight in Mexican-American War. While carrying a secret message from President Polk to General Winfield Scott, he is attacked and wounded. The Mexican general is also wounded and Dr. Kane saves his life and is befriended by the Mexicans. After the war, Kane becomes famous as an Arctic polar explorer

Mexican–American War (April 1846–February 1848)

This was a significant war for westward expansion of the United States. President Polk provoked the war, intending to expand US territory. After an easy victory, the United States took from Mexico half of its large territory, which then became the current US states of Texas, California, Nevada, Utah, New Mexico, and parts of Arizona, Colorado, and Oklahoma. A minor role in the war was played by Joseph Barnes, a Penn surgeon who became important later. Barnes was born in Philadelphia and got his MD from Penn in 1838, after which he trained for a year at Blockley and practiced for a year in Philadelphia. Enlisting in the Army, he served in Florida during the Seminole Wars and, in 1846, participated in the cavalry charge that captured Mexico City. During the Civil War, he became US surgeon general, serving from 1864 to 1882. He attended both Lincoln and Garfield when they were assassinated. His relationship with John Shaw Billings was important (see below).

The Civil War (1861–1865)

In the Civil War, chairman of Penn Surgery, Henry Hollingsworth Smith, was appointed surgeon general for Pennsylvania. His administrative accomplishments allowed efficient evacuation of wounded soldiers, for which he used a fleet of steamships. Agnew, Ashhurst, and John Shaw Billings all served as battlefield surgeons. More than

1861–1863
Agnew directs several Civil War hospitals in Philadelphia

Isaac Israel Hayes, graduate of Penn medical school and famous Arctic explorer, serves as director of surgical service at Satterlee Army Hospital

1,000 Penn alumni, faculty, and students fought in this war, 633 in the Union Army and 553 in the Confederate Army. Ten thousand military hospital beds were located in Philadelphia, the most in any city. Three Penn graduates became surgeons general of the Union army and two as surgeons general of the Confederate forces. Future chairman of Penn Surgery, D. Hayes Agnew, directed or served at three of the war's largest military hospitals which were in Philadelphia: Satterlee (4,500 beds), Mower (3,600 beds), and Hestonville (200 beds). Agnew became famous as a trauma surgeon, particularly for treatment of gunshot wounds. Because of this, he was called on to treat US President Garfield when he was shot by an assassin (see Chapter 7).

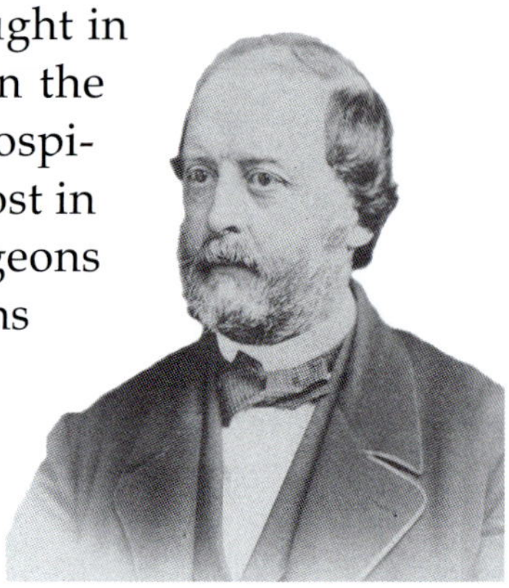
Henry Hollingsworth Smith

Battlefield Surgeons

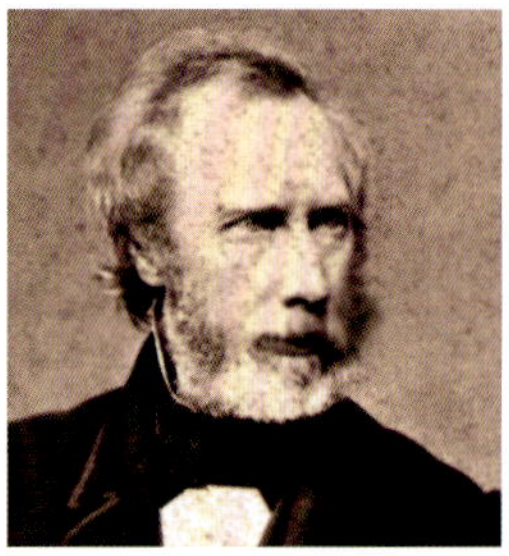
D. Hayes Agnew

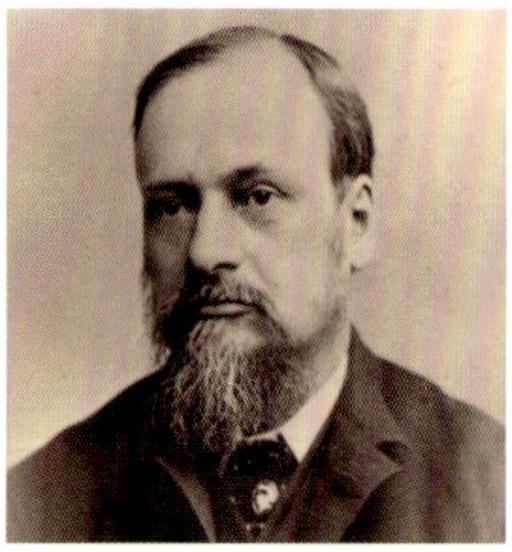
John Ashhurst, Jr.

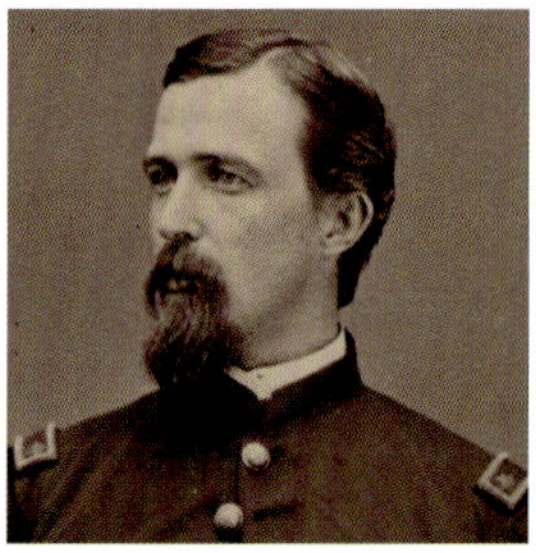
John Shaw Billings

Anesthesia had been famously demonstrated by William Morton and John Warren in 1846, and it was used frequently during the Civil War. Benefits of antisepsis were reported by Joseph Lister in 1865, too late for

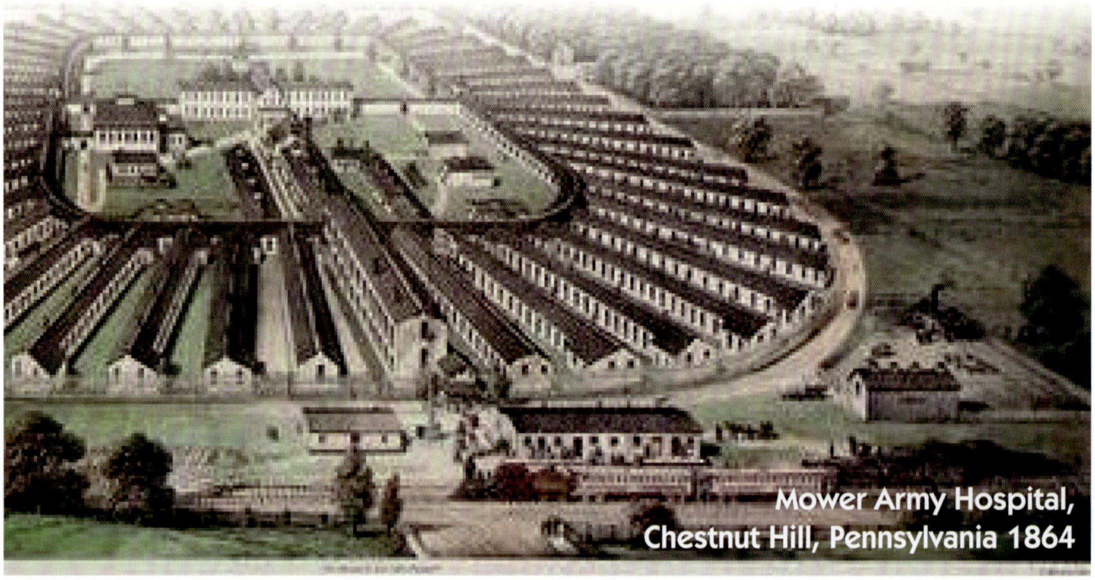
Mower Army Hospital, Chestnut Hill, Pennsylvania 1864

use during the Civil War. The most important medical contribution related to the war was made by a battlefield surgeon who later became HUP's director and a Penn department chair. Though he was not very successful in these roles, his story is well worth telling. He was one of the most influential surgeons this country has ever produced.

US Surgeon General Joseph Barnes is important in the establishment of the Surgeon General's library. In addition to appointing John Shaw Billings as director of the library, he strongly supports him throughout his career

Born in 1838, John Shaw Billings graduated from college at Miami University in Oxford, Ohio, and in 1858 from the Medical College of Ohio in Cincinnati.[4] Then as a Civil War battlefield surgeon, he participated actively in at least three major battles, including Chancellorsville and Gettysburg, and was said to be one of the Army's most skillful surgeons. When the Civil War ended, Billings stayed in the Army. He was assigned to the office of the surgeon general where he would remain until he retired from the Army thirty-one years later in 1895.

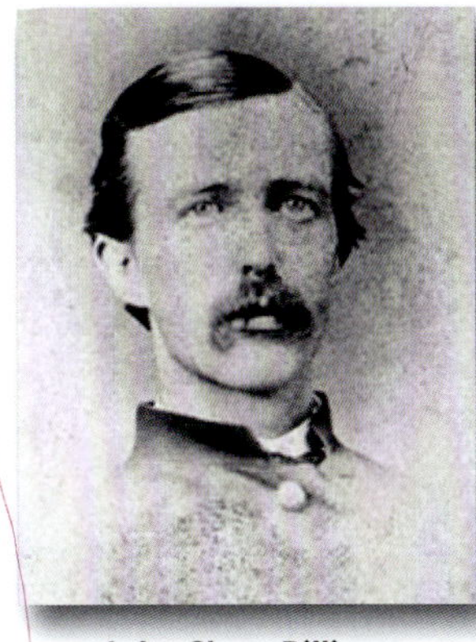

John Shaw Billings

In 1865, there were no guides to the medical literature, so a search for information required a personal visit to each library. Billings would change that. He was given the assignment of expanding the library of the surgeon general's office, a project that eventually led to the development of the National Library of Medicine. He was also assigned to visit and inspect the nation's Marine hospitals, and as a result of this study, he became one of the leading experts on

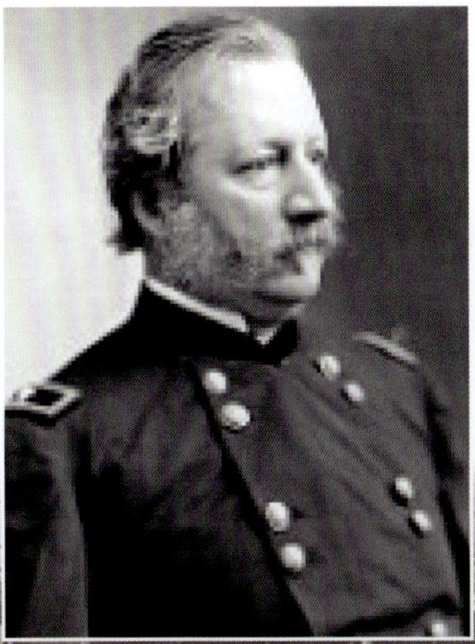

Major General Joseph K. Barnes

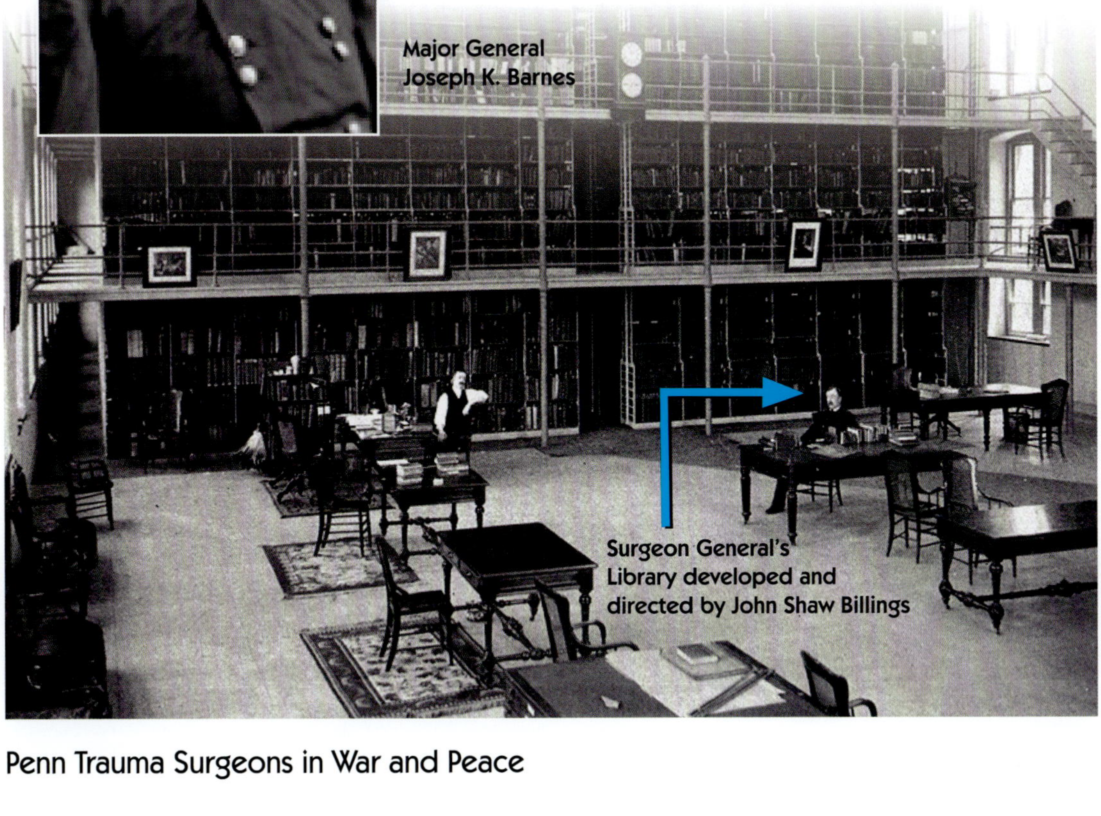

Surgeon General's Library developed and directed by John Shaw Billings

1865
Lincoln is assassinated, Barnes attends him

1881
President James Garfield is assassinated. Barnes and Agnew attend him

1889
John Hopkins Hospital opens, designed by Billings

hospitals, hospital construction, and public health. In 1867, he was assigned by US Surgeon General Joseph Barnes to work full-time at the Surgeon General's Library and to function as its director. He converted this small library into the world's largest and most complete library of basic scientific literature. Within six years, he had grown the library from 1,800 volumes to more than 25,000, and by the time he retired from the Army in 1895, the library had grown to nearly 90,000 volumes. The library was first known as the Army Medical Library and then the Armed Forces Library, but Billings made it available, not just to military personnel, but also to civilians. In 1956, it became the National Library of Medicine. As important as or more so than building the collection of volumes was Billings's creation of its index. It was arranged alphabetically by both authors and subjects and published monthly to include not only books but also periodicals and all new publications. Eventually this became Medline. It is recognized as one of the greatest contributions of the nineteenth century to the infrastructure of science and medicine.

At the same time as Billings was working on the library and its index, he was becoming one of the country's experts on hygiene and on hospitals and their construction. In addition, he designed and supervised the building of Johns Hopkins Hospital. Innovative aspects included its unique dome and its electrical and ventilation systems that were copied by many.

Billings was also crucially important in establishing the vision and goals of Johns Hopkins, recommending that the hospital should be part of the medical school and university, a concept unusual for the time. While he was visiting and studying European hospital designs, he met Dr. William Welch in Germany. He chose Welch as the first faculty member of Johns

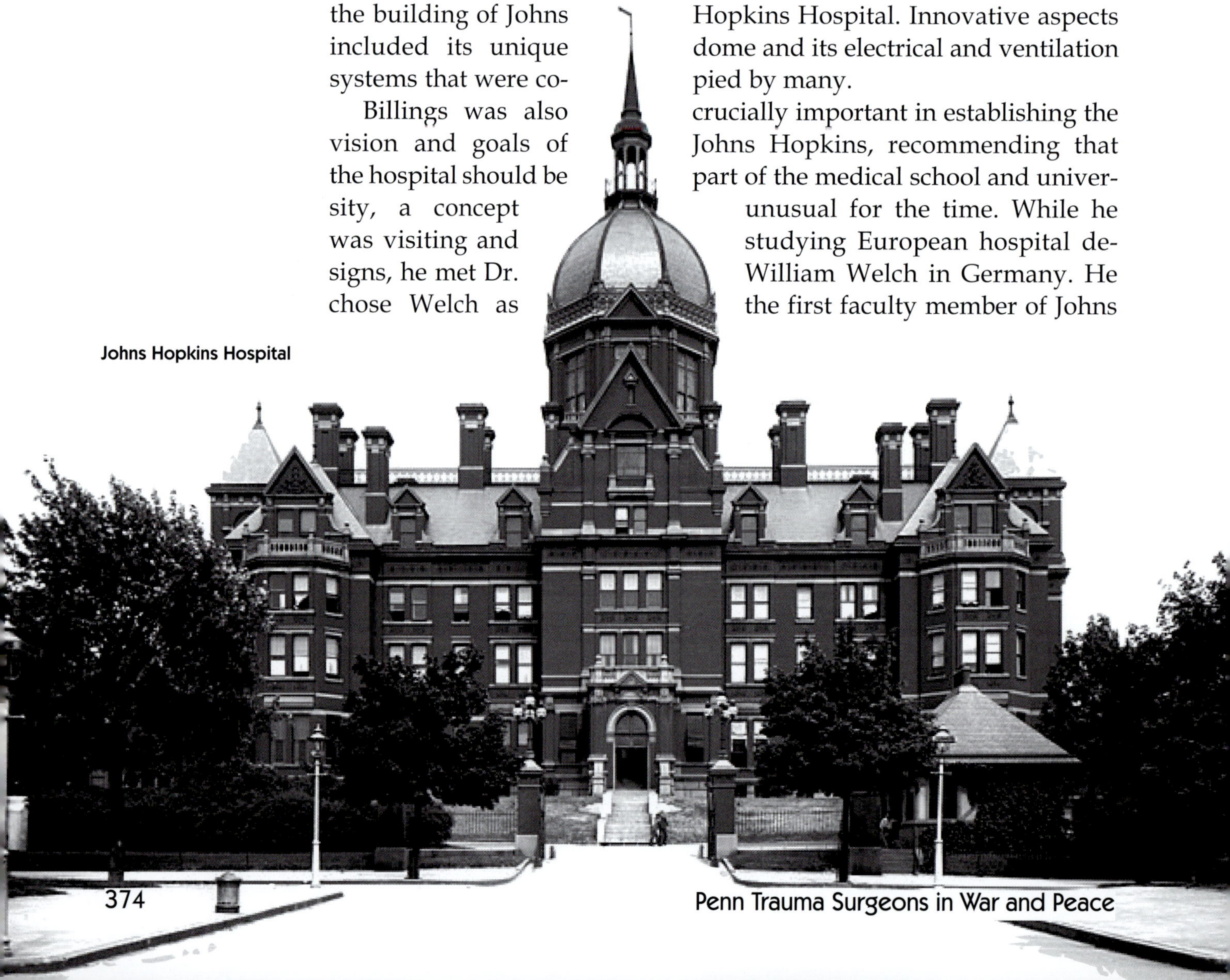

Johns Hopkins Hospital

Hopkins Hospital, chief of pathology, and subsequently the first dean when the medical school opened four years later. Billings and Hopkins University president Daniel Coit Gilman worked together in choosing the staff and faculty of the hospital, including William Osler, who left Penn in 1889 to become Hopkins' first chief of medicine. Welch then recommended William Halsted for chief of surgery.

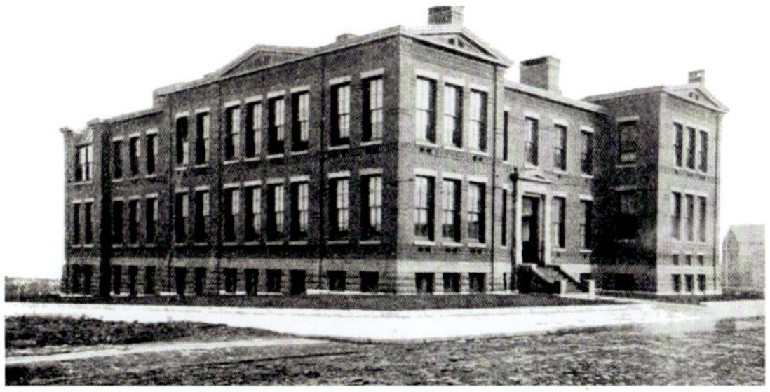

Penn's Hygiene Building designed by John Shaw Billings

In 1889, William Pepper Jr., Provost of the University of Pennsylvania, offered Billings a position as chairman of Penn's Department of Hygiene and director of the University Hospital (HUP). He also asked Billings to design a building to house the new Department of Hygiene. Pepper and Billings agreed that for the next three years, Billings would need to spend only one day a week in Philadelphia, and then from 1892 on, he would be required to work full-time in Philadelphia. Billings accepted the offer. The building he designed for the Hygiene Institute was opened in 1892, but Billings did not actually move to Philadelphia until 1895 when he officially resigned from the Army. In Philadelphia as director of the Institute for Hygiene, he delivered a series of lectures on public health. The curriculum also included biostatistics and epidemiology. Unfortunately, these were topics that interested few medical students of the day and few ever attended his lectures. Billings also designed a second building for clinical research called the Pepper Clinical Laboratory, named after William Pepper's father. It opened in 1895 for training investigators and conducting clinical research. Highly successful, it was the first such program in the country.

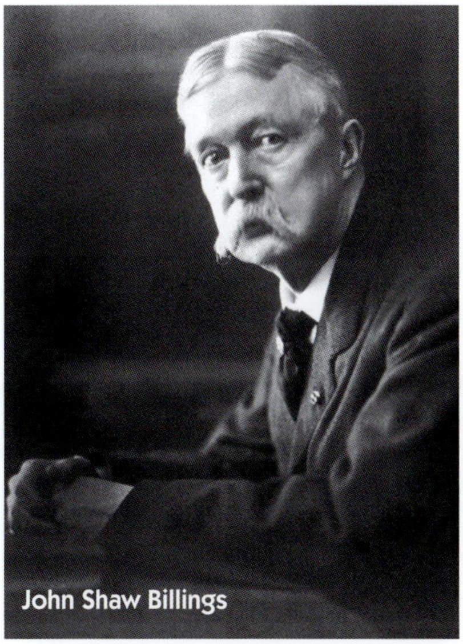

John Shaw Billings

Disappointed by his reception in Philadelphia after spending only eight months living there, he accepted a new challenge in New York City. The Philadelphia phase of Billings's career appears to have been his only failure.

Billings's New York challenge was to direct the New York Public Library and oversee construction of its building. He accomplished this by using the Samuel Tilden fortune to combine the great Astor and Lennox libraries. The famous building he designed for housing them remains a

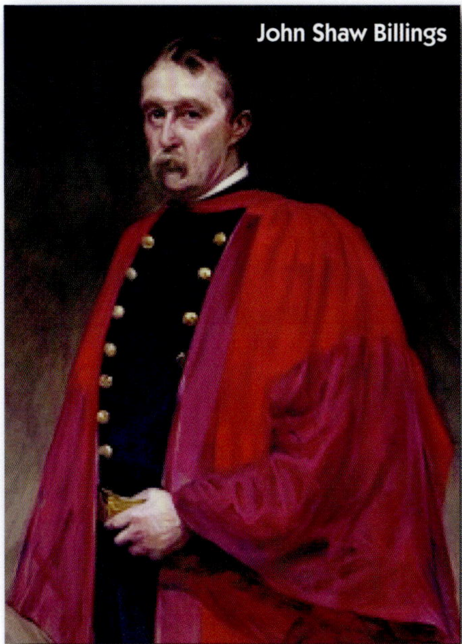

John Shaw Billings

1889
John Shaw Billings accepts Provost Pepper's offer of a Penn appointment as professor of hygiene and director of HUP

1892
Billings designs Hygiene Building, teaches course at Penn

1895
Billings designs Pepper Labs Building

1895
Billings moves to New York as director of New York Public Library and designs its famous building

1913
Death of Billings

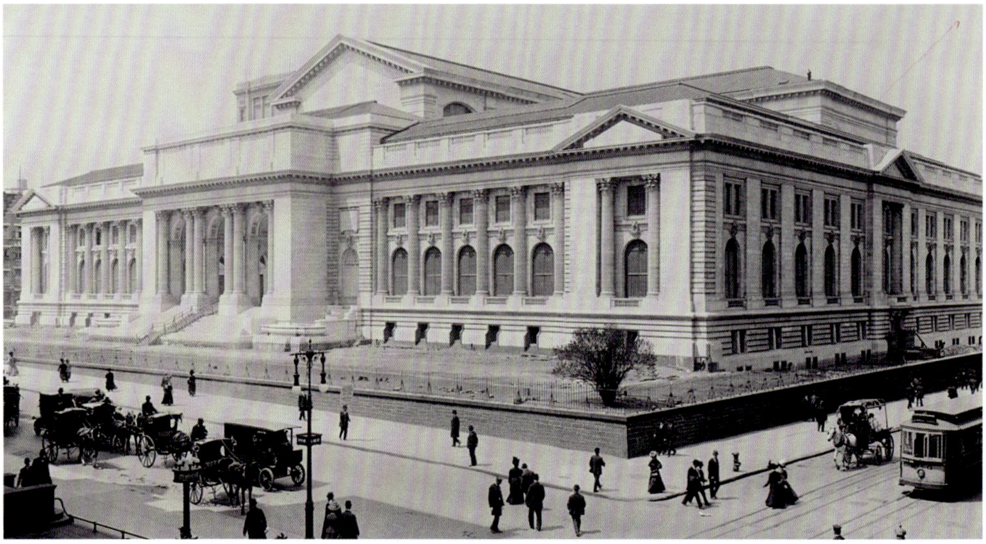

The New York Public Library during late-stage construction in 1908.

landmark on the corner of 5th Avenue and 42nd Street. Bringing order out of chaos, Billings created the New York Public Library system with its more than two million volumes and fifty branch libraries.

In 1913, Billings died of pneumonia after surgery for a urinary calculus. Many believe that Billings, with his many contributions—particularly the National Library of Medicine and the Index Medicus—was the most important surgeon this country has ever produced.

The Spanish–American War (April–August 1898)

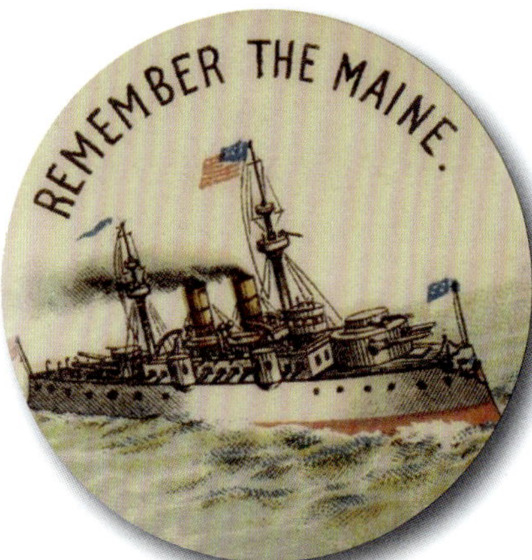

In the United States in 1898, there was a strong public sentiment in favor of Cuban and Filipino independence from Spain. On February 15, a mysterious (and still unexplained) explosion sank the USS *Maine* which was stationed in Havana Harbor. This helped propel the United States into war with Spain. Although President McKinley initially tried to smooth things over with Spain, the loss of 260 Americans on the *Maine* was inflammatory. Besides, he already had his sights on the United States' possession of Cuba. Yellow journalists of Hearst newspapers were quick to blame Spain for the explosion and called for war which ensued in April. "Remember the Maine" and Teddy Roosevelt charging up San Juan Hill with his Rough Riders rapidly became part of American legend.

As a result of American victory in what US Secretary of State John Hay called a "splendid little war," the United States acquired Guam,

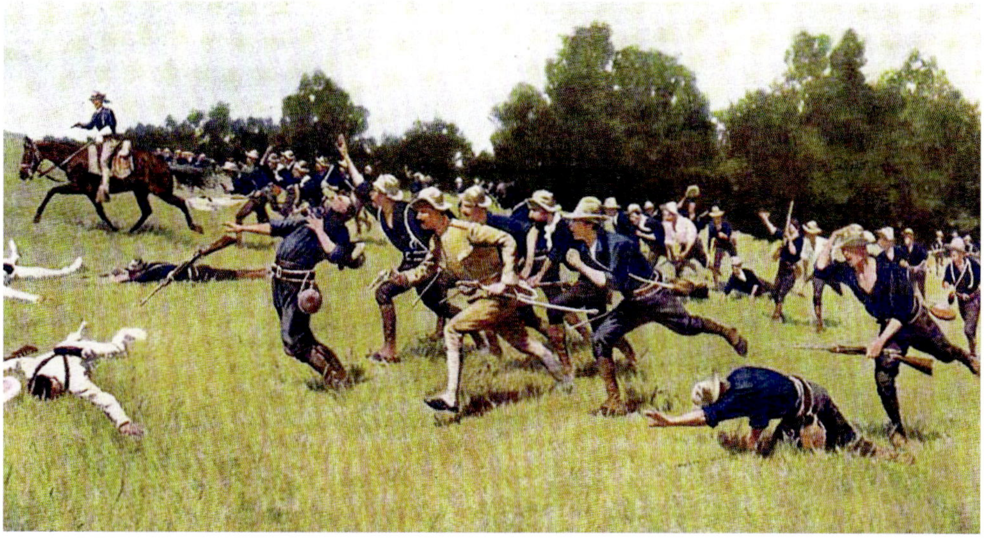

Charge of the Rough Riders at San Juan Hill

1898
(April 24–August 8)
The ten-week "splendid little war"

Three thousand Americans die in the war, mostly from typhoid

Puerto Rico, and the Philippine islands.

In this war, the doctors, including those from Penn, were very important. Three thousand Americans lost their lives in the war, 90 percent from typhoid and yellow fever rather than from battle wounds. Penn surgeon and future chairman, Edward Martin, had a prominent role in preventing more deaths. A battalion leader, Martin became one of the war's heroes by developing and enforcing sanitary precautions that stamped out the typhoid epidemic. He sent many of the severe cases to HUP for treatment by special train.

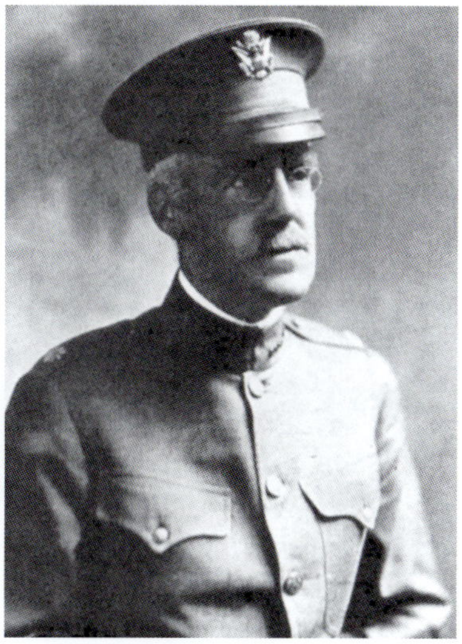

Edward Martin

World War I (1914–1918)

(US involvement: April 1917–November 1918)

The United States declared war on Germany in April 1917. Months before this, preparations had been made for the University of Pennsylvania's unit, Base Hospital 20. Chosen as director of Penn's Base Hospital 20 was John B. Carnett, associate in surgery. He appointed Eldridge Eliason, instructor in surgery, as the chief of the surgical service and George M. Piersoll, an associate in medicine, as chief of the medical service. All told, there were twenty-two medical officers, sixty-five nurses, and 153 enlisted men, essentially all Penn faculty, students, alumni, or healthcare professionals. They arrived in France in May 1918 and set up the hospital at Chatel-Guyon, a resort town that was halfway between Paris and Marseille. The hospital operated out of the

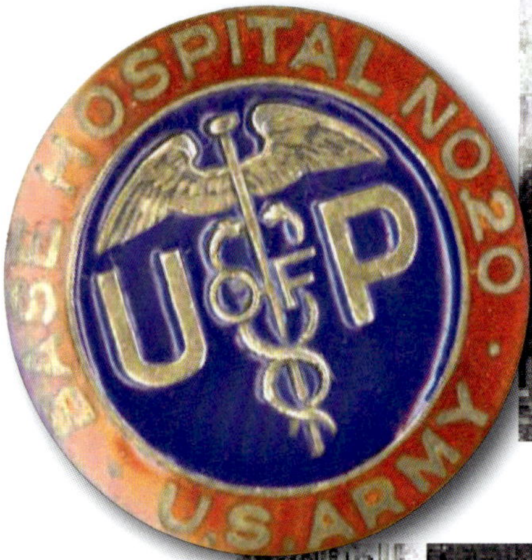

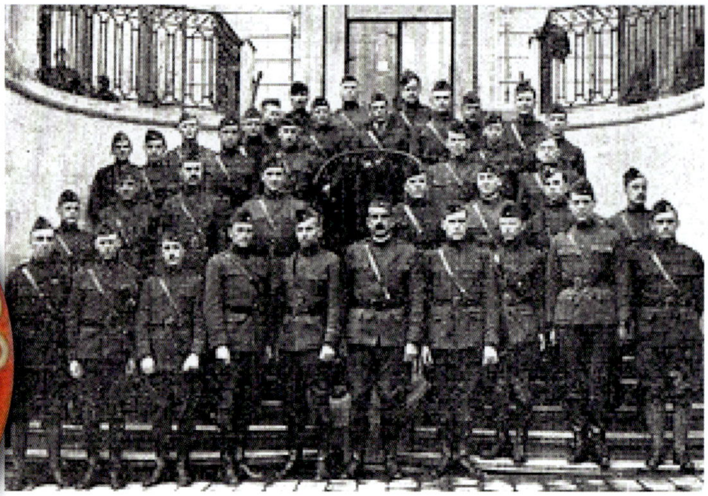

Penn Staff of Base Hospital 20

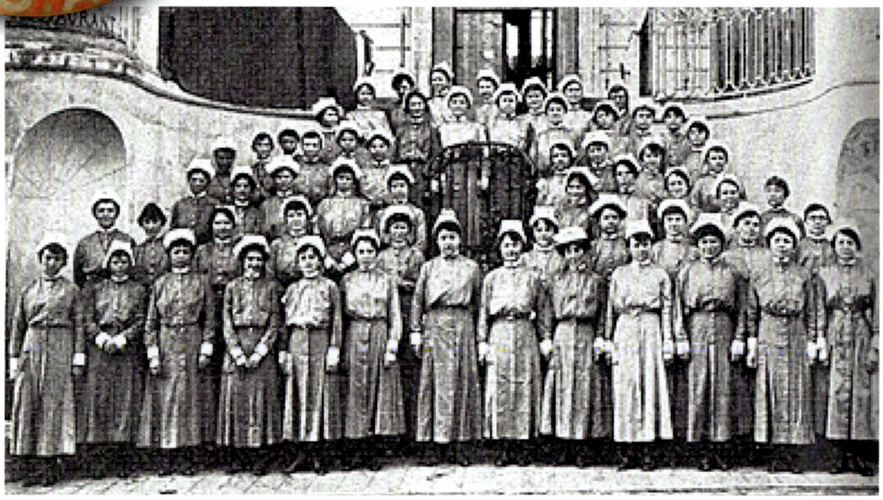

Penn Nurses of Base Hospital 20

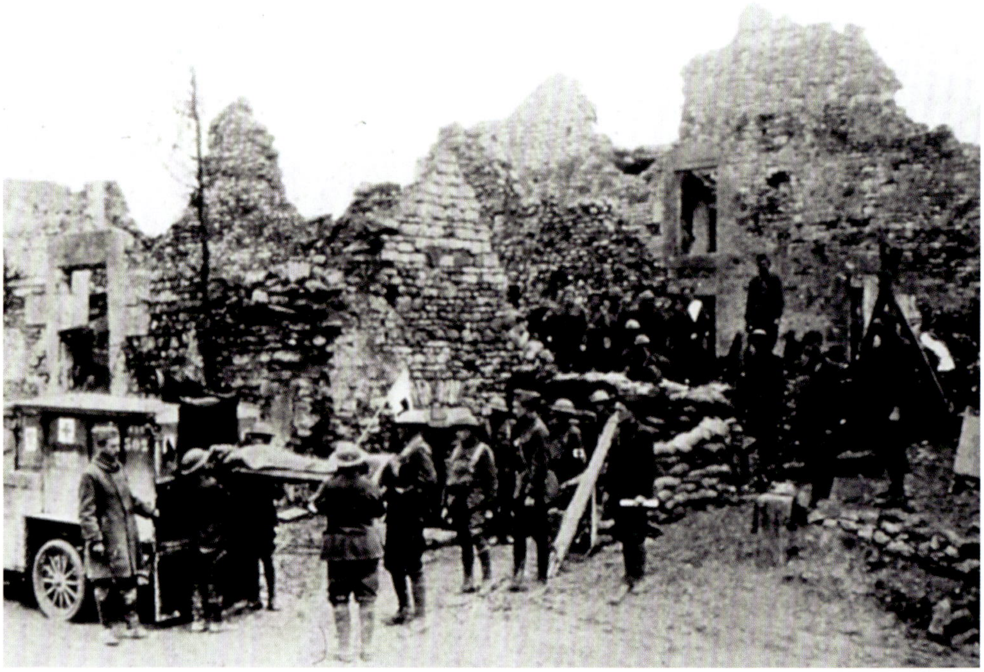

Transporting the wounded.

resort's hotels, occupying thirty-three buildings and eventually having 2,000 beds. During the eight months that Base Hospital 20 existed, there were 4,000 surgical cases, 3,500 medical and gas patients, and 1,500 others. Remarkably, there were only sixty-five deaths.[5] The hospital was particularly well-known for its treatment of tuberculosis and influenza.

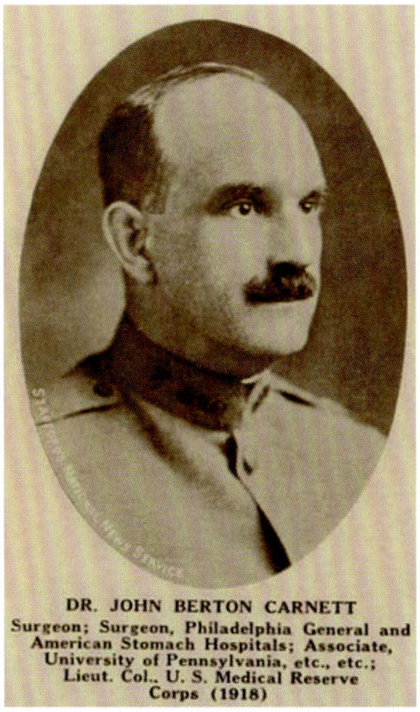
DR. JOHN BERTON CARNETT
Surgeon; Surgeon, Philadelphia General and American Stomach Hospitals; Associate, University of Pennsylvania, etc., etc.; Lieut. Col., U. S. Medical Reserve Corps (1918)

Commander of Penn's Base 20

John Berton Carnett, the hospital director, was one of the unsung heroes of the war.[6] As a Penn student, he was a well-known athlete, having been on the crew and for three years, a star of the football team. He supported himself during his education by writing for the newspapers. He graduated in 1899 with high honors. He served a two-year internship plus four months as chief resident at HUP where he became surgical assistant to J. William White and Edward Martin. He rapidly developed a big practice in part because he was so well-known locally as a football player.

When the US entered World War I, Carnett was appointed director of Base 20 Hospital. He had responsibility for organizing the hospital, recruiting its staff, and also for raising funds since during World War I, the government did not provide financial support for overseas hospitals. Soon after he established the hospital in France, Carnett, rather than remaining a hospital administrator, went to the front lines as part of an operating team and mobile hospital. When armistice came, he returned to the Base Hospital

1918
During the Spanish flu epidemic, 500 million people are infected worldwide. Twenty to fifty million die including 675,000 Americans. The epidemic's impact is minimized to maintain focus on the war

Within seventy-two hours of the epidemic's start, all thirty-one Philadelphia hospitals are filled. Schools and theaters are closed. In two weeks, there are 4,500 deaths

1919
President Wilson gets the flu and is impaired by it during the Paris Peace Conference. He never fully recovers

After his stroke, his wife manages many of the president's duties

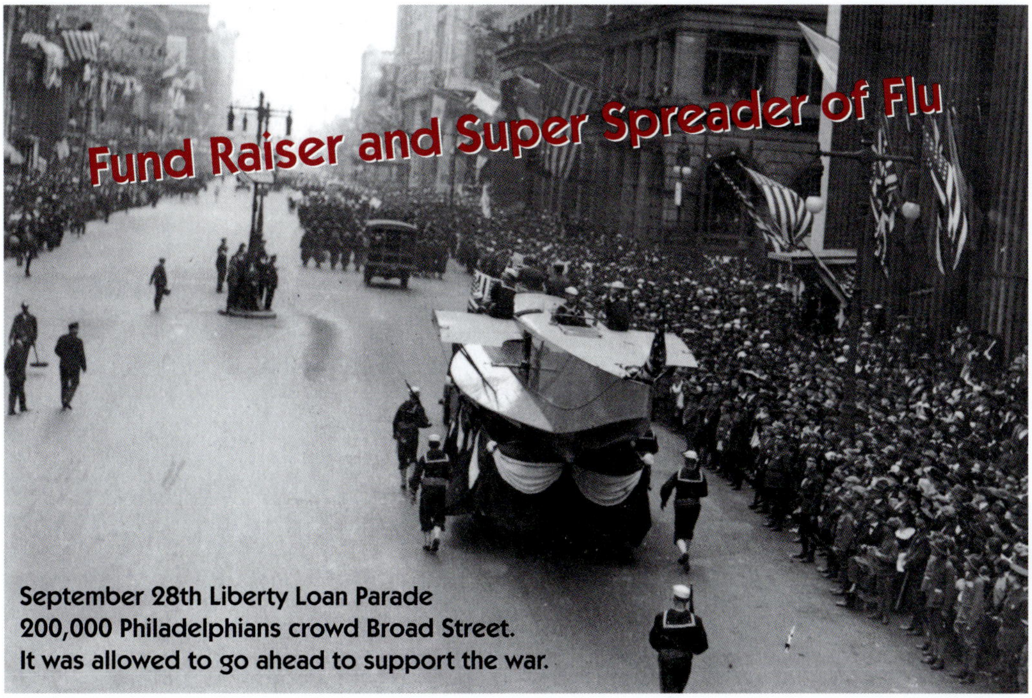
Fund Raiser and Super Spreader of Flu

September 28th Liberty Loan Parade
200,000 Philadelphians crowd Broad Street.
It was allowed to go ahead to support the war.

1934–1936
George Leib Harrison's $2.7 million endowment is originally intended for John Berton Carnett's research

Carnett dies before Harrison

Harrison dies and endowment is redirected to Penn Surgery research

where he was in charge of organizing the unit to go home.[7] Remarkably, when he returned to HUP, expecting to be welcomed as a hero and reappointed to the staff, Penn Surgery chairman John B. Deaver refused to take him back.[8] This was almost certainly because Carnett had been an assistant to J. William White with whom Deaver had an extremely bitter relationship (see Chapters 9 and 11).

Near the end of the war, retired surgery chairman J. William White organized a 180-bed American Ambulance Hospital in Paris. Charles Frazier directed a 950-bed military hospital at Cape May, New Jersey. The young I. S. Ravdin served briefly there in a minor role.

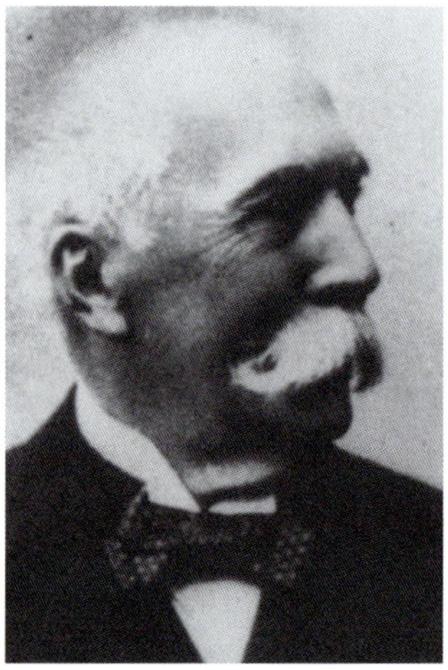

George Leib Harrison

Deprived by Deaver of a HUP appointment, Carnett was allowed to practice at Graduate Hospital. He soon became a professor in the Graduate School as well as vice dean. His interests in surgery included hernias, and he was considered a specialist in sliding hernias. He also developed a reputation for treating subdeltoid bursitis and intercostal neuralgia. He was known to be ruggedly honest and straightforward. He belonged to local but not national societies and divided all his attention between his practice and his family. He was the personal physician of the wealthy George Leib Harrison. Harrison was so grateful and fond of Carnett that he named him as the recipient of a $2.7 million endowment for research.[9] This plan did not work out because Car-

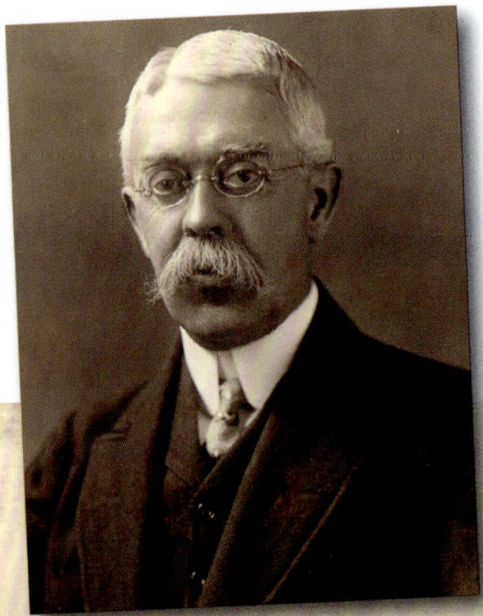

J. William White
Although terminally ill, he funds and directs the American Hospital.

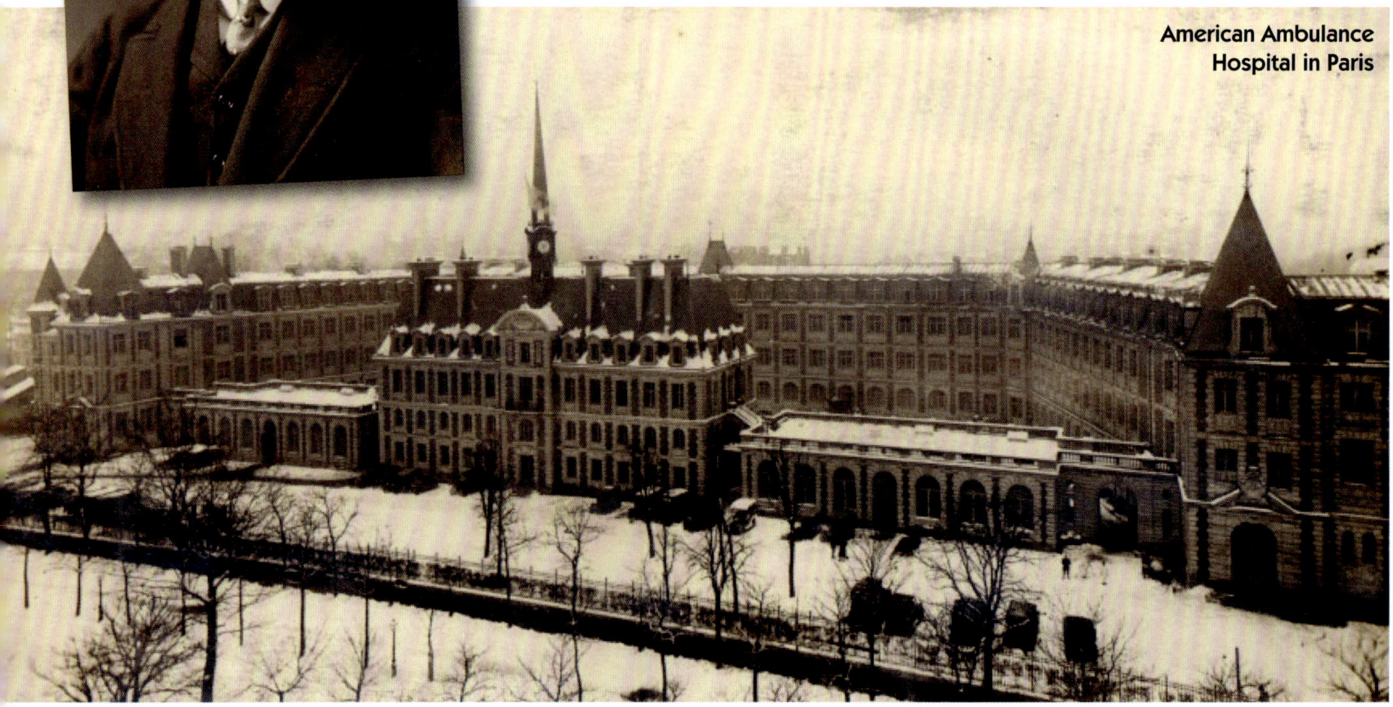

American Ambulance Hospital in Paris

nett died in 1934 before Harrison, who lived for another year. Therefore, the endowment was redirected to the research of the Department of Surgery of the University of Pennsylvania where I. S. Ravdin, as director of research, took control of it (see Chapter 14).[10]

1941 (Dec. 7)
Japanese bomb Pearl Harbor

Secretaries of the Army and Navy send I. S. Ravdin to size up status of medical facilities and care of US soliders

Ravdin travels on a small plane navigated by the stars. In a rush to leave, it is forgotten to load water. Ravdin gets by on a bottle of whiskey

He finds the medical facilities first rate

World War II (1939–1945)

(US Involvement: 1941–1945)

On December 8, 1941, the day after the Japanese brought the US into the war by bombing Pearl Harbor, I. S. Ravdin was sent there to evaluate the care of the wounded.[11] He found that they were receiving good care by General Heaton and his colleagues. Making friends with Heaton was useful later when the two of them shared in the care of President Eisenhower who had developed intestinal obstruction from Crohn's disease.

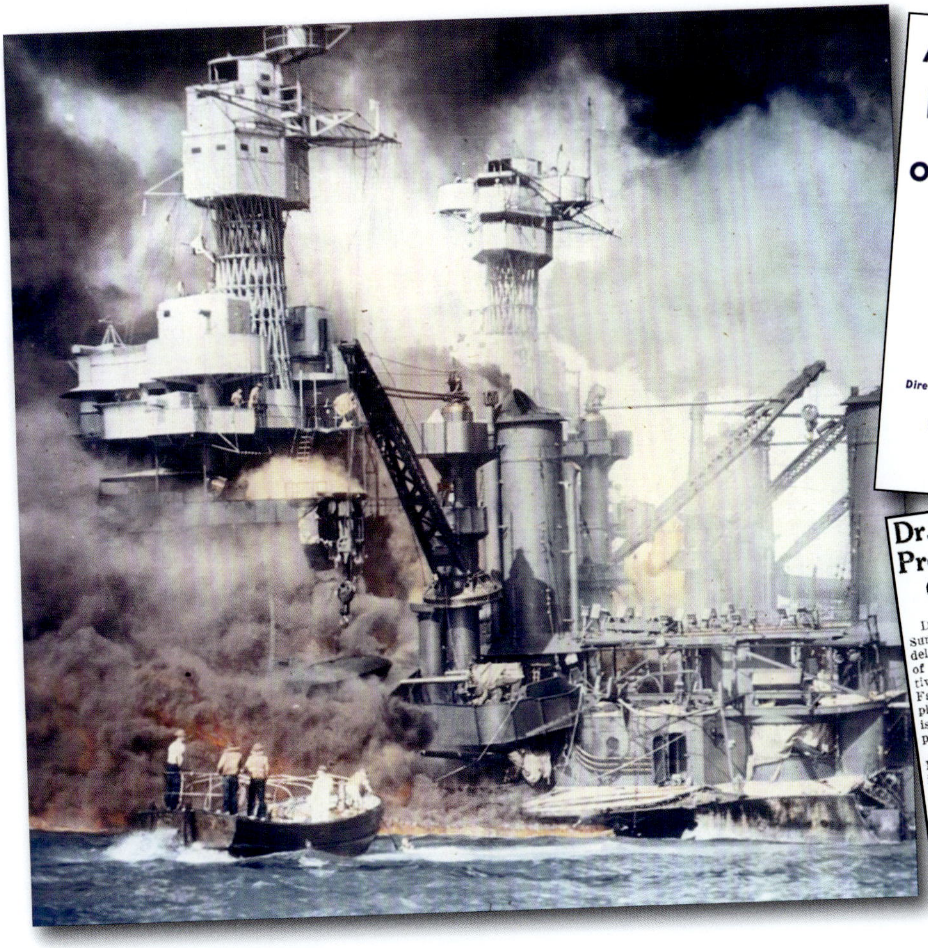

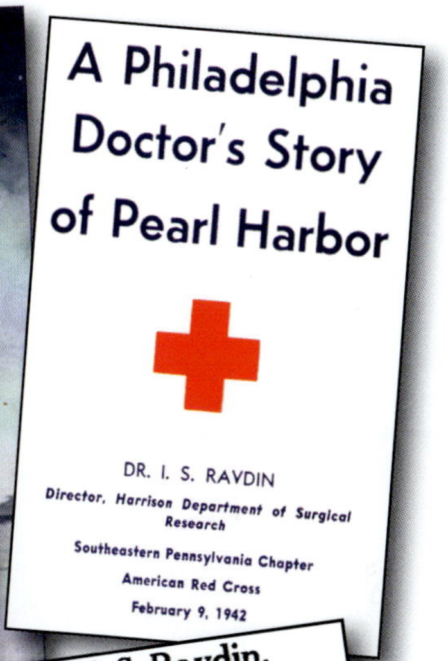

A Philadelphia Doctor's Story of Pearl Harbor

DR. I. S. RAVDIN

Director, Harrison Department of Surgical Research

Southeastern Pennsylvania Chapter

American Red Cross

February 9, 1942

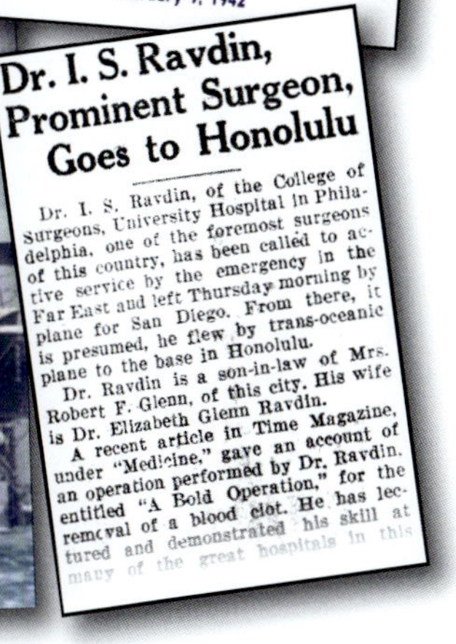

Dr. I. S. Ravdin, Prominent Surgeon, Goes to Honolulu

Dr. I. S. Ravdin, of the College of Surgeons, University Hospital in Philadelphia, one of the foremost surgeons of this country, has been called to active service by the emergency in the Far East and left Thursday morning by plane for San Diego. From there, it is presumed, he flew by trans-oceanic plane to the base in Honolulu.

Dr. Ravdin is a son-in-law of Mrs. Robert F. Glenn, of this city. His wife is Dr. Elizabeth Glenn Ravdin.

A recent article in Time Magazine, under "Medicine," gave an account of an operation performed by Dr. Ravdin, entitled "A Bold Operation," for the removal of a blood clot. He has lectured and demonstrated his skill at many of the great hospitals in this

The story of HUP's World War II 20th General Hospital is extensively covered in Chapter 14. It was the war's largest military hospital. Its assignment was to support the US invasion of Japanese-occupied northern Burma and care for Army engineers wounded as they built a road through the jungle to supply Chinese allies over land, rather than by dangerous flights to China over the Himalayan Mountains.

Merrill's Marauders

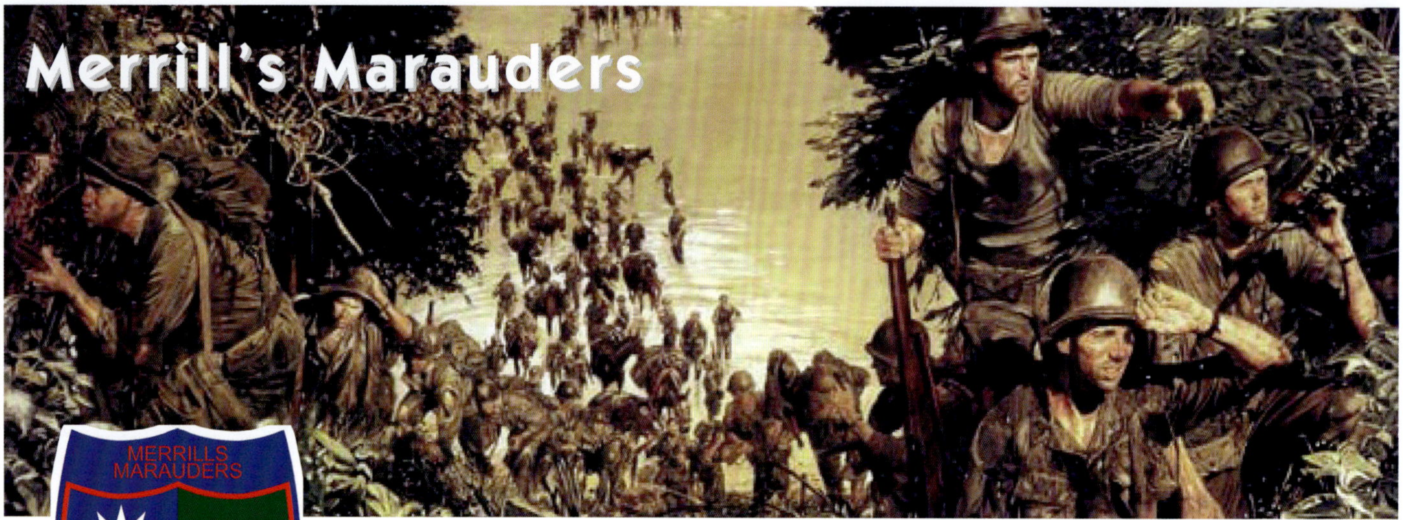

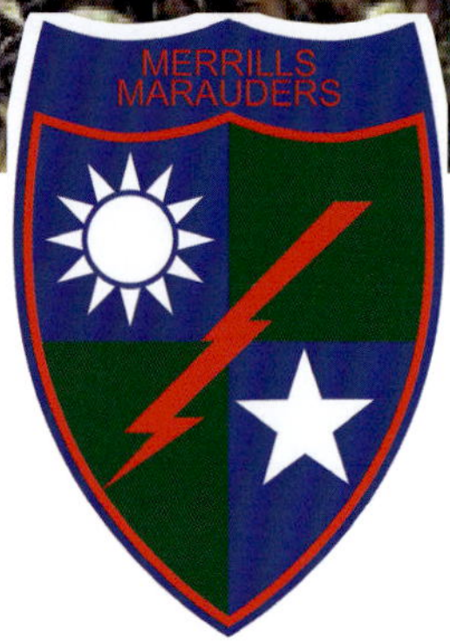

The famous Merrill's Marauders, a US commando force, fought behind enemy lines to protect the road and its builders and to harass the Japanese. The Marauders suffered almost 100 percent casualties. When wounded, they were cared for at the 20th General Hospital. The American commander Joe Stillwell, the Supreme Allied Commander Lord Mountbatten, and General Merrill himself all become patients at the hospital.

1943–1944
Ravdin's wartime staff after the war become HUP's leaders in Surgery and other departments

Also described in Chapters 13 and 14 is the extensive service in both the Army and Navy that was provided by Penn surgeons and Eliason and Ravdin residents.

In part due to Ravdin's mastery of stagecraft, the story of his 20th General Hospital captured most of the newspaper and subsequent coverage of Penn medicine's World War II history. Ravdin and his unit were certainly entitled to much praise. But the stories of many others deserve mention. Credit was due not only to professors of surgery and generals, but also to nurses, soldiers, sailors, and airmen, as well as to their leaders.

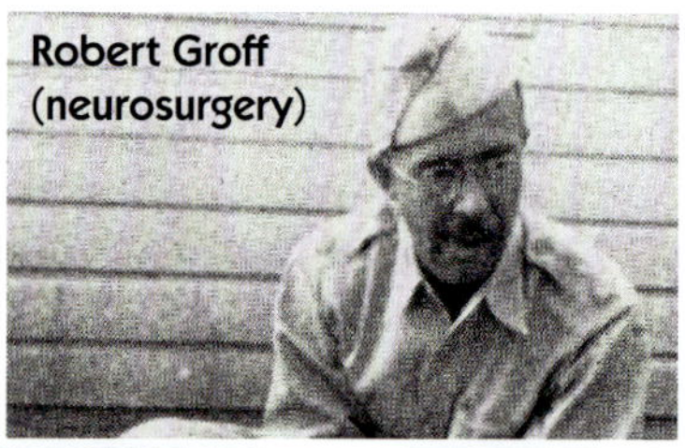
Robert Groff (neurosurgery)

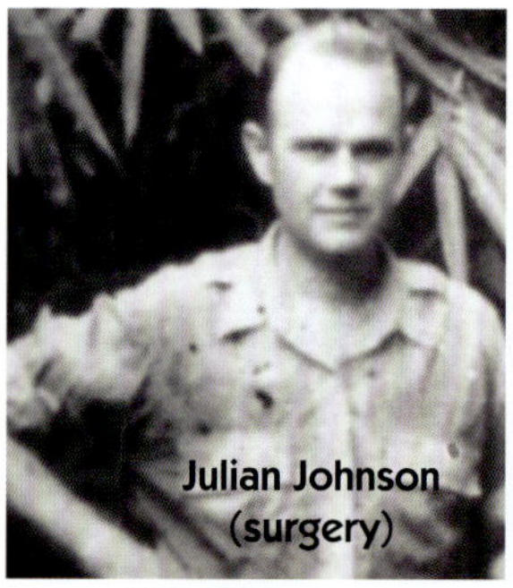
Julian Johnson (surgery)

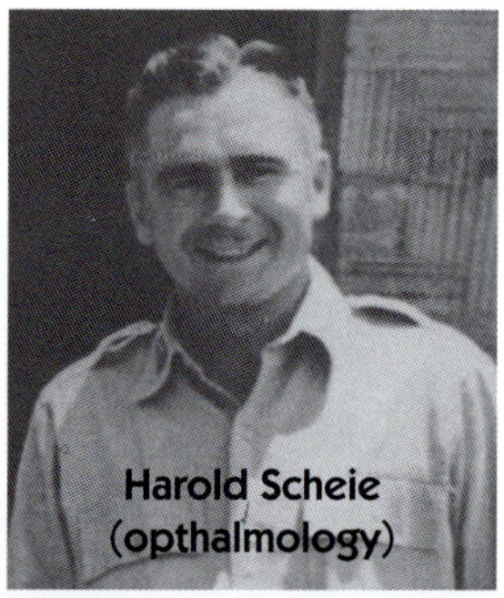
Harold Scheie (opthalmology)

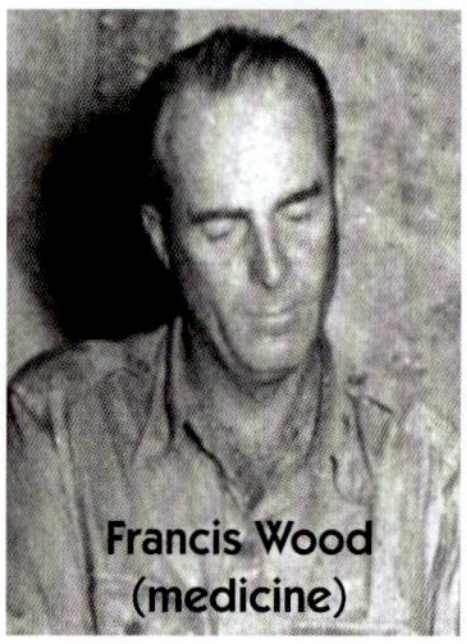
Francis Wood (medicine)

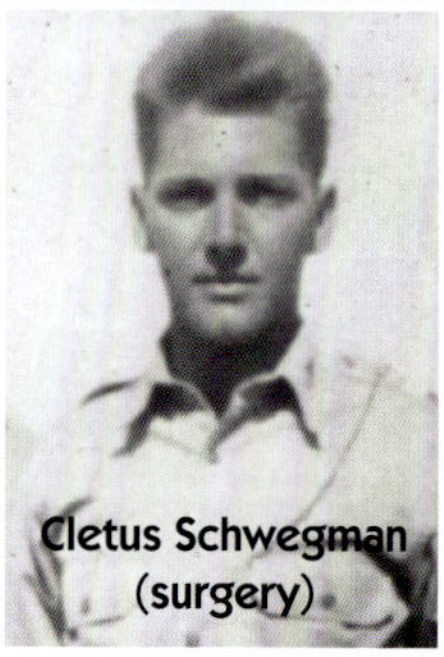
Cletus Schwegman (surgery)

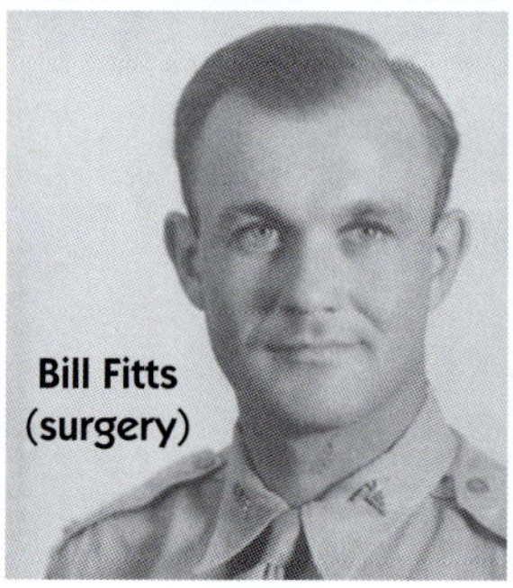
Bill Fitts (surgery)

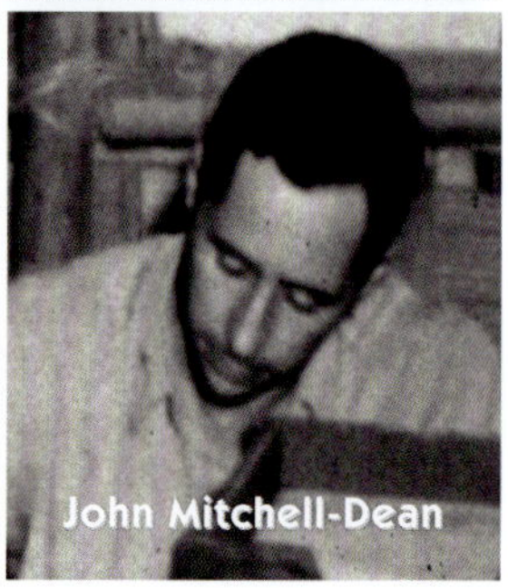
John Mitchell-Dean

John Gibbon

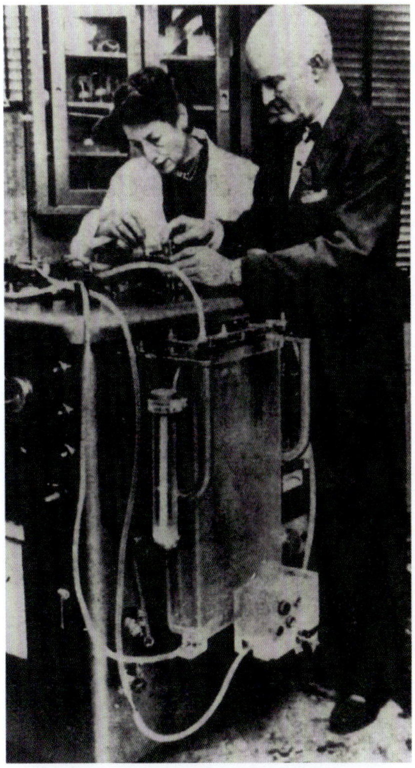

Gibbon and his wife Mary ("Maly") Gibbon with the newer version of the heart–lung machine (IBM II). This was the second and more refined model that Dr. Gibbon used on his first patients.

1941
John Gibbon surprisingly volunteers for military service at age thirty-eight. He is probably the first HUP doctor to see action in World War II

The war experience of John Gibbon, another future Philadelphia surgery department chairman, deserves a place here. Gibbon is usually remembered as a Jefferson man since it was at Jeff that he carried out the world's first successful open-heart operation in a human. Usually forgotten is that more than half the time he spent inventing his heart-lung machine took place in the Harrison Department of Surgical Research. The inspiration for the machine and the beginning of its development took place while he was a fellow at the Massachusetts General Hospital. But after that, from 1936 to 1941 in the Harrison Department, he improved it to the point that he could stop a cat's heart, keep the animal alive with his bypass machine, and expect prolonged survival. He reported this in a 1939 paper given to the American Association of Thoracic Surgery.[12] Reviewers Clarence Craford and Leo Eloesser compared it to a Jules Vern dream come true.[13]

In the spring of 1941, as he was making good progress toward using the machine in human patients, Gibbon surprised everyone by volunteering for the Army. This was not mandatory for a thirty-eight-year-old doctor with four young children, but he chose to do it even over the protest of his wife who was bitterly opposed.[14] Perhaps he was influenced by family tradition of military leaders including several generals and West Point graduates going back through the Spanish-American War, World War I, both sides of the Civil War, all the way to the Revolutionary War.[15] Whatever the reason, it would take him away from his research for a full four years. We will never know whether in these four years he might have carried the heart-lung project to its conclusion. If so, open-heart surgery would have begun at Penn. Probably not, though, since success eventually required the help and

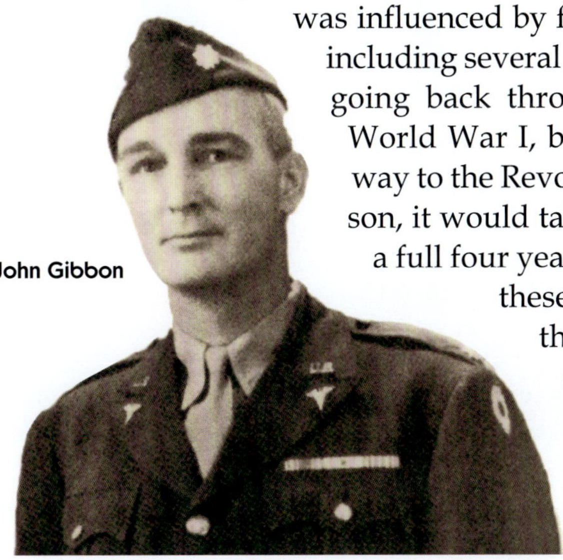

John Gibbon

1941–1944
John Gibbon's overseas wartime service

1944–1945
Gibbon develops painful herniated lumbar disc. Serves in Army hospitals in the United States for the rest of the war

expertise of IBM engineers who became available to him when he moved to Jeff after the war. Uncharacteristically, Dr. Ravdin did not recognize the interest and importance of Gibbon's project (see Chapter 34).

The Army unit Gibbon joined was the 52nd Evacuation Hospital, staffed mainly by personnel from Pennsylvania Hospital. It was the first medical unit to be activated and leave the United States. By January 20, 1942, Gibbon and 4,300 soldiers were on their way via the Panama Canal to the South Pacific, first to Melbourne, Australia, and then on to Bora Bora. The voyage was not without its dangers since their ill-equipped ship had only one workable lifeboat. A nearby ship was attacked by a submarine.

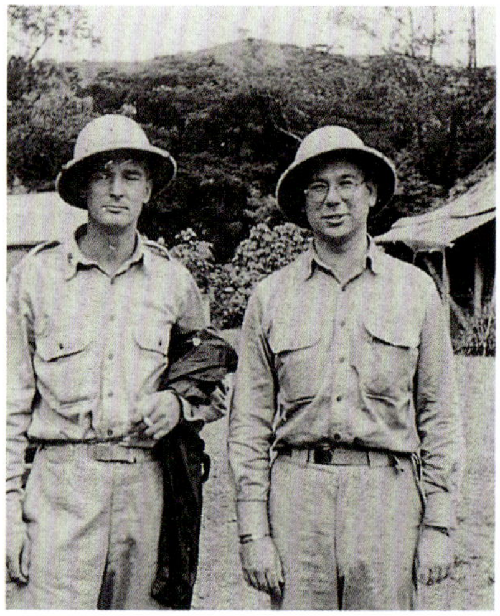
John Gibbon and another officer

By March 1942, the 52nd Evacuation Hospital, though uncomfortable and ill-equipped, was taking care of wounded soldiers in tents and thatched huts in Nouméa, New Caledonia, an island in the Coral Sea. Nouméa was also the headquarters of the South Pacific fleet, with Admiral "Bull" Halsey in command. By the time of the Battle of the Coral Sea in May and the Battle of Midway in June, the hospital was admitting as many as 100 wounded every day.[16] From Guadalcanal, the USS *Solace,* staffed by Penn surgeons Ferguson and North, delivered many more wounded to Gibbon's hospital. From August to December 1942, it had taken care of 9,000 patients.

In May 1943, Gibbon's hospital moved to the southwest tip of New Guinea and then to Woodlark, one of the Solomon Islands. There, a 5,000-foot fighter airstrip was constructed by the Seabees. By October 1943, a 700-bed hospital had been built, which frequently accommodated up to a thousand patients. The hospital was now vulnerable to Japanese bombing raids because of its proximity to the airstrip but fortunately escaped.

In the spring of 1944, Gibbon developed a painful herniated lumbar disc, causing him to be sent home to the United States. After he recovered, for the next year as a colonel, Gibbon served as chief of surgery at the Army Mayo General Hospital in Galesburg, Illinois.

Forgotten Fragments and Untold Stories of the War

Not everyone from Penn Medicine who served in World War II was a future department chairman. At a dinner of HUP doctors and their wives years after the war, I sat with Penn internists Al Sellars and Fred Goldwine. I learned they had been enlisted men—combat infan-

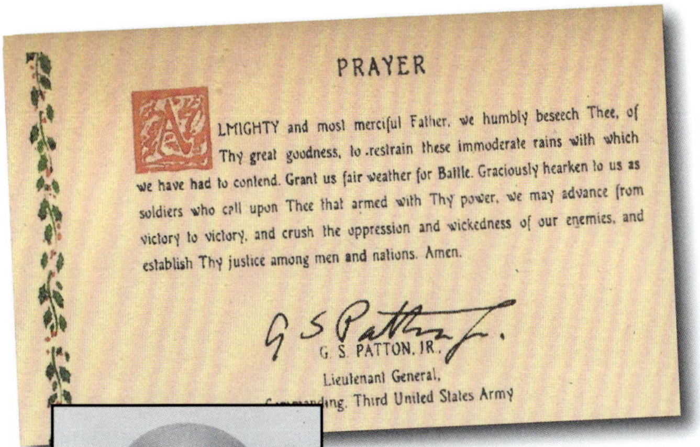

PRAYER

ALMIGHTY and most merciful Father, we humbly beseech Thee, of Thy great goodness, to restrain these immoderate rains with which we have had to contend. Grant us fair weather for Battle. Graciously hearken to us as soldiers who call upon Thee that armed with Thy power, we may advance from victory to victory, and crush the oppression and wickedness of our enemies, and establish Thy justice among men and nations. Amen.

G S Patton Jr.
G. S. PATTON, JR.,
Lieutenant General,
Commanding, Third United States Army

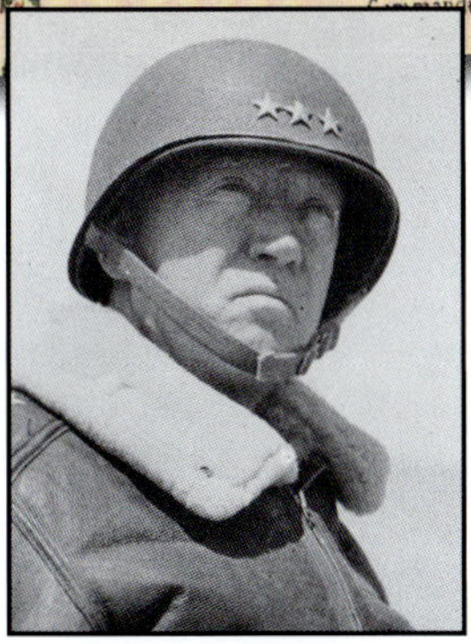

General George Patton and his prayer card.

trymen—in General George Patton's 3rd Army. Sellers had been at the Battle of the Bulge. He showed me a copy of a prayer that since then he had always carried in his wallet. It was on a card that Patton had sent to every member of his 250,000-man 3rd Army. This prayer was written by Patton's chaplain at the general's orders. It asked for clearing the skies and stopping the rain and mud that had impeded the fuel trucks, resulting in Patton's tanks being pinned down. The skies soon cleared, and Patton's army moved on.

Dec. 16. Jan. 25,
1944–1945
Battle of the Bulge. This German offensive late in World War II temporarily reverses the series of allied victories

I learned many years after the war that Marvin Sachs, a mild-manned HUP internist, had piloted a bomber in dangerous daylight raids over Germany.

It was a family story that Jim Hardy, Archie Fletcher, and my brother, Hal Barker—three Ravdin residents—together accompanied Patton's 3rd Army as it chased the Germans toward Berlin near the end of the war.

The Eliason residents of Chapter 13 also had a marvelous war record, now too little remembered. One of them was Charles McLaughlin, who was later professor at Nebraska and president of the American College of Surgeons. He served in a ship that was hit by Japanese kamikaze airplanes.

Ravdin Residents in Patton's Army

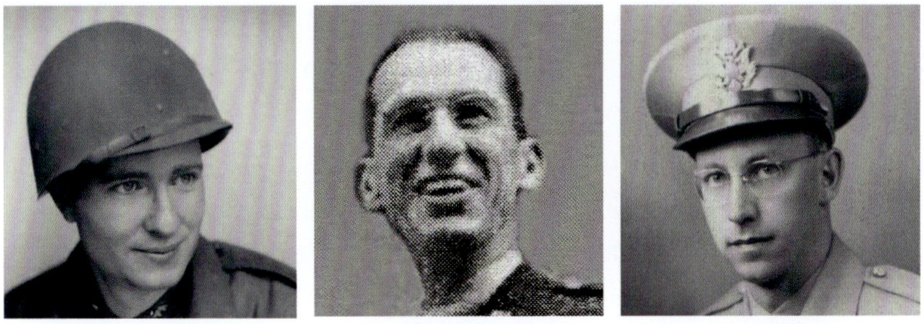

Jim Hardy | Archie Fletcher | Hal Barker

The USS *Solace*

The story of the hospital ship *Solace* is worth telling.[17] It was built in 1927 as a luxury liner named the *Iroquois.* It was the largest (894 feet long) and fastest (17 knots) of ships that carried vacationers up and down the East Coast between New York and Miami. When war came in 1941, the ship was converted to a floating hospital. It had 450 beds, two fully equipped operating rooms, and a fracture room. It happened to be anchored at Pearl Harbor on December 7, 1941. It escaped damage as its crew watched in horror while the American battleships were

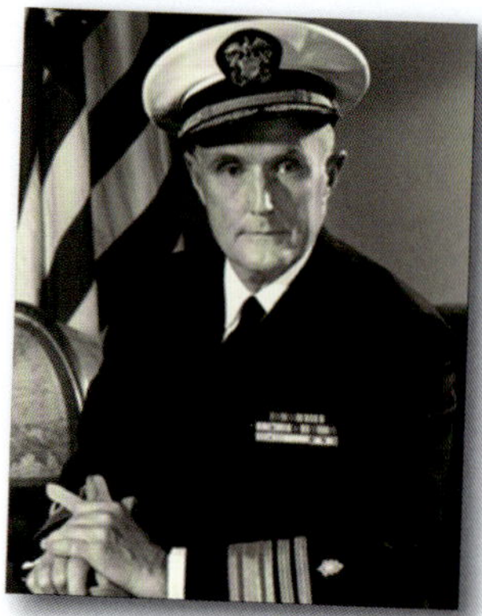

Robert Brown HUP surgical resident 1936-1941 and surgeon general US Navy 1965–1969

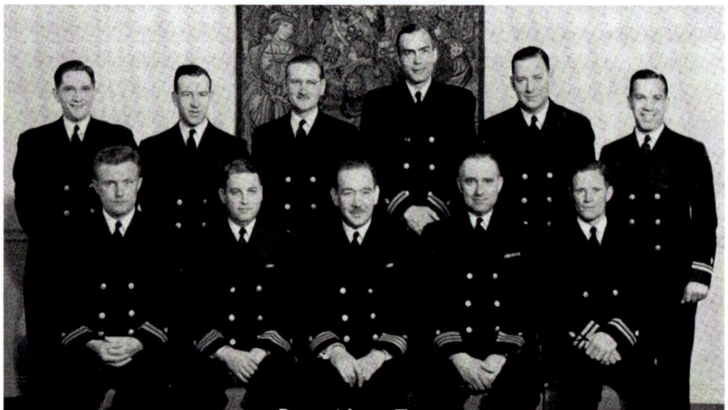

Penn Navy Team
FRONT ROW (l to r): Robert Brown, Kraeer Ferguson, Kern, Schenck, Nicholson, SECOND ROW: Wigton, Godfrey, Rode, Montgomery, Farnsworth, Silcox

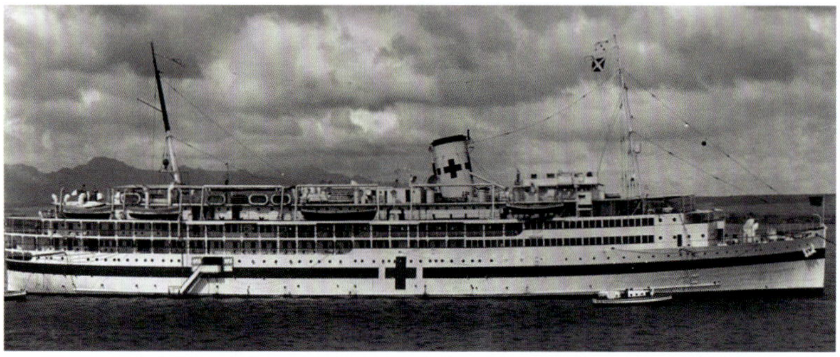

The hospital ship USS ***Solace*** was commissioned into the Navy on August 9, 1941, and in December she was at Pearl Harbor, where she would see her first action.

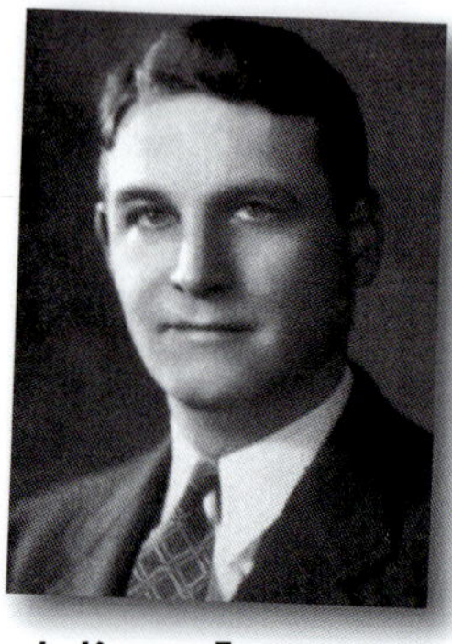

L. Kraeer Ferguson chief of surgery on the ***Solace***

torpedoed and sinking. For the next year, the *Solace* was the only hospital ship serving in the South Pacific, and for the rest of the war, it moved from one battle site to the next. It was especially busy during the Battle of Midway.[18] It also evacuated the wounded from action in Guam, Guadalcanal, and Iwo Jima.

Kraeer Ferguson, an Eliason resident and later a Penn professor of surgery, was chief of surgery on the *Solace.* Another Eliason resident on the *Solace* was Bob Brown, who later became the Navy's surgeon general. On one day, these two Penn surgeons operated on twenty-six wounded sailors. All told, during the war the *Solace* took care of 4,039 wounded soldiers and sailors. The mortality rate was only 7 percent.

Penn Medical Student and Father of Frogmen

Christian Lambertsen's career could easily serve as the plot for a gripping adventure novel or film. The *New York Times* began his obituary: "When American commandos slipped into the sea off the coast of Burma in World War II and swam underwater to attach explosives to Japanese vessels, Captain Christian Lambertsen often led them. After all, he had trained them to dive and had invented the breathing device that allowed them to stay under the waves."[19]

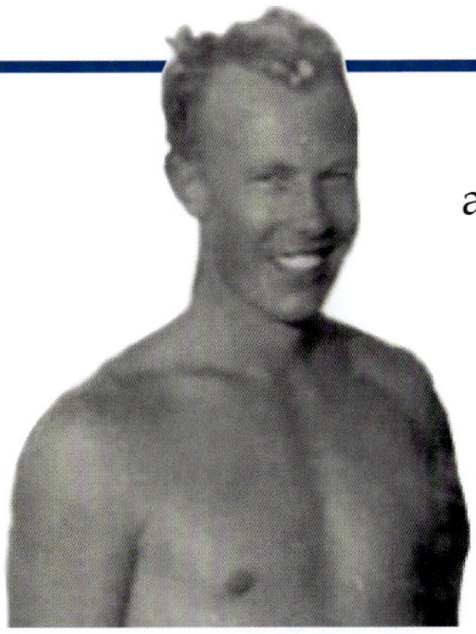

Penn medical student Christian Lambertsen

During World War II while Chris Lambertsen was a Penn medical student, he invented SCUBA, the self-contained rebreather equipment for prolonged underwater swimming.[20] The invention was at first termed LARU (Lambertsen Amphibious Respiratory Unit). Lambertsen later gave it the name SCUBA, by which it is now universally known. Lambertsen tested his invention in a pond on the Penn campus. He was then recruited by the Army and the Office of Strategic Services (OSS) to train US frogmen and later Navy Seals in underwater swimming. His training and equipment enabled them to conduct covert missions, such as preinvasion survey and clearing of enemy coastlines and underwater demolition.[21]

One of World War II's most interesting stories is that of a hero who was in medical school at the time

1941–1943
Chris Lambertsen invents SCUBA and trains frogmen to use it

Lambertsen's inspiration for inventing SCUBA was a medical school course in respiratory physiology. Students studied adverse respiratory conditions, such as hypoxia which they produced by holding their breath, and reduction of blood levels of CO_2 which they induced by hyperventilating. During medical school vacations at the Jersey shore, Lambertsen with his two cousins devised related experiments while diving and swimming underwater. At first, they attempted to prolong underwater swimming with a homemade rebreathing rig consisting of a mouthpiece and bag connected to the surface by a long garden hose. Through the hose, his cousins used a bicycle pump to deliver fresh air to Lambertsen while he swam. Later, this primitive air delivery system was replaced with a cylinder of compressed oxygen. This too proved unsatisfactory because exhaled CO_2 was trapped and accumulated in the air bag. With the advice of his physiology professor, Lambertsen solved

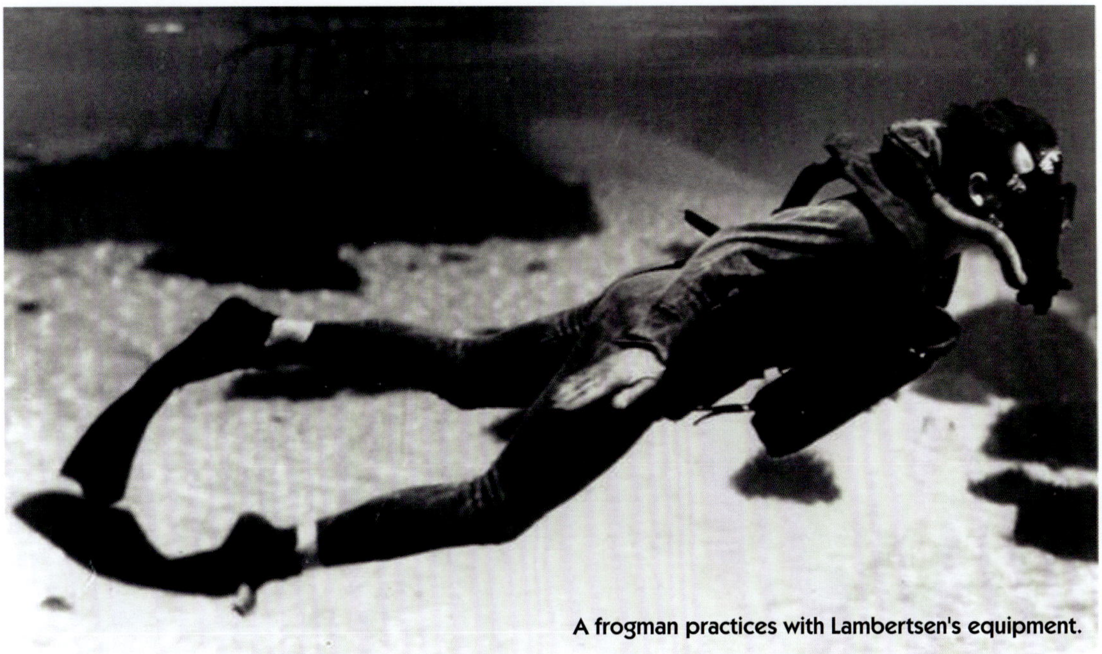

A frogman practices with Lambertsen's equipment.

1941
Lambertsen borrows anesthesia equipment to absorb CO_2

1942
Lambertson tests SCUBA in Lake Erie

1942
Lambertsen's research with SCUBA and oxygen toxicity causes him to suffer periods of unconsciousness and seizures

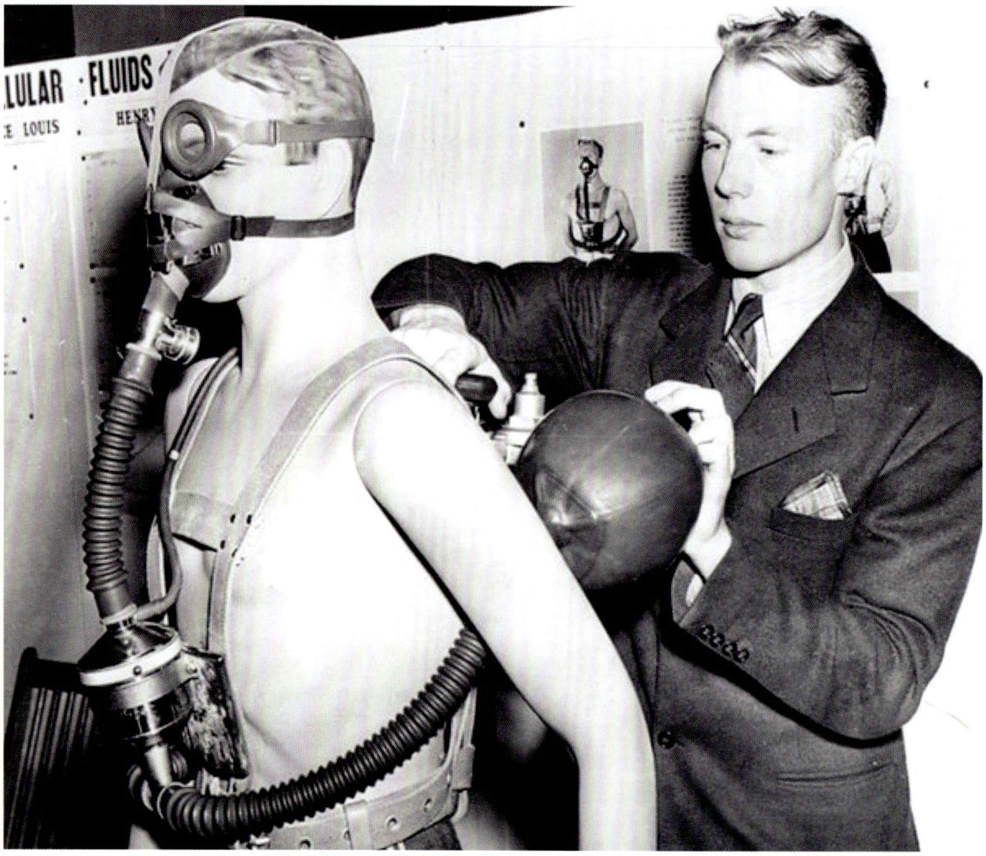

Christian Lambertsen—Inventor of SCUBA, Father of Underwater Combat

this problem by obtaining anesthesia equipment that contained a CO_2-absorbent device between the mouthpiece and the breathing bag.

Lambertsen then performed underwater tests of his device in Lake Erie. His equipment allowed him to do thirty minutes of light work while submerged at a depth of sixty feet. Remaining underwater for that long without a heavy diving suit and helmet was a feat unheard of at the time. But there were inherent dangers. In related experiments performed in an airtight chamber rather than underwater, Lambertsen experimented with his equipment on a canary, a dog, and himself. After a few minutes, the canary and the dog became unconscious, and when Lambertsen leaned over to check on the dog, he fell unconscious to the floor. Fortunately, help was quickly on hand to save his life. Other close calls were four episodes of oxygen toxicity including one that induced a seizure.

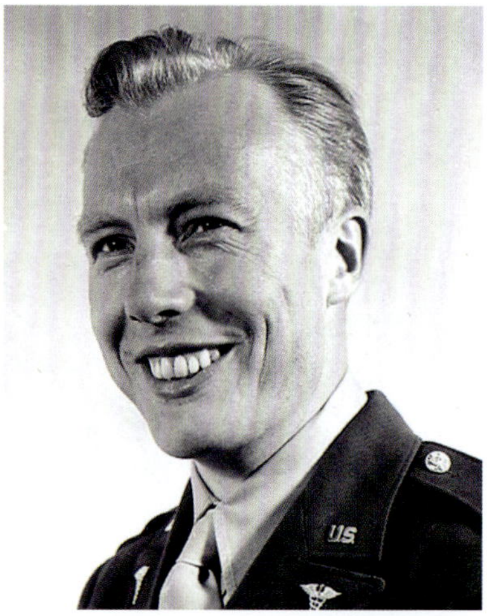

Dr. Lambertsen was transferred from the Army to the OSS. He participated in combat in Ceylon and Burma.

Only the dean of the medical school knew of Lambertsen's activities. But the remarkable feat of deep-water diving was too spectacular to keep secret. Lambertsen was encouraged to publish his experience. This made him a local celebrity and also attracted national attention.

In 1941 and 1942, because of the obvious promise of his invention for wartime military use, Lambertsen was invited to conduct trials for the US Navy, the Office of Strategic Services (OSS), and the British Admiralty. Surprisingly, the Navy was not interested, choosing to continue using conventional heavy diving suits and helmets. An aspect of the Lambertsen device that was unique and particularly attractive to the OSS was that the CO_2 scrubber (absorbent) not only allowed safe reuse of the oxygen in the self-contained system, but in addition left no telltale exhaust air bubbles to betray the presence of a diver to observers on the surface. As a result of the trials, Lambertsen was recruited by the OSS for training military divers in its use.

1943
Lambertsen graduates from medical school and is commissioned in the Army

1944
Model 10 of Lambertsen's LARU system used by frogmen of OSS

1944
While a HUP intern, Lambertsen meets with OSS to plan underwater maneuvers

1944–1945
Lambertsen and his frogmen swim underwater for pre-invasion clearance of coastlines

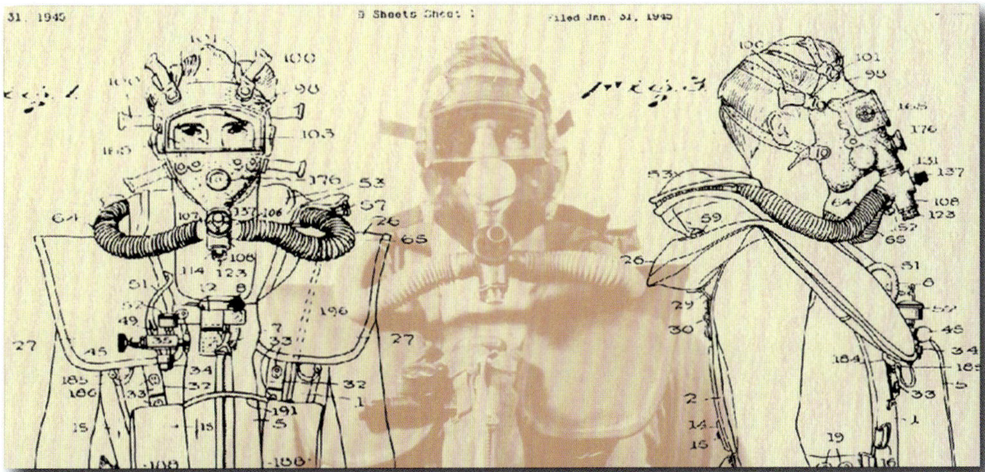

The LARU system used by OSS. Unlike the earlier systems, the Model 10 had a waterproof compass mounted on the front by the gas cylinder.

Fifty years later at a medical school class reunion, Lambertsen told his classmates more of the story. After he was recruited to train US frogmen (and later the Navy Seals) to use his device in covert underwater missions, he was given a letter by the medical school dean, William Pepper. It stated that for secret reasons he could be absent from medical school classes for any period of time with no questions asked. Lambertsen said that he almost failed Ob-Gyn because his professors wouldn't believe his cover story.[22]

As a HUP intern in 1944, Lambertsen met in the hospital's maternity waiting room with OSS and British personnel to plan undersea maneuvers. Then Lambertsen and his frogmen were sent to England and Europe and to the China, Burma, and India war theaters where, in the dark, they swam underwater for preinvasion clearance of coastlines and to attach explosives to enemy ships. They also ferried supplies and weapons to resistance fighters and rescued downed fliers.

1946–2006
Lambertsen is pharmacology faculty member at Penn School of Medicine

As a physician, Lambertsen was not expected to go on these dangerous missions. But as a superb young athlete and swimmer and a person never satisfied to let others do his job, Lambertsen became an active participant in these harrowing maneuvers and others, such as piloting a one-man submarine. He was also the first to exit and reenter a submerged submarine.[23] For these activities, he was awarded the Legion of Merit and the OSS Distinguished Service Award. In 2000, the Navy Seals designated him the "Father of US Combat Swimming."

As the war ended and back in civilian life, Lambertsen began a distinguished faculty career at Penn that was to last six decades. Since he was not only professor of pharmacology (his home department), but also professor of medicine, he was a familiar figure in the halls of the university hospital. Surgical residents including me were privileged to become his friends and colleagues as we had the somewhat questionable pleasure of diving with him through several atmospheres in his artificial submarine to help him and his team employ hyperbaric oxygen in treatment of patients with gas gangrene. Sometimes I think I can still feel the pain and hear popping in my ears. In experiments conducted in his high-pressure chamber, he studied the effects of hyperbaric O_2 and inspired CO_2 on cerebral blood flow and O_2 consumption.

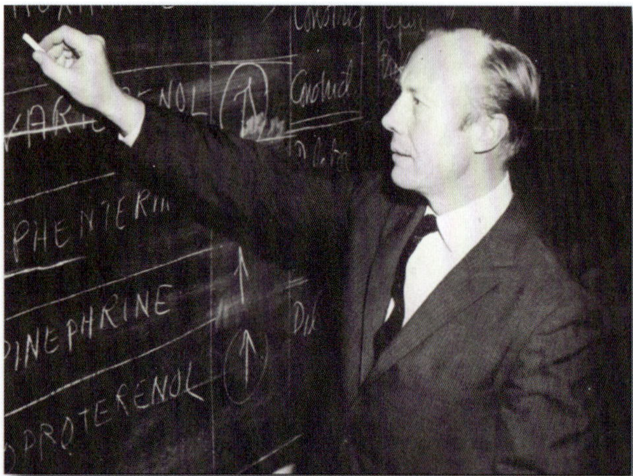

Professor Christian Lambertsen

Dr. Lambertsen's versatility is apparent from casual perusal of his more than 100 publications, most of them in high-impact journals. One that caught my eye was titled *From Submarines to Satellites.* In the 1950s and 1960s as the United States moved into exploration of space, because of Lambertsen's expertise in respiratory physiology under adverse conditions, he became a leader in the initial planning for our country's manned space flights.

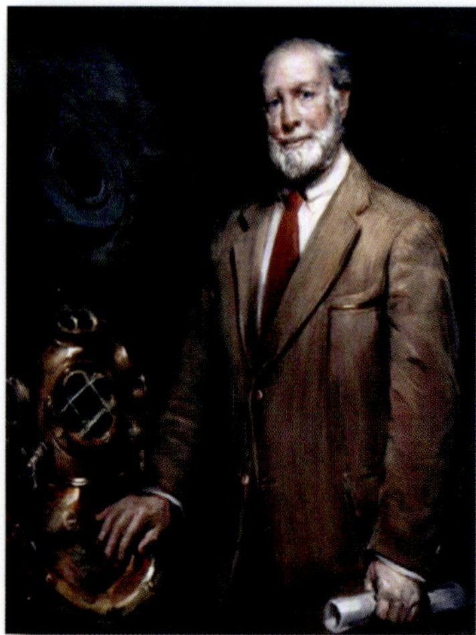

Christian Lambertsen

In 1968, Dr. Lambertsen was appointed director of Penn's newly established Institute for Environmental Medicine, where he continued his fundamental research and teaching and, in addition, supervised the use of hyperbaric oxygen therapy in clinical medicine. Since then, the use of hyperbaric oxygen therapy (HBOT) in clinical medicine has grown substantially in the number of conditions treated and treatment centers. In addition to its use in preventing or treating decompression sickness of divers (the bends), HBOT is effective in preventing or reducing delayed neurological sequelae from carbon monoxide poisoning. It is also widely used in the treatment of diabetic ulcers, radiation injury, and severe infections.

1950–1960
After the war, Lambertsen assumes a more conventional academic career, though one that is also spectacularly successful

Lambertsen became one of the most honored American physicians and scientists. A small sampling of his more than thirty awards and honors include:[24]

- Membership in the National Academy of Engineering
- The Meritorious Service Award and the Military Oceanography Award from the Secretary of the Navy
- Public Service Medal Awards from the US Coast Guard and from the Department of Defense
- US Navy SEAL Association Lifetime Achievement Award
- US Special Forces Green Beret Award
- A Lifetime Achievement Award from the US Naval Academy

2010
The John Scott Award is Lambertsen's last

Several years ago, I was privileged to present Chris Lambertsen with his last major honor, the John Scott Award, a lifetime achievement award from the City of Philadelphia. From his wheelchair, he talked about his continuing fascination with oxygen, its uses, and its toxicity. At age ninety-three, this larger-than-life character could still command an audience.

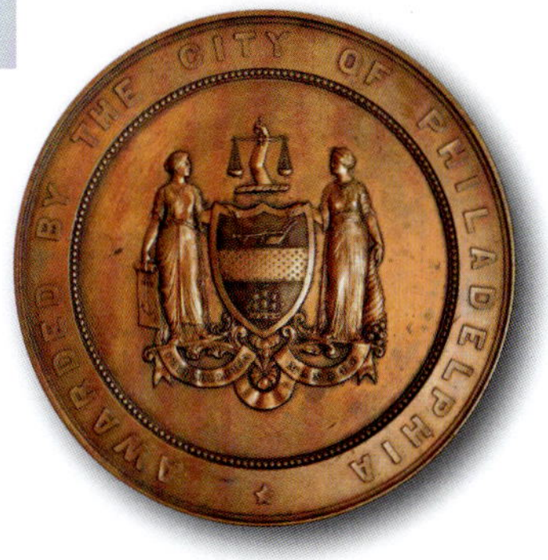

Penn Surgery's Chief Administrator Stars in *A Bridge Too Far*

Everybody knows what is meant by "a bridge too far." The Oxford English dictionary made it official in 2020, defining it as, "a step beyond what is safe, sensible or desirable."[25] But few know how this idiom entered our language and fewer still know that Penn Surgery's administrator, Henry Keep, had a lot to do with it.

Henry Keep was a year old when his Army officer father died in the Argonne Forest, the last great battle of World War I. Young Henry's mother later married Charles Biddle, a World War I air ace, who had shot down eleven German planes.[26] Henry and his mother moved into the Biddles'

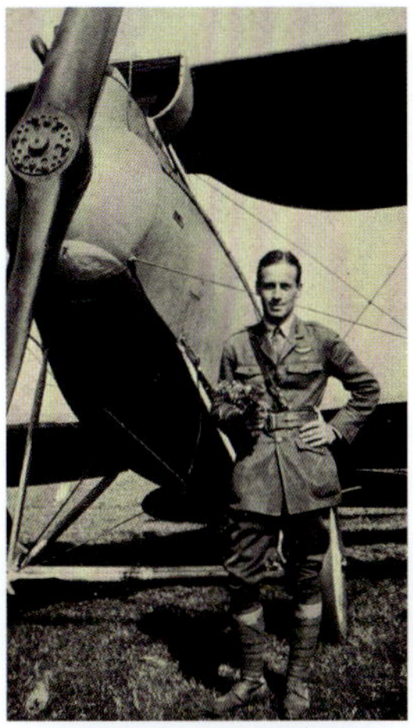
Henry's stepfather Charles Biddle

1918
Henry Keep's father dies. His mother marries into Philadelphia's wealthy Biddle family.

1944 (Sept. 17–25)
Operation Market Garden. Henry Keep has a prominent role

1944 (Sept. 20)
Waal River Crossing. The stuff of legend

1974
Cornelius Ryan's book *A Bridge Too Far*

legendary eighteenth-century estate, Andalusia, where Henry grew up as a beloved member of the wealthy Biddle family.[27]

After graduating from Princeton in 1941, Henry enlisted in the Army and volunteered for the paratroopers. Assigned to the 82nd Airborne, he jumped with his famous unit in Sicily, Italy, the Netherlands, Belgium, and Germany. In Sicily, he was wounded in a firefight with a German tank, earning him his first Silver Star.[28]

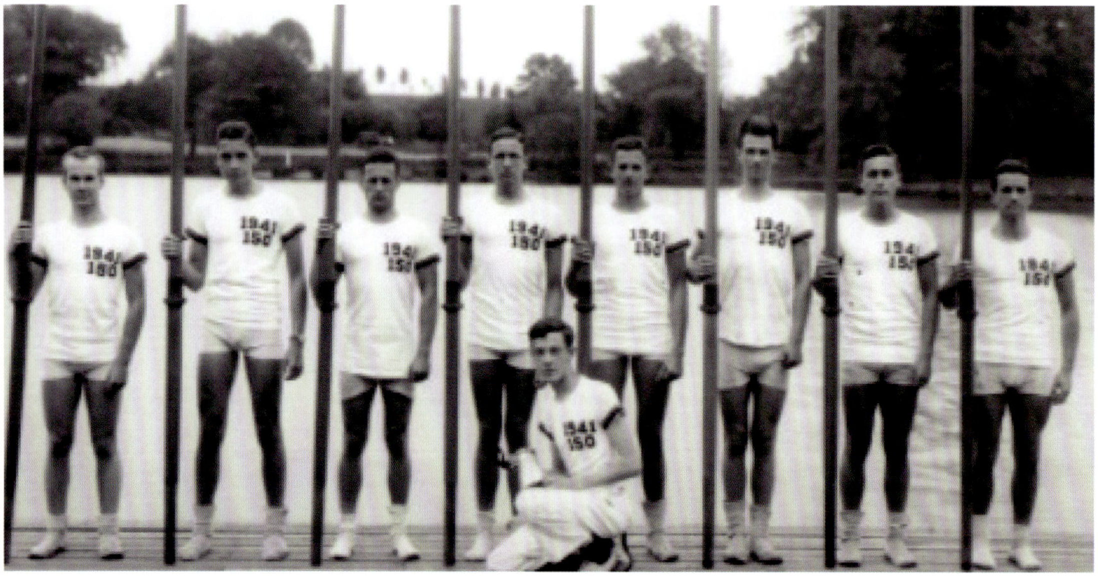

Henry Keep on the Princeton rowing team in 1941 (3rd from the left)

On September 17, 1944, Keep was dropped with 35,000 other paratroopers and 1,000 gliders into Holland, sixty miles behind enemy lines. It was the largest and most daring airborne attack in history. Called Market Garden, this campaign was designed to shorten the war by forcing open a narrow corridor through Germany's heartland for attacking and disabling the enemy's manufacturing center, the Ruhr.

To accomplish the mission, a series of nine bridges would need to be taken. To maintain an open road and reach the bridge at Arnhem (the last bridge, aka, The One Too Far), the next to last bridge at Nijmegen needed to be captured intact. Access to this bridge required crossing the Waal, one of Europe's widest rivers. This was a feat assigned to Keep's battalion. As the battalion's operations officer, it was Keep's job to plan the assault on the bridge, presuming the paratroopers could get across the river first. To assess the

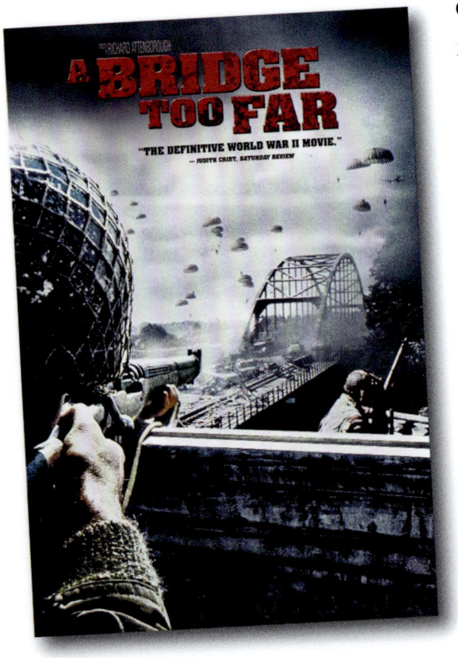

***A Bridge Too Far*, the classic history of Operation Market Garden, one of World War II's great campaigns—unfortunately, one that failed.**

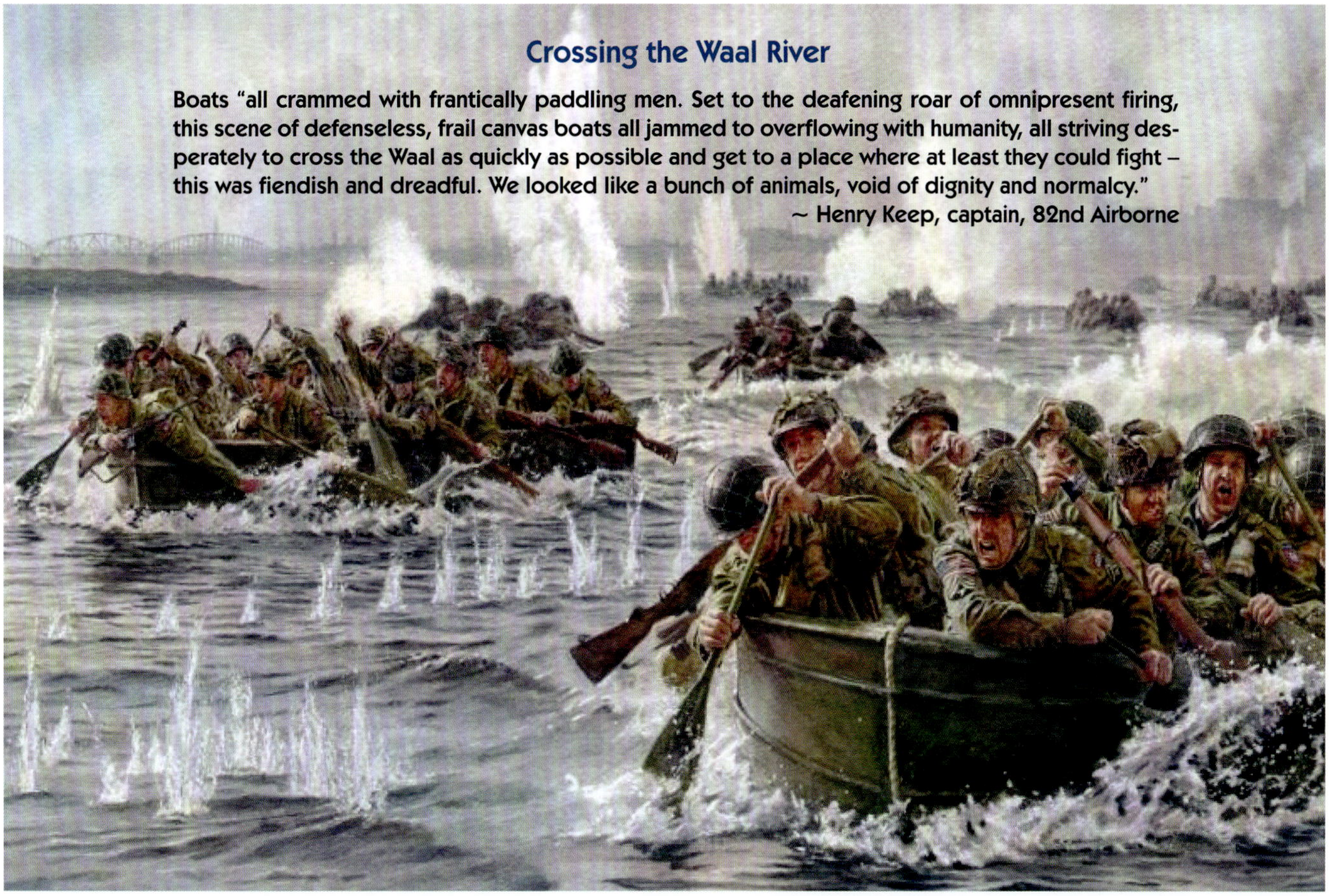

Crossing the Waal River

Boats "all crammed with frantically paddling men. Set to the deafening roar of omnipresent firing, this scene of defenseless, frail canvas boats all jammed to overflowing with humanity, all striving desperately to cross the Waal as quickly as possible and get to a place where at least they could fight – this was fiendish and dreadful. We looked like a bunch of animals, void of dignity and normalcy."

~ Henry Keep, captain, 82nd Airborne

bridge's defenses and formulate his plan, Keep climbed an abandoned tower to view the opposite shore. When he saw the enemy's extensive pillboxes, machine-gun emplacements, and mortars, Keep—despite his reputation for somewhat reckless courage—felt a little sick.[29] Because timing was crucial, the paratroopers couldn't wait for the cover of nightfall. Instead, they would need to cross the 400-yard-wide river in broad daylight under withering enemy fire.

1977
Movie of
A Bridge Too Far

To carry them across, the paratroopers had only defenseless, frail boats made of canvas.[30] There were too few paddles so they would use their rifle butts to row. Keep later wrote that they were like sitting ducks on a suicide mission. In the lead boats were Captain Keep and Major Julian Cook, who in the film, *A Bridge Too Far,* was portrayed by Robert Redford. If you have seen the movie, you will remember what happened. More than half of the troopers were killed crossing the river. Of twenty-six boats that started out, only eleven reached the opposite bank. Despite its frightful price, Keep's plan worked. The surviving paratroopers captured the bridge.[31] However, the British then delayed pushing on to the last bridge (at Arnhem), giving the Germans time

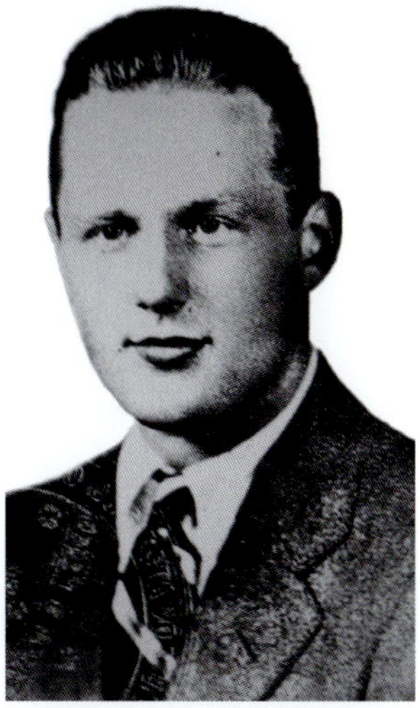

Henry Blair Keep Jr.

2000
Richard Davis's book, *Yours D*^{3}, is based on Henry Keep's experiences during World War II

to bring up an overwhelming force, causing the entire campaign to fail. The Allies suffered 17,000 killed or wounded in the effort.

Market Garden and the Waal River crossing have become the stuff of legend.[32] On Amazon, we counted thirty books that have been written about these events. Henry Keep is featured prominently in many of them. His contribution was recognized by a Bronze Star and a Silver Star.

Worth reading is a fictionalized account of Henry Keep's story in a 2012 novel published by Keep's friend, Dick Davis, a HUP neurosurgeon. Included in Davis's novel is an account of the Waal River crossing based on Keep's description. It is virtually the same as what happened in the movie and in real life.[33]

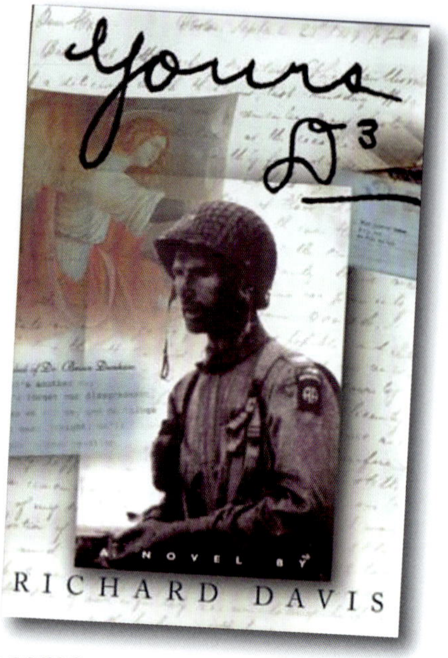

***Yours D*^{3} a novel by HUP neurosurgeon Dick Davis**

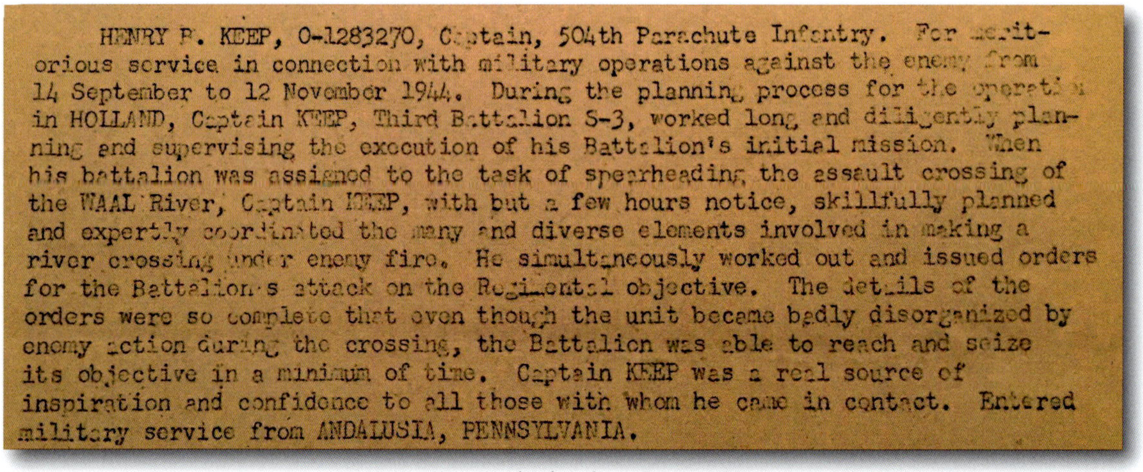

HENRY P. KEEP, 0-1283270, Captain, 504th Parachute Infantry. For meritorious service in connection with military operations against the enemy from 14 September to 12 November 1944. During the planning process for the operation in HOLLAND, Captain KEEP, Third Battalion S-3, worked long and diligently planning and supervising the execution of his Battalion's initial mission. When his battalion was assigned to the task of spearheading the assault crossing of the WAAL River, Captain KEEP, with but a few hours notice, skillfully planned and expertly coordinated the many and diverse elements involved in making a river crossing under enemy fire. He simultaneously worked out and issued orders for the Battalion's attack on the Regimental objective. The details of the orders were so complete that even though the unit became badly disorganized by enemy action during the crossing, the Battalion was able to reach and seize its objective in a minimum of time. Captain KEEP was a real source of inspiration and confidence to all those with whom he came in contact. Entered military service from ANDALUSIA, PENNSYLVANIA.

Henry Keep's citation for a Bronze Star

After the war, Henry served in the State Department as a military attaché in US embassies in India, Formosa, Japan, and the Philippines. Later, he worked for his friend, Bill Fitts, as our department's administrator and as a Philadelphia civic leader, philanthropist, University trustee, and member of boards and committees of organizations including those of United Way, the University Museum, the Philadelphia Art Museum, and the Philadelphia Orchestra.

Henry died in 1983 at age sixty-five during open-heart surgery at HUP. He was friendly with the younger members of our department of surgery. We knew nothing of his war record at the time. When his ashes were interred at Andalusia, the Biddle family estate on the Delaware River, a bus full of our department members made the trip to be there.

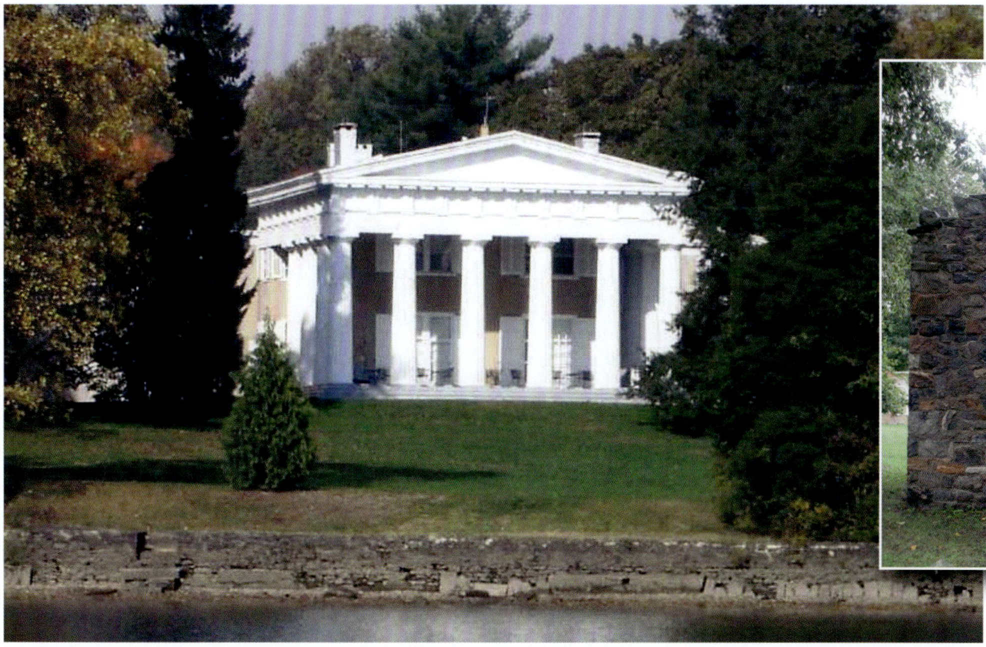

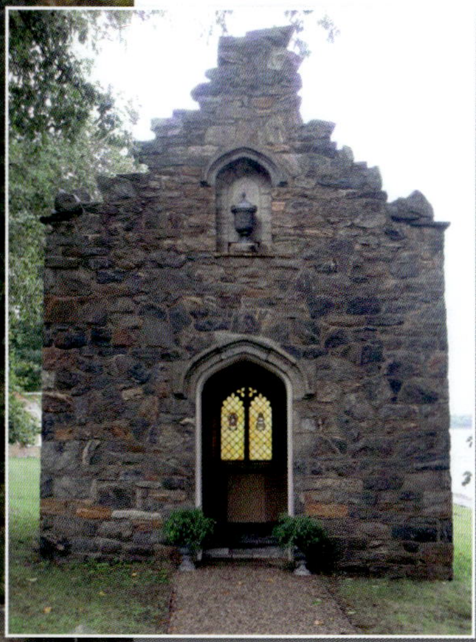

Andalusia Estate

The Korean War (1950–1953)

In the Korean War, mobile Army MASH units evolved to provide surgical treatment as close as possible to the wounded soldiers' site of injury. Ravdin's resident, John Howard, was probably the nearest prototype of Hollywood's and TV's *M*A*S*H* hero, Hawkeye Pierce. Howard had finished his HUP residency only six months before the start of the war and, at first, was one of only two board-certified surgeons in the Korean theater. In addition to commanding his MASH unit, Howard was assigned to organize and direct the US Army's research team in Korea.[34]

Howard was given two major research assignments. The first was to set up army dialysis units in Korea. The second was to solve the problem that was causing repaired arteries to fail from thrombosis even though vascular anastomoses initially appeared satisfactory. This was in the early days of vascular surgery. During World War II, the officially prescribed method of treating an arterial injury had been to ligate the artery. If it was a major artery, this led to amputation 50 percent of the time.[35] In the 1950s, the experience of Alfred Blalock and a few others at civilian hospitals was limited to subclavian to pulmonary artery shunts for blue babies[36] and operations for coarctation of the aorta.

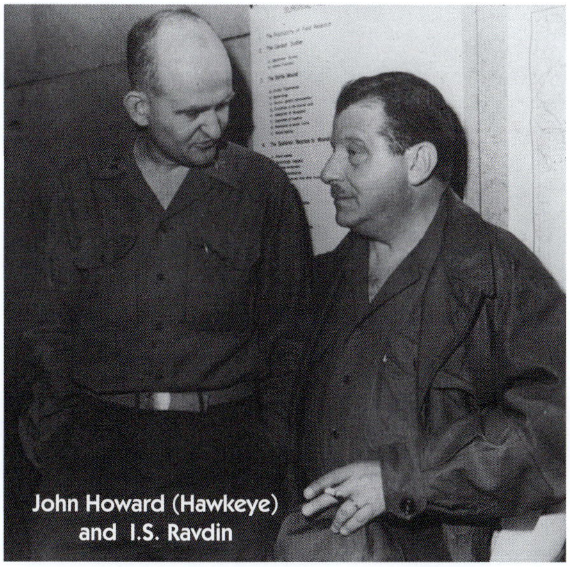

John Howard (Hawkeye) and I.S. Ravdin

1983
Henry Keep dies during heart surgery. Interred at Andalusia, the Biddle estate

1950
North Korea crosses 38th parallel and attacks South Korea, starting the Korean War

1950–1953
Ravdin resident, John "Hawkeye" Howard, directs US Army's research unit. Organizes dialysis units and pioneers repair of arterial injuries

1951
Successfully repairs arterial injuries by obtaining noncrushing vascular clamps

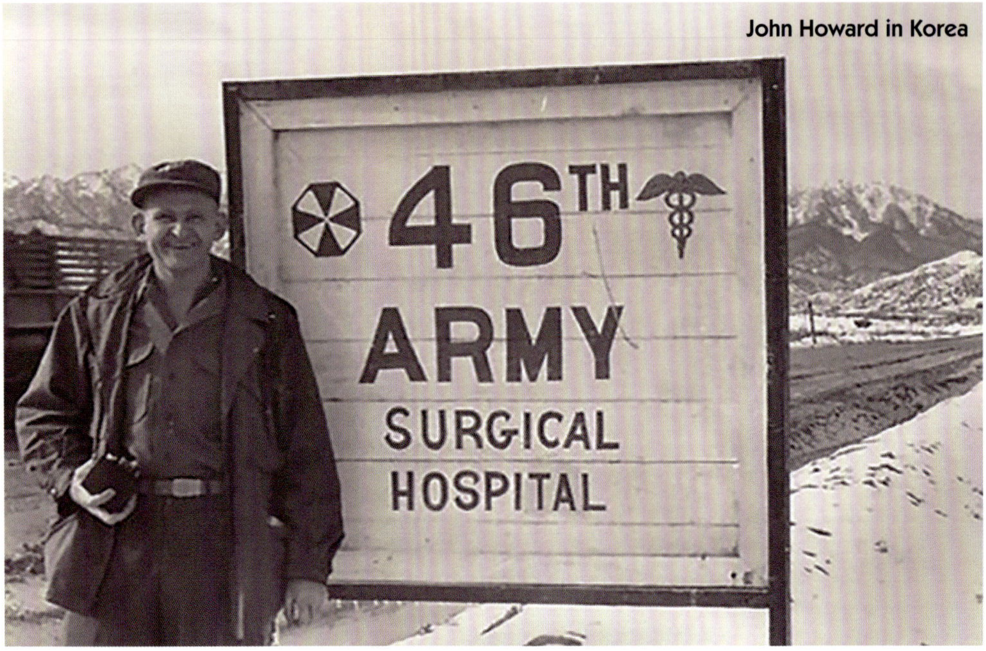

John Howard in Korea

This was about the only arterial surgery being done. In Korea, the equipment necessary for repair of injured arteries was unavailable. At first, Howard used ordinary hemostats to clamp arteries before they were sewn together. The teeth of the hemostats opposed each other, crushing the artery and causing it to thrombose even if on examination, the repair looked perfect. Howard's attempts at modifying the hemostats proved unsatisfactory. He then attempted to obtain Potts vascular clamps, which were available but scarce even at civilian hospitals in the United States. His request for them was greeted only by Army red tape and delays that were predicted to last months. Howard persuaded his commanding general to threaten the company making the clamps with breaking their patents if they did not respond to his urgent request. This promptly brought seven of the vascular clamps to Korea. With their use, the rate of thrombosis of repaired arteries suddenly fell from 50 percent to 7 percent.[37] Howard then brought together surgeons from all of Korea's MASH units. Most of them had only a year or two of residency training, but in one day, he trained

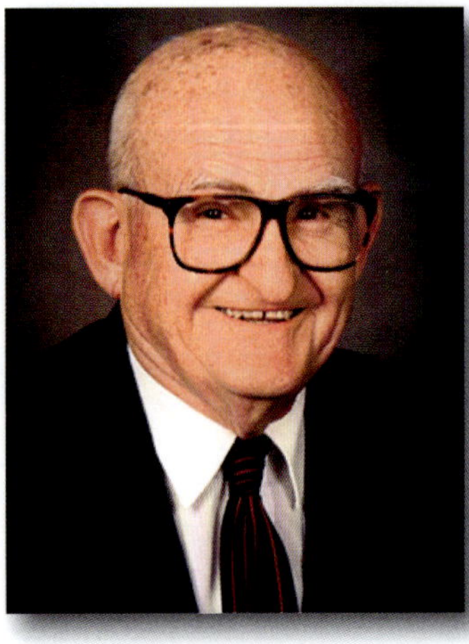

John Howard

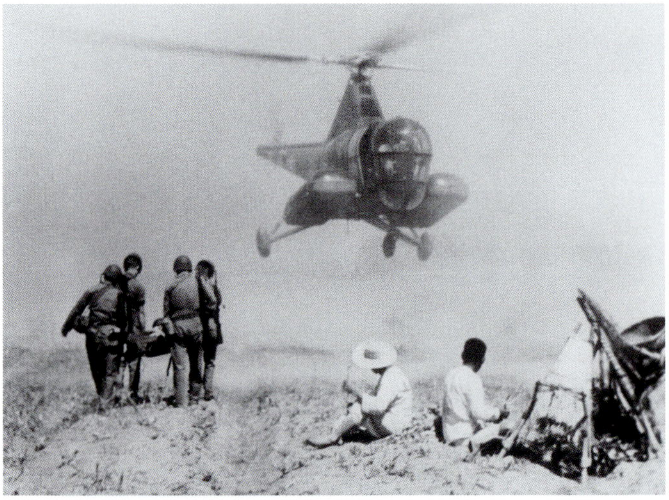

In Korea, a wounded soldier is brought to a helicopter from the battlefield for transport to MASH hospital.

these fledgling surgeons to perform vascular anastomoses in experimental animals using his small collection of noncrushing clamps. Suddenly, the results of vascular repairs in Korea became satisfactory. For these and other innovations in Korea, Howard was given the Medal of Honor by President Eisenhower.

Sept. Sept.
1967–1968
HUP resident
Jim Finnegan in Vietnam

2009
Jim Finnegan's account of the Vietnam War

The Vietnam War

Surgical experience in the Vietnam War is described in a book written by Jim Finnegan.[38] Jim Finnegan, HUP chief resident in 1971–72, also completed a residency in cardiothoracic surgery at HUP under Julian Johnson. He later received a master's degree in health administration from St. Joseph's University.

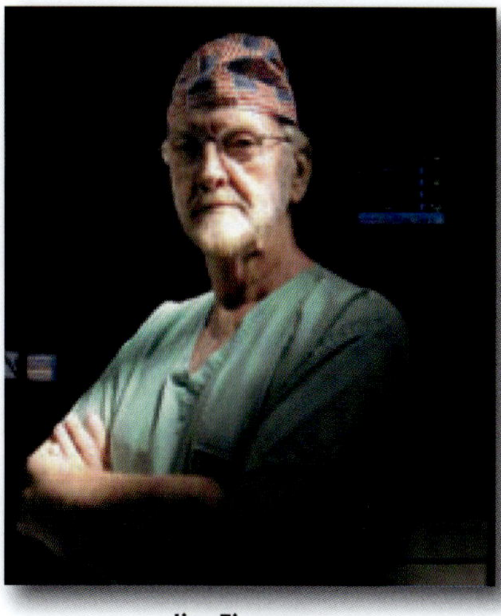

Jim Finnegan

Perhaps the most interesting and certainly the most intense period of Jim's career was the two years he served as a volunteer in the Marine Corps, after his second year of HUP residency. From September 1967 to September 1968, he was a combat surgeon in Vietnam. During the unrelenting enemy siege of Khe Sanh from January through April of 1968, he was the commanding officer of a surgical team that treated over 2,500 wounded marines. Jim sustained shrapnel wounds from an incoming mortar explosion and was awarded a Purple Heart. He was also awarded the Bronze Star with a Combat V for valor.

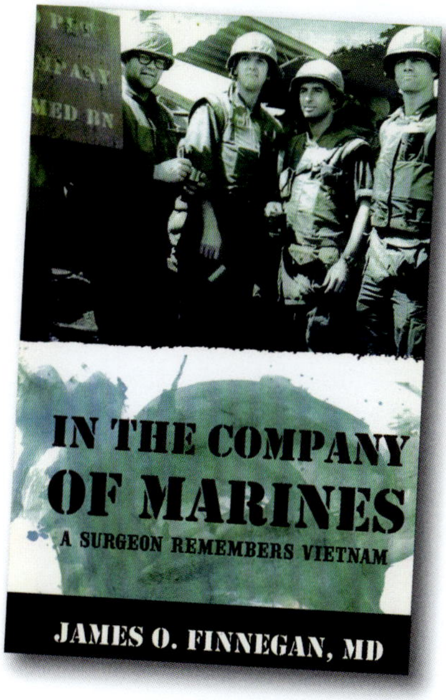

When I learned of Jim Finnegan's death in 2013, I searched for and found the book he had sent me when it was published in 2009. The cover of the book tells part of the story of his service in Vietnam. In one graphic passage that attracted considerable newspaper coverage, Jim tells how he closed a hole in the heart of one Marine, and for another who had been pronounced dead, he massaged the heart until his patient came back to life.

Rereading this account of Jim's harrowing experiences as a combat surgeon evoked half-forgotten memories of our country's attitude in the 1960s about the Vietnam War and the somehow unappreciated or forgotten heroism of our soldiers. It also brought back to me memories of Jim as a surgical resident. Jim was a character never likely to be forgotten. But to reinforce my recollection, I consulted the department's archives. Just as I had remembered, several of the more conservative faculty members criticized Jim, considering him somewhat too independent and aggressive for a HUP resident of that era. I dare say that these were positive attributes in Vietnam. Another letter in his file indicated that Julian Johnson, our department's master surgeon and one not given to hyperbole, rated Jim as a talented surgeon. In fact, Julian bragged a bit about his trainee's performance in Vietnam. I concluded that the praise Jim was given by the media was justified.

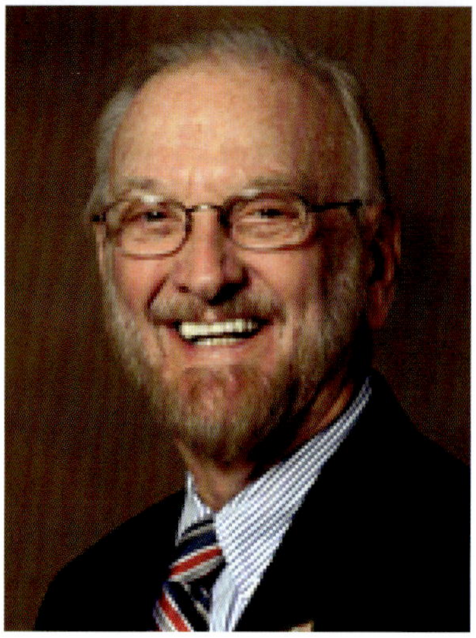

James Finnegan

After his tour in Vietnam, Jim returned to HUP and finished his training in general and cardiothoracic surgery. Subsequently, during his long career, he served as chief of cardiothoracic surgery at several of the area's institutions, including the Medical College of Pennsylvania, St. Agnes Medical Center, and Crozer-Chester Medical Center.

Jim's book, *In the Company of Marines,* is worth reading.

The War in Afghanistan (2001–2021)

Ron Fairman was one of the first to volunteer to contribute his expertise in endovascular techniques to improve the care of soldiers airlifted from Afghanistan to the Army hospital in Landstholl, Germany.[39]

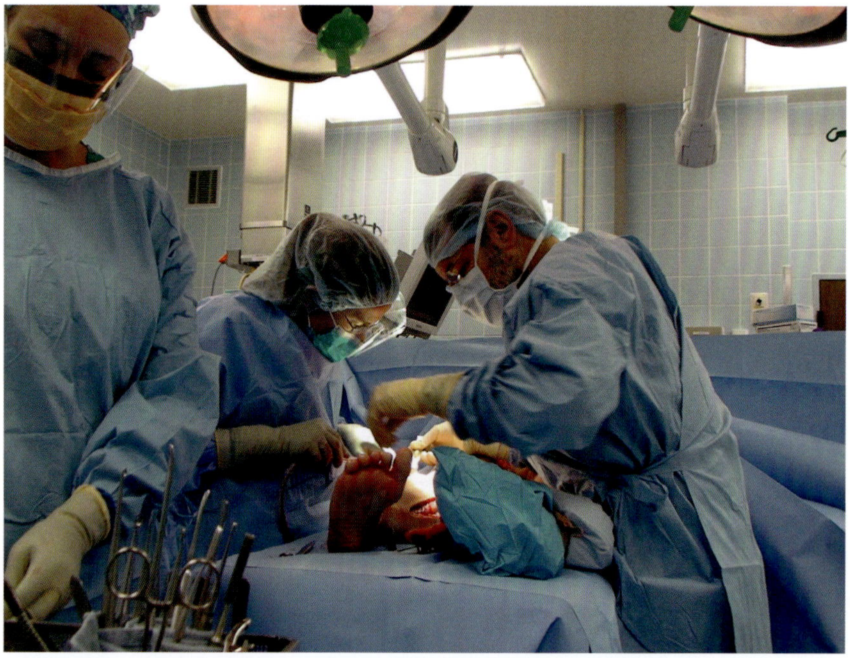

In Landstuhl, Ron Fairman operating on wounded soldier.

A particularly versatile Penn surgeon is Sloane Guy, who served two tours as an Army trauma surgeon in Afghanistan and another in Iraq. He graduated from college at Wake Forest where he played varsity football. After obtaining his MD at Penn and internship and several years of residency at HUP, he had further experience as a general surgery resident and faculty member at Walter Reed and UCSF before returning to HUP for his chief residency (2002) and CT fellowship. Since then, he has pioneered and directed minimally invasive and robotic cardiac surgery at Temple, Cornell, and Jefferson. He completed his prolonged military obligation in 2010 with a rank of lieutenant colonel.

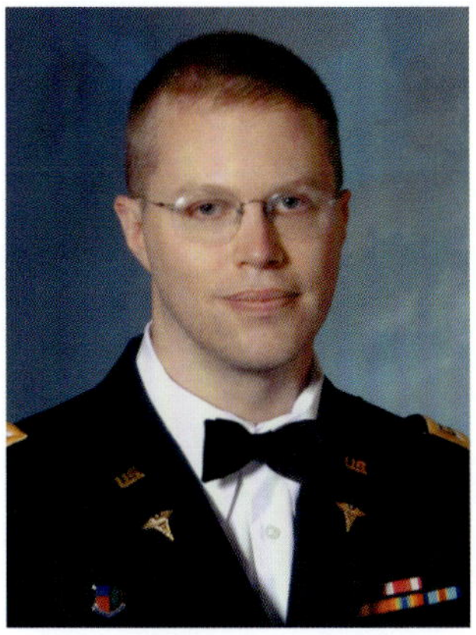

Sloane Guy

The Iraq War (2003–2011)

The story of John Pryor is not so much a part of the history of the Department of Surgery as a personal account of the life and patriotic motivation of a gifted Penn surgeon. John Pryor was in his second tour as a combat surgeon in Mosul when on Christmas morning in 2008, he was killed by an enemy rocket.

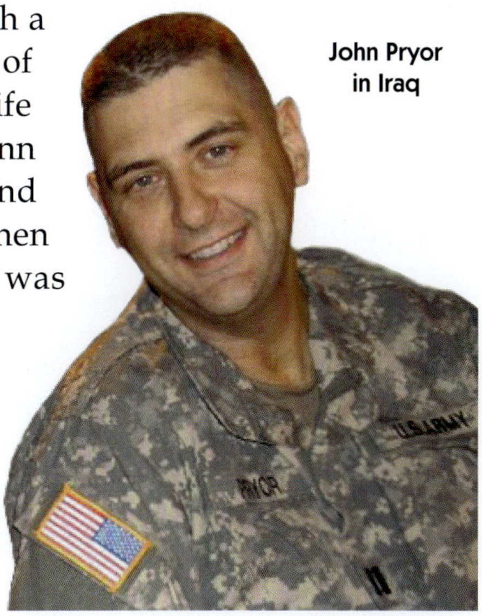

John Pryor in Iraq

Growing up in upstate New York, he was a Boy Scout and high school football star. Undistinguished college grades caused him to be rejected for medical school. Not willing to give up his desire to be a doctor, he marked time as an EMT and a brief period in a foreign medical school at Granada. He then transferred to medical school at SUNY—Buffalo where he was an AOA student and outstanding surgical resident. After a trauma fellowship at HUP, he accepted an invitation to join the faculty at the University of Pennsylvania. Within a few years, he was appointed as director of the trauma program at Penn. His prospect for an outstanding academic career was obvious.

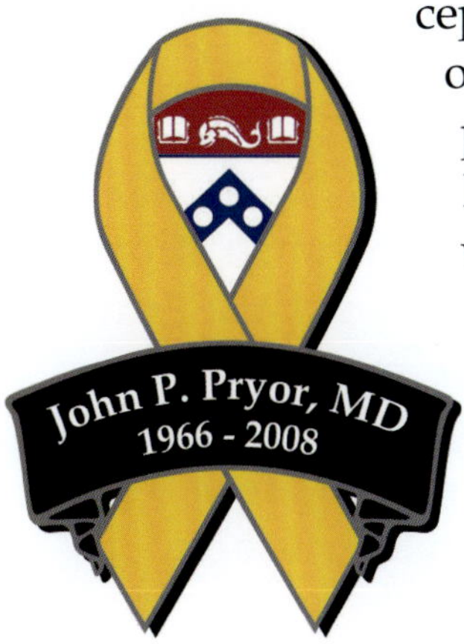

John's biography, *Alright, Let's Call It a Draw,* is a deeply personal account of his tragically short life, written by his brother, but largely pieced together from John's diary, essays he wrote, and family conversations with his brother,

1988
John Pryor graduates from State University of New York Binghamton

1992
Pryor attends St. George's University School of Medicine in Grenada, West Indies

1994
Pryor obtains MD from State University of New York Buffalo

1999–2001
HUP trauma fellowship

2001
HUP faculty appointment

2001 (Sept. 11)
Terrorist attack on World Trade Center in New York City

2008
John Pryor killed on Christmas morning

2009
John Pryor's biography

some real and some imagined. They talked about the meaning of life and how John saw his place in it.

Emotionally painful to read are graphic accounts of John's exhausting three-month tour as a combat surgeon in Iraq. He wrote about wounded soldiers he saved or lost with detailed descriptions of their injuries.

Reminiscent of John Gibbon interrupting his development of a heart-lung machine by volunteering for military service in World War II are Pryor's thoughts about volunteering to enter the Army, leaving behind his promising academic career, his wife, and three children.

After viewing on TV the collapse of the Twin Towers on 9/11, John was compelled to offer his services. In his remarkable account of his experience driving to New York that same day, he describes his struggle to overcome police barriers to reach Ground Zero. Then, as a trauma surgeon, he was welcomed by the first responders to remain and provide them with expert help. It became surprisingly eerie that there was nothing for him to do. There was no need for a trauma surgeon. Victims of this terrorist attack were not wounded but dead.

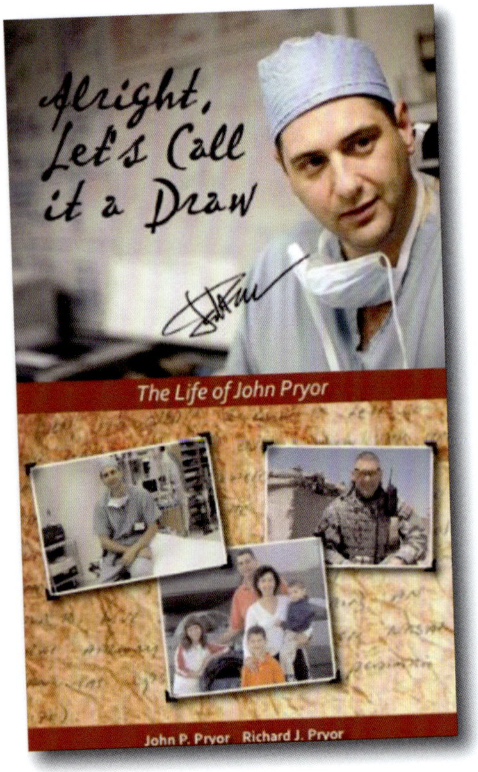

The experience on 9/11 was the inspiration for John to volunteer for the Army, anticipating that in that setting, he would be useful in Iraq as a combat surgeon. Not surprisingly, his wife and family and friends were bitterly opposed. He attributed his disregard of their protests to a conviction that the good life he had experienced as an American somehow obligated him to give back something. In an attempt to explain his decision, he wrote in his diary, "I'm a trauma surgeon. It's who I am . . . risky or not, the place for a trained trauma surgeon during war is in combat."[40] Whatever the reason, the rest of us should be grateful that there are men like John Gibbon and John Pryor.

Trauma Surgery at Home

In civilian aspects of trauma, Penn surgery chairmen Jonathan Rhoads and Bill Fitts were important leaders. Both were founders of the American Association for Trauma Surgery. Fitts became president of this association and longtime editor of the *Journal of Trauma.* He was an enthusiastic teacher of the principles of trauma surgery, in spite of being handicapped, because in his time, HUP had no trauma service and few trauma patients. One of Fitts's trainees, trauma surgeon Carter Nance, quipped that HUP had a Quaker-style trauma program, that is, there wasn't any trauma.

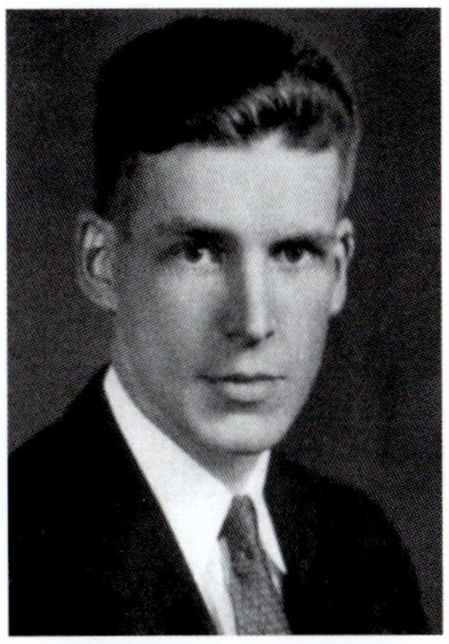

Jonathan Rhoads

1980–1983
Fitts resident, Gene Cayten, is trauma division chief. Lack of institutional interest and support for a trauma program is a handicap for him

Penn's trauma program is really only thirty years old, dating to its founding by Bill Schwab. Before that at HUP, there was not much interest in trauma care. It was almost as though there was an unstated policy to minimize HUP's trauma admissions. The hospital's administrators would have been content with this since many trauma victims were uninsured and most of the surgeons were happy not to be bothered with emergency admissions in the middle of the night.

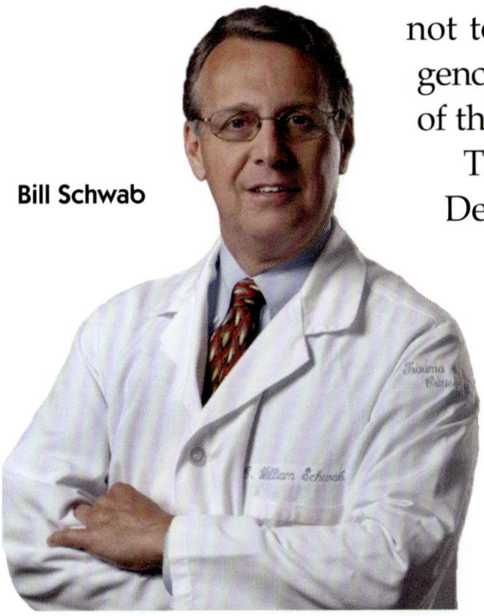

Bill Schwab

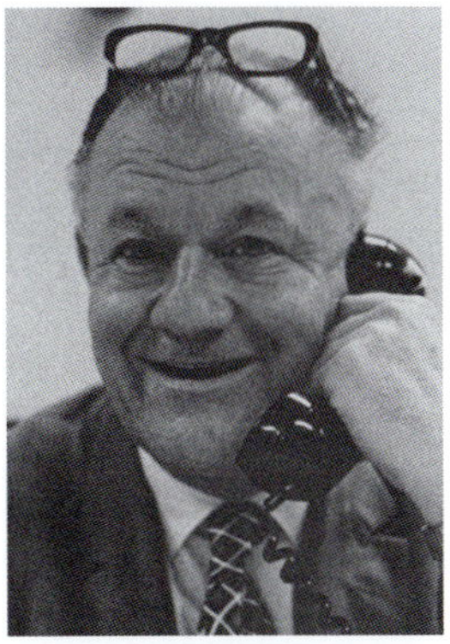

Bill Fitts

This changed in 1987, when Dean Edward Stemmler became aware that other Philadelphia hospitals were seeking accreditation as trauma centers. Stemmler, not liking the idea of HUP being left out of anything, approached me as the chairman of surgery and strongly suggested that I establish a trauma center. I have to admit that my enthusiasm for the idea was lukewarm. But since Stemmler agreed that the institution and not the Department of Surgery would cover any anticipated financial losses, I set out to follow his instructions. At first, it didn't seem that it should be difficult. Larry Stephenson, one of our department's cardiac surgeons, was a colonel in the Army reserves, so I appointed him as the trauma chief. I was annoyed to learn that for accreditation by the State and the American College of Surgeons, there were some additional requirements. For example, the center's surgeons must have ATLS (Advanced Trauma Life Support) accreditation. None of us had it, so a bunch of us went to Washington and took a two-day course to be certified. Filling out the application to be recognized as a center was another time-consuming nuisance, but we got it done and submitted it, assuming we would be approved. After all, we were the University of Pennsylvania.

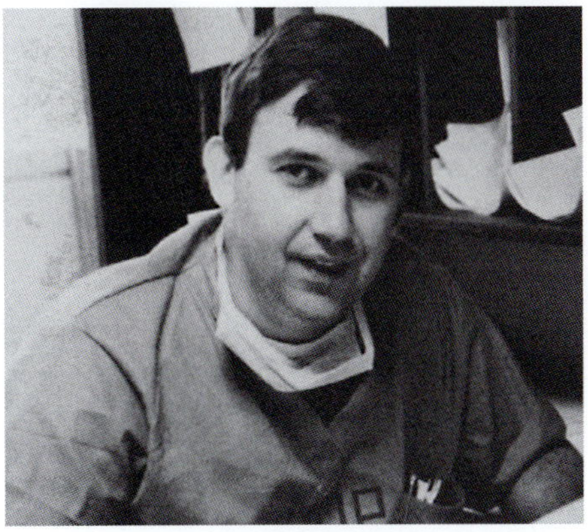

Larry Stephenson

1987
Dean Stemmler mandates a trauma center at HUP

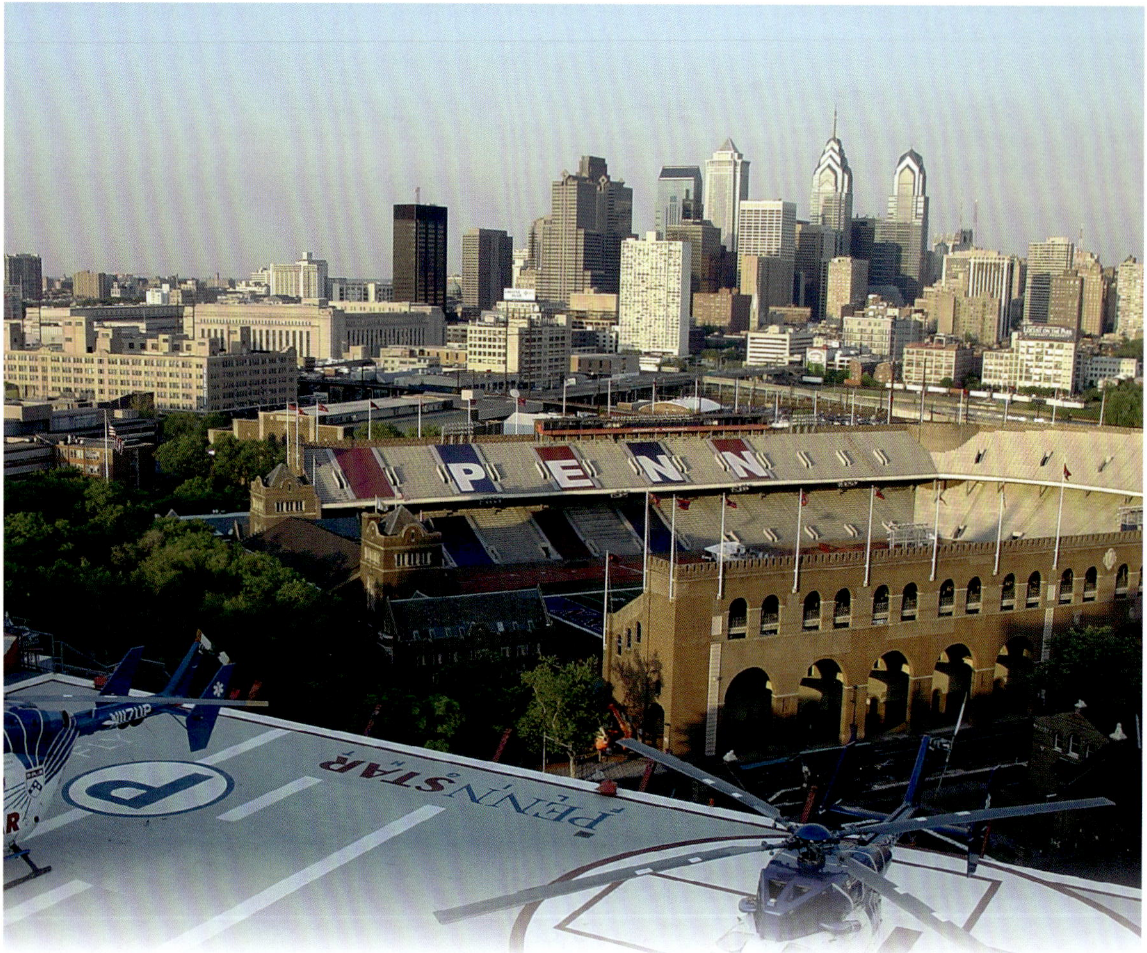

During a site visit, we were then evaluated by a team of trauma experts and, to my embarrassment, abruptly turned down. In retrospect, this was entirely appropriate. Our faculty members had neither the experience nor interest to qualify as trauma surgeons. Then it got tough. I realized that I needed someone with experience and expertise in this field as a leader. It wasn't easy to find someone like that, especially if you only looked at candidates from Harvard, Penn, Hopkins, and other predominantly research-focused institutions where, like at ours, there wasn't much interest in trauma. I interviewed a few candidates, but none seemed right. Then Larry Stephenson (our Army reserve colonel and temporary trauma center chief) suggested Bill Schwab, a young surgeon who was at Cooper Hospital in Camden. After his training in the Navy, he had directed trauma programs there and at Norfolk General Hospital. Although he had faculty appointments at the medical schools associated with these hospitals, his CV was missing the awards, prizes, and elite society memberships I was accustomed to scrutinizing in faculty candidates. There was one award I should have paid attention to—*Esquire* magazine's designation of Bill Schwab as "One of the Best of the New Generation, Men and Women Under 40 Who Are Changing America." Although skeptical, I invited him for an interview.

HUP's application for state certification of trauma center is declined

In less than five minutes, I knew that Bill Schwab was our man. His energy, knowledge, experience, confidence, and leadership qualities were obvious. After a few minutes more, he took me to the roof of the Ravdin Building to show me where the helicopters would land. I hadn't known we were going to have helicopters, but he had already named them PennSTAR.

The rest is history, summarized here only briefly. Bill Schwab quickly got HUP accredited as a trauma center and before long, built his trauma program into the best in the United States and probably the world. But what about those academic credentials, those trappings I was so narrowly focused on? How has he measured up to Penn standards in that respect? Well, after coming to Penn, it looks like he has surpassed us all. Bill Schwab easily got elected to membership in surgery's elite societies including the Society of University Surgeons and the American Surgical Association. He has been awarded honorary fellowships of the Royal College of Surgeons of England and Royal College of Physicians and Surgeons of Glasgow. He has won the highest awards of the surgical societies of the Netherlands, Sweden, and the European Society for Trauma and Emergency Surgery and of the Association of Trauma and Military Surgery of the Royal College of Surgeons of England.

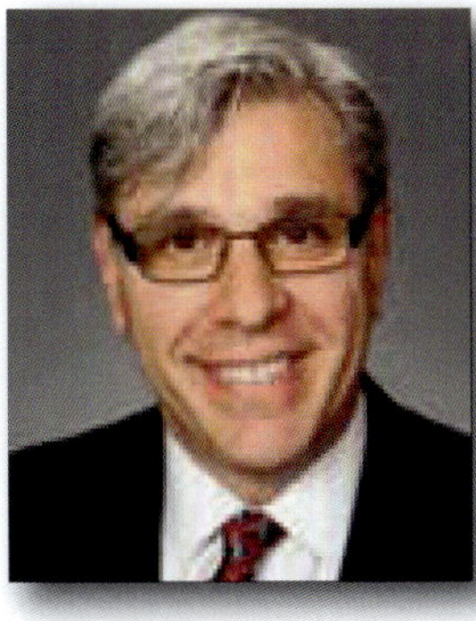
Michael Rotondo

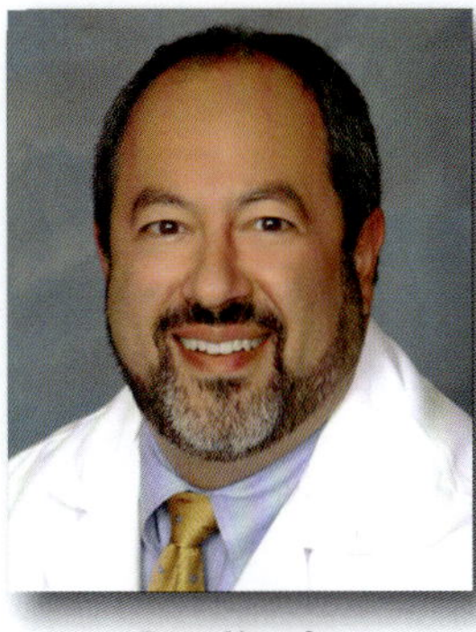
Don Kauder

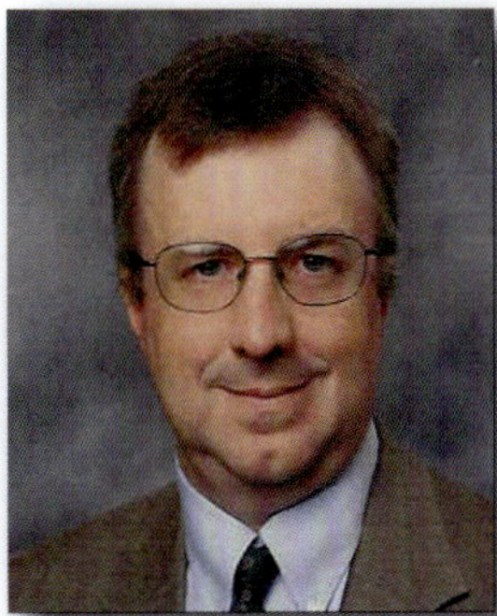
Pat Reilly

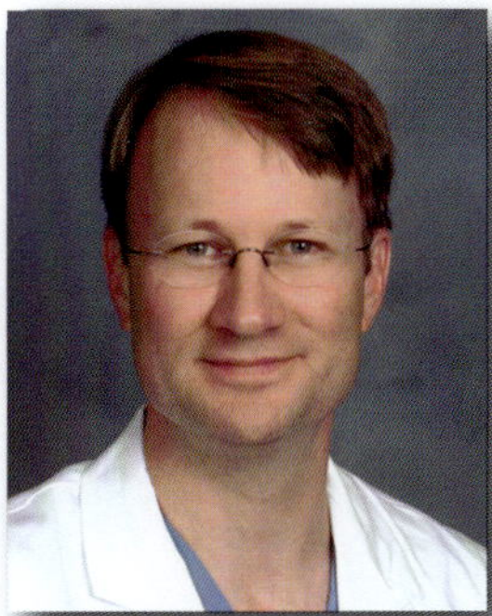
Mike Nance

Bill has served on the editorial boards of the *Journal of Trauma*, the *Archives of Surgery*, *Surgery*, the *Annals of Internal Medicine*, and the *New England Journal of Medicine*. He has been awarded an honorary degree from his alma mater, Ithaca College, where he has also chaired the Board of Trustees. He has been president of the Eastern Association for the Surgery of Trauma, the American Association for the Surgery of Trauma, and the International Association for the Surgery of Trauma. He has trained dozens of the world's trauma surgeons, many of whom have started their own trauma programs. He has been a visiting professor at over a hundred universities and medical centers and given the most prestigious named lectures in his field. He has published 250 peer-reviewed

1993
"Damage Control" emerges as a new paradigm

papers. The Institute of Medicine has sought his help in addressing problems with firearm injury and control.

More importantly though, how about Bill's professional accomplishments? Starting with a 1993 landmark paper in the *Journal of Trauma and Acute Care Surgery*, Dr. Schwab, Michael Rotondo, and other faculty colleagues have been responsible for a surgical paradigm shift. Borrowing a term from Bill's Navy background, they called it "damage control."[41] Patients with severe penetrating abdominal injury and bleeding were operated upon promptly without a delay for resuscitation, as had traditionally been advocated. The initial laparotomy was limited to rapid control of bleeding and contamination, and then, without further delay, expeditious temporary closure. This was followed by transfer to the ICU for resuscitation to restore normal physiology. Later, the stabilized patient was returned to the OR for anatomic reconstruction and definitive abdominal closure. After Bill and his team demonstrated that this strategy saved lives, it was widely adopted by military and civilian trauma surgeons. In addition, for selected patients whose physiology is severely compromised by nontrauma conditions, it can be useful and is not uncommonly employed.[42]

By pioneering with his faculty colleagues the concept of "damage control," a term now part of the surgical lexicon, Bill Schwab has changed the world of surgery, not just trauma surgery, and not just in America (like *Esquire* magazine predicted for him), but the world of surgery. It is entirely fitting that Bill's colleagues and friends have endowed a professorship of trauma surgery in his name.

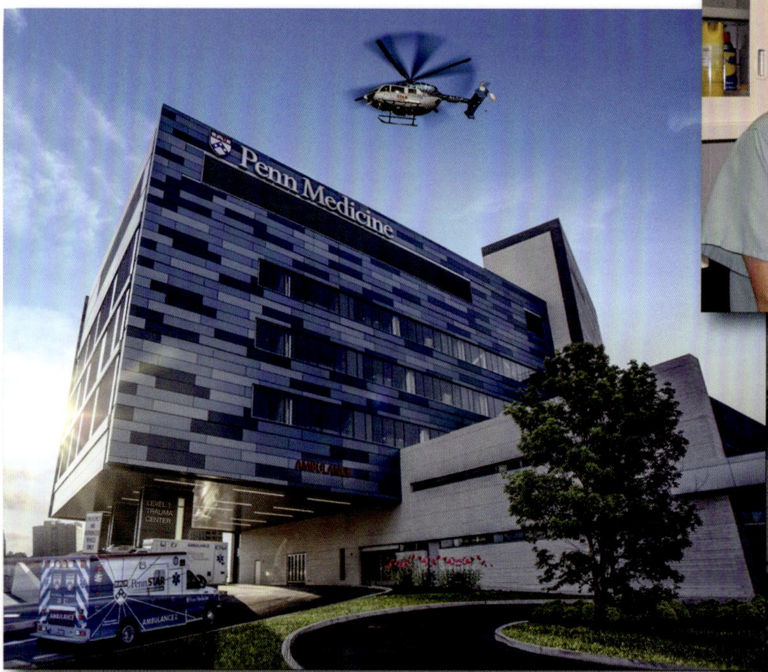

Trauma Center at Penn Presbyterian Medical Center

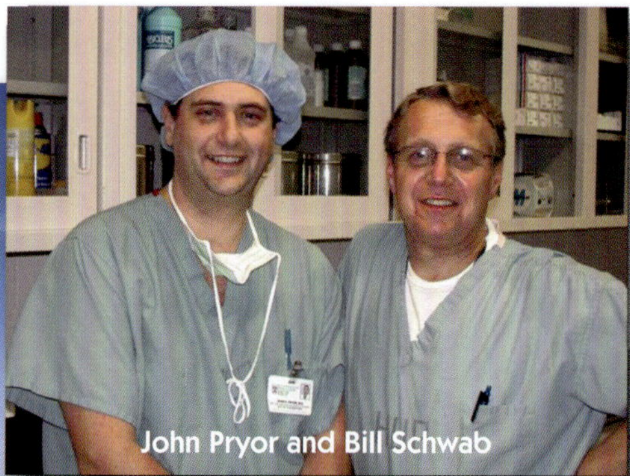
John Pryor and Bill Schwab

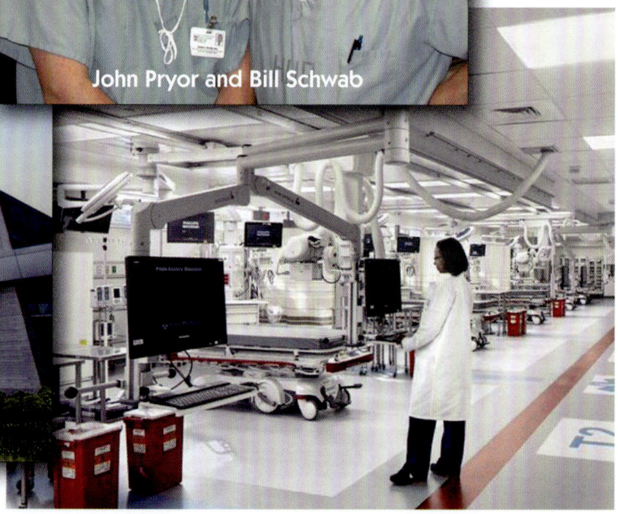
John Pryor Shock and Resuscitation Unit

Notes

[1] Flexner, JT. *The Traitor and the Spy: Benedict Arnold and John Andre* (New York: Harcourt Brace, 1953).

[2] Bell, Whitfield J. *John Morgan: Continental Doctor.* University of Pennsylvania Press (1965) p. 211.

[3] Bell, Whitfield J. *Patriot-Improvers: Biographical Sketches of Members of the American Philosophical Society Volume Three 1767–1768* (American Philosophical Society, 2010) pp. 13–14.

[4] Cameron JL. Early contributions to the Johns Hopkins hospital by the "other" surgeon: John Shaw Billings. *Ann Surg* (2001) 234(3):267-278. doi:10.1097/00000658-200109000-00001.

[5] Lloyd, Mark Frazier. Penn's Base Hospitals in World Wars I and II. Penn University Archives and Record Center. https://archives.upenn.edu/exhibits/penn-history/base-hospitals.

[6] Memoir of John Barton Carnett. *Transactions of the Philadelphia Academy of Surgery* (1932–33) Vol XXVI, pp. xxxiv-xxxivi.

[7] Ibid, p. xxxiv–xxxivi.

[8] *The Reminiscence of Isidor Ravdin.* Columbia University Oral History Collection Part II No 156. Isidor Ravdin, Saul Benison, Barbara Land, Columbia University Oral Research Office, New York Times Oral History Program (1971) p. 64.

[9] Cooper III, David Y and Ledger, Marshall A. *Innovation and Tradition at the University of Pennsylvania School of Medicine, An Anecdotal Journey* (Philadelphia: University of Pennsylvania Press, 1990) pp. 150–151.

[10] Ibid, pp. 151–153.

[11] *The Reminiscence of Isidor Ravdin.* Columbia University Oral History Collection, Part II No 156, pp. 144–152.

[12] Gibbon, JH Jr. The Maintenance of Life During Experimental Occlusion of the Pulmonary Artery Followed by Survival. *Surg Gynec + Obst* 69:602 (1939).

[13] Shumacker, Harris B. *A Dream of the Heart, The Life of John H. Gibbon, Jr. Father of the Heart-Lung Machine* (Santa Barbara: Fithian Press, 1999) p. 128.

[14] Ibid, p. 130.

[15] Ibid, pp. 87–100. In fact, two full chapters of Schumacker's biography of Gibbon are devoted to his family's military backgrounds (pp. 87–100, 224–252).

[16] Shumacker, Harris B. *A Dream of the Heart, The Life of John H. Gibbon, Jr. Father of the Heart-Lung Machine,* p. 138.

[17] USS *Solace* (AH-5). *Wikipedia,* Wikimedia Foundation, 22 Jan. 2022 https://en.wikipedia.org/wiki/USS_Solace_(AH-5).

[18] *Scope* University of Pennsylvania Medical School Yearbook (1943).

[19] Christian Lambertson, Inventor of Scuba Precursor, Dies at 93. *New York Times* (Feb. 25, 2011).

[20] *Scope* University of Pennsylvania Medical School Yearbook (1943).

[21] Cooper III, David Y and Ledger, Marshall A. *Innovation and Tradition at the University of Pennsylvania School of Medicine, An Anecdotal Journey,* p. 264.

[22] Personal recollection of Lambertson's medical school classmate, my brother Harold G. Barker.

[23] Cooper III, David Y and Ledger, Marshall A. *Innovation and Tradition at the University of Pennsylvania School of Medicine, An Anecdotal Journey,* p. 264.

[24] Christian J. Lambertsen. *Wikipedia,* Wikimedia Foundation (22 Jan. 2022). https://en.wikipedia.org/wiki/Christian_J._Lambertsen.

[25] New words list January 2020. *Oxford English Dictionary* (22 Jan. 2022). https://public.oed.com/updates/new-words-list-january-2020/.

[26] Mrs. C.J. Biddle of 'Andalusia,' Dies. *The Philadelphia Inquirer* (24 May 1973).

[27] Henry Blair Keep Jr. *Find a Grave* (22 Jan. 2022). https://www.findagrave.com/memorial/192763819/henry-blair-keep.

[28] Letter from Henry Keep to his father.

[29] McManus, John C. *September Hope: The American Side of A Bridge Too Far* (Penguin Publishing Group, 2012) p. 273.

[30] Ryan, Cornelius. *A Bridge Too Far* (New York: Touchstone, 1995) p. 460.

[31] Nordyke, Phil. *All American, All the Way: The Combat History of the 82nd Airborne Division in World War II* (Zenith Press, 2005).

[32] McManus, John. Operation Market Garden: 'hail Mary' in Holland. HistoryNet (July 5, 2012). https://www.historynet.com/operation-market-garden-hail-mary-in-holland/.

[33] Davis, Richard. *Yours, D^3* (White Plains, NY: Alliance House, 1999).

[34] Howard JM. Historical vignettes of arterial repair: recollections of Korea 1951-1953. *Ann Surg* (1998) 228(5):716-719. doi:10.1097/00000658-199811000-00012.

[35] Debakey ME, Simeone FA. Battle Injuries of the Arteries in World War II: An Analysis of 2,471 Cases. *Ann Surg* (1946) 123(4):534–579.

[36] Blalock, Alfred and Helen B. Taussig. The Surgical Treatment of Malformations of the Heart: In Which There Is Pulmonary Stenosis or Pulmonary Atresia. *JAMA* 128 (1945): 2123–2138.

[37] Howard JM. Historical vignettes of arterial repair: recollections of Korea 1951-1953. *Ann Surg* (1998) 228(5):716-719. doi:10.1097/00000658-199811000-00012.

[38] Finnegan, James O. *In the Company of Marines: A Surgeon Remembers Vietnam* (Lulu.com, 2010).

[39] Fairman RM. Measuring the worth of a vascular surgeon: Making it personal through a career of service. *J Vasc Surg* (2018) 67(5):1321-1327. doi:10.1016/j.jvs.2018.02.007.

[40] Pryor, Richard J and Pryor, John P. *Alright, Let's Call It a Draw: The Life of John Pryor* (lanxnal: Delmar, New York, 2012) p. 427.

[41] Rotondo MF, Schwab CW, McGonigal MD, et al. 'Damage control': an approach for improved survival in exsanguinating penetrating abdominal injury. *J Trauma* (1993) 35(3):375–383.

[42] Stawicki SP, Brooks A, Bilski T, et al. The concept of damage control: extending the paradigm to emergency general surgery. *Injury* (2008) 39(1):93–101.

CHAPTER 33

A Collection of Educators

Institutions like HUP are called teaching hospitals. Thus, all faculty members are expected to teach. For most, this is considered a privilege, not an onerous duty. But there have been some teachers who stood apart. This chapter sketches the careers of a dozen Penn surgeons who were acclaimed for their teaching, won the most teaching awards, or for whom teaching awards were named.

William Y. Inouye (1920–1985)

Bill Inouye

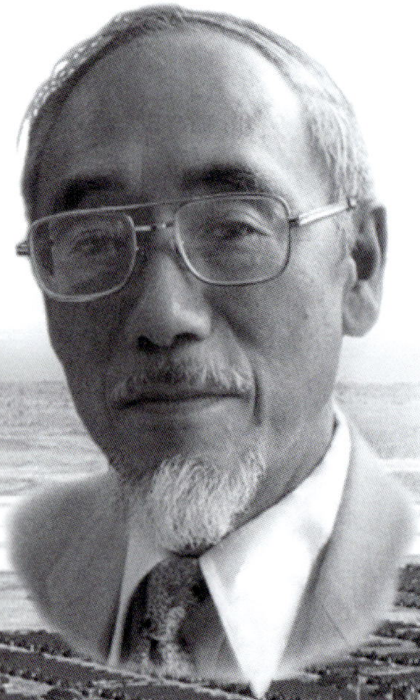

Each year the Department recognizes excellence in teaching by a surgical resident with the William Y. Inouye Award. Winners of this award can no longer appreciate why it was named for this beloved surgical faculty member who died before they were born.

Bill Inouye grew up in Sacramento, California. At the onset of World War II in 1941, the presumed threat to national security led to the imprisonment of Bill and his family with other Americans of Japanese descent at a camp at Tula Lake, California. In 1944, the Inouyes were allowed to move to Philadelphia where, for the rest of the war, they managed a hostel that served as a halfway house, helping to re-

Tule Lake Segregation Center, 1946

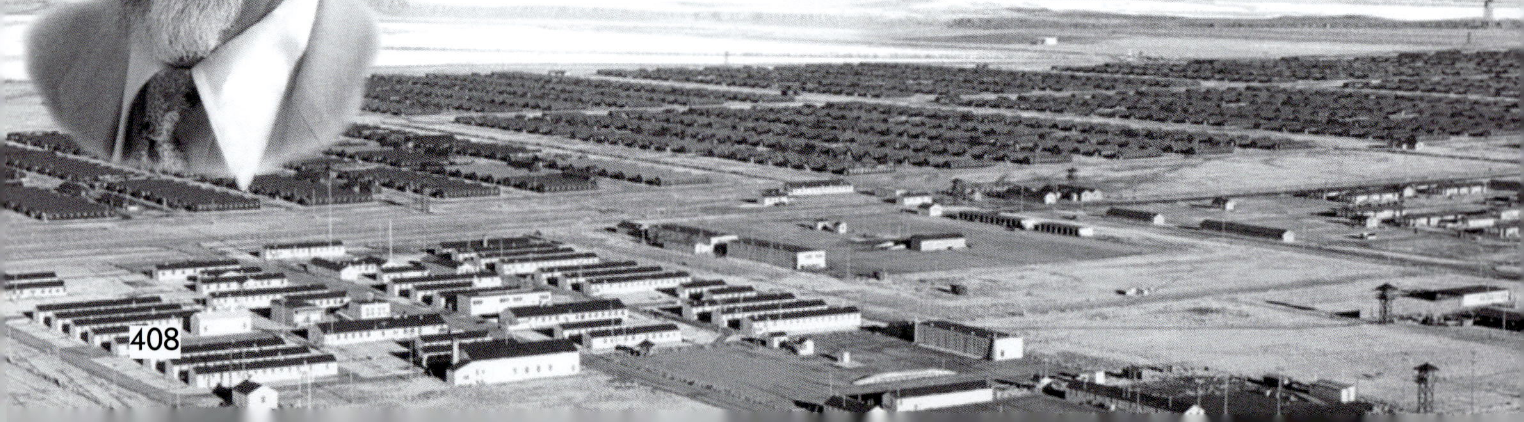

locate and aid more than 1,000 Japanese Americans from other parts of the United States. Twenty-five years after the war ended, Bill's mother was awarded the Order of the Sacred Treasurer by the Japanese Emperor for bettering relations between the United States and Japan.

Relocation to Philadelphia allowed Bill to attend Swarthmore College where he was Phi Beta Kappa, graduating in 1944. His plans to attend medical school were delayed by the economic losses suffered by his family during their imprisonment. For the next five years, Bill worked as a chemist in an asbestos factory.[1] Then, having saved enough money, he entered Penn Medical School in 1949, graduating AOA in 1953. While he was a medical student doing research in the Harrison Department of Surgical Research and in nephrologist Bill Bluemle's lab, he devised the first coil hemodialysis machine. He made this from screening material and cellulose tubing purchased from a hardware store. The ingenious device was enclosed in a standard Presto Pressure Cooker for distribution of the dialyzing fluid and to provide a closed system that allowed for ultrafiltration by using negative pressure.[2] Bill first described his dialyzer in the 1953 Surgical Forum.[3] It was used at HUP in nine patients,[4] some of the earliest successful hemodialyses.

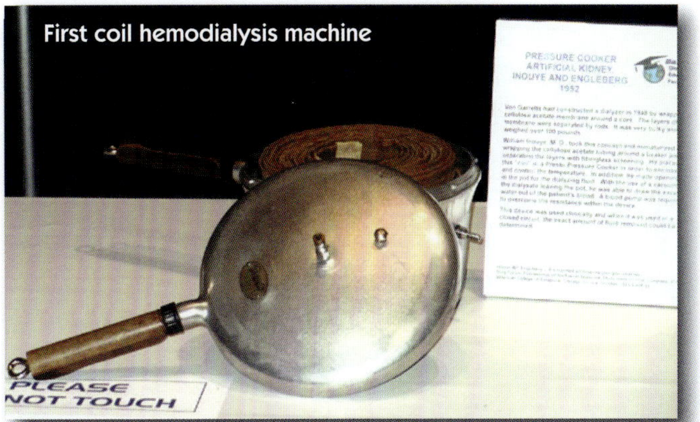

First coil hemodialysis machine

During this time, Willem Kolff visited Penn and was shown Bill's dialysis machine. Soon after, Kolff produced a similar model, failing to credit Inouye for the design. Former HUP nephrologist, Lee Henderson, contends that the coil dialyzer should have been named for Inouye. It soon became standard because it was a great improvement over the cumbersome drum model originated by Kolff. Years later, Kolff belatedly acknowledged Inouye's contribution, but earlier, many others had recognized its seminal importance. Inouye received the National Kidney Foundation's Dialysis Pioneer Award for design of the forerunner of the twin coil artificial kidney. His prototype is now exhibited in several museums, including the Smithsonian Institution.

After finishing the HUP surgical residency in 1961 and two years in the Army, Bill was appointed to the Penn Faculty. He developed a large clinical practice that he conducted mainly at Jeanes Hospital, which at that time, largely because of Bill, was a popular site of HUP surgical resident rotations. Although outstanding in his early years as a scientist and later as a clinician, it was as an educator that Bill Inouye particularly excelled. He was appointed chief of the Penn Service at Philadelphia

General Hospital and chief of the Residents Ward Teaching Service at HUP. Since he worked at several hospitals, he often traveled back and forth across town several times a day, making sure that every patient was covered. He was considered the best teacher by the residents and also by the medical students who dedicated their yearbook to him.

In the fall of 1982, while he was at the peak of his powers as a clinical surgeon and educator and shortly after his promotion to full professor, Bill noticed that he was short of breath. He was found to have a pleural effusion. This soon led to the diagnosis of mesothelioma, which seems certainly to have stemmed from his exposure to asbestos during the time he was working to earn money for medical school. As his disease progressed, his activities were more and more limited. His courage and dedication to teaching allowed him to continue some professional activity, and fortunately, he somewhat outlived predictions based on the usual natural history of his disease, perhaps because of an extensive pleural resection by his colleague, Alden Harken. Although in considerable pain, he continued to make teaching rounds with the residents until a few months before his death. When his physical limitations precluded this activity, he turned his attention to raising money for the residents' fund, pursuing this activity to within a few days of his death. He contacted every former HUP resident, urging each of them to contribute. Many generously did so, with the result that for years, this fund provided most of the support of resident travel to meetings. Bill donated the stipend he received for his teaching activities plus a sizable personal contribution to support this fund. He also endowed annual teaching awards to be chosen by the residents, one for a resident and another for a faculty member. Until his death, the residents refused to designate anyone but Bill as the recipient of the faculty teaching award.

Shortly after Bill's death in 1985, I was surprised to receive a brief note from him, obviously written in anticipation of his impending death. In it he said, "By the time you receive this note I will have passed on to wherever one goes on the great adventure. Life foreshortened by asbestos problems has denied some of the anticipated joys and luxuries of an extended postretirement phase. However I feel it has been my privilege to pursue the active life of a teaching surgeon, working with residents who seem to grow younger each year, to watch them develop and share with them the ever expanding knowledge of our profession. My best wishes to you. William Y. Inouye."[5]

Leonard D. Miller (1930–1997)[6]

Leonard Miller was born July 8, 1930 in Jersey City, New Jersey. After early education in the Jersey City public schools where he was a distinguished scholar and an All-City high school basketball player, he attended Yale University, graduating in 1951. At Penn's medical

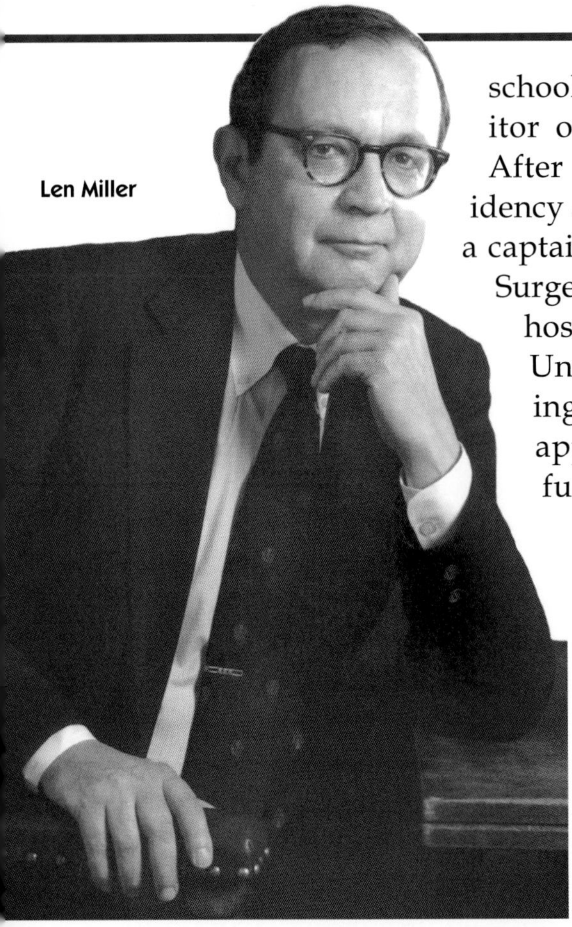

Len Miller

school, he was president of his class and editor of the yearbook, graduating in 1955. After internship and a year of surgical residency at HUP, he served from 1957 to 1959 as a captain in the US Air Force and as Chief of Surgery and commander of a large Air Force hospital in England. After returning to the University of Pennsylvania and completing his surgical residency in 1964, he was appointed to the faculty and became a full professor only five years later.

During his entire professional life, Len's greatest commitment was to education.

After finishing his tour as department chairman, Len took on the responsibility as chief of the teaching service. For the next fourteen years, he closely supervised the patients on this "ward" service by attending all the residents' operations, including those at night and on the weekends. Students and residents schemed to be on his teaching service, in his quiz sections, and his other classes. He was recognized with many awards: a Lindback Award; an honorary faculty membership in AOA; designation as the best clinical teacher by the medical school classes of 1992, 1993, and 1996, and by the surgical residents five times as their best teacher of the year. His national recognition as an educator was confirmed by his appointment as chair of the Surgical Education Committee of the Society of University Surgeons.

During his thirty-three years as a faculty member, Len assumed many important administrative roles. After several years as acting chairman of the Department, he succeeded William T. Fitts Jr. in 1978 as John Rhea Barton Professor and Chairman of the Department, and served in this role until 1983. See Chapter 23 for his experience as chairman.

For more than forty years, Len Miller was an important force at the University of Pennsylvania and especially in its Department of Surgery. Even as a resident, he was recognized by medical students and junior residents as an outstanding teacher. Later, his teaching skills would become almost legendary. He was more broadly knowledgeable about surgery than anyone can remember, and he was eager and effective in sharing this knowledge. But more so than his professional accomplishments and contributions to his school and department, it was Len's personal qualities which endeared him to his students and colleagues.

Over the last decade of his life, and particularly in his last illness, he exhibited great courage and resilience. Teaching had become his mission and almost totally occupied his waking hours. It was a tragic irony that his terminal illness from laryngeal cancer robbed him of his ability to speak and thus his lifelong passion, teaching. He confronted his final illness with a stubbornness and apparent good cheer that should serve as a lesson to everyone.

Julius A. Mackie Jr. (1927–2003)

The department's Distinguished Graduate Award is named for Julius Mackie, one of its most acclaimed teachers.

"Jack" Mackie was a native of Winston-Salem, North Carolina, and a graduate of the University of North Carolina and of the medical school of the University of Pennsylvania. While he was a surgical resident at HUP, his fellow residents recognized that he was unusually gifted and efficient. Dr. Ravdin, the chairman, became aware of this and promoted him to chief resident after only three years. After two years as chief of surgery at Ft. Hood Army Hospital in Texas, he returned to the Penn faculty for the rest of his life.[7]

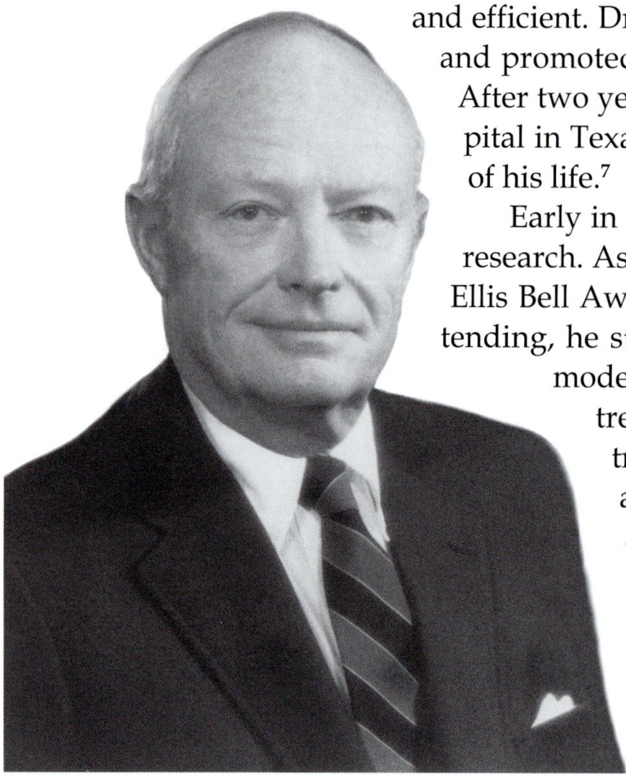

Jack Mackie

Early in his career, Jack showed promise in laboratory research. As a medical student, he was awarded the Mary Ellis Bell Award for research. As a resident and young attending, he studied gastrointestinal physiology in animal models of peptic ulcer disease as well as the surgical treatment of hypertension. Later his major contributions were in the clinical practice of surgery and in teaching. He maintained a broad interest and expertise in general surgery throughout his career. But because of an early interest, he became a cancer specialist before the era of "super-specialists." He developed a practice focused on breast cancer, gastrointestinal cancers, and cancer of the pancreas. Most of his publications were on those topics, many of them coauthored with Jonathan Rhoads with whom he collaborated in practice for many years.

From 1970 to 1980 as the education officer of the Department, Jack was in charge of the teaching of surgery to medical students and surgical residents. Both before and after this, he was considered by generations of surgical residents to be one of their most important mentors. In 1987, the HUP residents designated him as their most valuable teacher.

Dr. Mackie was prominent in medical and surgical circles, both locally and beyond. From 1972 to 1988, he was an associate editor of the *Journal of Trauma*. He was a member of the Philadelphia Academy of

Surgery, the Eastern Surgical Society, the American College of Surgeons, and the International Society of Surgery. He was also elected to membership in the Southern Surgical Association (a rare honor for a northerner). Perhaps his favorite society was an exclusive group of Philadelphia's leading physicians, the "Medical Club." Most others of this small group limited to thirteen members were chiefs of surgery or medicine, hospital directors, or university provosts and presidents. Sir William Osler and several generations of the Pepper family were once members. A tribute to the respect in which Dr. Mackie was held by these important colleagues was his election to the position of executive officer of this group.

Dr. Mackie was considered exceptionally gifted technically. Students, residents, and fellow faculty members (including the several department chairmen during his faculty career) sought his advice on clinical problems and asked for his help in difficult operations.

For over a half a century, through the tenures of six successive chairmen, Jack was a mainstay of the Department, a supportive and steadying influence. In a sense he was the Department's unsung hero. Before, during, and after Dr. Rhoads was the chairman, he owed much of his success to Jack. Without Jack, he could never have managed his huge clinical practice while traveling incessantly and devoting much of his time to local and national leadership activities.

I was not alone in observing that Jack had the skills and qualities that would have led to greater national, research, and academic prominence if he had devoted less time to Dr. Rhoads's clinical practice. But for whatever reason, national office and self-aggrandizement were never a focus for Jack. His real interests and greatest satisfaction came from patient care and teaching. At these activities, he was a master.

In pre- and postoperative care, Jack was obsessive, some thought to a fault. Many HUP residents were at first impatient and annoyed by Jack's attention to the details of patient care. After making complete rounds with the residents, he would often double back to satisfy himself that a sump drain was working or that a nasogastric tube was properly positioned. A fruitful example of Jack's attention to detail was recalled by his fellow faculty surgeon, Clete Schwegman. Dr. Schwegman vividly recalled how Dr. Mackie had saved his life after Clete had undergone surgery for cancer of a vocal cord. Though Jack had not performed the surgery, he feared that Clete might need more careful observation than was being provided. Late at night, Jack went to Clete's bedside to check up on him. He found that Clete, who was receiving oxygen, was blown up like a balloon because of an oxygen leak that threatened to cause a fatal tension pneumothorax. "Jack stuck a needle in my chest and deflated me, saving my life," said Dr. Schwegman.

Patients never complained of Jack's redundant attention. Many of his residents eventually acknowledged that their own habits in pre- and postop care followed Jack's pattern. Ted Copeland, in his presidential addresses to the American College of Surgeons, paid tribute to Jack for this aspect of his teaching.

Emulating Jack's performance in the operating room was harder. Most of us recognize that the technical aspects of operative surgery are a craft that can be learned by most individuals, given the proper environment and enough effort. Occasionally one sees, for want of a better term, a "born surgeon," whose skills surpass those of his mentors and colleagues. Jack Mackie was one of those few.

Jack worked hard at teaching residents to operate. During the 1960s, only Jack and one other HUP attending, Jerry Peskin, allowed the residents to operate on their patients (under appropriately careful supervision). The others usually performed the entire operation themselves, presumably with the assumption that watching them was the optimal learning experience for residents. Because of Jack's efforts, some of his skill rubbed off on even the less gifted.

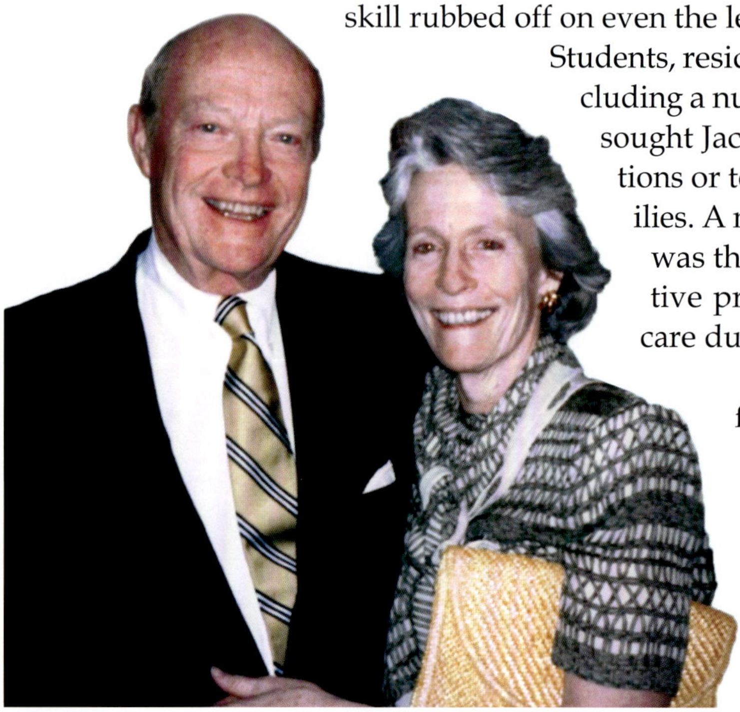

Jack and Joan Mackkie

Students, residents, and fellow faculty members (including a number of future department chairmen) sought Jack's advice and help in difficult operations or to take care of themselves or their families. A notable and most appropriate example was that even after Jack had retired from active practice, Dr. Rhoads called on him for care during his final illness.

Jack was lucky that during his own final illness, and for many years before, he had the love and support of his wife Joan. The department is grateful for Joanie's generosity in endowing the annual Mackie Distinguished Graduate Award and Lecture as well as for making it possible for a conference room in his name.

Alden Harken (1941–)

Before he went on to a distinguished career as a department chairman at two other institutions, Alden Harken was a Penn surgeon. Alden was the son of Dwight Harken, a Harvard surgeon who was one of the first to perform mitral valve surgery. Following college at Harvard and graduation from Case Western Reserve Medical School in 1967, Alden completed surgical and pediatric cardiovascular surgical residencies at the Peter Bent Brigham Hospital and Boston Children's Hospital. After three years as an investigator at the Walter Reed Army Institute of Research, he joined the faculty of the University of Pennsylvania in 1975.

During his eight years on the Penn faculty among a collection of fine educators, he stood out as the most charismatic and perhaps the most effective teacher I can ever remember. He was also successful in other areas. While at Penn, he had two NIH grants and published 100 papers. He pioneered the surgery for ventricular tachy-arrhythmias and won a Lindback Award for his teaching. He would have been a spectacular chairman at Penn, as he was at two other university institutions.

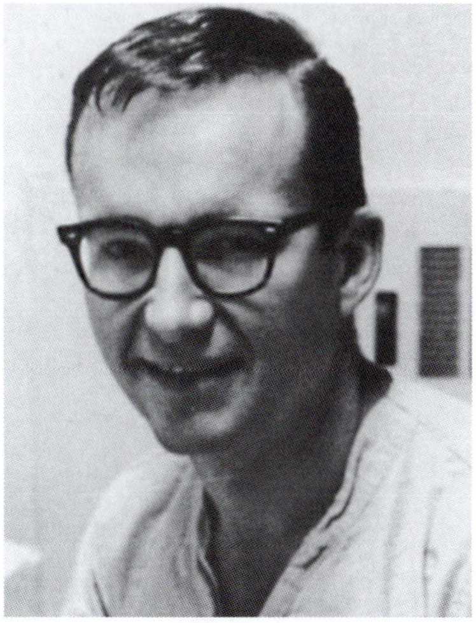

Alden Harken

HUP residents flocked to work in his lab. He was assigned to organize and moderate surgical grand rounds and as a prelude, he organized his own conference that met at 7:00 a.m. Saturday mornings. The format of this conference was a debate of controversial issues in surgery. Every week, he selected two residents and pitted them against each other, one for and one against a particular operation or other treatment. It didn't matter what their own opinion was; they were expected to build the strongest case for the side they had been assigned. The residents were given a week to organize their presentation and select current and historical references for support. It was a great learning experience for the residents and frankly for senior faculty members who attended. Attendance was not required, but the room was always full. Everyone had fun.

Although it had been obvious that Alden would be offered chairs at other institutions, he was such a valuable faculty member that I tried to keep him at Penn as long as possible. In 1983, Alden accepted the invitation to become chairman of the Department of Surgery at the University of Colorado. When he left, it was not surprising that several Penn residents and students chose to go with him.

After two successful decades in Denver, he moved to the University of California, San Francisco East Bay, as chairman of the Department of Surgery. It was not surprising that Alden won the top teaching awards in every institution he attended. Nor was it surprising that he became president of the Society of University Surgeons (and its lifetime achievement awardee) and president of the Association of Academic Surgeons.

He has authored more than 500 scientific publications and been awarded ten NIH grants. He has served as a director of the American Board of Surgery and the American Board of Thoracic Surgery and as a regent of the American College of Surgeons. None of this was unexpected, but in my mind, Alden's greatest gift is as a teacher.

Leonard J. Perloff (1940–1993)[8]

Each year, the department remembers Leonard Perloff by awarding a prize in his name to a resident for outstanding teaching.

Leonard J. Perloff lived his entire life in Philadelphia, except for a short time in the Army. In college at Penn, he was Phi Beta Kappa and a member of the fencing team. After medical school at Penn, internship at PGH, and residency and vascular fellowship at HUP, he spent two years on the transplant service at Walter Reed hospital, rising to the rank of lieutenant colonel. He then returned to Penn for the rest of his career, becoming professor of surgery in 1989. At HUP, he was associate chief of transplantation and assistant chief of vascular surgery. In 1993, Len died suddenly while jogging.

Dr. Perloff was a versatile academic surgeon. Although he said that basic research was not his long suit, the respect he was accorded by others to his status as an experimentalist was indicated by his appointment as chairman of the VA National Merit Review Board for Surgery. Several of the studies supported by his NIH ROI grant contributed substantially to the understanding of allograft rejection. He defined the importance of the transplant site in the fate of thyroid allografts. Using his skills as a microsurgeon, he compared in rodent models the survival of transplanted whole pancreas with isolated islet allografts.

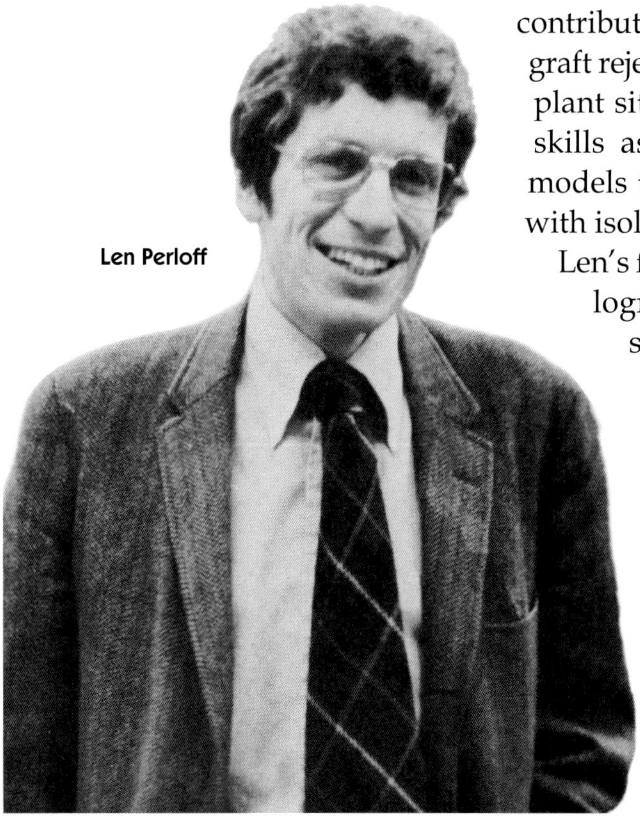
Len Perloff

Len's favorite experimental topic was the venous allograft. He was a foremost authority on this somewhat esoteric subject. A paper he presented to the Society of Vascular Surgery contained the best description to date of blood vessel allograft rejection. He, along with Craig Reckard, demonstrated for the first time that venous allografts would succeed if immunosuppression was used to prevent rejection. Len's expertise as a microsurgeon allowed him to study venous homografts, even in small rodents. This topic fascinated Len throughout his career, and he returned to its study many times, jokingly referring to this long series of papers as "The Venous Homograft," "The Return of the Venous Homograft," "The Son of the Venous Homograft," and so forth. In his last few months, Len was organizing a trial of venous homografts in patients.

Despite his considerable accomplishments as an experimentalist, Len was primarily a clinical surgeon, and a superb one. Trained by Brooke Roberts, a master vascular surgeon, Len became one of HUP's most active vascular surgeons. He was also an experienced transplant surgeon, and many of the 100 entries in his bibliography were clinical papers on this subject. At Walter Reed, he studied kidney preservation injury, a phenomenon he showed to be caused by antibodies in the plasma contained in the perfusate. Later at HUP, he described a previously unrecognized syndrome of soft tissue calcinosis in transplant recipients with ognized syndrome of soft tissue calcinosis in transplant recipients with secondary hyperparathyroidism. With Don Dafoe, Bob Grossman, and Ernie Ring, he defined percutaneous transluminal angioplasty as the preferred method of treating transplant renal artery stenosis. He was also the director of HUP's pancreas transplant program, the first in the region.

Len was a skilled and extremely popular teacher with a gift for developing rapport with students and residents. He directed the department's clerkship and chaired the school's Student Standards Committee. The medical students elected him to honorary membership in AOA, and in 1992 named him the school's Outstanding Teacher. In 1994, the Penn Medical School Yearbook was dedicated to him. The surgical residents named an annual teaching award in his honor.

Leonard's national and international recognition were confirmed by his election to many prestigious academic societies, including the International Transplantation Society, the Society for Vascular Surgery, and the Society of University Surgeons. An unusual honor was his posthumous election as a member of the American Surgical Association.

Len Perloff's greatest talents were not in the research laboratory, nor were they in the operating theater or the classroom. His people skills and sense of humor were his most widely recognized assets and through them, he contributed much to his patients, his colleagues, and his school. Only Larry the Barber knew more jokes than Len. In conferences, Len was called on frequently because his discussions were not only informative but always entertaining. However, verbal fencing with Len was dangerous. He was never at a loss, and one could always count on a clever response to a question even if Len didn't know the answer. Those who tried to best him found his wit so quick and riposte so sharp that the laugh was usually at their expense.

For a busy academic surgeon, Len had an unusually well-developed appreciation for life outside of medicine. Walter Hagen, the golfer, said, "You're only here for a short visit. Don't hurry, don't worry. And be sure to smell the flowers along the way." Len had some worries, but he always handled himself with style and grace. After his untimely death, most of the letters received from his friends, former fellows, and students commented on his talent for smelling the flowers, enjoying life, and sharing a joke. This is what we continue to miss the most about Len Perloff.

Gordon P. Buzby (1948–2003)

Shortly before Gordon Buzby's untimely death in 2003, he and his wife Karen met with Jim Mullen and established a fund that provides for an annual lecture and award in surgical leadership. This award in Gordon's name is presented to a surgical resident or faculty member chosen for interests and expertise similar to Gordon's, including a devotion to exploring vital issues of surgical management and leadership, that is, teaching, patient care, and administration. Gordon personally chose the first recipient. When asked how we should pick subsequent winners, he smiled and said, "I will leave you a note." Using that note, Jim Mullen chaired the annual selection committee for many years. The much-prized award is a fitting tribute to Gordon Buzby, one of the department's most beloved members as well as one of its most valued leaders and teachers.

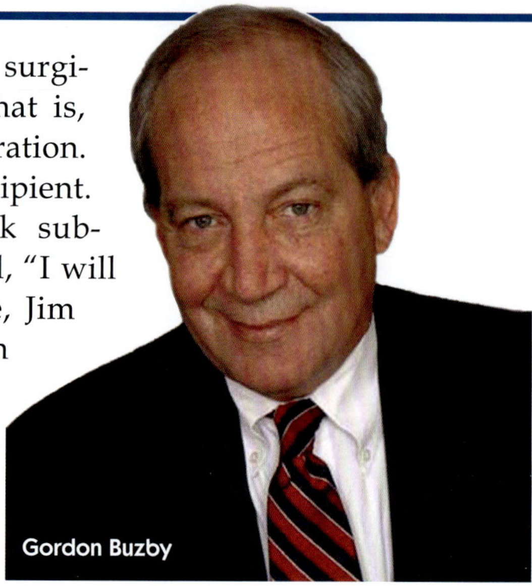
Gordon Buzby

Gordon was a lifelong Philadelphian, growing up in Abington and graduating from Abington High School. As a Penn undergraduate, he was Phi Beta Kappa and for three years, an All-American intercollegiate champion in sailing, a hobby that he continued to pursue throughout his life. Gordon also went to medical school at Penn, graduating in 1974 as an AOA. He then interned and was a general surgery resident at HUP, finishing as Chief Resident in 1981. He won the 1979 Meade Johnson National Research Forum Resident's Prize. At that time, he and his mentor, Jim Mullen, developed a prognostic nutrition index to define the interactions of nutrition and proteins in relation to operative morbidity and mortality and to pre- and postoperative nutritional support.[9] This and other studies were products of twenty important publications while Gordon was still a resident.

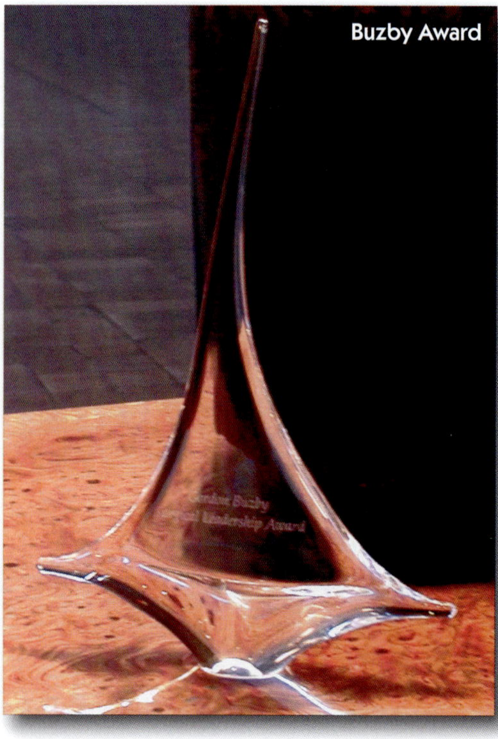
Buzby Award

In 1981, Gordon joined the faculty at Penn and the clinical staff at HUP and the Philadelphia VA Medical Center. In addition to building an active practice, Gordon became an independent investigator in both clinical and basic studies in the nutrition/metabolism field. He was codirector of the nutrition support service at HUP from 1981 to 1986 and director of the Surgical Metabolic Unit at the VA from 1985 to 1987. He was particularly active in the American Society of Parenteral and Enteral Nutrition, serving on its board of directors and in 1981 as director of its post graduate course. His research was consistently funded through extramural sources. Of particular importance was his role as study chairman and principal investigator of a randomized clinical trial of TPN in surgical patients, a multicenter study conducted at ten national academic medical centers. The results of this landmark termining the appropriate use of TPN in pre- and postoperative care of surgical patients. Gordon's work in the nutrition field resulted in many other publications totaling almost 100.

Despite his many other accomplishments, it was as a teacher and mentor of students and residents that Gordon was at his best. From 2001 until his death, he was the director of the department's general surgical residency. During that time, students and residents uniformly praised him. The Penn medical school class of 1992 selected him for their teaching award. Despite his many accolades, he was most proud of his ability to keep his life in balance with a clear focus on Karen, his children, and hours spent on the ocean.

His colleagues were devastated to learn that he had an incurable lung cancer. He confronted his last months with great courage and dignity.

The department continues to think of him often and to remember him with the annual named lecture and award.

James Mullen (1942–)

Jim Mullen is a native Philadelphian. Following graduation from Harvard College where he played baseball, he came to Penn as a medical student in 1963. He remained at Penn as a HUP intern and resident, and except for two years in the Air Force, has been here as a faculty member for the rest of his career.

In 2013, Jim Mullen was designated by the School of Medicine as the Robert D. Dripps awardee for excellence in graduate medical education. This award is named for one of the University of Pennsylvania's major educators and leaders, the founder of the Department of Anesthesia and vice president of the University for Medical Affairs. The award is specified to be for excellence in education of residents and fellows in clinical care, research, or administration. It might have been designed for Jim Mullen. Over his five decades at Penn, Dr. Mullen has developed an outstanding record in all of these diverse fields.

With regard to clinical care, he has been an active and highly respected surgeon at HUP since 1975. He originated and for many years directed the clinical nutrition support service. He has been chief of surgery at the VA Hospital and in 2008 to 2009 and 2017 was acting chairman of the Department of Surgery.

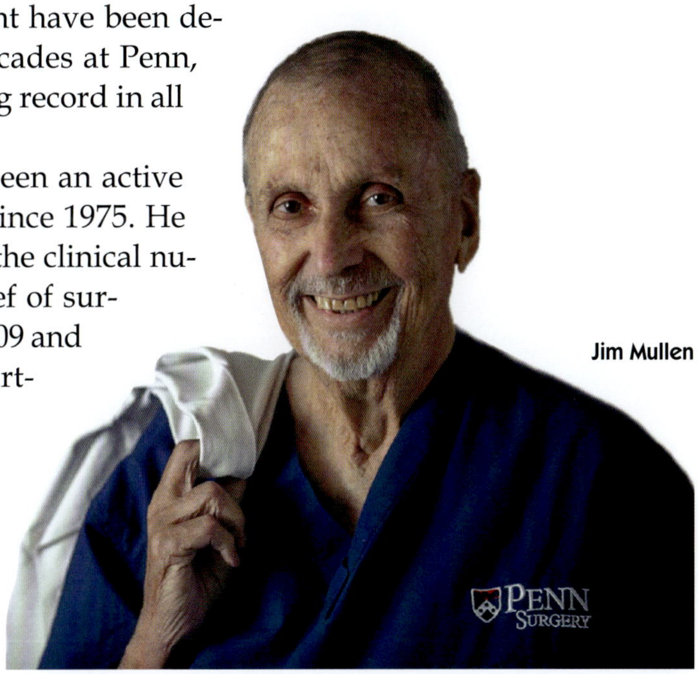

Jim Mullen

Dr. Mullen's basic research interest is in nutrition and metabolism. For many years, he was a productive and well-funded basic investigator in this field, and he continues to be a nationally field, and he continues to be a nationally prominent senior figure and advisor in this area.

Dr. Mullen has served as the Department of Surgery's director of teaching for medical students and as program director for the surgical residency. He also has directed the Department's program for continuing education, which he originated.

As an administrator, Dr. Mullen has been director of the Division of Surgical Education from 1976–98 and since then as vice chairman of the Department for Education. Since 1996, he has been medical director of the HUP operating rooms and coleader of perioperative services until a few months ago.

As distinguished a career as Dr. Mullen has had in these fields, his contributions to the Department of Surgery and to Penn Medicine have been greatest as an educator. It would not be an exaggeration to say that he has been the department's most important educator over the last four and a half decades. During much of that time, he was the program director of the surgical residency. His outstanding performance in this role was a key factor in the development of the department's overall reputation as one of the nation's best. The residency, as reorganized and managed by him since 1976, is widely regarded as one of the top two or three in the country. Most of its graduates have become faculty members at other universities. Sixteen chairs of university departments and dozens of division leaders at other universities are graduates of the Penn residency and fellowship programs. These academic surgeons have recognized Dr. Mullen as perhaps their most important mentor.

Since turning over the directorship of the residency program to younger department members, Dr. Mullen has continued to supervise the department's administrative and teaching programs as vice chairman, as acting Department chairman from 2008 to 2009, and then as head of the department's continuing education activities. In recent years, he has spearheaded the department's educational program by initiating innovative methods of teaching at the Clinical Simulation Center, an important educational asset not only for surgery but for other departments as well.

At the party that acknowledged Jim's Dripps Award, many of the residents asked to speak. In praising him as their teacher, they said a lot of nice things about Jim. Some of them attempted to characterize his unique style, struggling to explain why and how he has been so effective as an educator. Summarized below are a few of the things they said.

1. An organizational genius, comfortable with all aspects of the educational mission.
2. A larger-than-life mentor with an inimitable style.
3. Unshakeable loyalty for the department and ambition for its trainees.
4. Willingness to be unpopular in pursuit of what he believes is right.

5. A master of nonlinear planning that allows him to dominate from behind the scene.
6. Can speak to different people at all levels in their own language.
7. Believes that both surgery and life are contact sports.
8. The glue that holds the department's educational programs together.
9. A rare ability to serve effectively under six different department chairs.

The residents' remarks were all close to their target. Each of them got a piece of it. But the whole explanation of Jim Mullen remains elusive.

Jon Morris (1957–)

For Jon Morris to receive an award for teaching is hardly a surprise. Since his arrival at HUP in 1990, Jon has made medical student and surgical resident education a focus of his activity. While also maintaining an active practice of general surgery and authoring over 100 scholarly articles in the surgical literature, his performance as a teacher has resulted in his compiling a list of awards and prizes that is probably unequaled.

For the Department of Surgery, Jon has served in many educational roles including director of Medical Student Education (1993–1998), director of Housestaff Education (1999–2001, 2003–present), and program director of the surgery residency. For the School of Medicine, he was associate dean for clinical education (1997–2001) and since 2004 has been associate dean for student affairs.

In the Department of Surgery, Jon has received the faculty teaching award seven times. At the School of Medicine, he has twice received the medical students' award for teaching, the Penn Pearls Award for outstanding clinical teaching three times, the Christian R. and Mary F. Lindback Foundation Award for teaching and a special Dean's Award in recognition of outstanding service to the medical students. In addition, he was inducted into the Alpha Omega Alpha national medical honor society as a faculty member.

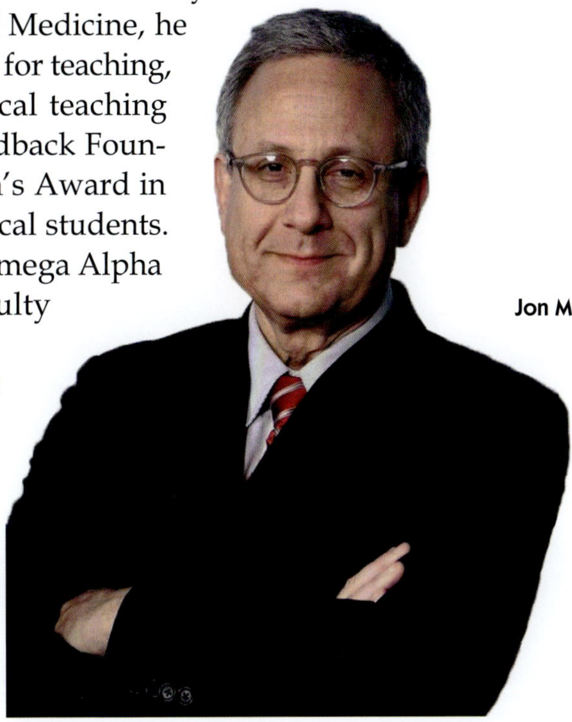

Jon Morris

Nationally, Jon is certainly one of the most recognized surgical educators. He was president of the Association of Program Directors in Surgery from 2014 to 2015. He is a member of the American Surgical Association. In 2014, he became the inaugural Ernest F. Rosato–William Maul Measey Professor of Surgical Education.

formal educational honors. He moderated the M&M conference, skillfully bringing the residents into the discussions. In another very valuable conference, he met weekly at 7:00 a.m. with the residents and selected faculty to review interesting cases as they were presented to him.

In 2018, Jon stepped down as program director of the Penn general surgery residency, a position he had held for fourteen years. He was succeeded by Cary Aarons but remains the department's vice chair of education, overseeing the Division of Surgical Education. In January 2018, Jon was appointed as the first director of the Center for Student Life. In 2019, he received the Robert D. Dripps Award for excellence in graduate medical education.

Ernest Rosato (1936–2012)

In communications to the department's newsletter, former residents all praise his teaching. Virtually every one indicates that Ernie Rosato was their most important teacher.

Ernie grew up in Philadelphia where his father was a busy community physician. He graduated from St. Joseph's University summa cum laude and in 1962 from the University of Pennsylvania School of Medicine with the election to AOA. After completing his surgical residency at HUP under Jonathan Rhoads, he remained at Penn as a faculty member for his entire professional career of more than fifty years.[11]

His first faculty assignment was at the VA hospital where he was chief of the Penn Surgery service from 1972 to 1978. During these years, he was active in basic research, studying GI physiology in primate models with Penn's chief of gastroenterology, Frank Brooks. Later, as his focus shifted to clinical surgery, his practice was conducted at HUP, and he continued to contribute importantly to the literature. His bibliography eventually included 189 papers on topics ranging from nutrition, malignancies of the pancreas and esophagus, inflammatory bowel disease, and breast disease. He served on the editorial boards of the *Journal of Surgical Gastroenterology*, the *Journal of Laparoendoscopic Surgery*, and the *Yearbook of Gastroenterology*.

In 1975, he was promoted to full professor and from 1988 to 2004 he was chief of the Division of Gastrointestinal Surgery. He contributed extensively to administrative activities of his school, hospital, and university. He was a member of the medical school's admissions committee, chairman of the postgraduate training committee, chairman of the hospital's medical faculty senate, chairman of the hospital's operating room committee, and vice president of the Medical Alumni Society.

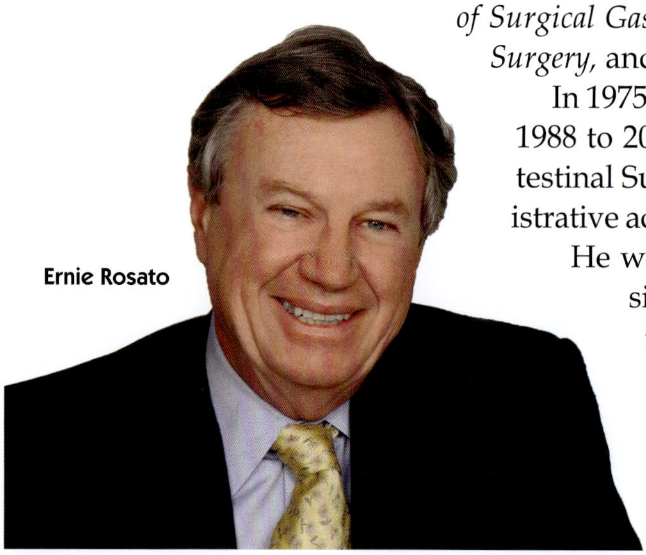

Ernie Rosato

faculty senate, chairman of the hospital's operating room committee, and vice president of the Medical Alumni Society.

For many years, Dr. Rosato was acknowledged to have the largest practice of surgery in the Philadelphia area. His extensive experience and skill as an operator, encyclopedic knowledge of general surgery, and superb judgment made him the "go-to surgeon" for the most challenging cases. Penn Medicine recognized these attributes with the 2008 I. S. Ravdin Master Clinician Award, the most prestigious clinical award that the institution can bestow on a faculty member.

Dr. Rosato was widely recognized beyond Penn by multiple listings in the Top Doctors edition of *Philadelphia Magazine* and a remarkable seventeen-year consecutive run as one of the Best Doctors in America. In recognition of the thousands of cancer patients who benefited from his compassionate care, in 2007 he was the recipient of the Humanitarian Award from the Philadelphia Chapter of the American Cancer Society. He also received the Physician of the Year Award of the National Foundation for Ileitis and Colitis.

Dr. Rosato's prominence in academic surgery was indicated by his long list of professional society memberships. They included the American College of Surgeons, the Society of University Surgeons, the American Surgical Association, the Halsted Society, the Association for Academic Surgery, the Society for Surgery of the Alimentary Tract, the Surgical Biology Club III, the Collegium Internacionale Chirurgie, the Societe Internationale de Chirurgie, the American Society of Clinical Oncology, the Society of Surgical Oncology, the Philadelphia Academy of Surgery of which he was the secretary, the Philadelphia College of Physicians, the Eastern Surgical Society, the American Physiological Society, the International Society for the Study of Lung Cancer, and the Society of Laparoscopic Surgeons. Dr. Rosato was particularly active in the affairs of the American College of Surgeons, serving on its committee for self-education and self-assessment program (SESAP), the executive committee of the College on medical motion pictures, and its executive committee on surgical education. He was chairman of the College's 1981 postgraduate course on diseases of the liver, biliary tract, and pancreas. In 1983, he was presiding officer of the Cine Clinic session at the Clinical Congress and in 1985, coordinator and presiding officer of the Film Festival.

In addition to his research, clinical, and administrative activity, Dr. Rosato placed his highest emphasis on medical education, superbly integrating students and housestaff into the care of his patients. His abilities as a teacher resulted in an unprecedented array of teaching awards. He received the Mary F. and Christian R. Lindback Award for distinguished teaching, a place on the medical student government faculty honor roll, and the Penn Pearls Award from the students for excellence in teaching twice. In 1980, the Penn medical school yearbook was dedicated to him.

Dr. Rosato trained generations of academic surgeons. The William Inouye Award for teaching is given annually by the graduating chief residents. Dr. Rosato received this award a record number of eighteen times.

In 2010, as he reached age seventy-four, Ernie had not slowed up. He continued to relish his large practice, his many family and social activities, including attention to his golf handicap, and his apparent robust good health. But in November, he was diagnosed with inoperable pancreatic cancer. How tragically ironic that Ernie would be stricken by a disease he had treated with such expertise throughout his long career. Thereafter, for many months, while receiving initially effective chemotherapy, he courageously pursued his usual activities in the operating room, office, and on the golf course with his family and friends.

A celebration of Ernie's long career was held on February 12, 2011, at Philadelphia's Academy of Natural Sciences. More than 400 of his admirers including students, residents, colleagues, family, friends, and patients gathered to share conversation and Rosato stories. Formal tributes were delivered by eighteen speakers: Drs. Drebin, Morris, Barker, Mullen, Acker, Luketich, Glick, Fairman, Barbot, Markmann, Gorman, Savino, Wu, Kelz, Williams, Low, Dempsey, and Mariano.

The speakers focused on Ernie's unmatched legacy of teaching. Mentioned were his record as Philadelphia's most prolific surgeon and his status as the surgeon of last resort who often succeeded in solving seemingly impossible surgical problems. Mentioned also were his intellectual approach to these problems, his encyclopedic knowledge of surgery, his basic and clinical research, and his national prominence. Current and past residents attributed their experience and competence as surgeons to their time on Ernie's service more than to any other aspect of their training. Perhaps even more importantly, most of the speakers dwelt on the personal relationship that Ernie developed with each of his residents, making them feel almost like family members. There was also time to recite a few of Ernie's patented teaching aphorisms, time for some gentle parody of the distinctive Rosato Philadelphia accent, and time to watch David Low's cartoons, depicting Ernie as the operating surgeon in Thomas Eakins's *Agnew Clinic.* The conclusion to this remarkable program was Ernie's superbly crafted response, delivered with just the right amount of restrained emotion. No one fortunate enough to be there will ever forget this remarkable evening.

Ernie and Gerry Rosato

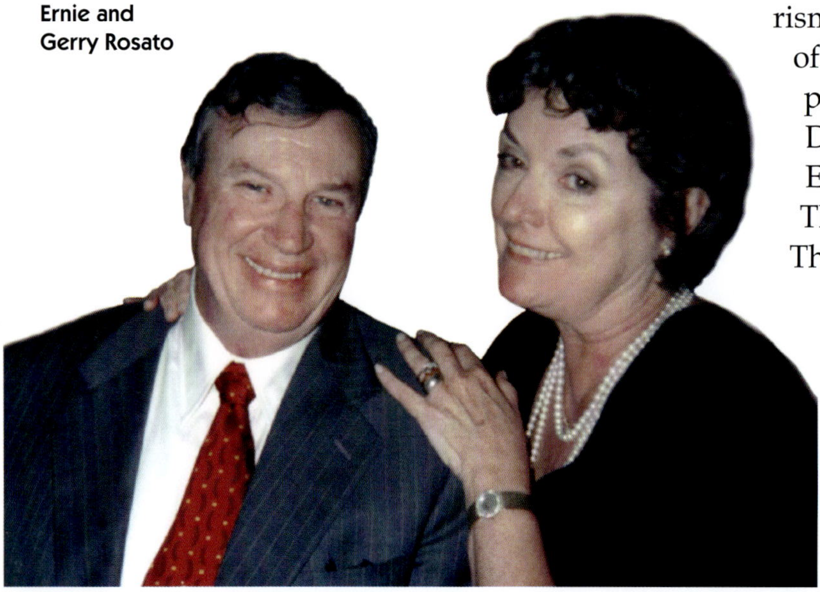

During the ensuing months, as symptoms overtook Ernie, it was fortunate that he was able to attend and enjoy the first in an annual lecture series that has been endowed in his name. He was also pleased to learn that an endowment had been secured for the University of Pennsylvania's Ernest E. Rosato Professorship in Surgical Education.

While Ernie accomplished great things professionally, his greatest pleasure and pride came from his wife, Gerry, and their nine children. It was fitting that at the end, he died in his home surrounded by his family and several close friends and colleagues. To paraphrase the conclusions from his white coat ceremony speech to the students, he was a physician, surgeon, and something more.

Doug Fraker (1956–)

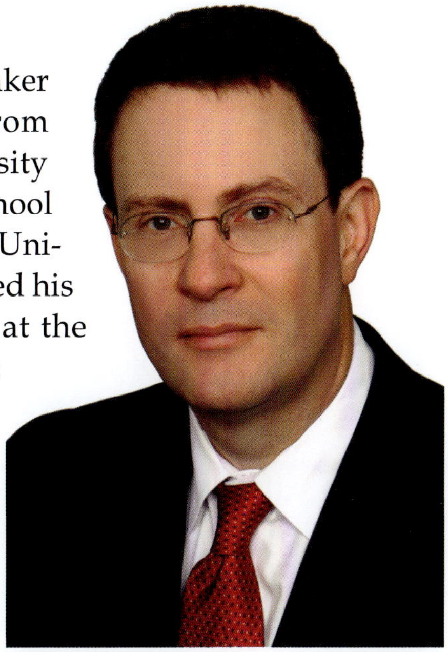

Doug Fraker

Of the department's active surgeons, Douglas Fraker is the longest-serving, having been recruited from the NIH in 1996. He is a graduate of the University of Wisconsin, after which he attended medical school at Harvard and trained in general surgery at the University of California, San Francisco. He interrupted his residency for a three-year research fellowship at the surgery branch of the National Cancer Institute where he worked in metabolism. After completing his chief residency at UCSF, he returned to the NCI as a senior investigator and soon as chief of the NCI's surgical metabolism section and head of endocrine surgery. He also became experienced in treatment of endocrine neoplasias and reoperative parathyroid surgery, as well as isolated limb perfusion for melanoma. At Penn, he has continued to lead in these areas. He has had a number of administrative roles, including vice chair for clinical affairs, deputy director of the Cancer Center, and surgery's vice chair for research. He has authored more than 300 peer-reviewed publications and serves on eight editorial boards. These and other aspects of his career are summarized in Chapter 37.

In every aspect of academic surgery, Dr. Fraker has been one of the department's stars. This brief summary touches only on his record as an educator. No faculty member has been a more consistent recipient of the department's or the school of medicine's teaching awards.

His generous mentorship has been particularly important to members of his division, including Brian Czerniecki, Frank Spitz, Rachel Kelz, Giorgos Karakousis, Robert Roses, Julia Chou, Heather Wachtel, and Frank Venuto. Dr. DeMatteo has acknowledged that his choice of oncology as his specialty was due to the influence of Dr. Fraker.

Robert Roses (1975–)

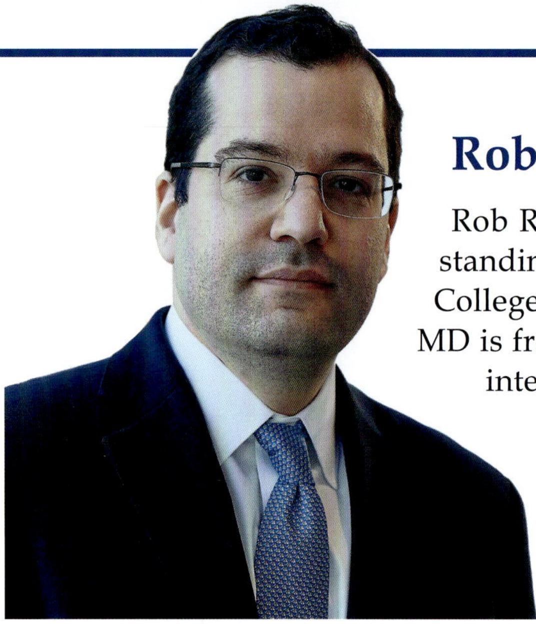

Robert Roses

Rob Roses, the youngest of this group of outstanding educators, is a graduate of Dartmouth College where he won high honors in music. His MD is from Tufts where he was AOA. He was an intern and resident at HUP from 2003 to 2010. During his residency, he had a two-year fellowship in oncology at Penn, and from 2010 to 2012, he was an oncology fellow at MD Anderson before joining the faculty at Penn in 2012. At HUP, he has been a very active clinical surgeon. He is the author of 166 publications and three books. He has been consistently acclaimed as an educator. During his ten years on the faculty, he has won ten named faculty teaching awards.

Sean Harbison (1960–)

Not all of the department's distinguished educators are chairs or endowed professors. One of the best was presented last year with the Blockley-Osler Award. For thirty-five years, this award has been given annually to a Penn faculty member for teaching clinical medicine at an affiliated hospital. It was created in 1987 by the Blockley Section of the College of Physicians, inspired by William Osler's initiation of bedside teaching at Philadelphia General Hospital (Blockley) from 1884 to 1889. This year's winner is Sean Harbison, professor of surgery and chief of the Division of General Surgery at Penn Presbyterian Hospital.

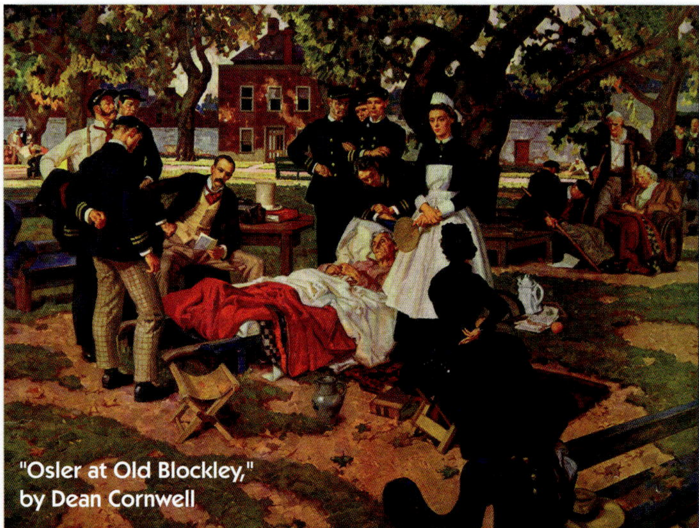

"Osler at Old Blockley," by Dean Cornwell

Sean Harbison's curriculum vitae has to be one of the most interesting I've read. Over the last three decades, Sean has had faculty appointments at six universities (Penn, Temple, Penn's Graduate School, Alleghany, Medical College of Pennsylvania, and Hahnemann). Sean earned his medical degree from Temple and completed a surgical residency at Graduate Hospital, a surgical oncology fellowship at Memorial Sloan Kettering, a master's degree in education from Penn's Graduate School, and a fellowship in education sponsored by the Association for Surgical Education. Prior to joining Penn Surgery in 1994, Dr. Harbison practiced general surgery at Graduate Hospital, Temple, Medical College of Pennsylvania, Hahnemann, and Alleghany. His leadership roles have included surgical residency program director at Graduate Hospital and Temple as well as student clerkship director at both institutions. He has been president of the Philadelphia Chapter of the American College of Surgeons and recorder of the Philadelphia Academy of Surgeons.

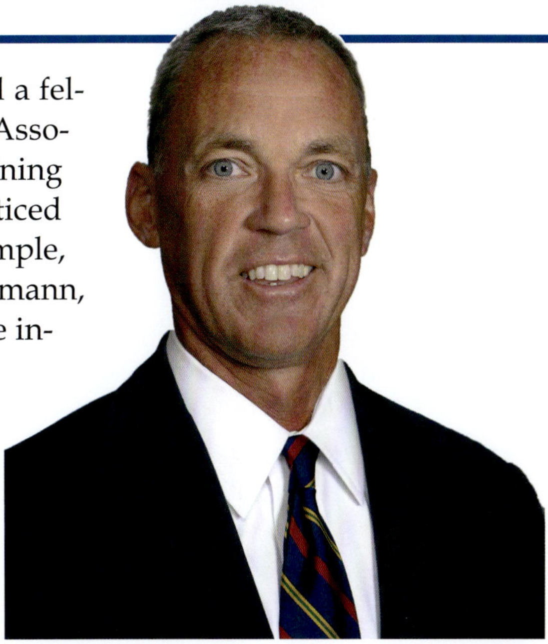

Sean Harbison

Pertinent to the Blockley/Osler Prize is Sean's remarkable list of twenty-five individual awards for teaching, including multiple Penn Pearls, Golden Apples, a yearbook dedication, and the University of Pennsylvania's coveted Lindback Award. Less interesting to me, but representing lots of work, is his list of seventy-seven academic committees on education, ethics, curriculum, governance, and leadership.

In 2003, Sean made an important career move. Dan Dempsey, then chairman at Temple, recruited him as head of the section of general surgery and vice chairman of the department. Dan recalls that Sean soon had Temple's largest surgical practice and that his unique style as a teacher reminded him of storied pied piper mentors of an earlier era. In 2013, he moved to his present position as head of surgery at Penn Presbyterian Hospital.

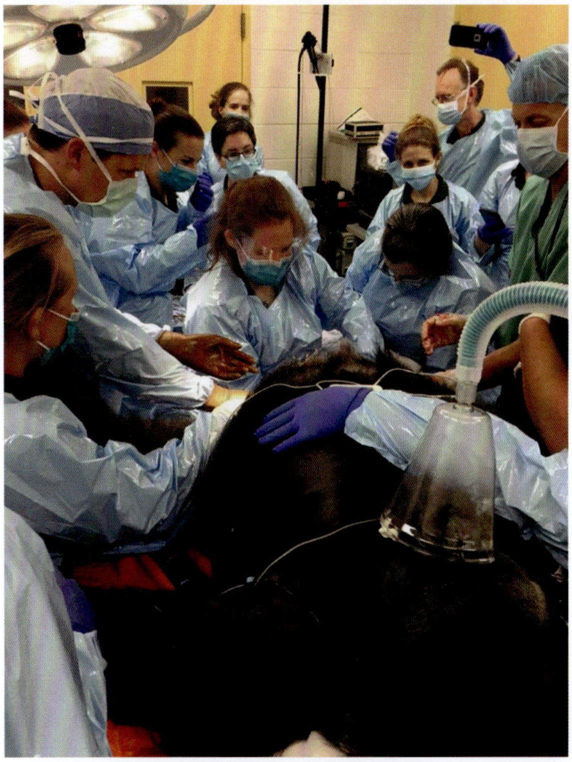

Sean Harbison operating on a western lowland gorilla.

Review of Sean's bibliography and lecture titles is also interesting. He writes and speaks about his extensive experience with reconstruction of the abdominal wall in patients with giant ventral hernias and of his electrostimulation (pacemaking) for diabetic gastroparesis (2016 report of 151 cases). On a personal note, he writes about teaching style and his love for the nearly extinct specialty of general surgery.

Not recorded in Sean's remarkable CV is his athletic career. At La Salle, he was an outstanding track star, excelling in the mile at college meets and in the Penn Relays. He has continued to participate in running events, such as the Broad Street Run and several marathons. He has also been a competitive swimmer and surfer. To stay in shape, he rows.

Sean has added another dimension in his several decades as a consultant in the primate program at the Philadelphia Zoo. On three notable occasions, he has had an active surgical role in care of one of the zoo's endangered species, its western lowland gorillas. His operations on gorillas have included a hysterectomy, an appendectomy, and a complex vaginal delivery in which his episiotomy avoided a Caesarian section after a gorilla's twenty-four hours of extended labor.

Notes

[1] Dr. William Y. Inouye; was professor at Penn. *Philadelphia Inquirer* (22 July 1985) B04.

[2] Inouye, W. and Engelberg, J., inventors. *Pressure cooker artificial kidney* (1953). Baxter (Travenol) Dialysis Machine Museum (virtual). Photo by Jim Curtis. https://icaot.org/virtual-collections/.

[3] Inouye WY, Engelberg J. A simplified artificial dialyzer and ultrafilter. *Surg Forum* (1953) 4:438–442.

[4] Inouye, WY. Construction and Performance of our Dialyser. *Transactions of Society of Artificial Organs* Vol 1 (1954) p. 36.

[5] Barker, Clyde F. Memoir of William Y. Inouye, M.D. *Transactions of the Philadelphia Academy of Surgery* Vol XXXIV (1981–1986) pp. 78–80.

[6] Barker, Clyde F. Memoir of Dr. Leonard Miller, Teacher and Surgeon. *University of Pennsylvania Almanac.* https://almanac.upenn.edu/archive/v44/n01/deaths.html.

[7] Barker, Clyde F. Memoir of Julius A. Mackie, Jr. *Transactions of Southern Surgical Association* Vol CXVI (2004) pp. 355–356.

[8] Wallace, Andy. Leonard Perloff, 52, Transplant Surgeon and Penn Professor. *Philadelphia Inquirer* (Feb. 16, 1993). Barker, Clyde F. Memoir of Leonard Perloff 1940–1993. *Transactions of the American Surgical Association* Vol CXIV (1994) pp. 375–376.

[9] Buzby GP, Mullen JL, Matthews DC, Hobbs CL, Rosato EF. Prognostic nutritional index in gastrointestinal surgery. *Am J Surg* (1980) 139(1):160–167.

[10] Veterans Affairs Total Parenteral Nutrition Cooperative Study Group. Perioperative total parenteral nutrition in surgical patients. *N Engl J Med* (1991) 325(8):525-532. doi:10.1056/NEJM199108223250801.

[11] Barker, Clyde F. Memoir of Ernest Rosato 1936–2012. *Transactions of the American Surgical Association* (2013).

CHAPTER 34

Surgeon-Scientists of the Department

1927
I.S. Ravdin spends a year abroad doing research. Nine years later in 1936, with the control of a $2.7 million endowment, he founds the Harrison Department of Surgical Research

Deciding which Penn surgeons to profile in this chapter was hard since so many of our trainees, alumni, and faculty have done important research. Early examples were Philip Syng Physick's development of absorbable sutures (1816), J. William White's discovery that castration shrank the prostate (1895), and Charles Frazier's demonstration that division of the sensory root of the fifth cranial nerve relieved trigeminal neuralgia (1930).

Surgical research has been disparaged by members of the cognitive disciplines, who claim that it is unlikely that clinical surgeons would be capable of or have time for meaningful investigation. James Thompson (HUP chief resident 1960) countered this assertion in his 1999 presidential address to the American College of Surgeons. He argued that in the last half-century, contributions of surgeons to medical science were at least as great as those made by others. He listed as advances: (1) cardiopulmonary bypass and cardiac surgery; (2) transplantation; (3) vascular surgery; (4) total parenteral nutrition; (5) metabolic response to trauma; (6) randomized controlled trials for cancer and effect of hormones on cancer; and (7) minimally invasive surgery.

In these areas, many Penn surgeons have contributed. An aid to the selection process was to consider the awards for innovation that have been won by Penn surgeons, such as the Lasker Award ("the American Nobel") that was given to John Gibbon in 1968 and to Bernard Fisher in 1985. Another was the Jacobson Prize for Innovation, the highest award of the American College of Surgeons. Since 1994, twenty-five of these awards have been made, five of them to Penn surgeons (Joel Cooper, Stanley Dudrick, Judah Folkman, William Pierce, and Bernard Fisher). This chapter highlights advances made by members of the Penn surgeons in each of the areas cited by Thompson.

John H. Gibbon Jr.: The Heart-Lung Machine

1927
Gibbon obtains MD from Jefferson

1928
Gibbon interns at Pennsylvania Hospital

1930–1933
In his research at Penn, Gibbon is mentored by professor of physiology, Eugene Landis

Many think that John Gibbon deserved the Nobel Prize for inventing the heart-lung machine and enabling open-heart surgery. Jefferson is justifiably identified as the venue for this achievement, since it came to fruition there. However, Penn deserves part of the credit. Of the eighteen years Gibbon worked actively on his machine, ten were spent in the Harrison Department of Surgical Research. Only the last seven were at Jefferson, but they were the ones leading up to and including Gibbon's first successful human open-heart operation under cardiopulmonary bypass.

John Gibbon was born in 1903 and spent most of his life as a Philadelphian.[1] He graduated from Princeton where he played on the soccer team and was more interested in studying literature and poetry than in science. Partway through medical school at Jefferson, he decided to quit and become a poet. Fortunately, his father talked him out of this. After he graduated in 1927 and interned at Pennsylvania Hospital, he spent a year as a research fellow under Dr. Churchill at the Boston City and Massachusetts General Hospitals (MGH). His research there was to measure blood pressure in the pulmonary artery. Assigned to help him was Churchill's experienced senior technician, Mary Hopkinson. They soon fell in love and married the next year.

At the MGH, Gibbon witnessed the tragic death of a young woman from a massive pulmonary embolus. Assigned to monitor her vital signs, Gibbon sat with her through a long night as her blood darkened and she struggled for breath. When her heart stopped, Churchill immediately carried out a pulmonary embolectomy, but she did not survive.[2] The experience stimulated Gibbon to consider whether he could oxygenate the blood and bypass the heart. This would not only rescue patients with pulmonary emboli but also allow a surgeon to open the heart and operate on cardiac defects under direct vision.

Returning to Philadelphia, for the next three years Gibbon spent mornings building his surgical practice at Pennsylvania and Bryn Mawr Hospitals and afternoons in the Harrison Department of Surgical Research. There he worked with the professor of physiology, Eugene Landis, on measuring capillary blood pressure. He learned a lot about basic research and laboratory techniques from Landis, whom he always considered to be his most important research mentor. Landis was one of the few who encouraged him to work on cardiopulmonary bypass.

Obsessed with the possibility of a heart-lung machine, he arranged to return to Harvard for another year of full-time research with Dr. Churchill, who had become chairman of Harvard's Department of Surgery.

During that year, his preliminary work on the heart-lung machine was greatly facilitated by Mary Hopkinson, who became not only his wife but also his lifelong research associate. Their experiments

1936–1941
John and Mary Gibbon work on the heart-lung machine at Penn

1942–1945
John Gibbon serves in the Army

1953
Moving to Jefferson, Gibbon performs the first successful open-heart operation in a human

progressed slowly, but by the end of the year, they were able to totally occlude the pulmonary artery of a cat and successfully bypass the circulation. Gibbon later recorded that they danced around the table with joy, realizing at this point that they would eventually be successful in their quest.

They then returned to Philadelphia where from 1936 to 1941, they worked at Penn in the Harrison Department of Surgical Research. This six-year period was important for adapting their machine to accommodate larger animals and in studying and overcoming complications of extended periods of bypass. At the end of this time, they were able to consistently bypass the heart with survival in dogs.

Soon after the Japanese bombed Pearl Harbor in 1941, Gibbon volunteered to serve in the Army. For four years, he was away from research, serving in the Pacific theater of war. As the war ended, he returned to the Harrison Department of Surgical Research as assistant professor of surgery at Penn. After a short time, he accepted the offer to become director of surgical research at Jefferson. There, he was fortunate to establish a relationship with Thomas Watson, president of IBM. Watson's interest and support, and the expertise of IBM engineers, played an indispensable role in the rest of the project. Watson and IBM generously funded the heart-lung research and equipment, helping adapt it so that it would support the circulation in large animals and then human patients.

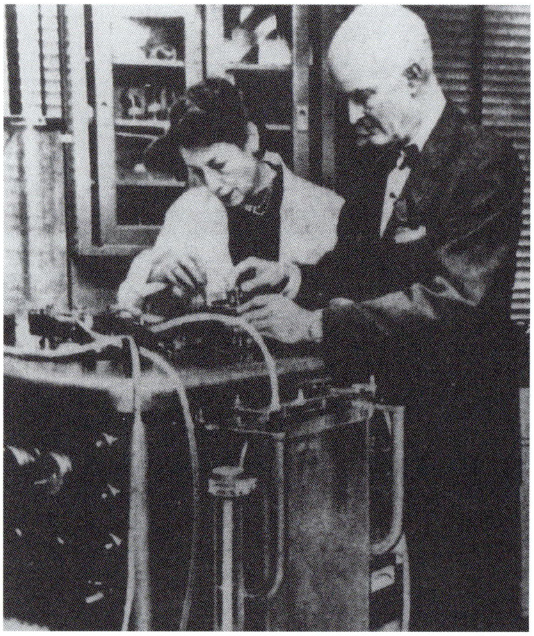

Mary and John Gibbon

On May 6, 1953, Gibbon carried out the first successful open-heart operation under cardiopulmonary bypass.[3] The patient, a young woman, survived the operation to close a large atrial septal defect. She lived for many years. Gibbon attempted two more open-heart operations with his bypass machine, but neither of these patients survived. He then elected to turn the open-heart program over to his young cardiac surgery colleagues. Three years later, he became Chairman of Jefferson's Department of Surgery in 1956 and served in that position until 1967. His clinical activity was mainly in noncardiac thoracic surgery.

Gibbon became one of the world's most honored surgeons. Among his many awards were the Strittmatter Award, the John Scott Award, the Philadelphia Award, and in 1968, the Lasker Award. He was President of the Philadelphia Academy of Surgery, the American Surgical Association, and the editor of the *Annals of Surgery.*

The first crucial success in Gibbon's work was not at Penn. In animals, it was at MGH and in the first human at Jefferson. But it is notable that Gibbon spent ten of his most important years working in the Harrison Department of Surgical Research. It is also interesting that neither Dr. Churchill at Harvard nor Dr. Ravdin at Penn gave him much encouragement, since they both thought that the idea of a heart-lung machine was too far-fetched. For once, Ravdin was not prescient in recognizing the promise of one of his young charges, but then, neither was Churchill. Only Penn's physiology professor, Landis, encouraged the Gibbons to pursue their dream.

Norman Freeman: The First Vascular Surgeon

The story of Norman Freeman, the Penn surgeon who pioneered vascular surgery, is a sad one. Among his forgotten accomplishments are the first resection of an abdominal aortic aneurism and the world's first treatment of hypertension by renal artery surgery.

Freeman was educated at Yale's college and medical school before coming to HUP for a two-year internship under I. S. Ravdin. Then during a two-year research fellowship in Harvard's department of physiology under Walter Cannon, he studied the influence of the sympathetic nervous system on shock, blood loss, and the peripheral circulation, authoring with Cannon many highly regarded basic research papers. After this, he completed a surgical residency at MGH and two extra years there as a surgical fellow.

In 1936, Ravdin recruited Freeman to Penn and assigned him to form and direct a vascular clinic.[4] For the next seven years as a member of Ravdin's surgical faculty, Freeman was productive both in clinical and basic research. His studies of peripheral circulation demonstrated that during shock, blood flow to vital organs was protected. In other studies, he was one of the first to show that renal artery constriction resulted in hypertension.

From 1943 to 1945, Freeman was a member of Ravdin's 20th General Hospital in India. Despite the primitive and hazardous conditions, Freeman produced multiple papers based on studies done on wounded soldiers. One such report was of his treatment by sympathectomy of 114 patients with causalgia caused by gunshot wounds.[5]

Freeman and Ravdin did not get along, and Ravdin did not reappoint his previously favorite protégé to his postwar faculty at Penn.[6]

After the war, Freeman was appointed as chief of surgery at DeWitt General Hospital in Auburn, California, one of the few US Army vascular centers. There he pioneered vascular reconstructions, such as direct repair of AV fistulas, eighteen successful examples of which he reported to the American Surgical Association in 1946.

In 1946, Freeman was recruited by Howard Naffziger, UCSF's surgery

1928
Norman Freeman receives MD from Yale

1928–1930
Freeman has two-year HUP internship

1930–1932
Freeman does two-year research fellowship at Harvard

1932–1936
Freeman is surgical resident and clinical fellow at MGH

1936–1943
Ravdin recruits Norman Freeman to Penn as J. William White Assistant Professor of Surgical Research. He develops the country's first vascular laboratory

1943–1945
In India, Major Freeman serves with Ravdin at 20th General Hospital

1945
Freeman quarrels with General Ravdin, is not reappointed to Penn faculty. After the war, he moves to California

February 1951
Freeman performs the world's first resection of an abdominal aortic aneurysm

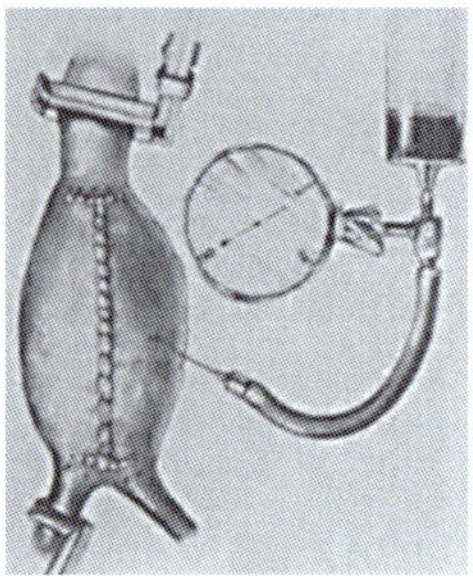

department chair, as associate clinical professor and chief of the vascular clinic. Among Freeman's innovations at UCSF were establishment of the first noninvasive vascular lab and routine employment of arteriography to define vascular lesions.[7]

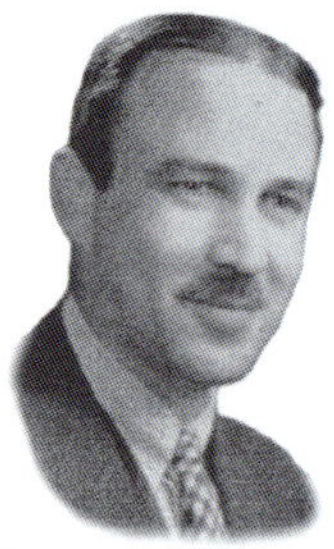

Norman Freeman

Before long, Freeman was at odds with Naffziger and moved to Franklin Hospital, a private institution. During this time, Freeman performed several novel operations that have been virtually forgotten. On February 26, 1951, he performed the first resection of an abdominal aortic aneurysm.[8] A month later, Charles Dubost in France performed the same procedure, which ever since has been unfairly regarded as the first.[9] A year later, Freeman's patient was alive and well.[10]

1952
Freeman performs first renal artery endarterectomy

In 1952, Freeman performed the first renal artery endarterectomy, curing the patient of hypertension.[11] In the same year, he did the first extra-anatomic bypass (a femoral-to-femoral artery bypass).[12]

Perhaps of more lasting importance than Freeman's technical innovations was the influence of his vision of vascular surgery as a distinct, independent specialty.[13] Others like DeBakey and Blalock saw it as part of cardiac, thoracic, or general surgery.

1953
Bill Inouye invents first coil dialyzer. Willem Kolff copies it. It is exhibited at the Smithsonian Institution

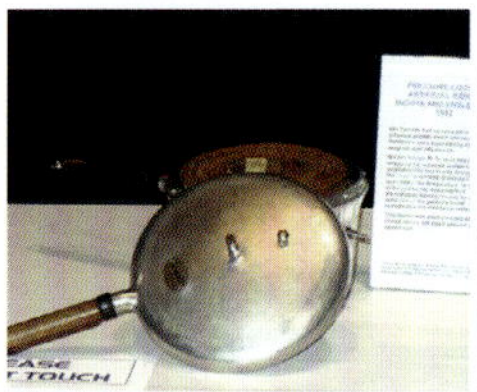

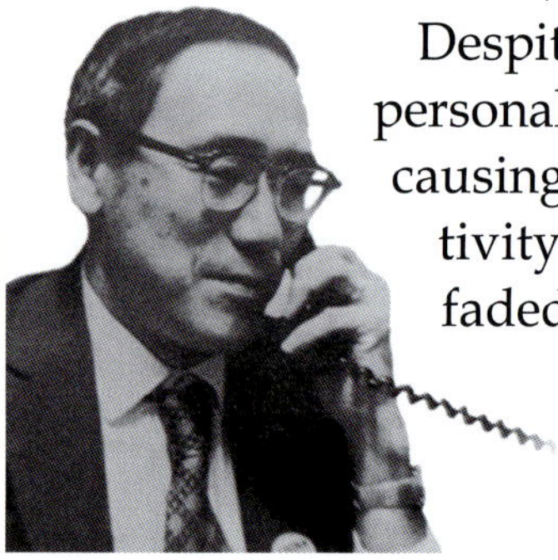

Despite his many accomplishments, Freeman's unusual personality and erratic behavior led to damaging conflicts causing his early retirement at age fifty-nine. With inactivity, his reputation in the expanding vascular field faded rapidly. At age seventy-two, he died from heart disease, virtually forgotten and unheralded as America's first vascular surgeon.

For a detailed account of Norman Freeman's sad story, see Chapter 15.

1963
Working in the Harrison Department, Penn Surgeon David Cooper defines role of the enzyme cytochrome P450

James Hardy: Pioneer of Lung and Heart Transplantation

1963
Jim Hardy performs world's first lung transplant. It functions for eighteen days

Of the forty-four failed lung transplants prior to Cooper's success in 1983, the most widely publicized was the very first one. It was carried out twenty years earlier by another Penn surgeon. On June 11, 1963, James Hardy (HUP chief resident, 1951) performed the transplant at the University of Mississippi where he was the chairman of the Department of Surgery. The patient died from renal failure after eighteen days, but the transplanted lung had functioned well throughout the postoperative course. This was a considerable achievement in these early days of transplantation. At the time, because immunosuppression was crude, only a few kidney transplant recipients had survived for as long as a year.

There was widespread criticism of Hardy's operation, which many deemed an unethical, publicity-seeking stunt with no chance of success.

Hardy acknowledged that the odds had been long. The patient had a resistant lung infection behind an airway-obstructing lung cancer and, in addition, substantial chronic renal insufficiency. Also fueling the negative outpouring was the fact that the patient was a prisoner, serving a life sentence for murder. Attracting even more attention to the story was the assassination of the well-known civil rights activist, Medgar Evers, which took place across town just at the time Hardy was performing the lung transplant. The stricken Evers was brought to the University Hospital. The chief resident who was assisting Hardy in the lung transplant broke out to attend Evers in the emergency room, but he soon died. Stimulating further hype in this era of civil rights turmoil was the unfounded rumor that it was Evers who had been used as the lung donor.

1964
Jim Hardy performs world's first heart transplant, using a chimpanzee donor. Failure of the heart and criticism of Hardy are both immediate

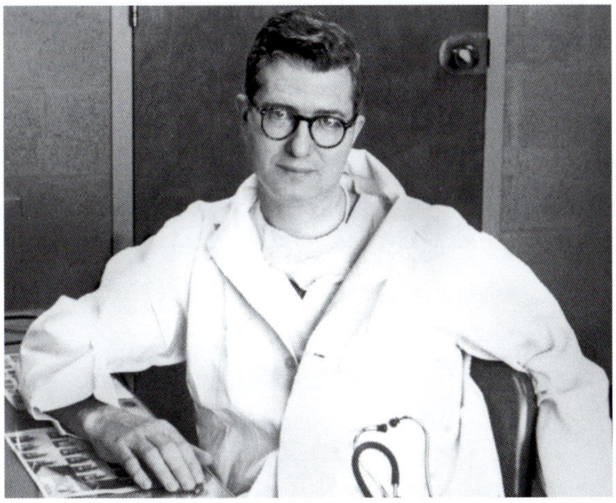

Jim Hardy

The force of the negative response was probably the reason Hardy did no more lung transplants. However, seven months later, he undertook a human heart transplant. Again, it was the world's first. Its failure within an hour engendered further criticism that it was premature and ill-conceived. Adding to the controversy was that a chimpanzee had been used as the heart donor when the prospective human donor suddenly became unsuitable after it was too late to abort the recipient operation.

Although in retrospect, Hardy's failed transplants appear to have had little chance of success, such attempts in otherwise doomed patients were not unusual in the early days of transplantation. Even in the simpler field of kidney transplants, only a handful had been successful. Since the concept of brain death had yet to be accepted, human deceased donors were difficult to obtain. In several centers, this had stimulated trials of primate donor kidney transplants. Their brief function had encouraged Hardy to fall back on the use of the chimpanzee heart. It would be another four years before the world's next heart transplant would be attempted by Christian Bernard. His "successful" first patient survived for only eighteen days.

Hardy's attempts were hardly spur-of-the-moment stunts. In the decade prior to his human cases, Hardy had perfected the surgical techniques and tested the day's crude immunosuppression in dogs. Of his sixty-eight canine lung autotransplants, thirty-three were long-term survivors. Of his 107 canine lung allografts, twenty functioned an average of twenty days and two for many months. Hardy had also performed large numbers of canine heart transplants with similar results. At the

1964
Criticism of Hardy's heart xenotransplant persists, blemishing his reputation

time, there were no IRBs to review research on humans, but Hardy's extensive experience in animals convinced the dean of his medical school that his trials of lung and heart transplantation in humans were justified.

Hardy's reputation was permanently blemished by these ill-fated transplants. To some extent, his professional life was ruined. This was unfortunate and not entirely fair. He was a thoughtful and totally moral individual. He was not just an irresponsibly bold investigator pioneering a previously unexplored field (perhaps prematurely). Instead, he was one of the most respected academic surgeons of his generation. Despite persistent criticism in the media, his surgical peers made him one of their most honored colleagues.

Known as a boy wonder, Jim Hardy was probably the most successful of Dr. Ravdin's many talented trainees. The first of his twenty-four books and many of his 605 papers were written while he was still a HUP resident. At age thirty-seven, he was appointed chairman of surgery at the University of Mississippi, a new school that he soon put on the surgical map. Among the many professional societies he served as president were the American College of Surgeons, the Society of University Surgeons, the American Surgical Association, the International Society of Surgeons, and the Society of Surgical Chairmen. He was editor of the *World Journal of Surgery.* An unvarnished account of Hardy's transplants is an essay he wrote for the Festschrift honoring Dr. Rhoads's eightieth birthday.[14] Hardy also told the story when he came to HUP in 1991 to receive the department's first Distinguished Graduate Award.

William S. Pierce: Mechanical Artificial Heart

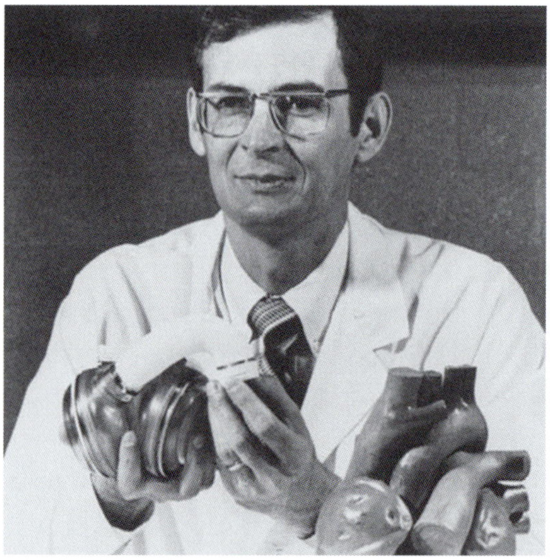
William Pierce

Long before John Gibbon's successful open-heart operation in 1953, surgeons talked about replacing the heart. A year later, the successful kidney transplant between twins suggested that transplantation was a feasible approach. But failure of early kidney allografts by French surgeons dampened enthusiasm. Other kidney allografts mostly failed until Starzl's breakthrough with immunosuppression in 1967. During this dark era of transplantation, an artificial mechanical heart seemed more promising to many than a heart transplant. As it turned out, the two methods would be complementary. Bill Pierce at the University of Pennsylvania was one of the earliest investigators to advance the artificial heart approach. He is often called the father of the ventricular assist device.[15]

1960–1970
HUP resident Bill Pierce builds one of the first artificial mechanical hearts

1970–2001
At Penn State, Pierce develops LionHeart pump first implanted in patients in 1976

Bill Pierce was born in Wilkes-Barre, Pennsylvania. He graduated from Lehigh University as a chemical engineer in 1958 and from Penn's medical school in 1962. While in medical school, he built his first model of an artificial heart. During his residency in general surgery and CT fellowship at HUP, he continued this research. In 1970, he was recruited by the department chair, John Waldhausen (former HUP surgeon) to the faculty of Penn State University and the Milton S. Hershey Medical Center where, joining forces with engineering associates, he designed and built the most advanced artificial heart in the world. One innovative feature was the seam-free surface of the chambers inside the pump. The smooth cavities helped prevent blood clotting that caused strokes in patients treated with earlier heart pumps. Another innovative feature of Dr. Pierce's pump was crucial; it was fully implantable. First implanted in patients in 2001, this pump has a battery-driven power source small enough to be worn outside the body. The need for transcutaneous wires connecting the battery and power source is obviated, eliminating this important source of infection. Dr. Pierce's LionHeart pump has been used to support transplant candidates who develop severe ventricular failure before a suitable donor heart is found. Versions and derivatives of the pump are now used at HUP and worldwide, both as a bridge to transplant and for temporary support of patients unable to come off bypass after open-heart surgery. Since its first clinical use in 1976, it has been implanted in more than 4,000 patients worldwide, saving thousands of lives.

A prolific scientific researcher and writer, Dr. Pierce has authored more than 300 peer-reviewed publications, more than ninety reviews and chapters, and two books. He has served on many editorial boards and holds nine patents. Dr. Pierce is a member of the American College of Surgeons, the American Association for Thoracic Surgery, the American Surgical Association, the Society for Vascular Surgery, the Society of Clinical Surgery, the Society of Thoracic Surgeons, the Society of University Surgeons, the National Academy of Medicine, the National Heart Lung and Blood Institute, the American Institute for Medical and Biological Engineering, the American Society of Artificial Internal Organs, and the International Society for Heart Transplantation.

Dr. Pierce's numerous honors include the Barney Clark Exemplary Humanitarian Award, the Wilkes-Barre Distinguished Service Award, the Monroe J. Rathbone Chemical Engineering Alumni Award, the International Historic Mechanical Engineering Landmark, and an Honorary Doctor of Science Degree from Lehigh University. After performing thousands of coronary artery bypass operations, including one in 1987 on Pennsylvania governor Bob Casey, Dr. Pierce retired from full-time clinical duties in 1996.

1965
Barker and Billingham design an artificial privileged site in guinea pigs

By proving the crucial importance of the lymphatic drainage in skin allograft rejection, they establish the principal of Immunologic ignorance (see Chapter 27)

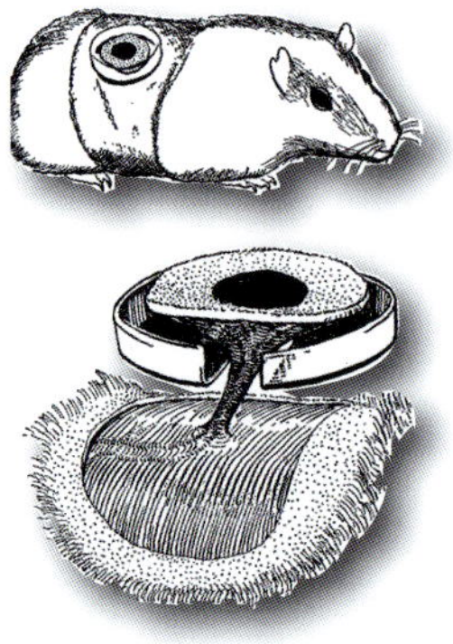

1966
Stan Dudrick succeeds with IV nutrition in humans by cannulating the subclavian vein (see Chapter 19)

In 2007, he received the Jacobson Innovation Award of the American College of Surgeons and in 2012, the distinguished graduate award of the University of Pennsylvania's School of Medicine, the institution's highest honor.

Stanley Dudrick and Jonathan Rhoads: Total Parenteral Nutrition

Stan Dudrick grew up in Nanticoke, a little town in Pennsylvania's coal mining country. His Polish immigrant grandfather worked in the mines, as did his father as a teenager before he graduated from college and bought a farm where Stan worked as a boy. Stan was a talented and ambitious kid who couldn't wait to spread his wings and get away from his hometown, which he remembered as being grimy, smoky, and smelling of the mines. He loved college at Franklin and Marshall, which was clean and attractive. There he was highly successful, Phi Beta Kappa, class president, and voted the outstanding member of his graduating class. Then during medical school at Penn, where he was also class president, he explored surgical research during a summer job by working for heart surgeon Charles Kirby.

As a surgical resident at HUP, Stan became interested in surgical metabolism and nutrition. He developed a close relationship with surgery chairman, Jonathan Rhoads, who had a similar focus on nutrition that he had inherited from his chief, I. S. Ravdin. For years, both of these legendary senior surgeons had dreamed of rescuing malnourished patients who were dying because they couldn't eat.[16] Their longstanding research goal was supplying these patients with sufficient calories by vein to sustain them until they could eat. Not surprisingly, this had also become the research assignment of a long list of HUP surgical residents who signed up to work in the lab of their chief, Jonathan Rhoads. Their attempts included administering potent diuretics to help the patients get rid of excess water in nutritional infusions of high volumes. In another approach, increasing the concentration of intravenous nutrients to provide more calories sclerosed the peripheral veins used for the infusions. These experiments resulted in numerous publications but never reached clinical usefulness.

As just one more of many surgical residents working on intravenous nutrition in Rhoads's lab, Stan was also at first frustrated by the same problems as his predecessors.[17] To follow every step of the way in Stan's own account of his research trail, read the sixty-six-page oral history he gave to the American Academy of Pediatrics.[18] One preliminary step was infusing hypertonic solutions to a vein in his own arm. To his remorse, he confirmed that this led to painful sclerosis. This experience confirmed Stan's conviction that concentrated nutritional solutions could be delivered only via high-volume, fast-flow central veins where they would provoke neither clotting nor sclerosis. He first threaded catheters from the jugular vein into the superior vena cava or right atrium. But the dogs soon displaced the catheters, preventing the long-term treatment that would be necessary.

1968
Dudrick and Wilmore keep a baby alive on IV feeding alone

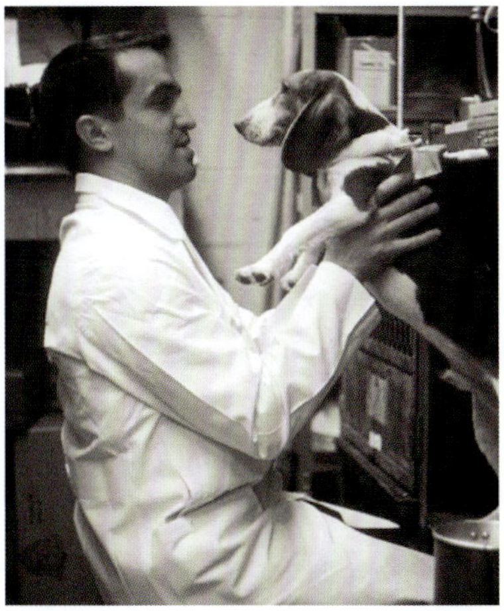

Stan Dudrick with puppy

In order to accomplish chronic treatment, an ingenious harness was designed that the dogs could wear while moving freely in their cages but not disturbing the flow of nutrients being administered 24/7. The harness secured and protected the intravenous cable with a swivel device that prevented tangling. Harry Vars, the surgery department's PhD biochemist, designed this device and also helped determine the optimal combination of essential amino acids, minerals, and vitamins necessary to keep the dogs healthy and growing.

Stan's continuous and almost sleepless attendance and care of the puppies over several months was essential to the success of the experiment that demonstrated normal growth of the pups nourished only by vein. It was a classic. Despite there being only four pups in the study, it was absolutely convincing. No statistics were needed.[19]

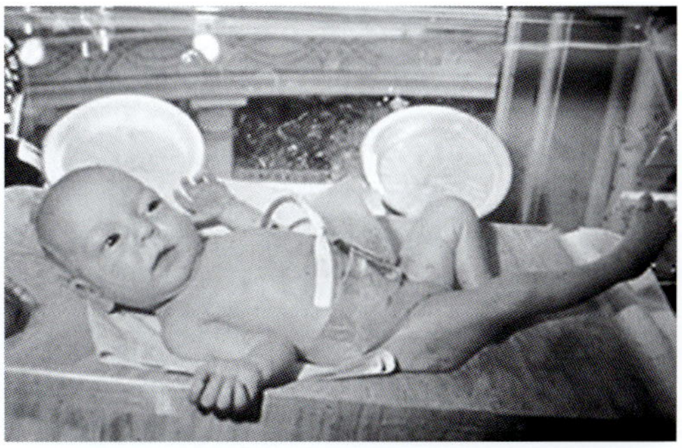

Baby whose only nutrition was by TPN

In April of 1968, while the puppy work was still in the early publication stage, a starving human infant showed up at CHOP. Intestinal atresia and two failed operations had left the baby with less than an inch of functional intestine. Death was inevitable and imminent. Working closely with HUP resident, Doug Wilmore, Stan succeeded in cannulating the central venous circulation. Intravenous nutrition kept the baby alive and growing normally for more than a year.[20]

The accomplishments of 1967 to 1968 alone would have been enough to place Stan Dudrick in the pantheon of surgical research. But there was more to come. Stan accessed the central venous circulation with a cannula introduced by infraclavicular percutaneous puncture of the subclavian vein. This was the key to long-term treatment in human patients. Other important contributions were the introduction of home TPN, treatment of renal failure patients, and promoting closure of intestinal fistulas.

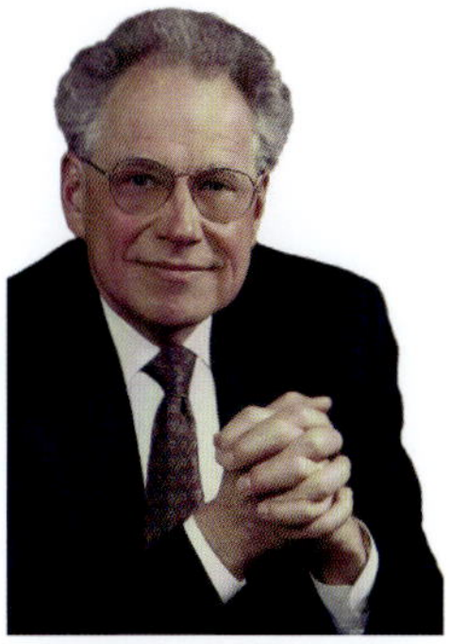

Doug Wilmore

Research Stanley Dudrick conducted while a HUP resident (1962–67) established total parenteral nutrition. TPN has saved millions of lives and is considered one of the twentieth century's most important contributions in all of medicine.[21] The importance of this research and Stan's

1979
Rhoads awarded ASA Medallion for Scientific Achievement for IV hyperalimentation

2009
Stan Dudrick awarded ASA Medallion for Scientific Achievement for IV hyper-alimentation

further contributions to nutritional science have been the basis of some 150 major awards and prizes including the most prestigious ones of the American Medical Association, the American Surgical Association, the American Academy of Pediatrics, and many other scientific societies. Penn's Department of Surgery and School of Medicine have both named him their distinguished graduate.

A Tale of Two Surgeon-Scientists

Total parental nutrition ranks close to the top of medical research accomplishments of the twentieth century. Because of its fame and importance, I suppose it was inevitable that there would be controversy over who was primarily responsible for TPN: Rhoads or Dudrick? In fact, over the years, ardent proponents of one or the other investigator have disagreed. An illustration of this can be seen by reviewing the sequence and timing of prizes that were awarded to them by the American Surgical Association (ASA), prizes honoring the same TPN work. In 1979, the ASA gave its highest award, the Medallion for Scientific Achievement, solely to Jonathan Rhoads. Thirty years later in 2009, the American Surgical Association gave the same Medallion for Scientific Achievement solely to Stan Dudrick. These and many other awards went to one or the other, and sometimes both, such as the ASA's Flance-Karl Award in 1997. But over time, the pattern of distribution changed. During the first decade and a half, TPN virtually always was attributed to the senior and much better-known Rhoads, while Dudrick was likely to be mentioned only as an afterthought as part of the Rhoads team. This wasn't fair!

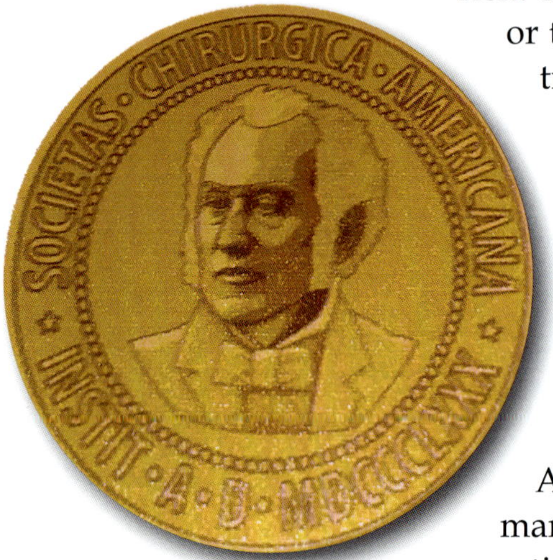

Later, after Rhoads retired and faded from the scene while Dudrick continued to work productively in the field, the two were likely to be credited as sharing the award. In the last few decades, it has been appreciated that it was Dudrick who performed the actual experiments. Thus, it is not surprising that Stan now dominates accounts of the TPN research. Rhoads is often not mentioned at all. This isn't fair!

The truth is that both Rhoads and Dudrick were indispensable in the creation of TPN. Without Rhoads, Dudrick, as a young resident working on his own, would never have had the opportunity or support to carry out the experiments and perhaps not even an interest in the nutrition field. Without Dudrick, the definitive experiments might never have been envisioned and accomplished. Fortunately, from the very beginning, the two surgeons recognized and were happy with their interdependence. While accepting the many prizes that came to each of them, they were unfailingly generous and gracious in crediting the other as a necessary partner.

1957
National Surgical Adjuvant Breast and Bowel meeting. Ravdin insists that Fisher get involved with randomized trials of treatment for breast cancer

Harry Vars: Unsung Hero of TPN

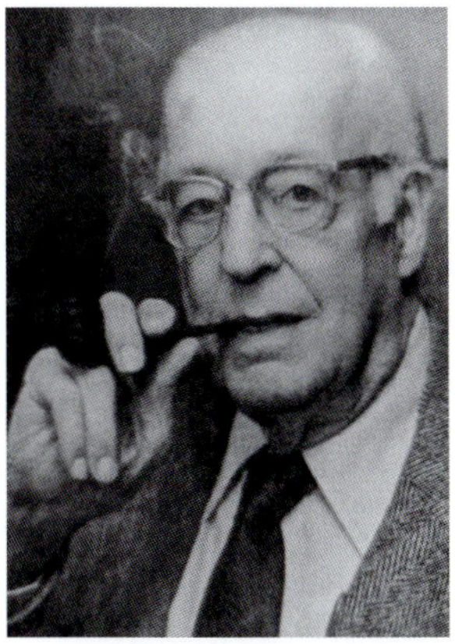

Harry M. Vars, PhD

Now almost forgotten, Harry Vars was the major mentor for generations of HUP residents working on nutrition in Rhoads's lab. He was a hands-on partner with Dudrick in perfecting the device that allowed continuous IV infusions in puppies. Although a member of the Department of Surgery, he was a PhD biochemist who had a secondary appointment in that department and was a popular teacher of Penn medical students in their biochemistry course. His major role in the TPN work led the American Society of Parenteral and Enteral Nutrition to name an annual award for him.

1961
Fisher's first report that chemotherapy delays recurrence of breast cancer

1967
Fisher becomes chairman of NSABP

Bernard Fisher: Randomized Trials of Cancer Treatment

In its 2017 obituary of Bernard Fisher, the *New York Times* praised him as one of the twentieth century's most important medical scientists.[22] Fisher went to college and medical school at the University of Pittsburgh, and after surgical residency there, served on that university's faculty for sixty-seven years. The *Times'* obituary omits that two of Fisher's most important years were spent as a HUP surgery resident and research fellow in the Harrison Department. After returning to the University of Pittsburgh as a faculty member, Fisher directed surgery's research program there, modeled after Penn's Harrison Department. His research led to his recognition as one of the most productive young leaders in the exciting new field of transplantation.

In 1957, Fisher was invited by Dr. Ravdin to a meeting at the NIH on breast cancer.[23] Ravdin organized this meeting to establish the National Surgical Adjuvant Breast and Bowel Project (NSABP) and set up randomized clinical trials for study of chemotherapy in treatment of breast cancer. Fisher was not interested in breast cancer or in clinical trials. But because Ravdin was so influential in academic surgery, he was afraid to decline. To his surprise, he was intrigued by what he heard at the meeting about tumor metastases and was struck by the potential power of multicenter, randomized clinical trials.

At the 1961 meeting of the American Surgical Association, Fisher reported the results of the first NSABP trials. Chemotherapy had delayed early recurrence of breast cancer.[24] In 1967, he become chairman of the NSABP and during the succeeding decades, he led the clinical trials that

Late 1960s
Fisher and NSABP prove radical mastectomy no more effective than simple mastectomy or lumpectomy

1990–1994
Fisher is accused of reporting false data and is fired by NIH

1994
Fisher sues NIH and Pittsburgh; accepts settlement after being found innocent of misconduct

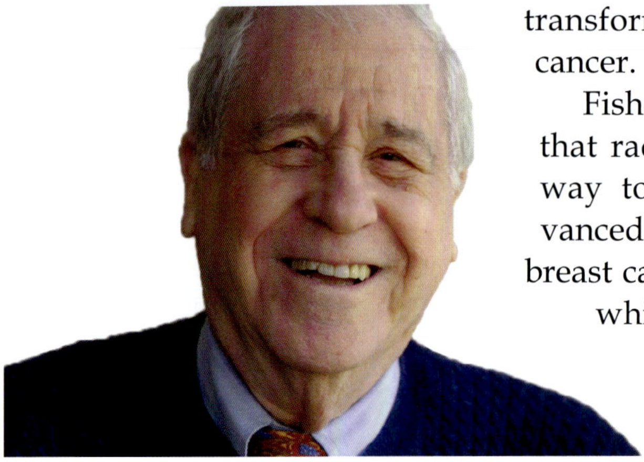

Bernie Fisher

transformed the treatment of breast cancer.

Fisher began to question the dogma that radical resection was the logical way to treat breast cancer and advanced the alternative hypothesis that breast cancer was a systemic disease in which tumor cells were disseminated throughout the body by the time of diagnosis. If this was so, he argued that more extensive regional therapy would not improve survival, and radical mastectomy should be abandoned. He was criticized for this view by many of his surgical colleagues. But by the late 1960s, his hypothesis was supported by the results of his NSABP trials that found radical mastectomy no more effective than simple mastectomy or even lumpectomy.[25] These findings were initially greeted with skepticism. But Fisher's data were so persuasive that eventually radical mastectomy was largely abandoned.

In 1990, a discrepancy was noted in the chart of an NSABP patient being treated by a researcher in Montreal who confessed that he had falsified data to get unqualified patients into the lumpectomy trial. After removing the falsified entry, Fisher reanalyzed the data, finding that the results were hardly changed and still valid. He notified the federal officials at the National Cancer Institute, but they accused him of publishing false data. Fisher was fired by NIH as head of the NSABP and abandoned by the University of Pittsburgh.[26] His reputation was ruined.

Fisher brought suit against both the NIH and the University of Pittsburgh for unfounded accusations. After investigation by the Federal Office of Research and a congressional committee, Fisher was found innocent of any scientific misconduct.

Bernard Fisher is now fully credited with transforming treatment of breast cancer. As important, perhaps, was the influence of his pioneering role in the use of multicenter, randomized clinical trials as the foundation of evidence-based medicine. The *New York Times* in its obituary forgot about Fisher's important years at Penn. But Bernard Fisher never forgot them or how much he owed to Penn and to Dr. Ravdin.

For the full story of Bernard Fisher, see Chapter 16.

Peter Jannetta: Cure of Tic Douloureux

Treatment of trigeminal neuralgia would seem more appropriate for a book on neurosurgery. I have included it here because the most important advances in the treatment of this disease were made by Penn surgeons. In 1921, Charles Frazier, chairman of Penn's Department of Surgery, with the neurologist Spiller, reported that in treatment of this disease, section of the sensory root of the fifth cranial nerve was as effective as resecting the gasserian ganglion and much safer.[27] Forty years later in 1970, Peter Jannetta, another Penn surgeon, discovered the cause of the disease and a treatment that usually cures it.

1963
Jannetta completes five-year HUP residency in general surgery. Begins training in neurosurgery at UCLA

At this time, neurosurgery is a division of Penn's Department of Surgery

Peter Jannetta died at age eighty-four in 2016. He was one of Penn Surgery's most illustrious members. How many others have discovered the cause of an important human disease and the cure for it? Since he was a neurosurgeon, it is ironic that the cause of his death was a brain injury stemming from a fall.

Even as HUP chief resident in 1962 to 1963, Pete was technically gifted and confident (sometimes almost to a fault). He was also good looking and athletic, having played college football and lacrosse for Penn. He was a jazz musician. He was charismatic, funny, and, in our tightly bonded group of residents, everybody's hero.

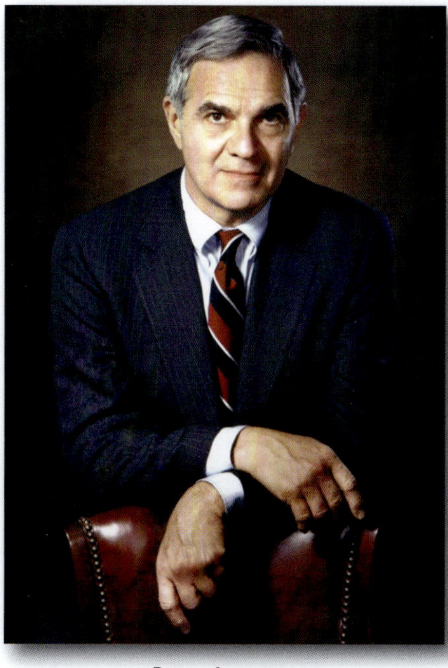
Peter Jannetta

After finishing HUP's general surgery residency and only two years as a neurosurgery resident at UCLA, Pete was appointed chief of neurosurgery at Louisiana State University. In 1971, he moved to the University of Pittsburgh where he remained Chairman of the Department of Neurosurgery for the next three decades. There he built one of the country's great academic neurosurgery programs. He trained more than 150 residents and fellows, many of whom became leaders in US and international neurosurgery. My son, now professor of neurosurgery at Harvard, was his fellow for a year.

Most responsible for Jannetta's wide and lasting reputation was the procedure he developed for trigeminal neuralgia (tic douloureux, a condition known since antiquity to be the cause of excruciating facial pain). Its cause was unknown. For patients whose symptoms were refractory to drug therapy, its only treatment had been cutting the trigeminal nerve or damaging it by injection, radiofrequency, or some other means. Because these treatments left the face numb, they weren't very satisfactory.

While he was still a neurosurgery resident at UCLA, Pete made an observation that would change this. While dissecting the cranial nerves of a cadaver, he noticed that impinging on the trigeminal nerve was a small blood vessel that had left an indentation on the nerve. Soon after this, he operated on a patient with trigeminal neuralgia. He looked for and found a similar relationship of the trigeminal nerve to a crossing blood vessel. He moved the vessel away and was elated to find that the

1970
Jannetta, a neurosurgery resident at UCLA, notes a blood vessel impinging on 5th cranial nerve in a patient with tic douloureux. By 1994, protection of the nerve has become standard treatment

1996
Report of Jannetta's 1,185 operations for tic douloureux in the *New England Journal of Medicine*

1972
Linton Whitaker founds first US craniofacial surgery program (see Chapter 37)

1972
Barker, Reckard, and Ziegler are the first to completely cure diabetes in animal model by transplantation of isolated pancreatic islets (see Chapter 27)

1982
Barker and Naji show that autoimmunity destroys islet allografts, even in recipients tolerant of the donor

patient's facial symptoms suddenly resolved. Over the next decade in successful operations on many patients, he refined this procedure. With the aid of a microscope, he was consistently able to relieve pressure on the nerve by dividing the impinging blood vessel if it was a vein, or if the culprit was an artery, by protecting the nerve from it with a tiny Teflon pad. At first, no one believed he was on to something, but eventually skeptics were convinced. In 1996, my son Fred, while Jannetta's fellow, was given the opportunity to report as first author in the *New England Journal of Medicine* his chief's twenty-year experience with this operation in 1,185 patients.[28] The paper is a citation classic, having been cited in other papers 1,636 times. The Jannetta procedure is now considered the standard treatment for trigeminal neuralgia. In most cases, it results in abrupt relief of the dreadful symptoms.

In 1995 to 1996, Jannetta served as secretary of health for the State of Pennsylvania. After retiring from the University of Pittsburgh in 2000, he joined the staff of Allegheny General Hospital where he remained active in research and writing right up until the time of his death.

His many honors included the Olivecrona Award of the Karolinska Institute, the Zulch Prize of the Max Planck Society for the Advancement of Science, and the Medal of Honor of the World Federation of Neurological Sciences. He was one of only a few neurosurgeons elected to membership in the American Surgical Association.

A Philadelphian by birth, educated at Penn and HUP, Pete often returned to his roots and never lost his feeling for his HUP mentors. On one such occasion in 1983, he gave the D. Hayes Agnew lecture. Pete Jannetta was one of Jonathan Rhoads's favorite residents and perhaps the one of whom he was most proud. In retrospect, it's not hard to see why.

Ali Naji: Pancreatic Islet Transplantation

The following section is taken from Ron DeMatteo's 2022 announcement appointing Ali Naji as the inaugural recipient of the Jonathan Rhoads II endowed chair. Previously, Dr. Naji held the J. William White chair for twenty-six years.

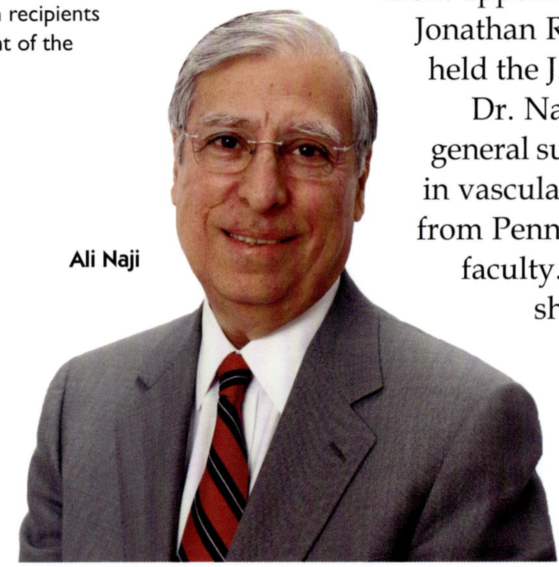
Ali Naji

Dr. Naji has been at Penn for fifty years. He did his general surgery residency at HUP as well as a fellowship in vascular surgery. He obtained a PhD in immunology from Penn in 1981, after which he was appointed to the faculty. He has held numerous departmental leadership roles, including vice chair of research and surgical director of the kidney-transplant program.

His research has focused on diabetes and immunological tolerance. On these topics, he collaborated for many years with me (see Chapter 27). This groundbreaking work on the immunology of diabetes unraveled new mechanisms of immune tolerance. For instance, Dr. Naji demonstrated that the thymus plays an essential role in regulating the maintenance and loss of immune tolerance to tissue-specific antigens, autoimmune diseases, and islet allografts.[29] In addition to this seminal work, Dr. Naji was one of the earliest and most successful in clinical islet transplantation for the treatment of Type 1 diabetes. He established the islet isolation facility at Penn. His extension of the Edmonton protocol for islet transplantation in animals and humans led to a successful Phase 3 clinical trial and a Biologics License Application to the FDA for approval of islet transplantation as a first line therapeutic option in Type 1 diabetes.[30] His recent demonstration that islets transplanted to the subcutaneous space can survive, function, and reverse rodent diabetes is another finding of fundamental importance.[31] Many of his publications are in *Science, Nature, PNAS,* and *Nature Medicine.*

1990
Naji and Posselt transplant islet allografts to thymus, inducing tolerance

2020
Naji successfully transplants islets to the subcutaneous space

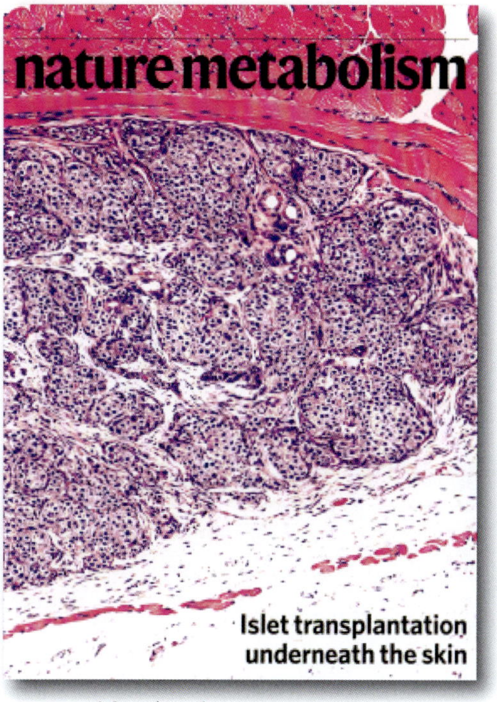

Islets in subcutaneous space

Dr. Naji has received a multitude of NIH grants and is currently the most federally funded surgeon in the country. He leads a U01 and a UC4, and is multi-PI on an R01 and another U01. Under Dr. Naji's leadership, the Human Pancreas Analysis Program was made possible by a $12 million grant from the National Institute of Diabetes and Digestive and Kidney Diseases (NIDDK). He has had uninterrupted funding from the NIH for over thirty years. His total cumulative funding is incalculable but is estimated at $80 million. He has published over 320 articles and has an H-index of 63. He has received numerous awards, including the prestigious Thomas E. Starzl Prize in Surgery and Immunology.

Dr. Naji's passion for teaching and research is boundless. He is an expert kidney, pancreas, and islet transplant surgeon, and an outstanding teacher in the operating room and on the floors. He is still an active participant in departmental conferences. Dr. Naji has been very involved in Penn's MD–PhD program. He has won two Penn Pearls. He has mentored many surgical trainees who have become prominent academic surgeons, including Jim Markmann, Ken Brayman, Andrew Posselt, Hooman Noorchashm, Howard Song, Jonathan Bromberg, John Odorico, Rob Redfield, and many others.

Overall, Dr. Naji is a superior clinician, outstanding investigator, and relentless teacher and mentor.

1983
First successful lung transplant by Joel Cooper in Toronto

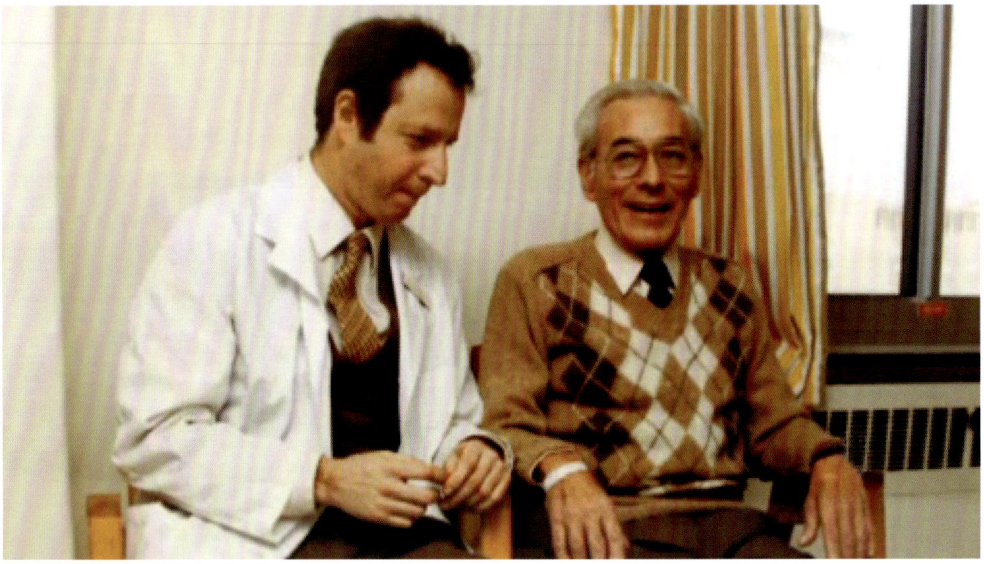

Joel Cooper with the first successful lung transplant patient, Tom Hall

Lung Transplantation: Joel Cooper

Joel Cooper performed the first successful lung transplants in 1983. His surgical training was not at Penn but at MGH and the University of Toronto. His breakthrough research and successful pioneering of lung transplantation also took place in Toronto. He belongs in this chapter because from 2005 to 2016, he was a highly valued and productive member of the Penn surgery faculty. He was the senior thoracic surgeon at HUP and an important mentor of younger members in this field.

On November 6, 2013, Joel Cooper traveled to Toronto to join 350 others in celebration of the thirtieth anniversary of the world's first successful lung transplant.[32] The success converted lung transplantation from a consistently fatal procedure into a lifesaving option for thousands of patients. In the early 1980s, Cooper conducted the basic laboratory experiments that were critical to his success. Over the twenty years before this, forty-four patients worldwide had received lung transplants, but all had died within days or weeks following the surgery, usually because the transplant's tracheal anastomosis refused to heal. In his animal experiments, Cooper found that immunosuppression with prednisone prevented the inflammation phase that is crucial to wound healing. He demonstrated that with cyclosporine-based immunosuppression, he could avoid prednisone and its adverse anti-inflammatory effects, thus allowing the tracheal anastomosis to heal. He also showed that wrapping the airway connection with omentum helped promote healing. He was then ready to proceed with a human transplant.

The next patient listed to receive a lung transplant was Tom Hall. Cooper recalled asking him, "Tom, there have been forty-four attempts so far and no one has survived. Are you sure you want to go ahead with it? He said, 'I am grateful to be number forty-five.' He was an upbeat person."[33] The transplant was successful, and Tom Hall lived for six years. The illustration shows him talking with Dr. Cooper while celebrating the fifth anniversary of his transplant in Paris.

After the first success, Cooper performed twelve consecutive successful single lung transplants, placing the procedure on a firmly accepted basis. In 1986, Dr. Cooper also performed the first successful double lung transplant. Additional aspects of his research in this field were also important, such as devising methods of preservation. In 1997, Cooper moved to Washington University in St. Louis. There he mentored Larry Kaiser, who later moved to Penn and started HUP's lung transplant program. Still later, Kaiser, as Penn chairman, recruited Cooper to Penn.

Credit for initiating lung transplantation and for its early development clearly belongs to Cooper, as recognized by his many awards and honors. In addition to the 1996 Jacobson Award (the American College of Surgeons' highest honor for innovation), in 2011 he was elected to membership in the Institute of Medicine. In 2013, he was awarded the Thomas E. Starzl Prize in Surgery and Immunology.

1985
Harvard student and future Penn chairman Jeffrey Drebin with Mark Green produces antibody to HER2/neu leading to first generation of monoclonal antibodies for treatment of breast cancer

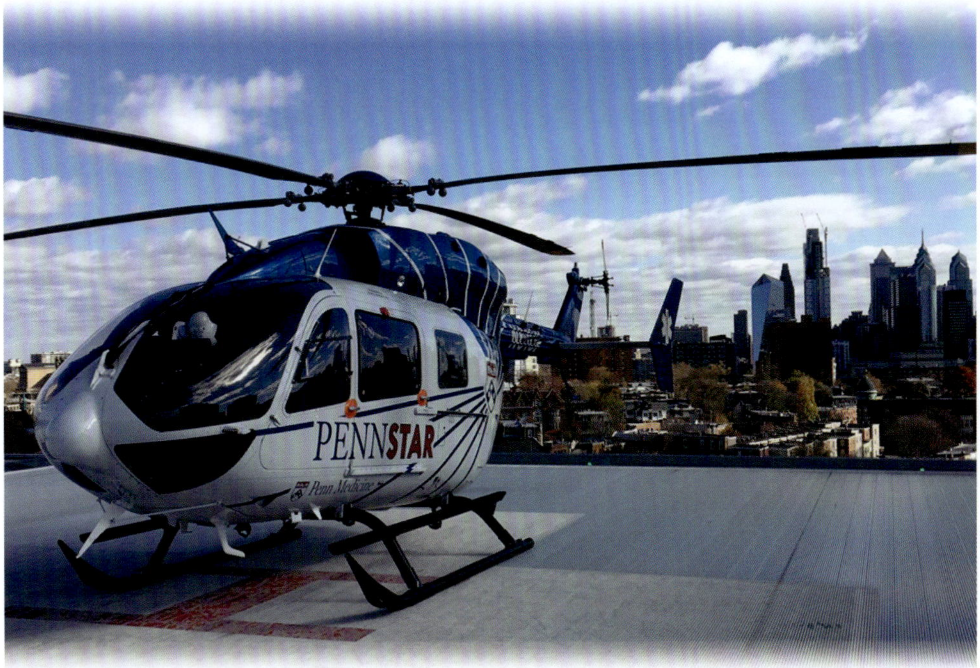

C. William Schwab: Damage Control for Trauma

Damage control may not be exactly the type of response to trauma that Jim Thompson envisioned when he made his list of scientific contributions by surgeons. It is probably aimed more at correcting abnormal physiology than abnormal metabolism. However, it fits with Thompson's

1987
Bill Schwab develops trauma program at HUP

list and this chapter because in saving lives, it is one of the most important surgical advances of recent decades.

Penn's formal trauma program and research in the field is only thirty years old, dating to Bill Schwab's arrival. Before that at HUP, there was not much interest in trauma care. It was almost as if there was an unstated policy to minimize trauma admissions. The hospital's administrators would have been content with this since many trauma victims were uninsured and most of the surgeons were happy not to be bothered with emergency admissions in the middle of the night.

This changed in 1987 when Dean Edward Stemmler became aware that other Philadelphia hospitals were seeking accreditation as trauma centers. Stemmler, not liking the idea of HUP being left out of anything, strongly suggested establishment of a trauma center. So I set out to follow his instructions.

During a site visit, we were evaluated by a team of trauma experts and, to my embarrassment, abruptly turned down. In retrospect, this was entirely appropriate. Our faculty members had neither the experience nor interest to qualify as trauma surgeons. I realized that we needed as a leader someone with experience and expertise in this field. Larry Stephenson (the department's Army reserve colonel)[34] suggested Bill Schwab, a young surgeon who was at Cooper Hospital in Camden. He directed trauma programs there and at Norfolk General Hospital. Although he had faculty appointments at the medical schools associated with these hospitals, his CV had yet to include the prizes and elite society memberships I was accustomed to scrutinizing in faculty candidates. There was one award I should have paid attention to: *Esquire* magazine's designation of Bill Schwab as "One of the Best of the New Generation, Men and Women Under 40 Who Are Changing America." Although skeptical, I invited him for an interview.

In less than five minutes, I knew that Bill Schwab was our man. His energy, knowledge, experience, confidence, and leadership qualities were obvious. After a few minutes more, he took me to the roof of the Ravdin Building to show me where the helicopters would land. I hadn't known we were going to have helicopters, but he had already named them PennSTAR.

Bill Schwab quickly got HUP accredited as a trauma center and before long, built his trauma program into the best in the US and probably the world. In addition, he quickly acquired academic credentials. He easily got elected to membership in surgery's elite societies, including the Society of University Surgeons and the American Surgical Association. He has been awarded honorary fellowships of the Royal College of Surgeons of England and Royal College of Physicians and Surgeons of Glasgow. He has won the highest awards of the surgical societies of the Netherlands, Sweden, and the European Society for Trauma and Emergency Surgery and of the Association of Trauma and Military Surgery of the Royal College of Surgeons of England.

Bill has served on the editorial boards of *Journal of Trauma, Archives of Surgery, Surgery,* and *Annals of Surgery.* He has been President of the Eastern Association for the Surgery of Trauma, the American Association for the Surgery of Trauma, and the International Association for the Surgery of Trauma. He has trained dozens of the world's trauma surgeons, many of whom have started their own trauma programs. He has been visiting professor at over a hundred universities and medical centers and given the most prestigious named lectures in his field. He has published 250 peer-reviewed papers. The Institute of Medicine has sought his help in addressing problems with firearm injury and control.

1993
Schwab, Rotondo, and others describe "damage control"

Rotondo later becomes Chair of Surgery at East Carolina University and is now CEO of University of Rochester Medical Faculty Group

1994
Kaiser, Smythe, and Albelda treat mesothelioma with gene therapy

Pertinent to this chapter, the importance of Bill's research accomplishments is as great as any on Thompson's list. Starting with a 1993 landmark paper in the *Journal of Trauma and Acute Care Surgery,* the research of Bill Schwab, Mike Rotondo, and their associates has been responsible for a paradigm shift in the management of trauma patients. Borrowing a term from Bill's Navy background, they called it "damage control."[35] Patients bleeding from severe, penetrating abdominal injury were operated upon at once without a delay for resuscitation, as had traditionally been advocated. The initial laparotomy was limited to rapid control of bleeding and contamination and expeditious temporary closure. This was followed by transfer to the ICU for resuscitation to correct hypothermia, acidosis, coagulopathy, and other abnormalities of physiology and metabolism. Later, the stabilized patient was returned to the OR for anatomic reconstruction and definitive abdominal closure. Studies in large numbers of trauma patients showed that patients managed by the damage control strategy had 77 percent survival, as compared to 11 percent survival in a matched group of patients managed by the previously recommended treatment.

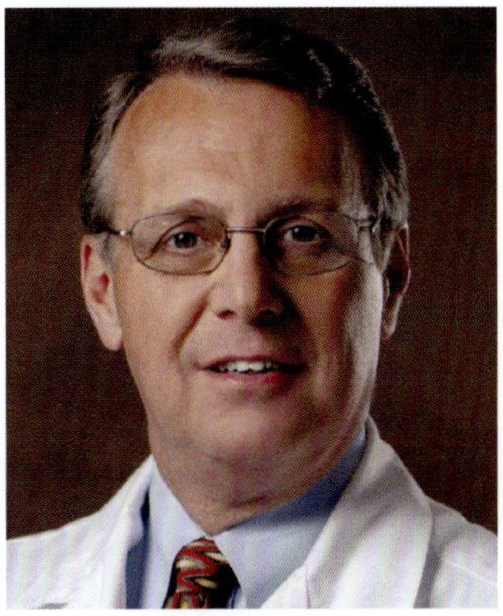

Bill Schwab

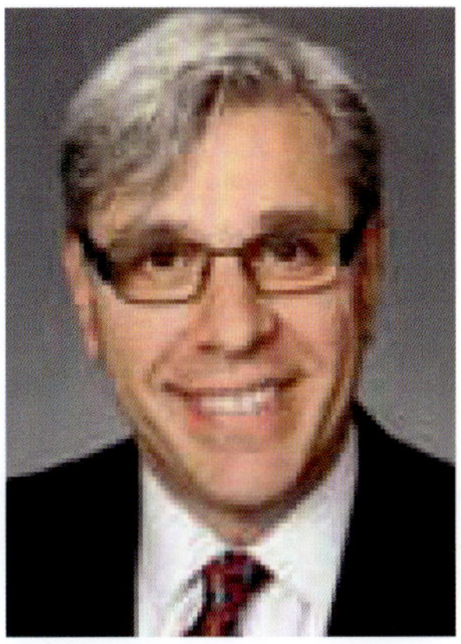

Mike Rotondo

After Bill and his team demonstrated that damage control saved lives, it was adopted by military and civilian trauma surgeons everywhere. In addition, for operations on selected patients whose physiology and metabolism are severely compromised by nontrauma conditions, damage control management can be useful and is not uncommonly employed.[36]

By pioneering with his faculty colleagues the concept of damage control, a term now part of the surgical lexicon, Bill Schwab has changed the world of surgery—not just trauma surgery, and not just in America (like *Esquire* magazine predicted for him), but the world of surgery.

1995–2016
Brian Czerniecki investigates breast tumor vaccines

1998
Ron Fairman introduces endovascular therapy to HUP

2001
Ronald DeMatteo establishes treatment of GI stromal tumors with Gleevec (see Chapter 38)

2015
Hand transplantation established by Scott Levin and Ben Chang

Brian Czerniecki: Breast Cancer Vaccines

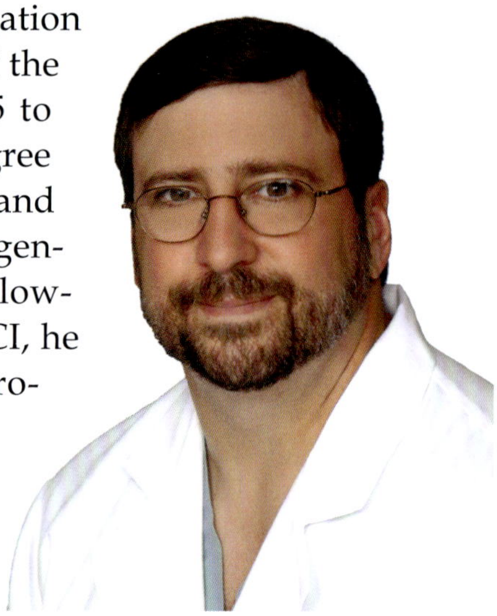
Brian Czerniecki

Brian Czerniecki's basic and clinical investigation of tumor vaccines was an important part of the department's research portfolio from 1995 to 2016.[37] Brian received his undergraduate degree from the University of Maine and his MD and PhD degrees from UMDNJ–Rutgers. After general surgery residency at Ohio State and fellowship training in surgical oncology at the NCI, he joined the faculty at Penn in 1995 and was promoted to full professor in 2012. He built a major research program in tumor immunology focused on breast cancer vaccines, as well as a successful surgical practice focusing on breast cancer and melanoma. His vaccine strategy targeted HCR-2/neu with potential for both prevention and treatment of early breast cancer. He was also a gifted educator and mentor who supervised the research experiences of a number of HUP residents who themselves went on to careers in surgical oncology, including Friederike Kreisel, Mark Faries, Isabelle Bedrosian, Laura Kruper, Anupama Sharma Saigal, Ken Lee, and Robert Roses. In 2016, Brian left Penn to accept the appointment as chairman of the Department of Breast Oncology at Moffitt Cancer Center and Research Institute, an NIH-designated Comprehensive Cancer Center in Florida on the campus of the University of South Florida in Tampa.

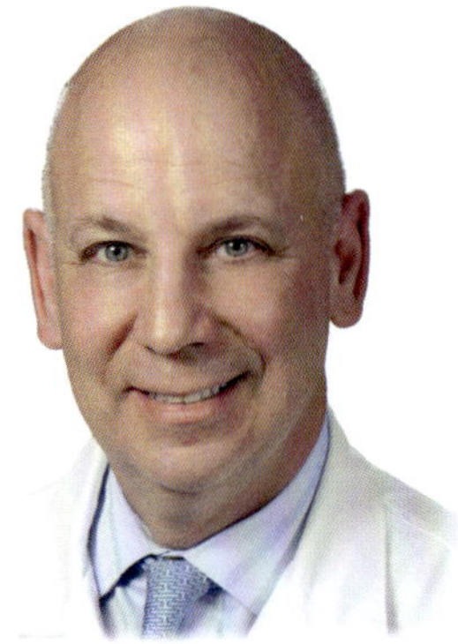
Scott Levin

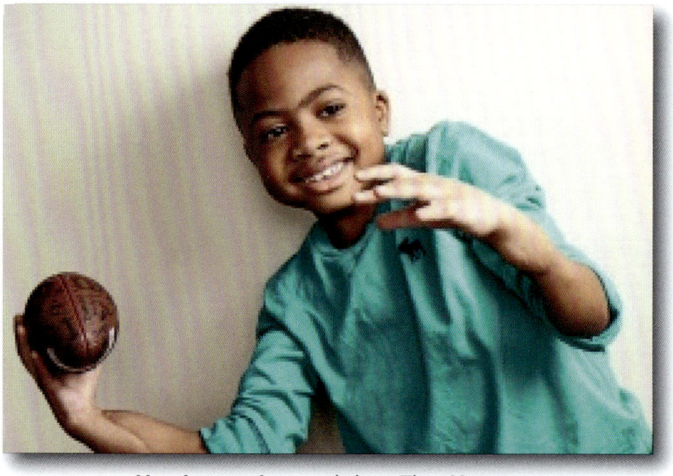
Hand transplant recipient Zion Harvey

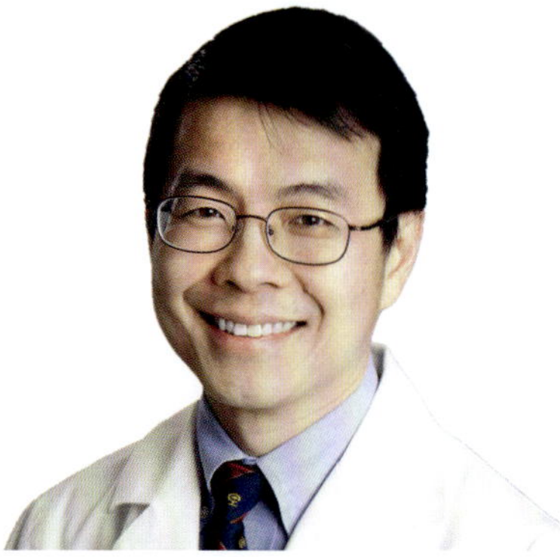
Ben Chang

Omaida C. Velazquez: Angiogenesis

Omaida C. Velazquez (HUP chief resident, 1997–98) was born in Cuba and moved to the United States at age eight, speaking no English. She obtained her BS from Stevens Institute of Technology and received her MD from the University of Medicine and Dentistry of New Jersey, where she graduated as valedictorian of her class in 1991. She trained in general surgery and vascular surgery at the University of Pennsylvania where she joined the faculty in 1999 and served eight years, becoming associate professor with tenure. In 2007, Dr. Velazquez was recruited to the University of Miami as associate professor of surgery, and chief of the Division of Vascular and Endovascular Surgery. She advanced rapidly, becoming chair of the Department of Surgery in 2015.

In her clinical practice, Dr. Velazquez focuses on endovascular and open-surgical treatments of vascular diseases. As a surgeon-scientist, she is the PI of two NIH R01 awards and has made seminal contributions in the area of angiogenesis, vasculogenesis, and wound healing. She reported in the *Journal of Clinical Investigation* three key discoveries: (1) diabetes results in decreased eNOS phosphorylation within the bone marrow, thus reducing mobilization of endothelial progenitor cells (EPCs); (2) diabetes results in downregulation of Stromal Derived Growth Factor 1 alpha (SDF-1α) within wounds, thus decreasing EPC homing to wounds; and (3) these two key diabetes-associated impairments in wound healing and neovascularization may be reversed by the combination of systemic hyperoxia and wound SDF-1α injections.[38] These novel findings may revolutionize the treatments for unsolved diseases, such as peripheral vascular disease, diabetic microangiopathy, and nonhealing diabetic, chronic wounds.

During its 2022 annual meeting, the National Academy of Medicine elected Dr. Velazquez to the Academy. The Academy provided the following citation:

> Omaida C. Velázquez pioneered research that identified E-selectin as a membrane-bound adhesion molecule that induces pro-angiogenesis and healing, in a vascular medicine field where previously only soluble factors had been considered therapeutic candidates. Her groundbreaking work ushered a paradigm-shifting platform to reverse tissue damage by arterial occlusion or diabetes.

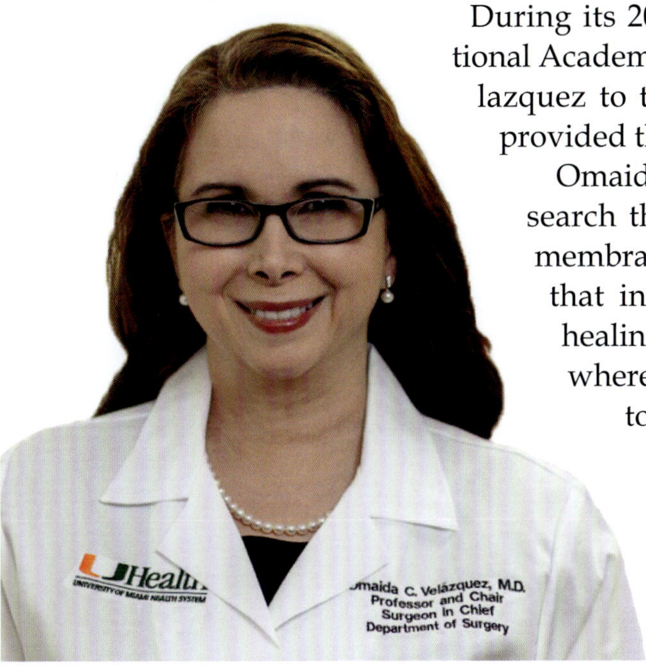

Omaida Velazquez

1994
Wilson and Raper perform first successful gene therapy in a patient with hyperlipidemia

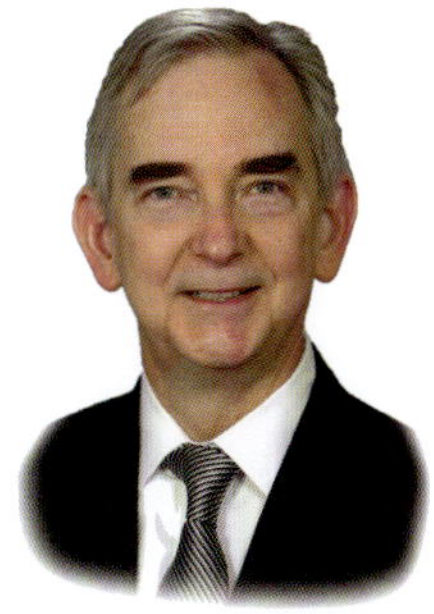

Steven Raper

1999
Wilson and Raper perform gene therapy for OTC deficiency. The patient dies. After the investigation of the death, the researchers and their institutions are criticized for inadequate informed consent

2000–2010
Gene therapy trials at Penn are shut down for ten years

2020
Paige Porrett performs at HUP one of world's first uterus transplants resulting in a successful pregnancy

1984
Hansell Stedman, as HUP resident, begins study of gene therapy for Duchenne Muscular Dystrophy

Omaida is one of a small number of surgeon members of the Society of Clinical Investigation as well as a member of the Society of University Surgeons and the American Surgical Association. In 2015, she was honored as a Distinguished Graduate of our department. Her latest honor is to have an endowed professorship at Miami named for her.

Hansell Stedman

Hansell Stedman's career proves that a clinical surgeon can also be a world-class basic scientist. While performing and teaching general and vascular surgery, Hansell has molded another full-time career as a molecular biologist pursuing the cure for a fatal disease that devastated his family.

Since his days as a HUP surgical resident (1984–1994), Dr. Stedman has searched for a cure of Duchenne muscular dystrophy (DMD), an X-linked, genetically determined disease that inevitably kills young boys from progressive weakness and failure of skeletal and cardiac muscle. Two of Hansell's brothers died from it.

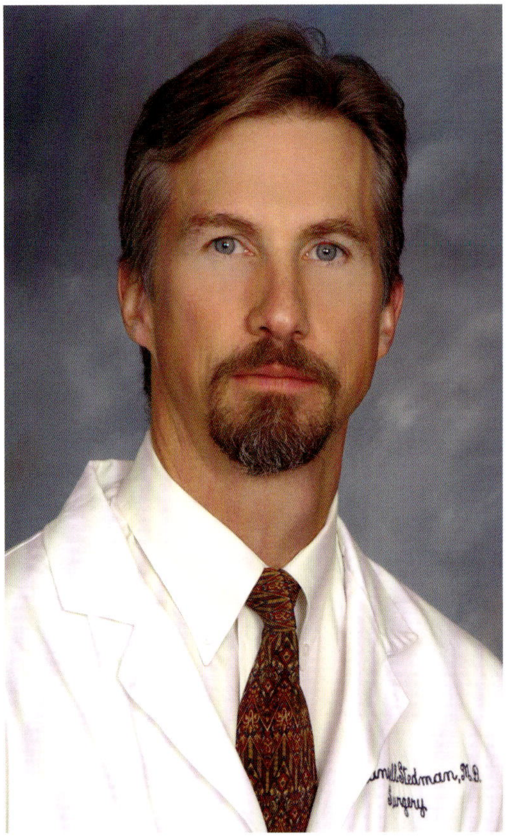

Hansell Stedman

The disease is caused by a mutation that prevents production of dystrophin, a protein required to protect muscle fibers from breaking down. Therefore, the approach of research has been to deliver and replace normal dystrophin. For many years, Hansell has pursued this strategy with promising results but never complete success. Recent findings suggest that he may be about to hit the jackpot.

The problem for gene therapy of DMD by delivering the dystrophin gene itself has been twofold: (1) the gene is enormous and requires removal of major portions for it to fit into an adeno-associated virus vector (AAV); and (2) clinical trials with the dystrophin gene have provoked an immune response, raising concern as to whether this would be safe. Therefore, Hansell has turned to the study of utrophin, a protein similar to dystrophin. During fetal development, utrophin localizes to the sarcolemma and over time is replaced there by dystrophin. It is smaller than dystrophin but still too large to fit into AAV. But by leaving out expendable sections of the protein, Dr. Stedman was able to fit it in. He found that the miniaturized utrophin was not immunogenic and safely stopped muscle deterioration and provided complete rescue in a mouse model of DMD. In a dog model, it also provided substantial improvement. Hansell's report of this in *Nature* demonstrated proof of principal and therapeutic potential in human patients.[39] Dr. Stedman believes human trials will soon be justified.

2016–2022
Stedman studies utrophin therapy in animal models of Muscular Dystrophy

Another example of Dr. Stedman's work was not specifically aimed at curing DMD, but of his many papers, it is my favorite. It illustrates Hansell's gift for recognizing the importance of an odd finding and the tenacity and versatility to pursue it. In 2004, while on the trail of genes connected with muscular disease, Dr. Stedman came across what appeared to be a new myosin gene—MYH16—that is predominantly expressed in muscles of the jaw. In studying the gene, he was surprised to find that it was different in humans than in related species.[40] In humans, MYH16, although coding correctly for 660 amino acids, had deleted two bases. To make sure of this, he tested people from Africa, Spain, Iceland, Japan, Russia, and South America, finding that the deletion was common in all of them. In contrast, he found in studying macaques, gorillas, chimpanzees, and five other nonhuman primates that the gene was intact and reliably did its job to make the complete MYH16 protein.

Then, by using genetic comparisons among species, he and his basic-science paleontologist colleague, Nancy Minugh-Purvis, calculated that the MYH16 mutation took place about 2.4 million years ago, just before human evolution began. The MYH16 protein is a key component only in jaw muscles. In humans, the mutated gene can build only a sliver of a jaw muscle compared to the same huge jaw muscles of nonhuman primates.

Humanoids that existed 2.5 million years ago had large jaw muscles, producing a strong bite. These muscles surrounded the head to anchor them on bony protuberances atop the skull. In one of these primates, Homo erectus, the jaw muscles shrank. At the same time, the fossil record showed that the skull expanded, making room for a larger brain. Dr. Stedman believes this would have been prevented by the large jaw muscles surrounding the heads of other primates.

Hansell's report in *Nature* of this scientific detective story and his fascinating but unprovable hypothesis attracted widespread attention. Within months, more than 100 papers in scientific journals and lay magazines retold the tale of a mutation that 2.4 million years ago changed the shape of the skull, provided more room for the brain, and was an important feature in human evolution.

But there was no Nobel Prize. Many scientists praised Hansell's work, but others objected, doubting that smaller jaw muscles would lead to enlargement of the brain or trigger evolution. Dr. Stedman stood by his results, though never suggesting that this mutation alone caused the development of Homo sapiens. At the very least, he should be credited

2020
Scott Damrauer's paper in *Nature Medicine* identifies eighteen novel genomic loci associated with risk of peripheral artery disease

2023
Damrauer elected rare surgical member of Society of Clinical Investigation

2010
Kelz founds Center for Surgery and Health Economics

with recognizing the first example of a defined protein difference between humans and great apes that might have had a functional consequence.

Rachael Kelz

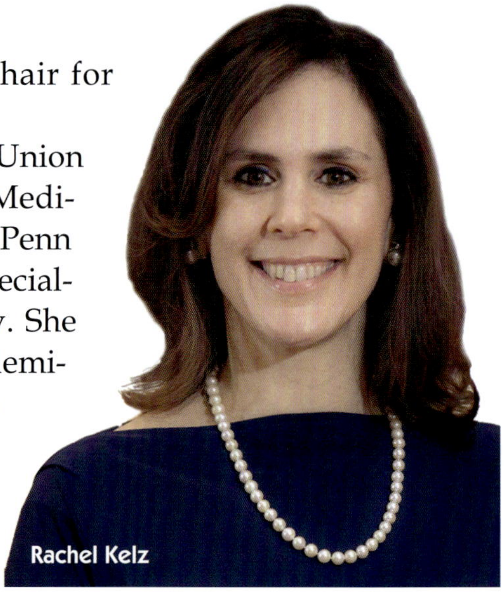

Rachel Kelz is the department's vice chair for clinical research.

Dr. Kelz graduated with honors from Union College and Yale University School of Medicine. After HUP residency, she joined the Penn faculty in 2004. In clinical practice, she specializes in thyroid and parathyroid surgery. She earned a master's degree in clinical epidemiology and biostatistics from the Perelman School of Medicine and an Executive MBA from the Wharton School. She was promoted to full professor in 2018. She is a member of the important surgical societies including the Society of University Surgeons and the American Surgical Association. In 2022, she was elected president of the Society of Clinical Surgery, the first woman to hold this important office..

Her research has been focused on innovations in education, surgical outcomes, and health-care disparities. Recently she has been recognized as a bridge investigator for her work uniting education with quality and safety. Her pioneering work on the integration of education and outcomes research has been funded by multiple organizations, including the NIH. Dr. Kelz is a senior fellow at the Leonard Davis Institute.

In 2010, Dr. Kelz founded the Center for Surgery and Health Economics. This center that she directs is affiliated with the Leonard Davis Institute at Wharton. Its mission is to work with collaborators within the Department and across multiple disciplines to improve the quality of surgical care delivered across the country through the use of novel techniques in education, clinical investigation, and health services research.[41] The Center maintains the infrastructure required to facilitate the academic mission of the Department in the clinical sciences. Since its inception, faculty of the Center have contributed to over thirty peer-reviewed publications related to the Center's mission, presented at multiple national and international surgical, health-services research, and educational meetings, and obtained grant support from public sources and private foundations.

Sunil Singhal

Sunil Singhal is the department's vice chair for translational research. He is responsible for overseeing the translational research portfolio of the department, increasing interactions of surgical investigators with other research programs in the university, and improving the education and research for the department's surgical trainees. Dr. Singhal is the William Measey Professor and chief of the Division of Thoracic Surgery. He graduated from Dartmouth College and Penn medical school. He completed his general surgery training at Hopkins and a fellowship in thoracic surgery at HUP. He has three RO1s and a Department of Defense grant and is a project leader on a PO1. He has published in the *Journal of Clinical Investigation*, *Cancer Cell*, and *PNAS*. He is one of the few surgeons who has been elected to the American Society for Clinical Investigation. He recently received the Luigi Mastroianni Clinical Innovator Award at Penn. Dr. Singhal also directs the Thoracic Surgery Research Laboratory, which is developing the next generation of intraoperative imaging by pursuing multiple approaches that will allow more complete resection of primary micro metastatic and lymphatic disease, while minimizing unnecessary tissue resections.

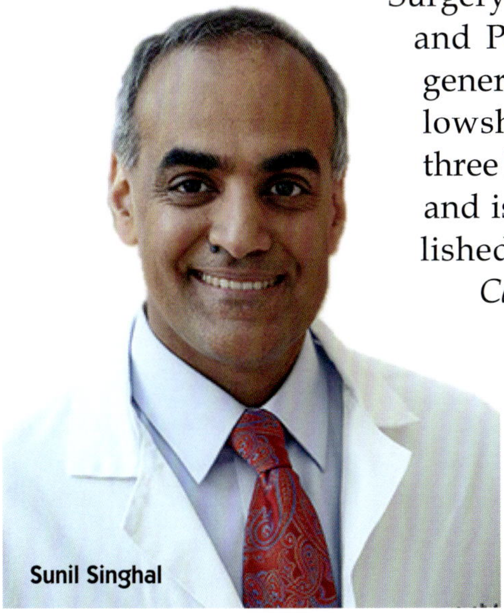

Sunil Singhal

2016
Sunil Singhal founds and directs Center for Precision Surgery and studies methods of making tumors glow

Dr. Singhal is also the founder and director of the Center for Precision Surgery within the Abramson Cancer Center. This center is based on a novel imaging technique devised by Dr. Singhal. The goal has been to make hidden tumors glow, thus allowing precise real-time intraoperative visualization of tumor margins and detection of other tumors or metastases not visible to the naked eye.[42]

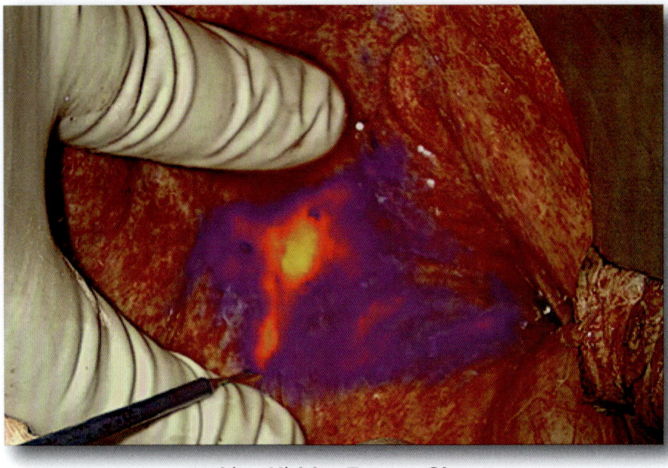

Making Hidden Tumors Glow

In as many as one in four lung cancer operations, there is incomplete resection of the tumors or failure to recognize and remove tumor implants or involved lymph nodes. Sunil's technique is changing this and should lessen the chances of tumor recurrence. His method employs an injectable dye specially engineered to be taken up by cancerous tissues more so than by normal tissues. Before surgery, patients are injected with the dye. Then, during the operation when exposed to near infrared light, tumors glow.

The impressive success of extensive NIH-supported animal experiments resulted in approval of human trials. Many hundreds of patients have now undergone these clinical trials with very encouraging results.

In a number of them, cancerous tissue has been identified that would otherwise have been overlooked. Originally, the method was used in patients with lung tumors, but it is now being tested also in patients with bladder, breast, head and neck, endocrine, brain, and other tumors. It may be particularly useful to neurosurgeons who, in resecting brain tumors, must identify tumor margins precisely so as to avoid removing or damaging important areas adjacent to the tumors.

Other Scientists

We had trouble limiting the list to a manageable number. Other Penn surgeons clearly belonging are not included because they have their own full chapters (DeMatteo, Drebin, Kaiser, Koop). Others are placed in the timeline (Raper) or are reviewed in Chapter 37 (Edmunds, Fairman, Whitaker, Adzick, Fraker, Rombeau). There have been many more. Probably everyone who reads this will have their own set.

Timeline of Research by Penn Surgeons

1756–1762 William Shippen trains in England with John Hunter, the father of scientific surgery; despite this, Shippen does no research in his forty-year career.

1816 Philip Syng Physick introduces absorbable sutures made from kid gloves and catgut.

1838 William Horner studies microscopic changes in small bowel of cholera victims.

1867–1895 John Shaw Billings directs surgeon general's library. It becomes the National Library of Medicine. He devises Index Medicus which becomes Medline.

1895 J. William White shows that castration shrinks the prostate in dogs and humans.

1901–1930 Charles Frazier and William Spiller find that dividing the sensory root of the 5th cranial nerve cures tic douloureux.

1911 At the second Clinical Congress of North America, Levi J. Hammond performs the world's first human kidney transplant. Because of twenty-four hours of warm ischemia, it could not have been a success. The same day, with possibly the same donor, he performs a testicle transplant, cooling the donor organ to avoid ischemic damage.[43]

1911 Edward Martin and William Spiller demonstrate that severing the anterolateral tracts of the spinal cord relieves lower body pain.

1927 During a research year in England, I. S. Ravdin investigates gallbladder function. For the next twenty years, he conducts research on nutrition and GI physiology.

1935 Jonathan Rhoads performs several peritoneal dialyses, probably the world's first.

1936–1941 At Penn, John and Mary Gibbon improve their heart-lung machine and succeed with heart bypass in cats.

1936–1943 At HUP, Norman Freeman studies shock and sets up the first non-invasive vascular laboratory.

1940s Chick Koop with Ravdin, Harry Vars, and others, studies blood substitutes and intravenous nutrition.

1943–1945 In India at the 20th General Hospital, Norman Freeman evaluates sympathectomy as treatment for causalgia.

1951 In California, Norman Freeman performs world's first successful resection of an abdominal aortic aneurysm.

1951–1953 In Korea, John Howard (Hawkeye) disregards Army regulations and, obtaining appropriate vascular clamps, successfully repairs arterial wounds; sets up dialysis in MASH units.

1953	William Inouye invents coil dialyzer; is copied by Willem Kolff.
1957	Ravdin initiates cancer chemotherapy program of NSABP (National Surgical Adjuvant Bowel and Breast Program); recruits Bernie Fisher to head it. Clinical trials eventually show that simple mastectomy or lumpectomy is as successful as radical mastectomy.
1960–1970	Bill Pierce, as Penn student and resident, builds one of first artificial hearts; first clinical use at Penn State in 1976.
1960–1970	Jonathan Rhoads, with a series of HUP residents, studies IV nutrition with large volume infusions (five-liter program); achieves positive nitrogen balance.
1961	Brooke Roberts determines cause of subclavian steal with hemodynamic laboratory studies.
1963	Ravdin resident David Cooper discovers the role of enzyme cytochrome P450.
1963	Ravdin resident Jim Hardy, after successful animal experiments, performs world's first human lung transplant at University of Mississippi. The lung functions for eighteen days.
1964	Jim Hardy, after successful animal experiments, performs world's first human heart transplant (using chimpanzee donor) at University of Mississippi. It fails at once.
1965	Clyde Barker and Rupert Billingham construct immunologic privileged site and establish principle of immune ignorance.
1966	Barker begins kidney transplant program at HUP; donors are selected by irradiated hamster histocompatibility test developed in Billingham's laboratory.
1966	Stan Dudrick, Jonathan Rhoads, and Harry Vars show that puppies nourished only with parenteral nutrition can survive and grow normally.
1967–1990	Ravdin resident Peter Jannetta at UCLA, Tulane, and Pittsburgh establishes that compression of 5th cranial nerve by crossing blood vessel is cause of tic douloureax; alleviation of pressure on the nerve cures the disease.
1968	Dudrick and Douglas Wilmore keep human infant alive and growing with TPN alone (for one year).
1970–1985	L. Henry Edmunds studies blood surface interactions and large animal models of heart valve and ventricular remodeling.
1972	Barker and HUP resident Craig Reckard are the first to completely and lastingly reverse animal diabetes by pancreatic islet transplantation.
1972	Linton Whitaker introduces cranialfacial surgery program at HUP and CHOP.

1974	Moreye Nusbaum and Stanley Baum catheterize mesenteric arteries to treat portal hypertension or to locate site of bleeding from small bowel.
1979	Alden Harken and Mark Josephson alleviate intractable ventricular arrhythmia by endocardial resection of the relevant electrophysiologically determined site.
1979	Brooke Roberts and Ernie Ring develop balloon angioplasty of stenotic arteries.
1980	Gordon Buzby and Jim Mullen develop prognostic nutritional index for GI surgery, one of Mullen's many contributions in nutritional research.
1982	Brooke Roberts dissolves clots in occluded arteries using streptokinase.
1982	Barker and Ali Naji show that in neonatally tolerant rodent recipients, autoimmunity alone destroys islet allografts.
1983	Future Penn faculty member Joel Cooper at University of Toronto is first to succeed with lung transplantation in humans.
1985	Mike Acker and Larry Stephenson show that electrical pulses can convert fast-twitch skeletal muscle into fatigue-resistant, slow-twitch muscle. Modified skeletal muscles could contract for years and might be used for replacing or augmenting parts of a failing heart.
1985	Future Penn chairman Jeffrey Drebin, as a Harvard medical student, and Michael Greene develop monoclonal antibodies against HER2/neu, the foundation of targeted treatment of cancer.
1990	Andrew Posselt, Naji, Jim Markmann, Michael Choti, and Barker induce intrathymic tolerance.
1993	Bill Schwab and Michael Rotondo establish damage control as improved method of treating severe trauma wounds.
1994	James Wilson and Steve Raper perform the first successful human gene therapy, demonstrating improvement in hypercholesterolemia.
1994	Scott Adzick initiates fetal surgery program at CHOP; in 2011, reports success of multi-center trial of fetal surgery for spina bifida.
1995	DeMatteo, Raper, and Markmann show that gene transfer to the thymus abrogates the immune response to adenovirus vector.
1995–2016	Brian Czerniecki studies vaccine for breast cancer.
1995	Larry Kaiser, Roy Smythe, and Steve Albelda report successful suicide gene therapy of mesothelioma with thymidine kinase/ganciclovir.
1996	Douglas Fraker conducts isolated limb perfusion for melanoma and studies intra-abdominal photodynamic therapy.

1996	Alan Flake at CHOP directs fetal surgery program; studies stem cells, gene therapy, in utero tolerance, and artificial uterus.
1998	Ron Fairman establishes endovascular surgery program at HUP with multiple clinical trials.
1999	Wilson and Raper attempt gene therapy in patient with ornithine transcarbamylase deficiency. Death of patient results in closure of gene therapy program at Penn for ten years.
1999	Omaida Velazquez studies angiogenesis and endothelial biology; shows that E-selectin induces healing.
2000	Robert and Joseph Gorman design novel heart valves and study post-myocardial infarction ventricular remodeling.
2001	Conducting clinical trials at Memorial Sloan Kettering, Ron DeMatteo establishes Gleevec treatment of GIST as worldwide standard of care. Employs mouse model for ongoing studies.
2003	Markmann, Naji, and Barker initiate human islet transplant program.
2004	Hansell Stedman discovers that MYH16 is mutated in humans, causing weak jaw muscles and possibly expansion of the skull.
2010	Rachel Kelz establishes Center for Surgical and Health Economics.
2011	Scott Levin and Ben Chang initiate hand transplantation at Penn.
2016–2022	Hansell Stedman in animals uses nonimmunogenic utrophin as substitute for dystrophin as treatment for muscular dystrophy.
2016	Sunil Singhal establishes Center for Precision Surgery; molecular imaging makes tumors glow.
2020	Paige Porrett performs at HUP one of first uterus transplants.
2020	Scott Damrauer studies genetic and molecular epidemiology of vascular disease; reports that eighteen novel genomic loci are associated with blood vessel disease.

Notes

[1] Shumacker, Harris B. *A Dream of the Heart, The Life of John H. Gibbon, Jr. Father of the Heart-Lung Machine* (Santa Barbara: Fithian Press, 1999).

[2] Churchill's pulmonary artery embolectomy was accomplished in less than seven minutes but failed to save his patient. At the time, no successful embolectomies for pulmonary emboli had been performed in the US and only nine worldwide.

[3] Prior to Gibbon's 1953 case, John Lewis at Chicago had succeeded in open-heart surgery carried out without bypass but instead with hypothermia. A few months before Gibbon's success, Clarence Dennis performed an open-heart operation with his heart-lung machine, but the patient died. Had it been successful, Dennis would probably be known as the father of open-heart surgery.

[4] Johnson, J. Obituary of Norman E. Freeman. *Trans American Surgical Association* (Philadelphia 1976) 94: 55–57.

[5] Connolly, John E. Norman Freeman, The "First" American Specialist in Vascular Surgery. *J Vasc Surg*, Vol 22, No 2, p. 189.

[6] Ibid., p. 129.

[7] Connolly, John E. Norman Freeman, The "First" American Specialist in Vascular Surgery, p. 190.

[8] Connolly, John E. Norman Freeman, The "First" American Specialist in Vascular Surgery, p. 191.

[9] Ibid., p. 192. Dubost C, Allary M, Oeconomos N. Apropos du traitement des aneurysnes de l'aorte. *Mem Acad Chir* (1951) 77:381–3.

[10] Ibid., p. 192.

[11] Ibid., p. 192.

[12] Ibid., p. 192.

[13] Freeman, Norman. Vascular Surgery. *California Medicine*, Vol 68, No 1, p. 43–44.

[14] Barker, Clyde F and Daly, John M, eds. *Jonathan E. Rhoads Eightieth Birthday Symposium* (Philadelphia: J. B. Lippincott Co, 1989) pp. 123–136.

[15] Snyder AJ, Pierce WS, Rosenberg G, Weiss WJ and Runt J. Progress in the development of an innovative ventricular assist system. *Am. Soc. Artif. Intern. Organs*, Abstracts 42(2): 13 1 (March–April, 1996).

[16] Barker, Clyde F. Jonathan Rhoads, MD. *Annals of Surgery* (2002 May) 235 (5) 740–744. Ravdin IS, Vars HM, Thorogood E, Schultz J, Johnson J. The Liver Glycogen and Lipid Concentrations Following Intravenous Administration and Diet in the Dog and Man in the Presence of Liver Damage. *Ann Surg.* (1941) 114(6):1018–1025.

[17] Barker, Clyde F. Memoir of Stanley Dudrick. *Transactions of the American Surgical Association* (2020).

[18] *Oral History of Stanley J. Dudrick, MD.* Interviewed by John R. Gosche, MD, Pediatric History Center, American Academy of Pediatrics (Dec 15, 2006). https://studylib.net/doc/18295607/stanley-j.-dudrick—md.

[19] Dudrick SJ, Wilmore, DW, Vars, HM and Rhoads, JE. Long-term Total Parenteral Nutrition with Growth, Development, and Positive Nitrogen Balance. *Surgery*, 64:134 (1968).

[20] Wilmore DW, Dudrick SJ. Growth and development of an infant receiving all nutrients exclusively by vein. *JAMA* 203: 142 (1968).

[21] Barker, Clyde F. Memoir of Stanley Dudrick. *Transactions of the American Surgical Association* (2020).

22 Gellene, Denise. Dr. Bernard Fisher, Who Revolutionized Breast Cancer Treatment, Dies at 101. *The Philadelphia Inquirer* (19 Oct 2019).

23 Travis, Kate. Bernard Fisher Reflects on a Half-Century's Worth of Breast Cancer Research. *JNCI: Journal of the National Cancer Institute,* Vol 97, No 22 (16 Nov. 2005) pp. 1636–1637.

24 Fisher B, Ravdin RG, Ausman RK, et al. Surgical Adjuvant Chemotherapy in Cancer of the Breast: results of a decade of cooperative investigation. *Ann Surg* 168; 337–356 (Sept. 1968).

25 Fisher B, Anderson S. Conservative surgery for the management of invasive and noninvasive carcinoma of the breast: NSABP trials. National Surgical Adjuvant Breast and Bowel Project. *World J Surg* (1994) 18(1):63–69.

26 Davidson, Nancy. Bernard Fisher, MD: In Memoriam (1918–2019). *Cancer Research.* 80. 3–4 (2020).

27 Frazier, Charles H. A Refinement in the Radical Operation for Trigeminal Neuralgia. *JAMA* (1921) 76(2):107.

28 Barker II, FG, Jannetta PJ, Bissonette DJ, Larkins MV, Jho HD. The long-term outcome of microvascular decompression for trigeminal neuralgia. *N Engl J Med* (1996) 334(17):1077–1083.

29 Posselt A, Barker CF, Tomaszewski JE, Markmann JF, Choti MA and Naji, A. Induction of Donor Specific Unresponsiveness by Intrathymic Islet Transplantation. *Science* 249:1293–1295 (1990).

30 Markmann JF, Deng S, Huang X, Desai NM, Velidedeoglu EH, Lui C, Frank A, Markmann E, Palanjian M, Brayman K, Wolf B, Bell E, Vitamaniuk M, Doliba N, Matschinsky F, Barker CF, Naji A. Insulin Independence Following Isolated Islet Transplantation and Single Islet Infusions. *Annals of Surgery* 237(6):741–9; discussion 749–50 (June 2003).

31 Yu M, Agarwal D, Korutla L, May CL, Wang W, Griffith NN, Hering BJ, Kaestner KH, Velazquez OC, Markmann JF, Vallabhajosyula P, Liu C, Naji A. Islet transplantation in the subcutaneous space achieves long-term euglycaemia in preclinical models of type 1 diabetes. *Nature Metab.* (2020 Oct.) 2(10):1013–1020. doi: 10.1038/s42255-020-0269-7. Epub 2020 Sep 7. PMID: 32895576; PMCID: PMC7572844.

32 Joel D. Cooper. Surgeon of the World's First Successful Lung Transplant. *ATS News* (Nov. 2013). https://news.thoracic.org/community/whos-who/joel-d-cooper-surgeon-of-the-worlds-first-successful-lung-transplantation.php. Joel D. Cooper. *Wikipedia,* Wikimedia Foundation (29 Jan. 2022). https://en.wikipedia.org/wiki/Joel_D._Cooper.

33 Personal conversations with Joel Cooper.

34 Larry Stephenson, who was head of our trauma program in the beginning, could have done the job well. But he was primarily a busy cardiac surgeon, and there were no other faculty with an interest in that field to back him up in trauma.

35 Rotondo MF, Schwab CW, McGonigal MD, et al. 'Damage control': an approach for improved survival in exsanguinating penetrating abdominal injury. *J Trauma* (1993) 35(3):375–383.

36 Stawicki SP, Brooks A, Bilski T, et al. The concept of damage control: extending the paradigm to emergency general surgery. *Injury* (2008) 39(1):93–101. doi:10.1016/j.injury.2007.06.011.

37 Koski GK, Roses R, Xu S, Cohen PA, Czerniecki BJ. Re-engineering dendritic cell-based anti-cancer vaccines. *Immunologic Reviews* 222: 256–276 (2008).

[38] Gallagher KA, Liu ZJ, Xiao M, Chen H, Goldstein LJ, Buerk DG, Nedeau A, Thom SR, Velazquez OC. Diabetic impairments in NO-mediated endothelial progenitor cell mobilization and homing are reversed by hyperoxia and SDF-1 alpha. *J Clin Invest* (2007) 117(5):1249–1259. doi:10.1172/JCI29710.

[39] Song Y, Morales L, Malik AS, Mead AF, Greer CD, Mitchell MA, Petrov MT, Su LT, Choi ME, Rosenblum ST, Lu X, VanBelzen DJ, Krishnankutty RK, Balzer FJ, Loro E, French R, Propert KJ, Zhou S, Kozyak BW, Nghiem PP, . . . Stedman HH. Non-immunogenic utrophin gene therapy for the treatment of muscular dystrophy animal models. *Nature Medicine* (2009) 25(10), 1505–1511. https://doi.org/10.1038/s41591-019-0594-0

[40] Stedman HH, Kozyak BW, Nelson A, Thesier DM, Su LT, Low DW, Bridges CR, Shrager JB, Minugh-Purvis N, and Mitchell MA. Myosin gene mutation correlates with anatomical changes in the human lineage. *Nature* (2004) 428(6981), 415–418. https://doi.org/10.1038/nature02358.

[41] Tong JKC, Akpek E, Naik A, et al. Reporting of Discrimination by Health Care Consumers Through Online Consumer Reviews. *JAMA Netw Open* (2022) 5(2):e220715. Published 2022 Feb 1. doi:10.1001/jamanetworkopen.2022.0715. Kelz RR, Tong J. Examining Quality Improvement in Medicine and Business. *J Am Coll Surg* (2021) 233(6):809–810. doi:10.1016/j.jamcollsurg.2021.09.006. Zhao C, Dowzicky P, Colbert L, Roberts S, Kelz RR. Race, gender, and language concordance in the care of surgical patients: A systematic review. *Surgery* (2019) 166(5):785–792. doi:10.1016/j.surg.2019.06.012.

[42] Azari F, Kennedy GT, Chang A, et al. Glycoprotein Receptor CEACAM5-Targeted Intraoperative Molecular Imaging Tracer in Non-Small Cell Lung Cancer [published online ahead of print, 2022 May 27]. *Ann Thorac Surg* (2022) S0003-4975(22)00731-7. doi:10.1016/j.athoracsur.2022.05.019. Kennedy GT, Azari FS, Bernstein E, et al. Targeted Intraoperative Molecular Imaging for Localizing Nonpalpable Tumors and Quantifying Resection Margin Distances. *JAMA Surg* (2021) 156(11):1043–1050. doi:10.1001/jamasurg.2021.3757. Azari F, Kennedy G, Bernstein E, et al. Intraoperative molecular imaging clinical trials: a review of 2020 conference proceedings. *J Biomed Opt* (2021) 26(5):050901. doi:10.1117/1.JBO.26.5.050901.

[43] Baron, Pamela; Schulsinger, David; Sheynkin, Yefim. Fri-09 The Curious Case of Dr. Levi Hammond: Transplantation Galore of 1911. *Journal of Urology* (Apr. 2015) Vol 193 No 4S p e1-e1118. doi: 10.1016/j.juro.2015.02.487.

CHAPTER 35

Distinguished Graduate Awardees

For a department of surgery, nothing is more important than the training of its residents. Success of this responsibility can only be assessed years later by examining the careers and accomplishments of the trainees. In 1991, the Department of Surgery began naming annually a distinguished graduate of the HUP residency. Their photographs are installed in a place of honor outside the Department library. The awardees are invited to come for several days as visiting professor and lecturer. They have not been chosen from the Department's current faculty, although a few were former faculty members. Their prominence had usually been attained elsewhere, and HUP residents had not had a chance to interact with them. Thus, this program is valuable in giving Penn residents, students, and faculty an opportunity to develop relationships with these important members of the Penn surgical family, some of them otherwise forgotten.

After 1998, this program was interrupted. When it was restarted in 2007, it was named for Julius Mackie, a recently deceased, beloved HUP faculty surgeon. From 1970 to 1980, Dr. Mackie was the Department's education officer and director of the residency program. In 1987, the Penn medical students voted him their most valuable teacher. He was also an exceptionally gifted technical surgeon who devoted much of his time to backing up Jonathan Rhoads. Without him, Dr. Rhoads could never have conducted his active surgical practice while devoting so much of his time to the national and international administrative responsibilities that made him famous. Dr. Mackie's wife, Joan, has generously sponsored the distinguished graduate program.

Listed here are the twenty-two distinguished graduates chosen between 1991 and 2023. They are quite a group! Four were presidents of the American College of Surgeons, three presidents of the American Surgical Association. One was US surgeon general, one a university president, thirteen were chairs of surgery at universities, and seven headed equally important academic specialty centers or programs.

Brief biographical sketches of each awardee are provided. For those who have been extensively described elsewhere in the book, only very abbreviated summaries appear, along with chapter references to more complete accounts.

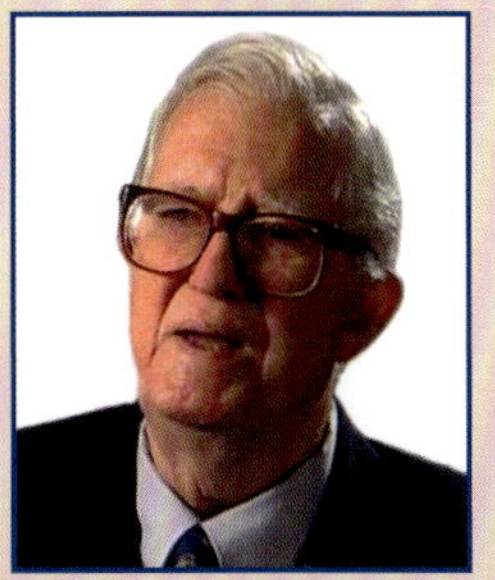

James D. Hardy 1991

HUP Chief Resident (1946–1947)

Jim Hardy was chairman of surgery at the University of Mississippi for thirty-two years. In 1963, he performed the world's first human lung and heart transplants (see Chapter 34). Their success was limited, but as if to compensate for this disappointment, his peers elected him to more positions of leadership than any academic surgeon of his time. He was president of the Society of University Surgeons, the American Surgical Association, the American College of Surgeons, the Society of Surgical Chairmen, and the International Society of Surgery. He was also editor of the *World Journal of Surgery*.

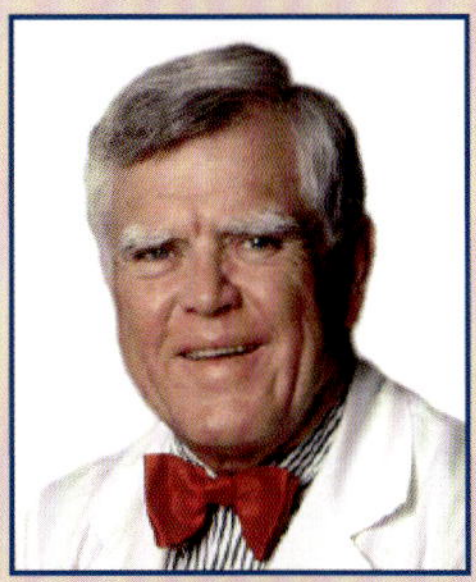

James C. Thompson 1992

HUP Chief Resident (1958–1959)

Jim Thompson was chairman of surgery at the University of Texas Medical Branch for twenty-five years. A highly productive basic researcher in GI physiology, he was president of the American Surgical Association and the American College of Surgeons. He was also a member of the National Academy of Medicine and the American Philosophical Society. In charisma and humor, he surpassed all others. See Chapter 14 for a more complete biography.

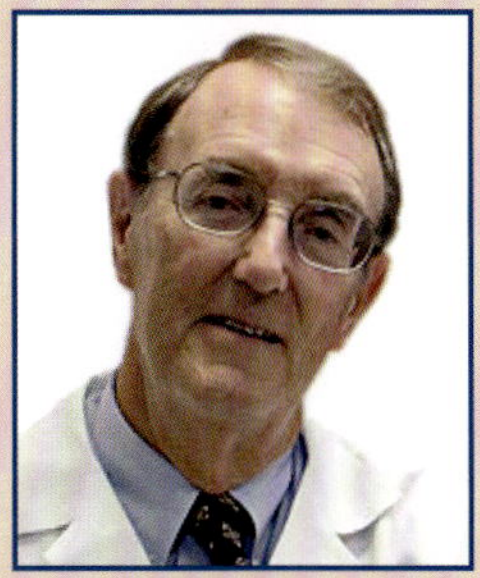

Edward M. Copeland III 1994

HUP Chief Resident (1968–1969)

Ted Copeland's early faculty career was at MD Anderson and the University of Texas, Houston where he was mentored by Stan Dudrick. He served as chairman of surgery at the University of Florida for twenty years. He was president of the American College of Surgeons, the Association of Academic Surgery, the American Board of Surgery, and the Halsted Society. His extensive research was in oncology and surgical nutrition, especially TPN.

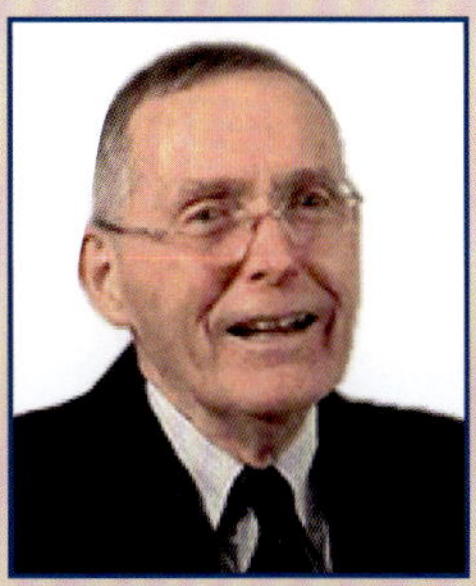

R. Scott Jones 1995

HUP Chief Resident (1966–1967)

A native Texan, Scott Jones went to medical school in Galveston. As a HUP resident, he spent a year studying GI physiology in the lab of Frank Brooks, chief of medicine's GI section. After residency, in addition to clinical surgery, he continued basic research, first as a fellow at

UCLA, then on the faculty at UCSF, and for ten years at Duke, where he was mentored by David Sabiston. From 1982 to 2002, he was chairman of surgery at the University of Virginia. Scott became one of surgery's most important leaders as president of the American Surgical Association and the American College of Surgeons. After his chairmanship, he worked full-time for the American College of Surgeons on its executive staff, promoting the quality improvement program and studying health-care policy.

1996

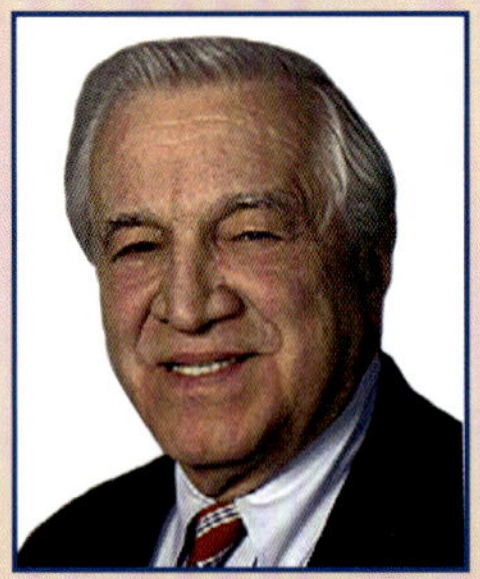

Stanley J. Dudrick

HUP Chief Resident (1966–1967)

Stan Dudrick was the inaugural chairman of surgery at the University of Texas, Houston. While a HUP resident, his landmark research with Jonathan Rhoads resulted in the success of intravenous hyperalimentation (see Chapter 34). Later, he was chief of surgery at Pennsylvania Hospital and then of Yale-affiliated St. Mary's Hospital, while also professor of surgery at Yale.

1997

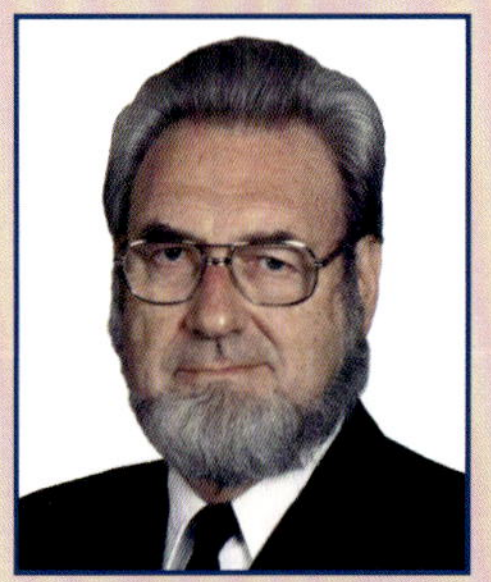

C. Everett Koop

HUP Chief Resident (1946–1947)

Although he had almost no training in children's surgery during his HUP residency, I. S. Ravdin appointed Chick Koop as the first chief of surgery at Children's Hospital of Philadelphia, a role in which he served for thirty-four years. With his colleagues, he developed many of the surgical treatments now standard in pediatric surgery. In 1986, he was appointed by President Reagan as US surgeon general. In this role, he was so successful and famous that he became known as America's doctor. See Chapter 31 for more complete biography.

1988

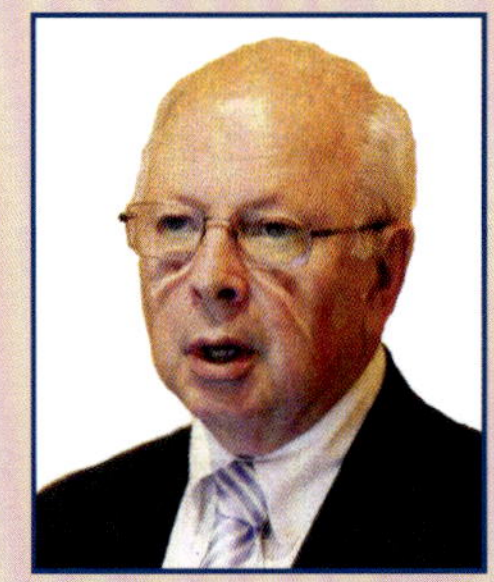

Moritz M. Ziegler

HUP Chief Resident (1973–1974)

Mory Ziegler, working with fellow resident Craig Reckland in my lab, was one of the pioneers of experimental islet transplantation. After training with Chick Koop in pediatric surgery, Mory was a faculty member at CHOP. At the same time, he served for several years as chief of HUP's kidney transplant program. Later, he became chairman of surgery of three of the nation's top programs in pediatric surgery at Cincinnati Children's Hospital, Boston Children's Hospital, and Children's Hospital of the University of Colorado. In 2017, he was awarded the Ladd prize, the highest honor in pediatric surgery. See Chapter 31.

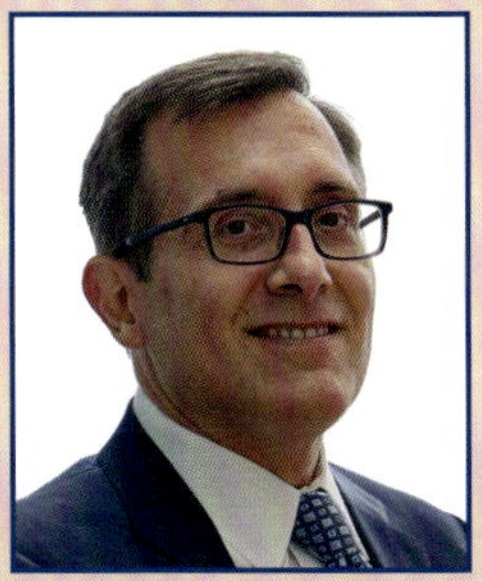

Ronald DeMatteo

2007

HUP Chief Resident (1996–1997)

In July 2017, Ronald DeMatteo become John Rhea Barton Professor and Chairman of the Department of Surgery of the University of Pennsylvania.

Ron is a graduate of Johns Hopkins University and of Cornell University Medical College. During his general surgery residency at HUP, he won the Jonathan E. Rhoads research award, the Leonard J. Perloff chief resident teaching award, and the British Journal of Surgery award for the outstanding surgical resident at HUP. While a resident, he spent four years in basic research studying molecular biology, virology, immunology, and transplantation, working with Jim Wilson, Steve Raper, Jim Markmann, and me. After completing a surgical oncology fellowship at Memorial Sloan Kettering Cancer Center and a research fellowship there under Murray Brennan, he was appointed in 1999 to the faculty at Memorial.

In 2006, he became head of the Division of General Surgical Oncology at Memorial and vice chair of the Department of Surgery. He also held appointments as professor of surgery at Weill Cornell Medical College. From 2012 to 2017, he represented Memorial Sloan Kettering as associate dean at Cornell.

Ron's large clinical practice at Memorial was focused on hepatic, biliary, and pancreatic diseases and also on abdominal sarcoma.

Ron is active in both basic and clinical research. His laboratory has been continuously funded by NIH since 2001. He currently leads R01 and T32 grants and is the faculty co-mentor of a K–12 grant. He has mentored more than thirty-five laboratory fellows, many of whom have since obtained NIH grants. He is a member of the Cancer Immunopathology and Immunotherapy Study Section of the NIH. Many of his 351 peer-reviewed publications have appeared in journals such as *Nature Medicine, Lancet, Lancet Oncology, Journal of Clinical Oncology, Journal of Clinical Investigation, Journal of Experimental Medicine,* and *Annals of Surgery.* He is a member of the editorial board of *Annals of Surgery*.

In clinical research, Ron has been the principal investigator of three national trials of adjuvant therapy with imatinib (Gleevec) following resection of gastrointestinal stromal tumors. One trial led to FDA approval and changed the standard of care worldwide.

Ron has devoted much effort to surgical education. From 2006 to 2013, he directed Memorial Sloan Kettering's Surgical Oncology Fellowship. He has mentored more than 100 clinical fellows in career development, research, and job acquisition. Many of his fellows have assumed leadership positions in academic institutions.

Ron is the recipient of many honors and awards. He was the inaugural recipient of the Leslie H. Blumgart Chair in Surgical Oncology. He has been elected to the American Society of Clinical Investigation, a rare honor for a surgeon. He is a member of the American Surgical Association, the Society of Clinical Surgery, The Surgical Biology Club I, the James IV Surgical Association, the International Surgical Group, and the National Academy of Medicine. See Chapter 38.

2009 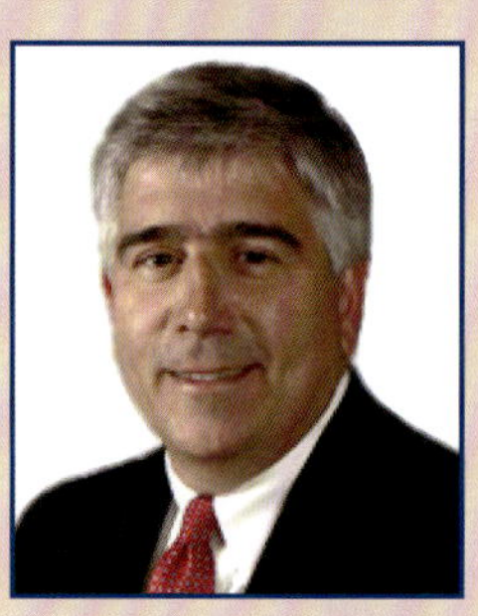

Stephen Bartlett

HUP Chief Resident (1984–1985)

Steve Bartlett graduated from the University of Chicago School of Medicine. During his HUP residency, he worked with Will Silvers in the Department of Genetics. Their important research finding was that pretransplant culture of pancreatic allografts could delete antigen-presenting cells and prevent their rejection. After fellowship in vascular surgery at Northwestern University, despite his transplantation experience being limited to mouse experiments, he was recruited to the University of California, Davis, as chief of transplantation. In 1991, he moved to the University of Maryland as chief of transplantation. Within five years, he had developed Maryland's kidney and pancreas transplant program into one of the largest and most successful in the world. He and his colleagues were leaders in the development of laparoscopic donor nephrectomy. Later, he and his associates performed the world's most complete face transplant. Their research finding that the inclusion of vascularized bone marrow as a part of face transplants decreased the requirement for immunosuppression was a fascinating clue in the search for tolerance that remains to be fully explored.

In 2003, Steve was appointed chairman of surgery at the University of Maryland. After serving in this role for fourteen years, in 2017 he became executive vice president and chief medical officer of the University of Maryland's fourteen-hospital system. In 2020, Steve resigned from the University of Maryland after twenty-eight years and turned his attention to vascular surgery. Steve is a member of all of the prestigious surgical societies including the American Surgical Association. He has been president of the International Pancreas Transplantation Association.

2010 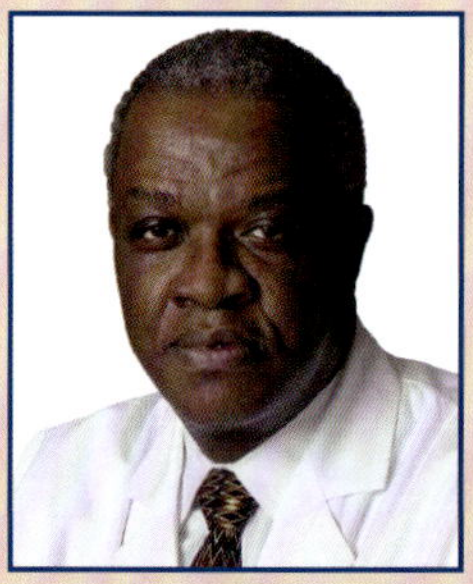

Danny O. Jacobs

HUP Chief Resident (1985–1986)

A native of a small town in rural Georgia, Danny attended part of his high school years at Phillips Exeter Academy. He graduated from Harvard College and obtained his MD from Washington University in St. Louis. After finishing his HUP residency, he returned to Harvard as a research fellow, remaining there for fourteen years, rising to associate professor of surgery and earning an MPH degree from the Harvard School of Public Health. He also served as the associate program director of the Brigham and Women's Hospital's clinical research center, chief of the hospital's metabolic support services and director of its laboratory for surgical metabolism and nutrition. He left Harvard in 2000 to join the faculty at Creighton University as chairman of the Department of Surgery. In 2003, he moved to Duke University as David Sabiston Professor and chairman of the Department of Surgery. In 2012, Danny went to Galveston as executive vice president, provost and dean of the school of medicine of the University of Texas Medical Branch. He also oversaw the institution's research programs and directed the school's successful completion of a $450 million capital campaign. In 2018, he moved from Galveston to Portland where he is now president of Oregon Health Services University.

In addition to his success as an administrative leader of top academic institutions, Danny has been an outstanding surgeon-scientist. His research has focused on the impact of critical illness and malnutrition on cellular bioenergetics, organ function, and metabolism. A prolific writer, he has published 300 peer-reviewed manuscripts. He has been a member of twelve editorial boards, including the *New England Journal of Medicine.* He is a member of many honorific academic societies including the Society of University Surgeons, the American Surgical Association, the American Physiological Society, the Society of Black Academic Surgeons, and the National Academy of Medicine.

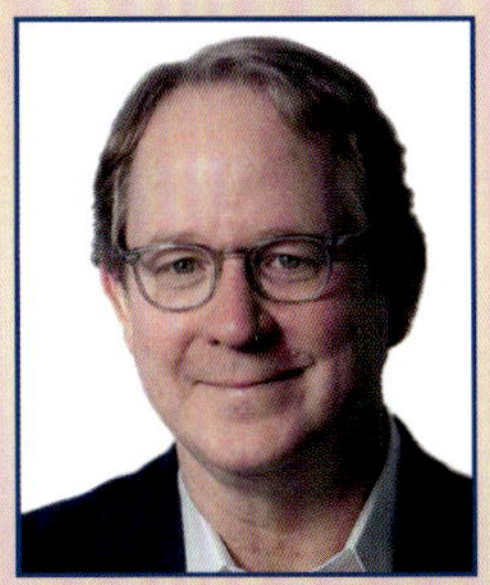

W. Roy Smythe 2011

(HUP Chief Resident 1995–1996)

Roy Smythe is a proud native of Texas. As a National Merit Scholar, he obtained his BS degree at Baylor University where he also starred on the school's Southwest Conference championship football team. He attended medical school at the Texas A&M College of Medicine where he was AOA and won the Raleigh White, Jr. Award as the top student in surgery. Roy also received the Salyer Medal as the school's Outstanding Graduating Student for Academic Achievement. While a medical student, he spent time at the NIH and a year at the University of Pennsylvania's Department of Surgery as a Charles A. Dana Foundation Scholar and at the Leonard Davis Institute of the Wharton School. During that year, he regularly attended HUP's transplant laboratory meetings and authored several research publications with Don Dafoe, Ken Brayman, and others.

From 1988 to 1998, Roy trained at HUP in general and then in cardiothoracic surgery and was also a postdoctoral investigator in the Harrison Department of Surgical Research and the Wistar Institute. His research in oncology and molecular biology with Larry Kaiser and Steve Albelda was the first to evaluate adenoviral vectors in transfer of genes for the treatment of cancer. Roy was the lead author on the important paper, describing this novel approach in laboratory models of cancer. This work became the basis for a clinical trial at HUP, which was one of the world's first human gene therapy trials for cancer and the world's first for mesothelioma.

In 1988, Roy joined the University of Texas MD Anderson Cancer Center where he was awarded the MD Anderson Institutional Physician Scientist Award. He also directed the University of Texas MD Anderson Cancer Center Mesothelioma Treatment and Research Program. In 2004, he left MD Anderson to become chairman of the Department of Surgery at the Texas A&M College of Medicine and the Scott & White Health System. There he was professor of surgery, molecular and cellular medicine. He was also a member of the

Physician Board of Directors for Scott & White, as well as the Health System Board of Trustees and the vice chair of the Scott & White Healthcare Foundation. The Scott & White Health System is the fifth largest group practice in the country with more than 1,000 providers, ten hospitals, and sixty-five regional clinics in Texas.

Roy's primary clinical interest was the treatment of mesothelioma and other complex thoracic cancers. His investigative efforts focused on the molecular pathogenesis and potential gene therapy of mesothelioma and other malignancies as well as on vascular permeability related to trauma and shock. A theme common to all his basic and translational research was dysregulated programmed cell death. His research was consistently supported through RO1 and other NIH grants. He also served on several NIH study sections and special emphasis panels. He is cofounder and vice president for medical affairs for Atumida, Inc., a biotechnology startup company developing novel biologic treatments for vascular permeability. He has been a prolific writer on diverse topics, having published more than 250 manuscripts, editorials, and essays related to his clinical and research activity, as well as other essays on surgical history, education, medical human interest, and the modern provision of healthcare.

Roy was the editor-in-chief of *Cell Death, Metabolism and Survival* and served on the editorial boards of *Gene Therapy and Molecular Biology,* the *Internet Journal of Cardiothoracic Surgery* and *Case Reports in Medicine.* Roy served as a governor of the American College of Surgeons and was a member of many professional societies, including the Society of Thoracic Surgery, the American Society of Gene Therapy, the Society of University Surgeons, the Society for Clinical Surgery, the Southern Surgical Association, the Surgical Biology Club II, and the American Surgical Association.

Having acquired all the important markers of success for a leader in academic surgery, he shifted his attention to a role as a health-care business entrepreneur. Following a period as global chief medical officer for strategy and partnerships at Royal Philips, in 2018 he became CEO of Somalogic, a global leader in health information.

2012

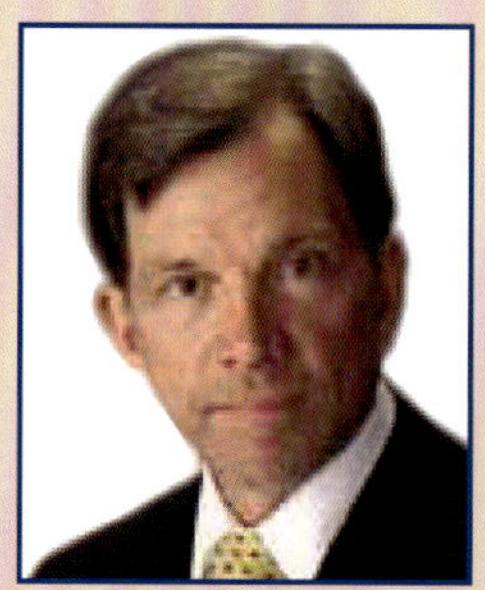

James D. Luketich
(HUP Chief Resident 1992–1993)

Jim Luketich received his bachelor's degree from Old Dominion University, his master's degree in biochemistry from Vanderbilt University, and, in 1986, his MD (AOA) from the Medical College of Pennsylvania. As a HUP resident and postdoctoral researcher in the Harrison Department of Surgical Research, he studied nutrition and metabolism with Jim Mullen. He was the 1993 Leonard Perloff Chief Resident Teaching Awardee.

After completing fellowships in thoracic and cardiothoracic surgery at the Cleveland Clinic, New York Hospital/Cornell University, and Memorial Sloan-Kettering Cancer Center, Jim joined the surgical faculty of the University of Pittsburgh. His leadership there resulted in the Division of Cardiothoracic Surgery growing to be one of the largest groups of academic cardiothoracic surgeons in North America. He now holds the prestigious Henry T. Bahnson Chair in Cardiothoracic Surgery. Jim is chief of thoracic and foregut surgery, director of thoracic surgical oncology, codirector of the Lung Cancer Center, and director of the Mark Ravitch/Leon C. Hirsh Center for Minimally Invasive Surgery. In 2010, Jim became the inaugural chairman of the Department of Cardiothoracic Surgery.

Jim has been consistently funded through NIH RO1 grants for his studies of the molecular staging of lung and esophageal cancer. He has become world renowned for minimally invasive surgery for esophageal cancer, a procedure he has performed on more than 1,500 patients. He has also organized and completed a multicenter trial to prospectively study clinical outcomes of minimally invasive esophagectomy with sixteen participating centers. Using minimally invasive techniques, he also performs other complex operations for gastroesophageal reflux, lung cancer, giant paraesophageal hernias, and achalasia.

Jim serves on the editorial boards of the *Annals of Surgery,* the *Journal of Thoracic and Cardiovascular Surgery,* and the *Journal of Gastrointestinal Surgery.* He is an associate editor for *Diseases of the Esophagus.* He has published 250 peer reviewed papers and 150 invited reviews, chapters, and editorials.

Jim directs the Cardiothoracic Surgical Residency Program at the University of Pittsburgh. He has trained more than fifty fellows in thoracic surgery and minimally invasive surgical techniques. He has also developed and directed over 100 national and international courses on esophageal disorders, minimally invasive esophagectomy, radio frequency ablation, and video-assisted thorascopic lobectomy.

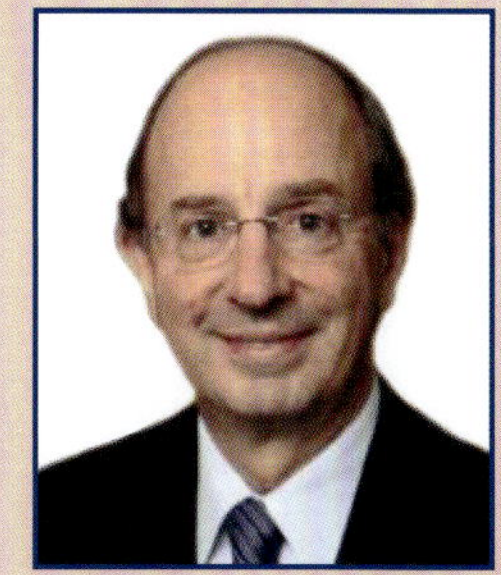

Michael A. Choti 2013

(HUP Chief Resident 1989–1990)

Mike is a graduate of Yale Medical School. During his HUP residency, he spent two years in my and Ali Naji's transplantation laboratory. From 1990 to 1992, he was a clinical fellow in surgical oncology at Memorial Sloan Kettering. In 1992, he was appointed assistant professor of Surgery at Johns Hopkins. In 2004, Mike obtained an MBA degree at Johns Hopkins University. He eventually held full professorships there in surgery, oncology, radiology, and computer science. He was director of the Colon Cancer Center, chief of the Division of Surgical Oncology, and Handlesman Professor of Surgery. In 1998, he was appointed vice chair of the Department of Surgery.

In 1998, he became program director of a very successful surgical oncology fellowship. His former fellows are now faculty members at more than a dozen university centers. In his laboratory, he has also mentored thirty-eight research fellows. He has served as visiting professor and invited speaker at 138 universities, medical centers, and national or international symposia.

Mike holds many leadership positions in national and international societies. He was a member of the Surgical Oncology Board of the American Board of

Surgery. He has chaired several study sections for the American Cancer Society. He served as the chair of the NCI-CTEP Hepatobiliary Task Force and was the director of the National Comprehensive Cancer Network Neuroendocrine Tumor database. He served on the American College of Surgeons' Commission on Cancer, the Gastrointestinal Committees of the National Surgical Adjuvant Breast and Bowel Project (NSABP), and the American College of Surgeons Oncology Group (ACOSOG). He has been on the editorial boards of the *Journal of Gastrointestinal Surgery,* the *Annals of Surgical Oncology,* the *Journal of Surgical Oncology* and the *American Journal of Surgery.* He is associate editor of the *Journal of Gastrointestinal Cancer* and section editor of the *Annals of Surgical Oncology.*

Mike's clinical practice specializes in the surgical treatment of hepatopancreatobiliary and gastrointestinal malignancies. In addition to his clinical role, he has pursued research in hepatobiliary, pancreatic, colorectal, and other gastrointestinal cancers. Specific aspects of his research are robotic and image-guided research in cancer therapy, molecular genetics, and biomarkers in colorectal and gastrointestinal cancer.

Mike is also active in conducting clinical trials in gastrointestinal cancer therapy. He has led a national cooperative randomized trial in cancer therapy and serves as the lead investigator in an international randomized trial for treatment of advanced colorectal cancer. He has authored more than 260 peer-reviewed research publications and over 100 review articles and book chapters.

Mike is a member of numerous professional societies, including the American Surgical Association, the Southern Surgical Association, the Society of University Surgeons, the Society of Surgical Oncology, the Halsted Society, and the Surgical Biology Club II.

Several months after he was our 2013 distinguished graduate, he left Johns Hopkins to accept an appointment as chairman of surgery at Southwestern Medical School. In 2018, Mike became division chief of surgery at Banner MD Anderson Cancer Center in Gilbert, Arizona.

2014

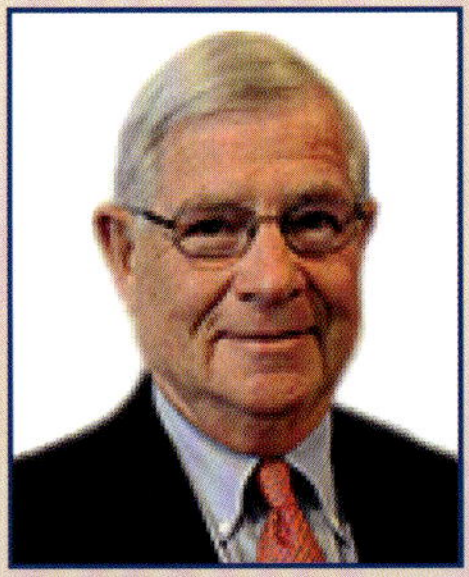

Howard A. Reber

HUP Chief Resident (1969–1970)

Howard Reber, a native Philadelphian, is a graduate of Temple University and the University of Pennsylvania School of Medicine. During residency, he began his research on the pancreas under the direction of Jonathan Rhoads and Frank Brooks (chief of the GI section in the Department of Medicine). After two years in the US Air Force, he joined the surgical faculty at the University of California, San Francisco, in 1972. There he was mentored by Larry Way in further study of the pancreas. In 1978, he moved to the University of Missouri, as chief of surgery at the Truman Veterans Administration Medical Center.

In 1986, he moved to UCLA as chief of surgery at the Sepulveda Veterans Administration Medical Center and became the chief of gastrointestinal surgery at UCLA in 1997. His other administrative activities there have included serving as Department vice chairman, chief of the Division of General Surgery, Director of Education, and codirector of the Surgical Residency Training Program. In recent years, he has devoted a significant portion of his administrative time to faculty mentoring, appointments, and promotions; he recently completed a term as the chair of the Council on Academic Personnel for the entire UCLA campus. His current position is distinguished professor of surgery, chief of gastrointestinal surgery, and director of the Center for Pancreatic Diseases at UCLA. He authored a book with John Howard on the pancreas which, through many editions, became standard in the field.

Howard has had important international leadership roles in surgery. He is a member of all major learned surgical societies, including the American Surgical Association, Society of Clinical Surgery, Society of University Surgeons, American Gastroenterological Association, Society of Surgical Oncology, and the Halsted Society. He has served as the president and for twenty years, secretary-treasurer of the American Pancreatic Association. He was elected as vice president of the Society for Surgery of the Alimentary Tract and was a member of its Board of Trustees.

Howard has established a world-renowned surgical practice focused on pancreatic diseases. Clearly recognized as one of the top five pancreatic surgeons in the world, he has been a named lecturer at many prestigious institutions throughout North America, Asia, and Europe. He was awarded the Vay W. Liang and Frisca Go Award for Lifetime Achievement in Pancreatology, was the Awardee of the Pancreas Club in 2012, and has won multiple teaching awards at UCLA.

Howard has conducted pioneering research in the study of benign and malignant pancreatic diseases. As a young investigator, he performed basic physiologic studies regarding the role of the pancreatic ductal epithelium in pancreatic electrolyte secretion. He then became interested in acute pancreatitis and developed a concept that became known as the pancreatic duct mucosal barrier. This work established that a variety of substances could increase ductal permeability and cause acute pancreatitis. He next took up the study of chronic pancreatitis, developing the hypothesis that the gland became severely ischemic in this disease and that this ischemia was responsible for the characteristic severe pain. Over the past decade, he has focused his work on pancreatic cancer. He has developed and directs a multifaceted translational research program at UCLA. His research has been continuously supported for over forty years by grants from NIH, the VA Administration, and the NCI. He is the author of more than 350 scientific manuscripts, over 100 book chapters, and is the editor of eight books. He serves on the editorial board of six medical journals.

Howard has been a mentor for a long list of trainees. His laboratory has hosted young surgical scientists from around the world. More than forty investigators have worked under his direction. Moreover, he has trained dozens of surgical residents in gastrointestinal and pancreatic surgical techniques. Residents uniformly agree that the rotation with Dr. Reber in the chief year is the most enjoyable of the residency and identify the time with him in the operating room as the pinnacle of their surgical training.

2015

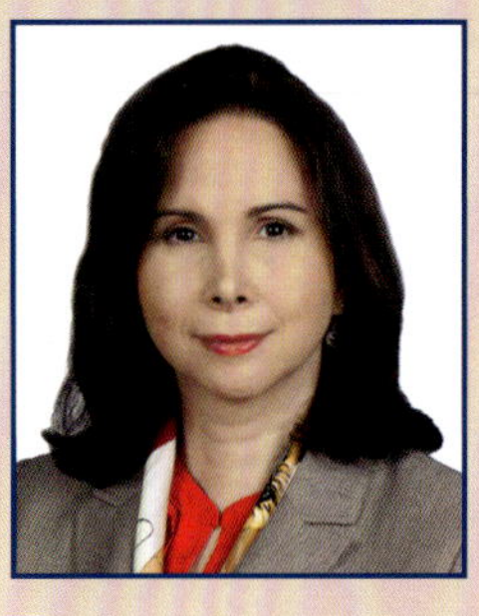

Omaida C. Velazquez

HUP Chief Resident (1997–1998)

Omaida Velazquez was born in Cuba. At the age of ten, she fled to the United States with her family. She spoke no English but learned quickly enough to be valedictorian of her high school class. In college, at the Stevens Institute of Technology, she received the award as the top student in chemistry. At UMDNJ Medical School, she was a Junior AOA, valedictorian, and won fifteen awards. During residency at HUP, she ranked at the top. For her studies of gene transfer to cells of the GI tract while in John Rombeau's laboratory, she won the department's 1997 Jonathan E. Rhoads Research Award and the Harry Vars Award of the American Society of Parenteral and Enteral Nutrition.

Following residency and vascular fellowship at HUP, she served for eight years as a faculty member in Penn's Vascular Division. During that time, she turned her research attention to endothelial cell biology, angiogenesis, vasculogenesis, wound healing, and atherosclerosis. Initially, she was mentored by Meenhard Heryln at the Wistar Institute and then established her own independent lab. For her work in this field, she received the Von Liebig Foundation Award for Excellence in Vascular Surgical Research (2001), and the University of Pennsylvania Center of Excellence Faculty Scholar Award (2002).

In 2007, Omaida moved to the University of Miami as chief of the Division of Vascular Surgery. She established an accredited vascular surgery fellowship and a preclinical vascular research team of fifteen members. She directs a highly successful basic research program supported by NIH R01 grants. Her sponsored clinical trials focus on novel treatments for lower extremity arterial occlusive disease, diabetes-related wound healing defects, and atherosclerosis-related occlusive and aneurysm diseases.

As a physician-scientist, Omaida's research findings include (1) the survival and differentiation of human microvascular endothelial cells into capillaries depend on their direct cell–cell contact with dermal fibroblasts; and (2) the signals mediating this fibroblastendothelial cross talk are dependent on a synergistic cell-matrix-cell interaction which is made possible by Vascular Endothelial Growth Hormone and the Integrin V 3, and further amplified via N-Ras and PI3-K intracellular signaling cascades.

In addition, Omaida has shown that growing capillaries *in vitro* using fibroblasts embedded in type I collagen has potential value as a vascularized substrate for covering wounds. She also began to study another key cell that participates in postnatal angiogenesis, the bone marrow-derived endothelial progenitor cell (EPC). She found that the recruitment of EPCs to hypoxic, ischemic cutaneous wounds is severely impaired, this being correlated with delayed wound healing. Recognition of the clinical importance of this work led to her being awarded the Joel J. Roslyn Research Award from the Association of Academic Surgeons.

More recently, Omaida reported that endothelial progenitor cells from the adult bone marrow can be released into the circulation by a nonphysiologic hyperoxia-stimulus that triggers an increase in bone marrow nitric oxide (NO). She showed that the diabetic impairments in NO-mediated mobilization and homing of EPCs to cutaneous wounds can be reversed by hyperoxia and Stromal Derived Growth Factor 1alpha. These findings are of potential importance in treatment of peripheral vascular disease and the chronic wounds of diabetics.

By all the traditional indices, Omaida is one of the most accomplished academic surgeons of her generation. She has been a member of an NIH study section. She has published more than 100 peer-reviewed articles. She is a member of the editorial board of the *Journal of Vascular Surgery.* She has been cited in Who's Who in the World.

Among the twenty-five distinguished professional societies Omaida lists are the Society of University Surgeons, the Society for Vascular Surgery, and the American Surgical Association. She has also been elected as a member of the American Society for Clinical Investigation ("The Young Turks"). Very few surgeons have ever become members of this prestigious society. In 2022, she was elected to the National Academy of Medicine.

At Miami, Omaida has served as executive dean of research, research education and innovative medicine. In 2015, she was appointed chair of the University of Miami Department of Surgery.

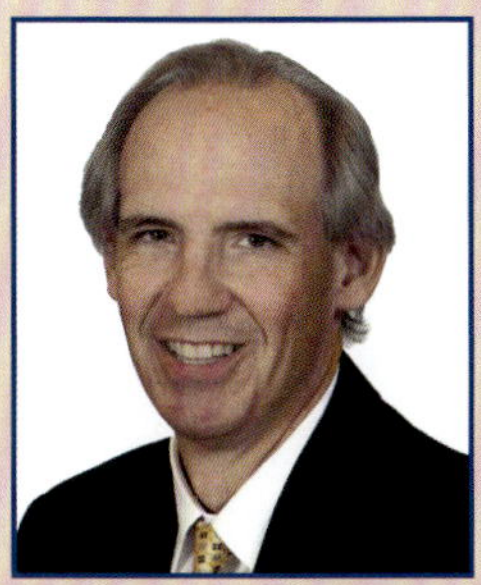

James F. Markmann 2016

HUP Chief Resident (1995–1996)

Jim Markmann is in some ways the most academically accomplished of the distinguished graduates. Other than Chick Koop who was at CHOP, Jim is the one who spent the most time at Penn. His twenty-six years in our department began when he was a high school student working as a laboratory assistant for Ali Naji (who later became his brother-in-law). This continued while he was in college at La Salle, resulting in his first three publications. By the time he finished medical school at Penn, his bibliography included thirty entries in journals, such as *Nature, Diabetes, Surgery,* and the *Journal of Immunology.*

Jim's early and most persistent research interest has been in transplantation of isolated pancreatic islets, not only as a treatment for diabetes, but also as a model to define the etiology of diabetes, the pathogenesis of autoimmune diseases, and an approach to transplantation tolerance. With Ali Naji, he elucidated the autoimmune pathogenesis of type 1 diabetes in an animal model of the disease. With Naji, Andy Posselt, Mike Choti, Niraj Desai, Jon Odorico, and Ron DeMatteo, he explored manipulation of the thymus as a promising method of developing transplantation tolerance.

After completing his MD and PhD in immunology at Penn, Jim declined the offer to remain on the faculty here and sought further training in clinical transplantation at UCLA, with a focus on liver transplantation. We were then fortunate to recruit him back to Penn where he spent the next nine productive years, during which he extended his bibliography to 140 publications, directed an independent laboratory funded by multiple NIH R01 grants, and with Ali Naji, started HUP's highly successful human islet transplantation program.

In 2007, he was recruited to Harvard and the Massachusetts General Hospital as chief of transplantation. As might have been predicted from his earlier record, he has been highly successful there. In the competitive setting of multiple New England clinical transplantation centers, he has greatly increased (almost doubled) MGH's clinical activity, especially in liver transplantation. Jim's efforts at the MGH have been well balanced between clinical work, basic and translational research, administration, and teaching. His research laboratory consists of eight to ten individuals, including students, technicians, visiting scholars, graduate students, residents, and fellows. This provides opportunity for what he finds to be the most rewarding setting for teaching. He has been the scientific mentor for thirty-six trainees, including six PhD students.

Jim's research has three main thrusts: developing tolerogenic strategies that permit graft acceptance without immunosuppression, isolated pancreatic islet transplantation, and *ex vivo* liver perfusion. The basic transplantation biology research has been supported by NIH R01 grants. Liver perfusion studies are supported by smaller grants and a large program project grant.

A top priority at the MGH has been developing a pancreatic islet transplantation program in human diabetics. In 2010, Jim performed his first human islet transplant at MGH and soon after performed seven allo islet transplants and more than thirty auto islet transplants.

Jim Markmann is one of the most productive and most respected surgeon scientists of his generation. As the Claude E. Welsh Professor, he occupies the endowed chair named for one of Harvard's and MGH's most beloved surgical heroes. Jim has been elected to Surgery's most prestigious societies: the Society of University Surgeons, the Halsted Society, the Society of Clinical Surgery, the Surgical Biology Club, and the American Surgical Association. In the fields of diabetes research, pancreatic and islet transplantation, and surgical immunology, he has had leadership positions in most of the important national committees and workgroups, such as NIH study sections, and various national and international societies. He serves on the editorial boards of *Transplantation, Surgery*, and the *American Journal of Transplantation.* His laboratory is funded by eight NIH grants, including two R01s, and has enjoyed NIH funding for more than fifteen consecutive years. His work is documented in nearly 250 peer-reviewed papers, most of them in high-impact journals such as *Science, Nature Medicine, JAMA, Diabetes,* and the *Annals of Surgery.* He has become an important spokesman for islet transplant research and clinical trials, as illustrated by his recent editorial in the *American Journal of Transplantation* which summarizes the field's current status.

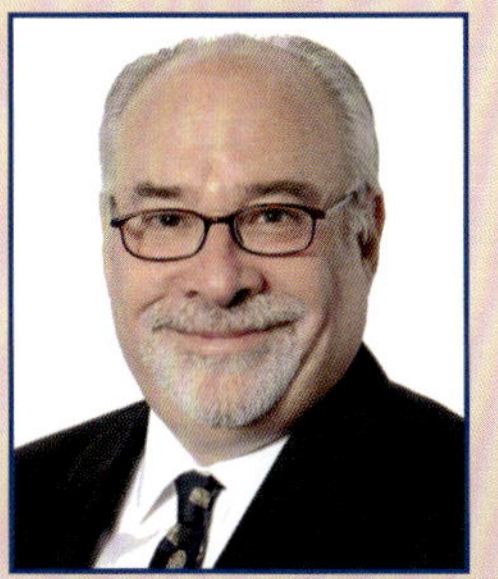

Kenneth L. Brayman

2017

HUP Chief Resident (1988–1989)

Ken Brayman is professor of surgery, medicine, and biomedical engineering at the University of Virginia School of Medicine where he is also the Nabi Professor of Transplantation.

Ken grew up in Massachusetts and attended college at the University of Massachusetts, obtaining his undergraduate degree summa cum laude in 1977, majoring in Biochemistry. Ken attended the University of Pennsylvania School of Medicine, where he was elected AOA and received his medical degree in 1981. Following medical school, Ken completed his internship and residency in general surgery at HUP. During that period, he spent three years in my and Ali Naji's research laboratory studying autoimmunity and beta cell replacement strategies for type 1 diabetes. He received the Jonathan E. Rhoads Research Award in 1987. Ken also took postdoctoral training in the Pathology Graduate Group at Penn and received his PhD in 1989.

Following general surgery training, Ken spent three years at the University of Minnesota as a transplant surgery fellow. He returned to the University of Pennsylvania in 1992 as an assistant and subsequently associate professor of surgery, medicine, and pediatrics. He was a member of the Transplantation Division, working closely with me and Dr. Naji and subsequently with Drs. Shaked and Olthoff. During that period, he directed the pancreas transplant program at HUP and the renal transplant program at CHOP.

In 2002, Ken was recruited to the University of Virginia as director of the renal, pancreas, and islet transplant programs. In 2009, he became division chief of transplantation and director of the Charles O. Strickler Transplant Center of the University of Virginia Health System.

Ken served as president of the University of Pennsylvania Medical Alumni Association from 2002 to 2004 and in 2011, was recognized by the University of Massachusetts with a distinguished alumni award for his contributions to diabetes research and transplantation surgery. Ken's current research interests include islet transplantation, bioengineering and 3D bioprinting, transplant immunosuppression and tolerance induction, xenotransplantation, regenerative medicine, and stem cell/gene therapy. He is responsible for developing and establishing the Islet Isolation GMP Facility at UVA and has overseen the allo- and autotransplantation of islets in more than forty recipients.

His bibliography includes 213 peer-reviewed papers and forty-six book chapters and reviews. He has been a visiting professor or invited distinguished lecturer at 259 universities, hospitals, and societies and has mentored thirty-four doctoral and postdoctoral students.

Ken is a member of many distinguished professional societies including the American Diabetes Association, the American Society of Gene Therapy, the American Society of Transplant Surgeons, the American Surgical Association, the Association for Academic Surgery, the International Pancreas and Islet

Transplant Association, the Societé Internationale De Chirurgie, the Society of University Surgeons, the Southern Surgical Association, and the Cell Transplant Society.

2018

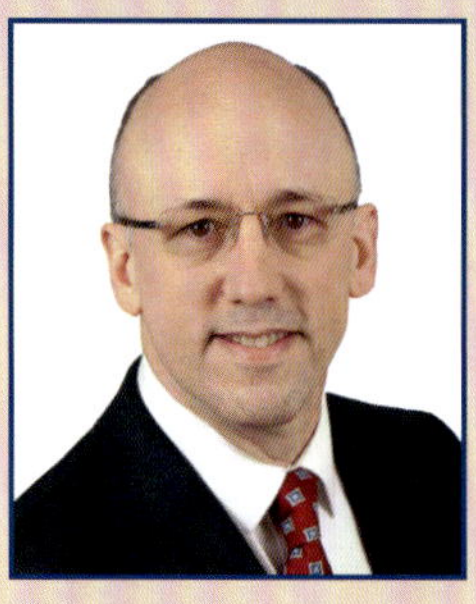

Steven J. Fishman

HUP Chief Resident (1991–1992)

Steven Fishman is professor of surgery at Harvard Medical School and the Stuart and Jane Weitzman Family Chair in Surgery at Boston Children's Hospital.

Born and raised in the Chicago area, Steve obtained his combined BS and MD degrees through the Honors Program in Medical Education at Northwestern University. After completing his HUP residency and in 1994 his fellowship in pediatric surgery at Boston Children's Hospital, he has remained on faculty at Boston Children's for his entire career. He is active in the practice and teaching of the broad spectrum of pediatric surgery with a particular clinical and research focus in the area of vascular anomalies. In 1999, he became codirector of the Vascular Anomalies Center at Boston Children's Hospital. Annually, this center's multidisciplinary group evaluates about 1,700 patients with hemangiomas, rare vascular tumors, and vascular malformations of all types. Steve is past president of the International Society for the Study of Vascular Anomalies. He also created and hosts an international registry of hepatic hemangiomas.

Over his career, Steve has authored over 200 scientific publications and chapters as well as two books, including a comprehensive reference work on vascular anomalies. He has a particular focus on developing an understanding and approach to visceral vascular anomalies. Though these anomalies are extremely rare, Steve's international referral practice has facilitated the recognition of patterns in their clinical presentation and opportunities for treatment. He has focused on developing evaluation and intervention techniques, including innovative operative procedures for the treatment of visceral vascular anomalies. Steve also has extensive experience with resecting, debulking, and reconstructing vascular malformations and associated overgrown tissues of the torso, genitalia, neck, and extremities. He has also studied the role of dynamic contrast lymphangiography of the thoracic duct which has led to the use of novel treatments and reconstruction of thoracic duct anomalies. Recognizing the limitations of surgical techniques, he is focusing on understanding the biologic mechanisms involved in the development and progression of these lesions.

In recent years, Steve has assumed a host of administrative leadership roles at Boston Children's. In 2015, he became the president of the Physicians' Organization and senior vice president for access and business services. He also serves on the hospital's Board of Trustees and the executive committee among many other strategic and operational responsibilities.

In 2019, Steve became chief of surgery at Boston Children's Hospital. See Chapter 31 for additional history of Steve and two other Penn surgeons at Boston Children's Hospital.

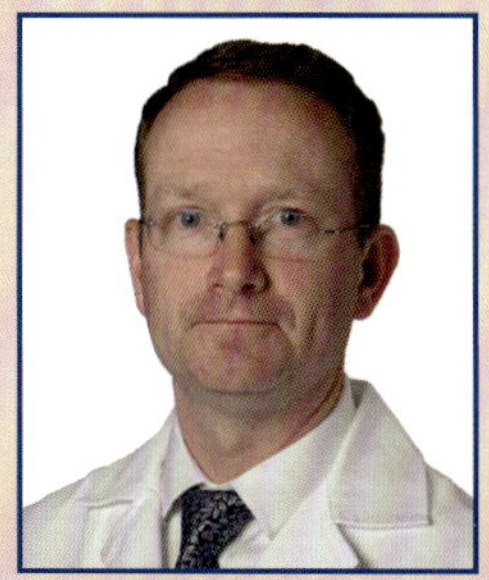

Mark Faries

2019

HUP Chief Resident (2001–2002)

Mark Faries obtained his BA degree from Haverford College where he wrote his thesis on medical history. After graduating from Cornell University Medical College as the top surgical student in the class of 1995, he returned to Philadelphia for internship and residency at HUP. He was honored with the 2002 Leonard Perloff Chief Resident's Award, which is chosen by the HUP residents as the "chief resident contributing most to their education." As a research fellow in Brian Czerniecki's laboratory, he studied dendritic cell function and cancer vaccines.

After residency, he was, for two years, a fellow in surgical oncology at the John Wayne Cancer Institute in Santa Monica, California. Since then, he has remained on the faculty at the John Wayne Cancer Center where his research has focused on melanoma and other malignancies. He has directed multiple clinical trials and pioneered work with sentinel node biopsy and minimally invasive inguinal lymph node dissection.

At John Wayne Cancer Center, Mark is professor of surgery, head of the Division of Surgical Oncology, and codirector of the Melanoma Program of the Angeles Clinic and Research Institute. He is also surgical director of Experimental Therapeutics and a member of the Samuel Orchin Cancer Center of Cedars Sinai Medical Center. He has also been director of the Donald Morton Melanoma Research Program and director of the Surgery Oncology Fellowship.

His research has been funded by multiple industrial sources and the NIH. He is at present the PI on an R01 grant for a selective lymphadenectomy trial. He has served as a guest lecturer or visiting professor at ninety-four institutions and authored 150 peer-reviewed publications and book chapters. He has served on the AJCC melanoma staging committee and the editorial board of the *Annals of Surgical Oncology,* the NASCO/SS0 Guidelines Committee for both surgical treatment and systemic therapy for melanoma, and the European Society for Medical Oncology Melanoma Consensus Committee. He has also served on multiple NIH study sections and committees.

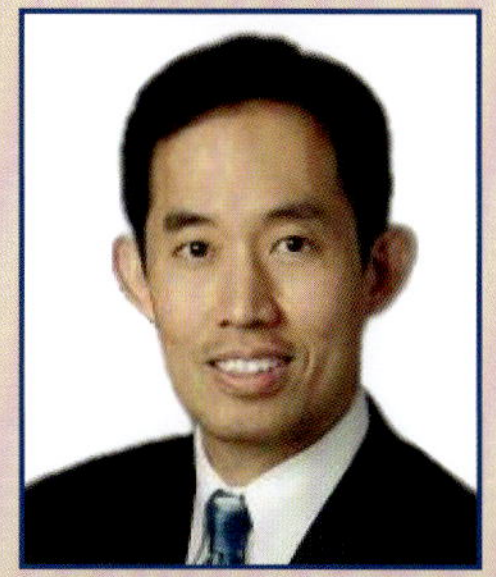

Joseph Woo

2021

HUP Chief Resident (1998–1999)

Joseph Woo is a 1988 graduate of MIT. He then attended the University of Pennsylvania School of Medicine, graduating in 1992 as a member of AOA and recipient of the I. S. Ravdin prize as the top student in surgery.

As a HUP surgery resident, he was outstanding. Among his accolades were the William Y. Inouye teaching award, which is voted by the medical students, and the Leonard J. Perloff chief resident teacher, chosen by his fellow residents. Additional honors as a surgical resident included the surgical scholar award for scoring 99 percent on the American Board of Surgery inservice exam, first place of the Pennsylvania Association of Thoracic Surgery Residents, and the American Heart Association's Vivien Thomas Young Investigator award.

Following residency, Joe remained at Penn for a cardiothoracic fellowship under Hank Edmunds, and then as a HUP faculty member. While an assistant professor of surgery, he was named by the Philadelphia Business Journal as an under-forty award winner, and by Philadelphia Magazine as one of twenty-one up and coming leaders of Philadelphia. He also won an American Society for Clinical Investigation travel scholarship. In 2012, he was the Luigi Mastroianni Clinical Innovator awardee.

After joining the Penn faculty in 2002, Joe quickly became a nationally respected clinician researcher and educator. He directed the department's minimally invasive and robotic cardiac surgery program and the cardiac transplantation and mechanical circulatory support program. He developed several new approaches to minimally invasive techniques for mitral and aortic valve repair and reconstruction. He also performed over 350 operations a year. He frequently had American and foreign cardiac surgeons visiting Penn to learn his techniques. He was also invited to perform operations in China, India, and Japan. His laboratory was funded by NIH and investigated new paths to myocardial repair through angiogenesis. He was the principal investigator for several clinical device trials and translational scientific clinical trials. He is a member of the editorial board of the *Journal of Thoracic and Cardiovascular Surgery.* Joe became a full professor at the University of Pennsylvania in 2013.

An exceptionally accomplished academic surgeon, Joe has more than 300 peer-reviewed publications. He is a member of the Society of Thoracic Surgeons, Society of University Surgeons, Society of Clinical Surgery, and the American Surgical Association. He has been the PhD thesis advisor for four candidates, has participated in more than ten NIH study sections, is principal investigator on several NIH grants and has mentored over fifty research laboratory trainees. In 2014, Joe was recruited to Stanford as the Norman Shumway Professor and chair of the Department of Cardiothoracic Surgery. At Stanford, he has had a spectacular career that is credited with increasing both clinical and research productivity and the reputation of the institution.

2022

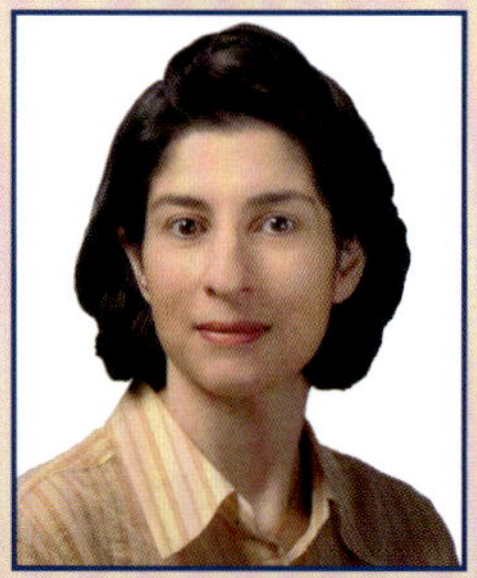

Isabelle Bedrosian
HUP Chief Resident (2000–2001)

Isabelle Bedrosian is a Phi Beta Kappa and summa cum laude graduate of Tufts University and received her MD AOA from Northwestern University Medical School in Chicago. After her chief residency at HUP in 2001, she completed a surgical oncology fellowship at the University of Texas, MD Anderson Cancer Center in Houston, Texas. She joined the faculty there in 2004 and is currently professor of breast surgical oncology. Isabelle's research program focuses on prevention of breast cancer. Her laboratory uses genomic approaches to characterize molecular pathways in early tumorigenesis that may serve as novel targets for prevention of breast cancer and approaches to finding biomarkers predictive of breast cancer risk. Her research has been supported by grants from the NCI, the Susan G. Komen for the Cure, the Avon Foundation, the Society of Surgical Oncology, and the American Society of Oncology. Isabelle has published more than 174 peer-reviewed papers in journals including *Oncogene, Clinical Cancer Research, Journal of the National Cancer Institute*, and *Proceedings of the National Academy of Sciences*. In addition, she has authored multiple invited reviews and book chapters. Isabelle is a member of many national societies and committees, including the Society of University Surgeons and the American Academy of Surgeons. She has also been cochair of the prevention committee for the Alliance Cooperative Group, a member of the NCI's Cancer Prevention Steering Committee, and cochair of ASCO's Expert Panel on Germline Mutation Testing in Breast Cancer.

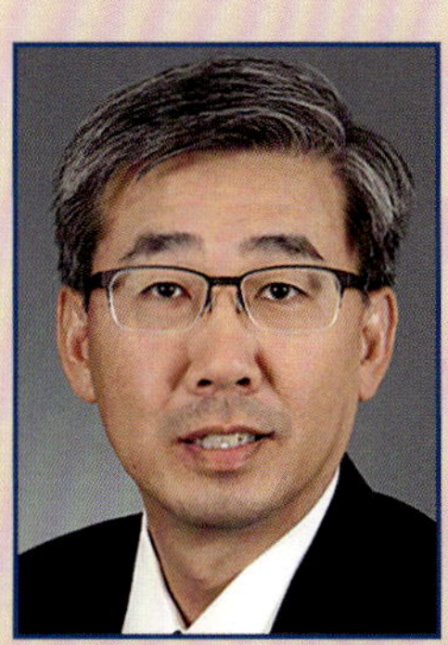

Heung Bae Kim **2024**

HUP Chief Resident (1999–2000)

Heung Bae Kim graduated from Yale in 1989 and Albert Einstein Medical School in 1993. His general surgery residency was at HUP (1993–2000) where he was a star, winning the Penn Pearls Teaching Award from medical students and the 2000 Keith Reemtsma Award as the HUP resident of the year. During two years of research with Alan Flake at CHOP, he studied in mice microchimerism and transplant tolerance induced by in utero bone marrow transplantation.

After his HUP chief residency, he took his fellowship in pediatric surgery at Boston Children's Hospital. He then spent two years as a fellow in liver transplantation at the Lahey Clinic while also working as a research fellow in transplantation biology at Massachusetts General Hospital. There he worked with David Sachs in developing a large animal model of *in utero* bone marrow transplantation that successfully induced tolerance to kidney allografts.

In 2005, Heung Bae returned to Boston Children's Hospital as a faculty member. There he has had a very successful career. He originated the serial transverse enteroplasty (STEP) procedure for patients with short bowel syndrome. In this operation, the bowel is stapled into V-shapes on alternating sides decreasing its width and increasing its length. Heung Bae's procedure has been widely adopted. It is now in use worldwide as the predominant intestine-lengthening operation for patients where standard surgery to correct short bowel syndrome is not feasible. More recently, he has developed an aortic-lengthening procedure for use in children with midaortic syndrome.

In addition to performing many STEP procedures himself, Heung Bae has developed an international registry to determine the long-term outcome of the procedure. Over 100 patients have been registered from thirty-seven different centers, including nineteen states and nine foreign countries. Data from the registry has shown that approximately 50 percent of patients undergoing STEP are able to be weaned from intravenous nutrition and avoid the need for intestinal transplantation.

Within three years of completing his transplant fellowship, Heung Bae was appointed surgical director of the Boston Children's Hospital's liver and kidney transplant programs. He also started the first successful intestine transplant program in New England. In 2004, he performed the first successful multivisceral transplant in New England.

In 2006, he formed a Pediatric Transplant Center at Boston Children's. Since 2008, he has been director of the Center with responsibility for the overall administration and management of all transplant related issues.

Heung Bae is also prominently involved on a national level as a member of several committees that are responsible for the maintenance of the national organ allocation system managed by the United Network for Organ Sharing (UNOS). He is now professor of surgery at Harvard and, at Boston Children's Hospital, is the director of transplantation and vice chair of surgery.

CHAPTER 36

Named Lectures of the Department

At HUP, the named lectureship is a fairly recent creature. Until the middle of the nineteenth century, American medical school curricula were limited to dissection of cadavers and large lectures usually given by the school's professor to an audience of the entire student body. Bedside teaching of small groups of students did not begin in this country until it was started at HUP by William Pepper in 1877. In the 1940s and 1950s, Dr. Ravdin expanded the curriculum by inviting many of the country's prominent surgeons to HUP as visiting professors, but the lectures they gave were not named. Not until 1960 did Dr. Rhoads, then a new department chairman, begin naming the lectures. Not surprisingly, he named the first one for the school's iconic figure, D. Hayes Agnew.

Additional named lectures were not necessarily established by careful consideration of a potential honoree's academic rank or accomplishments, but instead often spontaneously to memorialize a beloved colleague, suddenly lost through retirement or death. Indeed, only one of HUP's lectureships is named for a department chair, Dr. Agnew. Nevertheless, I believe that the priorities, values, and culture of the department are easily recognized by reviewing the names of the lectureships and the invited speakers. The list of Agnew lecturers is remarkable. It traces the very history of the field of surgery and its accomplishments over the last six decades.

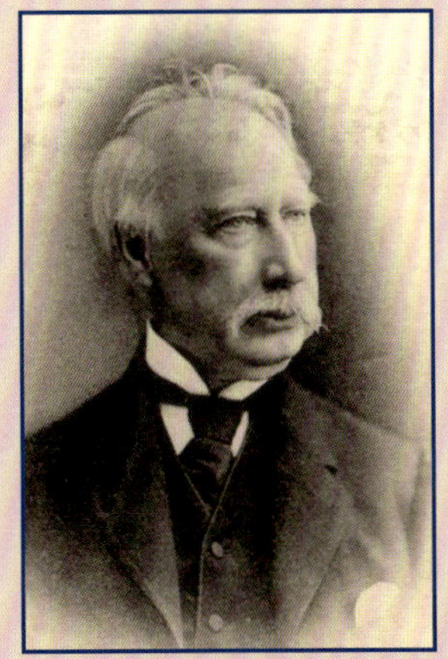

D. Hayes Agnew

D. Hayes Agnew Lecture

1960 William A. Altemeier
1962 Francis D. Moore
1963 John H. Gibbon Jr.
1964 Charles G. Child III
1965 Owen H. Wangensteen
1966 Charles G. Rob
1967 Denton A. Cooley
1968 J. Englebert Dunphy
1969 Norman E. Shumway
1970 William A. Altemeier
1971 David C. Sabiston Jr.
1972 Francis D. Moore
1974 Curtis P. Artz
1975 G. Tom Shires
1976 H. William Scott Jr.
1977 Marshall J. Orloff
1978 James C. Thompson
1979 Alexander J. Walt
1980 Ward O. Griffen Jr.
1981 W. Dean Warren
1982 M. Judah Folkman
1983 Peter J. Jannetta
1984 Samuel A. Wells
1985 Keith Reemstma
1986 Seymour I. Schwartz
1987 David B. Skinner
1988 John L. Cameron
1989 William P. Longmire
1990 Richard L. Simmons
1991 John A. Mannick
1992 Jonathan E. Rhoads
1993 Sir Peter J. Morris
1994 Edward M. Copeland III
1995 R. Scott Jones
1996 Stanley J. Dudrick
1997 Thomas E. Starzl
1998 James C. Thompson
1999 Andrew L. Warshaw
2000 John M. Daly
2001 Danny O. Jacobs
2002 W. Randolph Chitwood Jr.
2003 Michael J. Zinner
2004 Barbara L. Bass
2005 Ronald W. Busuttil
2006 Hiram C. Polk Jr.
2007 Richard K. Reznick
2008 Josef E. Fischer
2009 Professor the Lord Darzi
2010 Steven A. Rosenberg
2011 Robin S. McLeod
2012 Haile T. Debas
2013 Diana L. Farmer
2014 Keith D. Lillemoe
2015 Julie Ann Freischlag
2016 Fabrizio Michelassi
2017 Henri R. Ford
2018 Gary L. Dunnington
2019 Jennifer S. Lawton
2021 Susan Moffatt-Bruce
2022 Gretchen Purcell Jackson

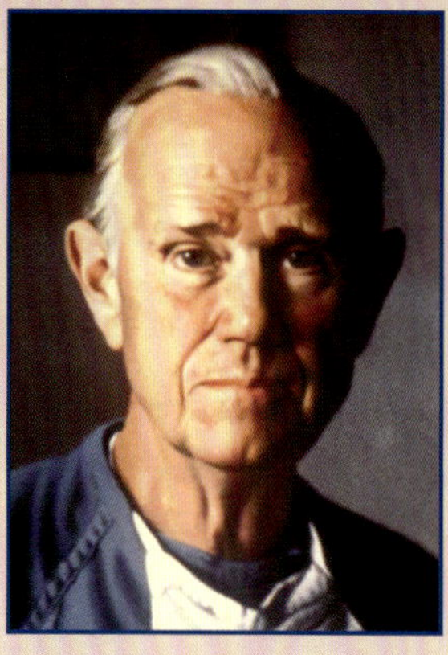

Johnson's Intimidating Stare

Julian Johnson Lecture

HUP's second named lecture was established in 1974 to honor Julian Johnson who had recently retired. Julian Johnson, one of the world's pioneers in cardiothoracic surgery, was a master surgeon, surely HUP's best. I loved the old SOB, but because he was such a perfectionist and strict disciplinarian, he was unpopular with many of the residents. Jim Hardy, HUP chief resident in 1949, was the first surgeon to perform human heart and lung transplants. In 1974, he was selected as the first Johnson lecturer. The next two decades were perhaps CT surgery's finest; its leaders virtually dominated academic surgery in America. The stars of that remarkable era all appear on the list of Johnson lecturers. Each of them paid tribute to Johnson's pioneering influence.

Penn's modern Department of Surgery had been founded in 1946 by I. S. Ravdin and his two partners, Jonathan Rhoads and Julian Johnson. Dr. Ravdin endowed the Johnson lecture through his Buckingham Foundation. Why a HUP lecture has never been named for I. S. Ravdin is hard to understand.

1974 James Hardy
1975 John W. Kirklin
1976 David C. Sabiston Jr.
1977 Norman E. Shumway
1978 Frank C. Spencer
1979 W. Gerald Austen
1980 Dwight C. McGoon
1981 E. Stanley Crawford
1982 Albert Starr
1983 Gordon K. Danielson, Jr.
1984 Denton A. Cooley
1985 Bruce A. Reitz
1986 Paul A. Ebert
1987 Henry T. Bahnson
1988 Joel D. Cooper
1989 William S. Pierce
1990 Aldo R. Casteneda
1991 Judah Folkman
1992 Victor Parsonnet
2003 Hartzell V. Schaff
2004 Alian Carpentier
2006 Tirone E. David
2007 Eric A. Rose
2008 Joseph S. Coselli
2009 Shaf Keshavjee
2010 Robert A. Guyton
2011 John B. West
2012 Frank Sellke
2013 Joel D. Cooper
2014 Mark Slaughter
2015 Clyde F. Barker
2016 O.H. Frazier
2017 Joseph E. Bavaria
2018 Samer A. M. Nashef
2019 Robert J. Cerfolio
2023 Joseph F. Sabik III

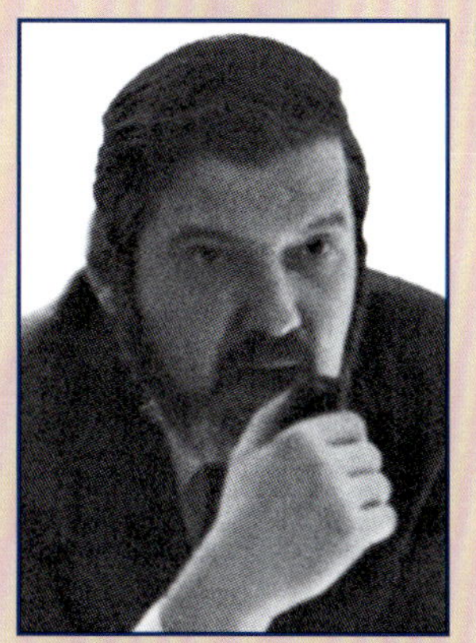

Robert Ravdin

Robert G. Ravdin Lecture

HUP's third lectureship was named after I. S. Ravdin's son, Bob. It began in 1974, the same year as the Julian Johnson lecture, but the two honorees could not have been more different. Johnson, famous as much for his intimidation of residents as for his preeminence as a surgeon, was feared by his trainees. In contrast, Bob Ravdin was beloved by the residents for his remarkably sensitive concern for them and for his patients. In fact, this quality was responsible for the lectureship. Money to endow it was raised by the residents to honor their favorite mentor. Bob Ravdin was a brilliant young surgeon who died too soon. He graduated from Harvard at age fifteen and from Columbia's medical school after only three years. After a HUP residency, his father appointed Bob to the faculty where I always thought too much of his time was consumed by managing his father's huge practice. His major professional accomplishment was initiating and managing HUP's cancer chemotherapy clinic, perhaps the nation's first. At age fifty, he suffered a fatal heart attack while playing bridge at Philadelphia's Union League. A staunch political liberal, Bob would have appreciated the irony of this site for his demise. Early speakers were chosen by the residents to reflect Bob's broad interests.

1974 Lewis Thomas
1975 Edmund D. Pellegrino
1977 J. Englebert Dunphy
1980 C. Everett Koop
1981 Daniel Hadlock
1982 Richard A. Selzer
1983 Francis D. Moore
1984 John Philip Sandblom
1985 Thomas J. Krizek
1986 Fritz Linder
1990 C. Rollins Hanlon
1992 Joseph Murray
1994 George Sheldon
1996 C. Everett Koop
2005 Michael Longaker
2006 David Bartlett
2007 Robert Udelsman
2008 Douglas S. Tyler
2009 James Pingpank Jr.
2010 Funda Meric-Bernstam
2011 Herbert Chen
2012 John A. Olson
2013 Monica Morrow
2014 Timothy Michael Pawlik
2015 Steven K. Libutti
2016 Nipun Merchant
2017 Richard Hodin
2018 David L. Bartlett
2019 H. Richard Alexander
2023 T. Peter Kingham

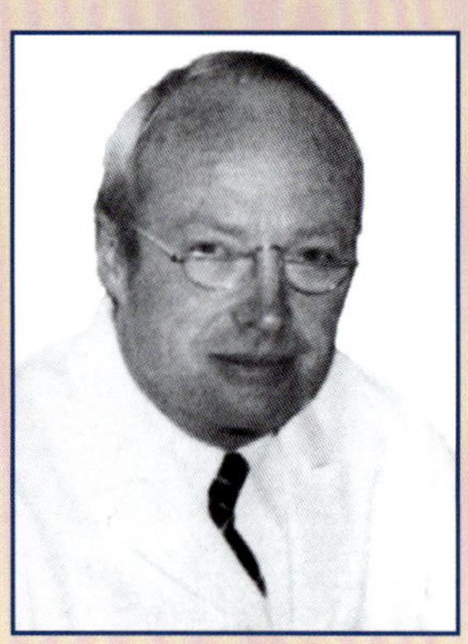

Julius Mackie

Julius A. Mackie Distinguished Graduate Award and Lecture

In 1991, the department began selecting from the list of former HUP residents a distinguished graduate of the year. This custom was interrupted in 1998. When it was resumed, the Distinguished Graduate Professorship and Lecture was given a name, that of Julius A. Mackie. Jack Mackie, a beloved HUP surgeon who died in 2003, was an unusually gifted technical surgeon. But it was his devotion to pre- and postoperative care of his patients that really set him apart. His attention to detail sometimes drove his resident staff crazy, but it saved lives. Its value was reinforced strikingly by one case. On a late-night check of his own and other patients, Jack discovered and treated a tension pneumothorax that had been missed on routine rounds by other surgeons and their staff. This otherwise fatal complication had taken place in Jack's faculty colleague, Clete Schwegman, who had been operated on by another surgeon. Jack's wife Joan's generous support of the lecture and the accompanying annual dinner have made the distinguished graduate celebration one of the department's most popular traditions.

1991	James D. Hardy	2012	James D. Luketich
1992	James C. Thompson	2013	Michael A. Choti
1994	Edward M. Copeland III	2014	Howard A. Reber
1995	R. Scott Jones	2015	Omaida C. Velazquez
1996	Stanley J. Dudrick	2016	James F. Markmann
1997	C. Everett Koop	2017	Kenneth L. Brayman
1998	Moritz M. Ziegler	2018	Steven J. Fishman
2007	Ronald P. DeMatteo	2019	Mark B. Faries
2009	Stephen T. Bartlett	2021	Joseph Woo
2010	Danny O. Jacobs	2022	Isabelle Bedrosian
2011	W. Roy Smythe	2024	Heung Bae Kim

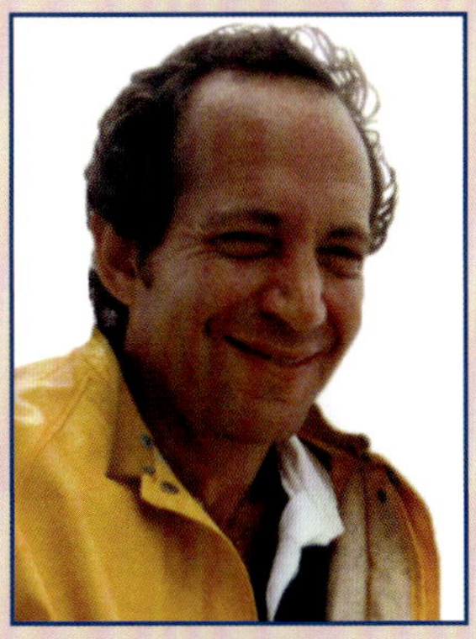

Gordon Buzby

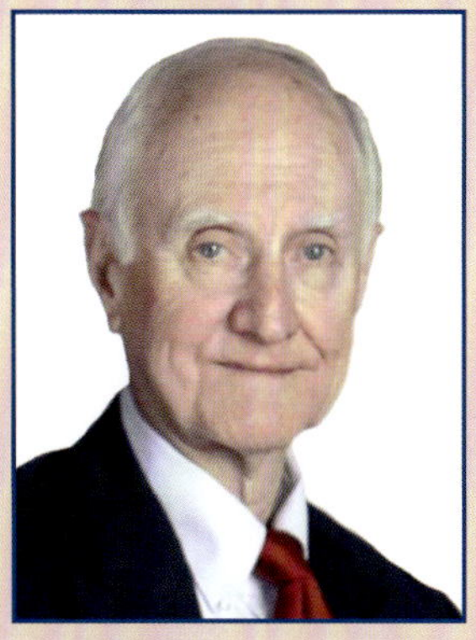

Linton Whitaker

Gordon P. Buzby Lecture on Leadership

Gordon Buzby, the director of HUP's surgical residency program, died in 2003 at age fifty after a battle with lung cancer. Gordon was an athlete. An expert sailor from childhood, he became national intercollegiate sailing champion. He was especially admired and respected by the residents for his leadership skills and style. Therefore, in endowing this lectureship, Gordon and his wife and family specified that leadership be a criterion for selecting speakers.

2004 Thomas J. Krizek
2005 Roch Parayre
2006 Michael Useem
2007 William N. Kelley
2008 Mario Moussa
2009 Layton F. Rikkers
2010 Ralph W. Muller
2011 Jennifer J. Deal
2012 Kenneth R. Feinberg
2013 Arthur H. Rubenstein
2014 Jack Devine
2015 Peter Bergen
2016 Dereck/Beverly Joubert
2017 Jane Golden
2018 Larry R. Kaiser
2019 Philip Mudd
2022 Julia Haller
2023 Patricia Turner

Linton Whitaker Lectureship

Linton Whitaker is one of the world's most important pioneers in craniofacial surgery. The spectacular results of these operations made him perhaps the most famous of HUP surgeons. He was chief of the Division of Plastic Surgery from 1987 to 2004. He also founded the unique Center for Human Appearance. In addition to the HUP lecture, the American Society of Craniofacial Surgery has established another an annual lectureship in his name.

2006 Fernando Monasterio
2007 Fu Chan Wei
2008 Paul N. Manson
2009 Jeffrey Fearon
2010 Scott P. Bartlett
2011 Robert J. Allen
2012 Fernando Molina
2013 John A. Persing
2014 Eric Arnaud
2015 Joseph E. Losee
2016 James Zins
2017 Stephen Baker
2018 Richard Warren
2019 Mirko Gilardino

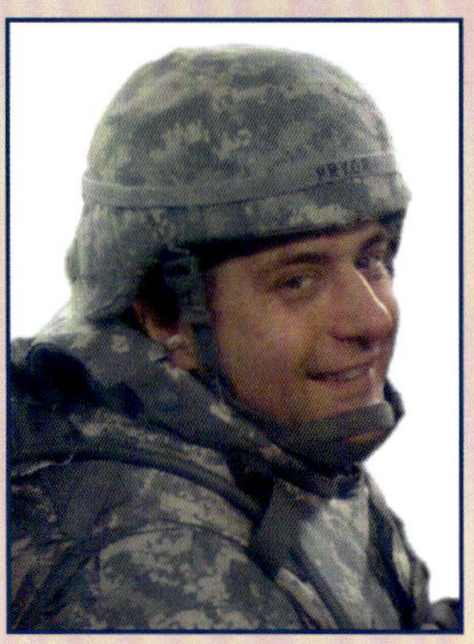

John Pryor

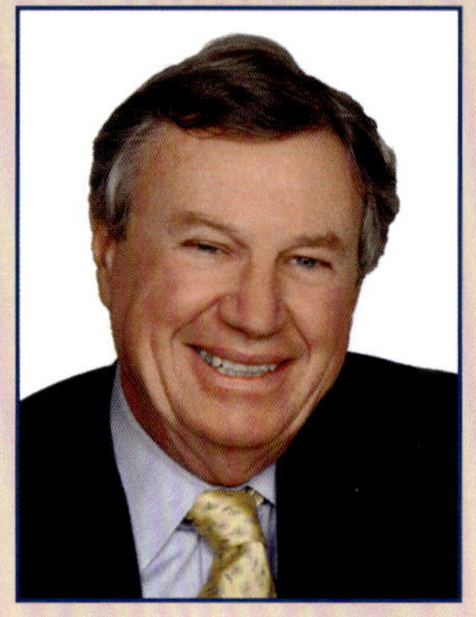

Ernie Rosato

John Paul Pryor Oration

John Pryor was serving his second deployment in Iraq when on Christmas Day 2008, he was killed by enemy fire. Prior to his military service, he had been director of Bill Schwab's trauma program at HUP. In the new trauma center at Presbyterian Hospital, the Shock, Trauma and Resuscitation Unit is named for John Pryor.

2009 David V. Feliciano
2010 Andrew B. Peitzman
2011 Arthur L. Kellermann
2011 Robert C. Mackersie
2012 Jay A. Johannigman
2013 Martin A. Schreiber
2014 Raul Coimbra
2015 Grace Rozycki
2016 Lenworth Jacobs
2017 Michael F. Rotondo
2018 Amy J. Goldberg
2019 John Efron
2022 Christine Gaarder

Ernest F. Rosato – William Maul Measey Endowed Lectureship in Surgical Education

Highly respected for his mastery of technical surgery and thoughtful patient management, Ernie Rosato was regarded by the residents as their most important role model in these areas. Shortly before Ernie's untimely death, The Measey Foundation established this lecture that is intended to emphasize surgical education. Fortunately, Ernie was able to attend the first lecture.

2011 Clyde F. Barker
2011 Stanley J. Dudrick
2012 Keith R. Erickson
2013 John R. Potts III
2014 L. D. Brit
2015 Ronald C. Jones
2016 John L. Tarpley
2017 Steven C. Stain
2018 Selwyn M. Vickers
2019 Michael L. Nance
2021 Jo Buyske
2022 Douglas Stewart Smink

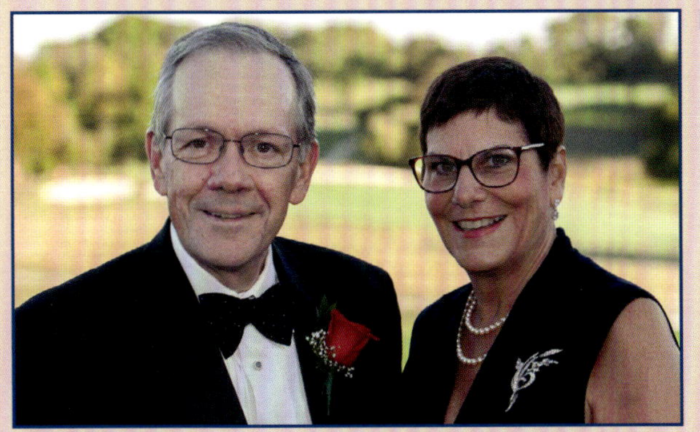

Dan and Barbara Dempsey

Barbara and Daniel Dempsey Gastrointestinal Surgery Research and Education Lecture

This annual lecture was endowed by Dr. Dempsey's patient, Professor Raghupathi. It honors Dr. Dempsey and his wife, Barbara, both graduates of Princeton and the University of Rochester (Barbara, MBA, and Dan, MD). Barbara was a career-long researcher for Johnson & Johnson. Dan (HUP chief resident 1986) was chairman of surgery at Temple (2000-2011), chief of gastrointestinal surgery at Penn (2011-2021), president of the Philadelphia Academy of Surgery, and the 2019 Strittmatter Awardee.

2022 Aurora D. Pryor	2023 Mark P. Callery

In addition to the nine HUP named lectures, described below are several other named lectures. They were not established by HUP and do not (usually) take place at HUP. Thus, these are not truly HUP lectures, but they are named for and given in honor of HUP surgeons. I confess there could be other named lectures of which I am not familiar, perhaps proposed by other societies or by Penn Surgery divisions. Examples are the Linton Whitaker Lecture of the American Society of Craniofacial Surgery and the new Herndon B. Lehr Lecture of the HUP Plastic Surgery Division.

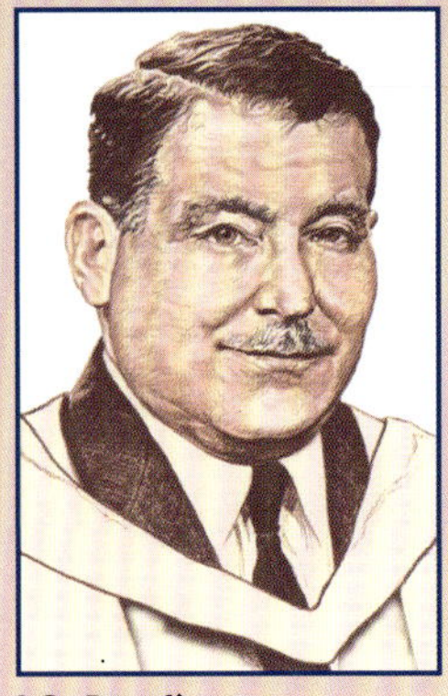

I.S. Ravdin

I. S. Ravdin Lecture in the Basic and Surgical Sciences

This distinguished lecture is given at the Clinical Congress of the American College of Surgeons, one of only ten named lectures of the College. It was established in 1964 by Dr. Ravdin's colleagues and trainees of the I. S. Ravdin Society. For reasons I never understood, this society and its successor, the Ravdin–Rhoads Society, were discontinued in 2001. Because of Dr. Ravdin's prominence and contributions to the College, this lecture continues to be given annually. It has a very illustrious cast, including eight Nobel Prize winners.

1964 R. E. Billingham
1965 J. H. Comroe Jr.
1966 P. A. Weiss
1967 R. A. Gregory
1968 D. V. Bates
1969 A. C. Kornberg
1970 G. F. Cahill Jr.
1971 R. A. Good
1972 H. B. Glass
1973 F. Story Musgrave
1974 Charles B. Huggins
1975 Arthur C. Guyton
1976 James Watson
1977 Norman C. Staub
1978 Paul Berg
1979 Alfred E. Harper
1980 Rosalyn Yalow
1981 Britton Chance
1982 John B. West
1983 C. G. Cochrane
1984 Charles A. Dinarello
1985 Howard Green
1986 John H. Exton
1987 Peter A. Ward
1988 Daniel Nathans
1989 Paul D. Hart
1990 Victor F. Weisskopf
1991 Joseph E. Murray
1992 C. Robert Valeri
1993 Salvador Moncada
1994 M. Judah Folkman
1995 Leroy E. Hood
1996 Douglas W. Wilmore
1997 Richard L. Simmons
1998 Frank A. Plummer
1999 A. Gerson Greenberg
2000 John A. Mannick
2001 Robert H. Bartlett
2002 James C. Stanley
2003 Steven A. Rosenberg
2004 Thomas E. Starzl
2005 Timothy G. Buchman
2006 Michael R. Harrison
2007 Joseph P. Vacanti
2008 David N. Herndon
2009 Michael T. Longaker
2010 Ian Frazer
2011 Robert D. Howe
2012 Richard S. Hotchkiss
2013 Roy A. J. Spence
2014 Piero Anversa
2015 Melvin J. Silverstein
2016 Andres M. Lozano
2017 John C. Alverdy
2018 John J. Fung
2019 Ronald V. Maier
2020 Nancy N. Baxter
2021 Melina R. Kibbe
2022 Carla M. Pugh

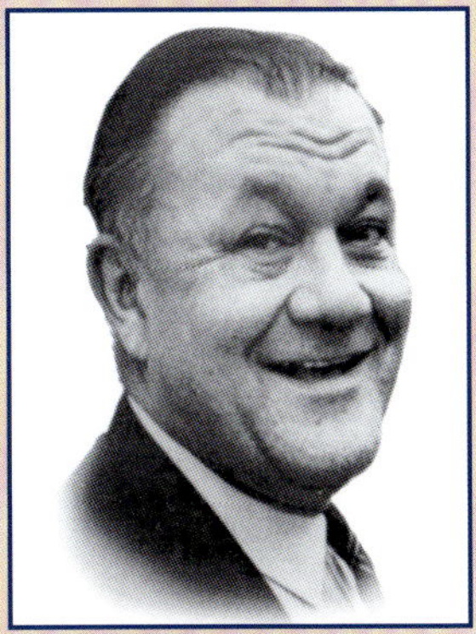

William Fitts

William T. Fitts Lectureship

The American Association for the Surgery of Trauma established the William T. Fitts Lectureship in 1975 to memorialize the many contributions made by Dr. Fitts as president and secretary of the Association and as editor of the *Journal of Trauma*.

1975 Curtis P. Artz
1976 Francis D. Moore
1977 G. Tom Shires
1978 Lloyd D. MacLean
1979 Mr. Peter S. London
1980 Carl T. Brighton
1981 John W. Kinney
1982 Thomas W. Langfitt
1983 Col. Robert Scott
1984 F. William Blaisdell
1985 Donald P. Becker
1986 Sheng Chih-Yong
1987 Paul Dudley Hart
1988 Roderick A. Little
1989 Prof. Martin Allgower
1990 Philip R. Lee
1991 Donald D. Trunkey
1992 Basil A. Pruitt Jr.
1993 John H. Davis
1994 John R. Border
1995 Jonathan E. Rhoads
1996 Susan P. Baker
1997 George F. Sheldon
1998 Leonard Evans
1999 Barbara Barlow
2000 Johannes A. Sturm
2001 Janet Reno (Cancelled)
2002 C. James Carrico
2003 Ellen J. MacKenzie
2004 Colonel John Holcomb
2005 Sylvia D. Campbell
2006 Sten E.V. Lennquist
2007 Thomas M. Scalea
2008 Charles E. Lucas
2009 Frederick P. Rivara
2010 Charles N. Mock
2011 H. Leon Patcher
2012 David B. Hoyt
2013 Frank R. Lewis Jr.
2014 Ronald G. Tompkins
2015 L. D. Britt
2016 M. Margaret Knudson
2017 Ronald Maier
2018 C. William Schwab
2019 Timothy C. Fabian
2023 J. Wayne Meredith

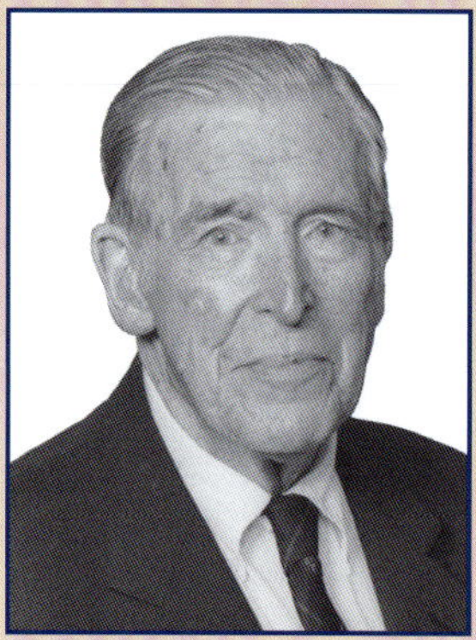

Jonathan Rhoads

Jonathan E. Rhoads Commemorative Lecture and Gold Medal

In 1996, this lecture was established by Herman Goldstine, Rhoads's close associate at the American Philosophical Society. Goldstine, a mathematician, was a member of the team responsible for developing ENIAC, the world's first electronic computer. He and his friends contributed all of the funds to endow this lecture. Goldstine specified that responsibility for the lecture should rotate between three of the institutions that had been headed by Rhoads: the American Philosophical Society, HUP's Department of Surgery, and the Philadelphia College of Physicians. The topic of lecture was intended to be relevant to the broad field of medicine rather than narrowly focused on surgery. The speaker is also given a solid gold medal. Every three years, Penn Surgery's chairman has the opportunity to pick the speaker and the site of the lecture.

Lectures given at HUP

2002 Thomas E. Starzl
2007 Clyde F. Barker
2010 John E. Niederhuber
2014 Jeffrey I. Gordon
2018 Timothy R. Billiar

Rhoads Prize Lectures—not given at HUP

US Senator Marie Kassebaum-Baker; surgeons Francis Moore, Judah Folkman, Michael DeBakey, Scott Jones; Nobel Laureate Joseph Murray; Lasker Awardees Aaron Beck and Mary Claire King; Assistant Surgeon General Ann Schuchat; NIH Director Elias Zirahouni; medical writers Lawrence Altman, Sherwin Nuland, and Abraham Verghese; Anthony Fauci; Drew Weissman and Kaitlin Karikó.

CHAPTER 37

Evolution of Specialties and Divisions

In the late twentieth century, the development of new surgical procedures and entirely new surgical fields led to specialization and enlargement of surgery departments. Initially, I was one of many who spoke emotionally about the dangers and disadvantages in fragmentation of general surgery. But it also became obvious that for progress in some areas, specialization would be necessary and divisions probably inevitable. Therefore, somewhat reluctantly, while I was chairman, I oversaw the formation of four new divisions in our Department of Surgery: surgical oncology, trauma, gastrointestinal surgery, and general thoracic surgery. Many of the leaders in these disciplines were as important, or more so, than the department chairman. In fact, quite a few eventually became department chairs at other universities. The scope of this book does not allow detailed histories of the divisions or full biographies of their leaders. This chapter briefly describes the origin of the divisions and contains abbreviated profiles of their important faculty members.

Surgical Oncology

The first of Penn Surgery's new divisions was surgical oncology. In 1986, John Daly was recruited from Memorial Sloan Kettering to direct this controversial division. He was born in Philadelphia and graduated from La Salle College and Temple Medical School. During medical school, he had a summer job with Stan Dudrick in Penn's Harrison department, where Stan's landmark research on total parenteral nutrition was just beginning in 1966.[1] Stan persuaded Daly to take his residency in surgery at the University of Texas at Houston where Stan

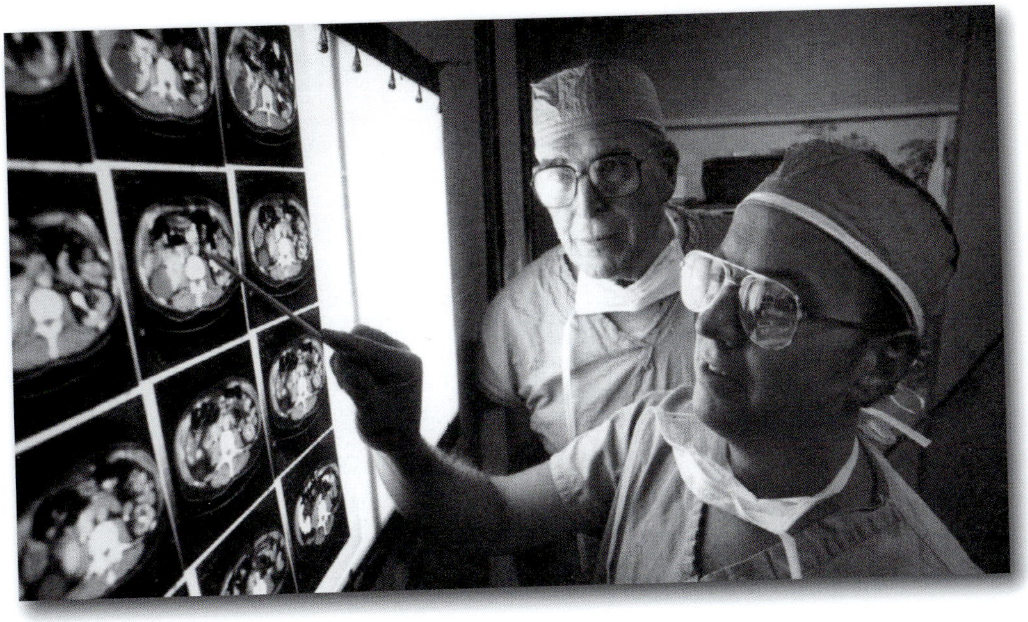

Jonathan Rhoads and John Daly

had become the inaugural surgical chairman. Daly followed this with a fellowship in surgical oncology at nearby MD Anderson Cancer Center where he worked with Ted Copeland, another Penn surgeon.[2] Daly then became a faculty member at Memorial Sloan Kettering in New York where he did some of the earliest work on intra-arterial chemotherapy for colorectal liver metastases. In 1986, he was recruited back to Philadelphia as the inaugural Jonathan Rhoads professor and chief of the new division of surgical oncology. This was HUP's first venture into specialization and fragmentation of the broad field of general surgery. There was serious resentment on the part of several general surgeons who saw themselves as the department's experts in cancer surgery. Fortunately, Daly's ability to get along with people allowed him to become friends with most of his competitors. For his next eight years at Penn, his clinical research and educational performance were exceptional. In addition to winning several R01 grants, he established NIH funding of a T32 training grant which supported research of HUP residents during and for several years after Daly left Penn. Daly's productive research and popularity as a mentor attracted many HUP residents to his laboratory. This group included Noel Williams, now director of the Metabolic and Bariatric Center at Penn, and Mike Lieberman, director of surgical oncology at New York Hospital and Cornell. In addition, Daly established relationships with surgical training programs in Ireland, attracting many young Irish surgical residents to come to Philadelphia for training in his laboratory.

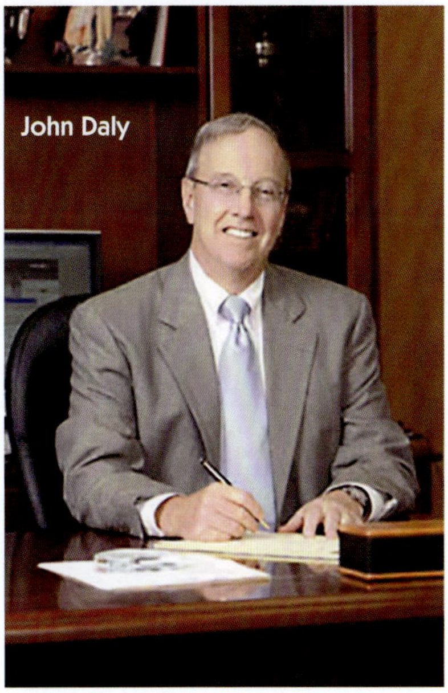

John Daly

This group included a number of individuals who have become academic surgery leaders in Ireland, including John Reynolds, now chief of surgery at Trinity College, Dublin; Paul Redmond, chair of surgery at University College, Cork; and Cathal Kelly, the CEO of the Royal College of Surgeons in Ireland.

In 1993, Daly left Penn to become professor and chairman of the Department of Surgery at Cornell and chief of surgery at New York Hospital. He soon became recognized as one of America's most successful and prominent academic surgeons. He was elected president of the Society of Surgical Oncology and the American Society of Parenteral and Enteral Nutrition, and vice president of the American College of Surgeons and the American Surgical Association. He was also awarded honorary fellowships in the Royal College of Surgeons of Glasgow and the Royal College of Surgeons in Ireland. He authored more than 250 peer-reviewed publications and served on the editorial boards of more than a dozen journals.

In 2002, Daly was called back to his alma mater in Philadelphia as the dean of Temple's medical school. Several months later, he developed severe liver failure and underwent a liver transplant at HUP for cirrhosis caused by hepatitis C. He recovered quickly and his liver function remained normal the rest of his life. As Temple's dean, he was successful in enhancing the educational performance of the school and in raising money for a state-of-the-art teaching and research building. In 2011, he stepped down as dean and for several years practiced surgery at Fox Chase. In 2018, he was asked to become Temple's interim dean and a short time later, the interim was dropped, and he was fully at the helm in Temple's medical school at the time of his untimely death from an accident in 2021.[3] In recognition of his contributions, Temple, with help from the Measey Foundation, has established an endowed professorship of medical education in his name.

Douglas Fraker was recruited in 1996 from the NIH to succeed Daly and continues to serve as chief of the Division of Surgical Oncology. Dr. Fraker is a renowned endocrine and oncologic surgeon who has decades of NIH-funded research experience and one of the largest endocrine surgery practices in the country.

Dr. Fraker received his BA in molecular biology from the University of Wisconsin. After medical school at Harvard, he trained in general surgery at the University of California, San Francisco. He interrupted his residency for a three-year research fellowship at the Surgery Branch of the National Cancer Institute where he worked in surgical metabolism. After completing his chief residency at UCSF, Dr. Fraker returned to the NCI as a senior investigator and was later named chief of NCI's Surgical Metabolism Section and head of endocrine surgery for the National Institutes of Health. For the next four years, he studied a variety of endocrine conditions, such as gastrinomas and insulinomas. He also gained experience with surgery for multiple endocrine neoplasias (MEN-1 and MEN-2) and reoperative parathyroid surgery.[4] He also conducted extensive preclinical and clinical research on regional therapies for cancer, including trials of TNF for isolated limb perfusion for melanoma and sarcoma.[5]

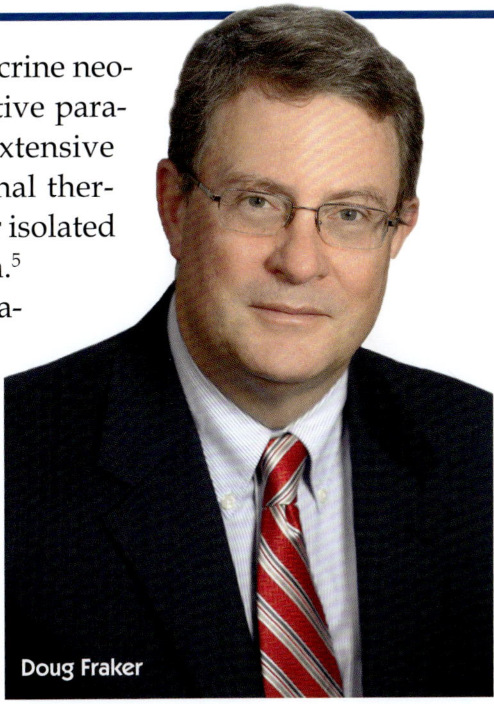
Doug Fraker

After joining the University of Pennsylvania in 1996, Dr. Fraker continued his work on regional perfusion[6] and conducted a trial of photodynamic therapy for treatment of intraperitoneal malignancies.[7] Because of Dr. Fraker's interest in and large experience with endocrine surgery, his division was renamed the Division of Endocrine and Oncologic Surgery. He has had a number of leadership roles at Penn, including vice chair for clinical affairs, deputy director of the University of Pennsylvania Cancer Center, and surgery's vice chair for research.

Dr. Fraker has authored more than 265 publications and currently serves on eight editorial advisory boards of journals, including the *Annals of Surgical Oncology* and *The Laryngoscope.* He is a member of the American Surgical Association and multiple professional associations in which he has held leadership roles on boards and committees.

A number of universities have courted Dr. Fraker to become chairman of their surgery departments, including Indiana University and the Robert Wood Johnson Medical School of Rutgers University. Fortunately for us, he has thus far preferred to remain at Penn.

At present, members of his division include Ari D. Brooks; Oluwadamilola Fayanju (director of the breast center); Rachel Kelz (vice chair of clinical research and director of the Center for Surgery and Health Economics); Giorgos Karakousis; Robert Roses; Dahlia Sataloff; Julia Tchou; Heather Wachtel; and Chairman Ron DeMatteo.

General Thoracic Surgery

The genesis of the general thoracic surgery division was the perception of Hank Edmunds that Penn should have a program in lung transplantation, not a particularly common procedure at the time. Hank strongly suggested that we recruit Larry Kaiser, who had been on the faculties of the institutions that pioneered the field: the University of Toronto[89] and Washington University in St. Louis.[10] Kaiser arrived at Penn in 1991 and promptly started a successful lung transplant program. He soon became more interested and active in general (noncardiac) thoracic surgery than in transplantation and turned most of his

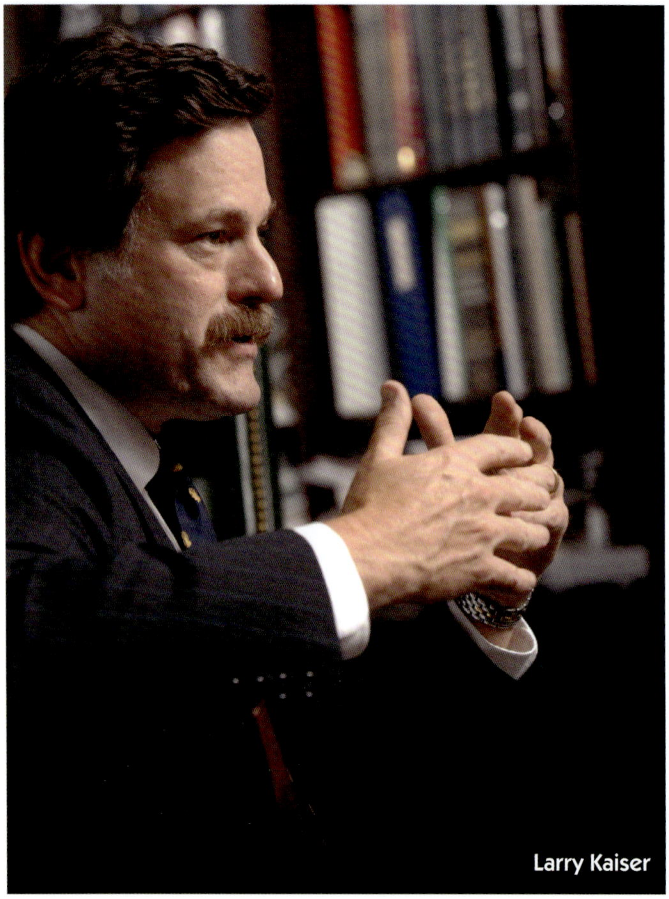
Larry Kaiser

attention to this broader field, which soon evolved into an official division. The leadership in lung transplantation was assumed by members of the CT division where it is presently listed.

Although Julian Johnson, Hank Edmunds, and other CT surgeons had been perfectly competent at pulmonary and other thoracic procedures, Kaiser's broader experience and expertise allowed him to dominate the field at HUP and achieve national and international recognition. He was also productive in research, especially with trials of suicide gene therapy.[11]

Kaiser was very effective in stimulating the interest of many HUP residents in thoracic surgery and encouraged faculty appointments of them and other young thoracic surgeons. These included Joe Shrager, a HUP resident and MGH fellow, who after several Penn faculty years in 2008 became and remains chief of thoracic surgery at Stanford. Another was Joe Friedberg, an MGH resident who, after thoracic fellowship at the Brigham and several faculty years under Kaiser at Penn, has led thoracic surgery at the University of Maryland and now at Temple.

Joel Cooper

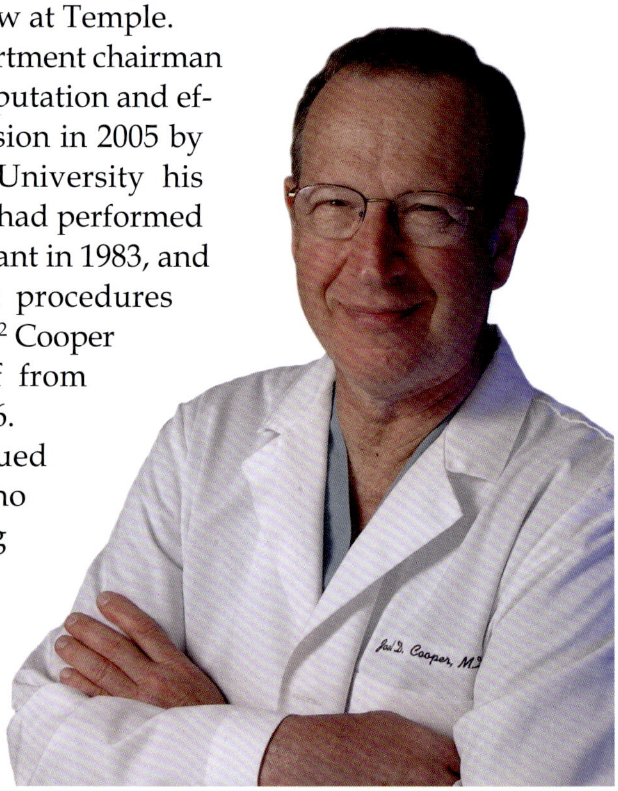

After becoming Penn's department chairman in 2001, Kaiser enhanced the reputation and effectiveness of the thoracic division in 2005 by recruiting from Washington University his own mentor, Joel Cooper, who had performed the first successful lung transplant in 1983, and invented other novel thoracic procedures such as lung reduction therapy.[12] Cooper served as the division's chief from 2005 until his retirement in 2016.

As chairman, Kaiser continued to train thoracic surgeons who have become leaders, including Blair Marshall at Georgetown and Penn's two most recent thoracic division chiefs, John Kucharczuk and Sunil Singhal.

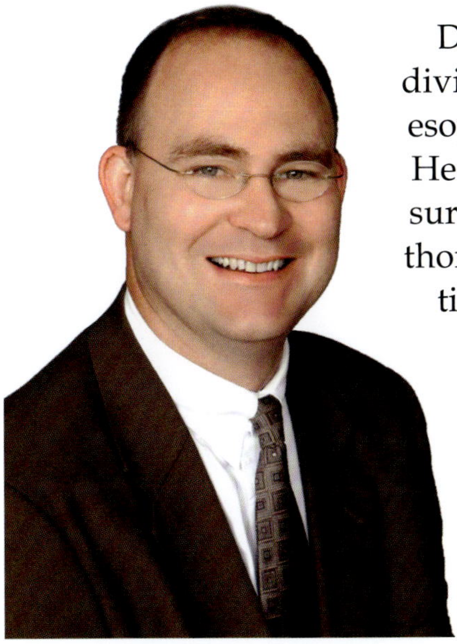

John Kucharczuk

Dr. Kucharczuk, who was chief of the thoracic division from 2011–2021, is a master surgeon in esophageal, pulmonary, and mediastinal diseases. He is responsible for positioning Penn thoracic surgery as a dominant referral center for expert thoracic surgical care both regionally and nationally. Among other divisional achievements, Dr. Kucharczuk established the thoracic oncology service line, a model for the health system's streamlined approach to accessible and comprehensive cancer care. He has expanded the division from three to nine clinical locations. After retiring as division chief in 2022, Dr. Kucharczuk is expanding his leadership role as director of the thoracic oncology network of the Cancer Center, while continuing to lead the thoracic oncology service line.

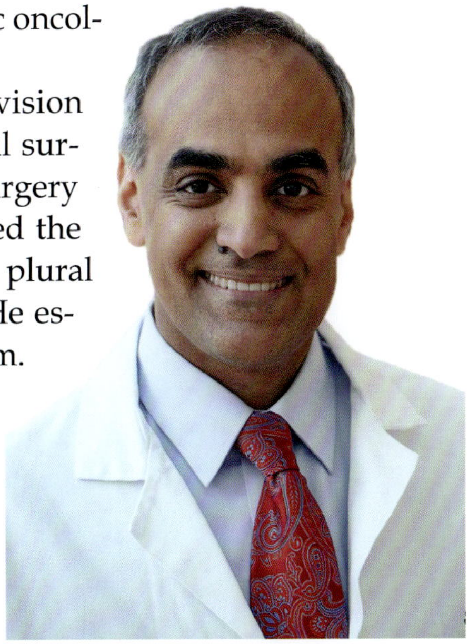

Sunil Singhal

Sunil Singhal succeeded Dr. Kucharczuk as division chief in 2022. After medical school at Penn, general surgery residency at Johns Hopkins, and a thoracic surgery fellowship under Kaiser at Penn, Dr. Singhal joined the faculty in 2008. His active practice is in lung cancer, plural mesothelioma, and congenital chest wall defects. He established the HUP robotic thoracic surgery program. He received an MBA from Wharton in 2018.

Dr. Singhal's research interests include intraoperative molecular imaging for thoracic malignancies and neoadjuvant immunotherapy for advanced lung cancer (see Chapter 34). His clinical molecular imaging program is the largest in the United States, and he has been the principal investigator of over $14 million in federal funding including multiple R01s, an NCI Biomedical Research Partnership, and grants from the Department of Defense, the Veterans Administration, and the State of Pennsylvania. His work resulted in the first multi-institutional, randomized phase 3 clinical trial of intraoperative molecular imaging in lung cancer. Dr. Singhal has published over 250 peer-reviewed articles, including papers in *Science, Translational Medicine, Cancer Cell, PNAS, Clinical Cancer Research,* and the *Journal of Clinical Investigation.* He is a member of the American Society of Clinical Investigation, the Society of Clinical Surgery, the American Surgical Association, and the editorial board of the *Annals of Surgery.*

Other members of the division include Christian Bermudez, director of thoracic transplantation and ECMO; Ed Cantu, director of ex-vivo lung perfusion and associate director of lung transplantation; Taine Pechet, chief of surgery at Penn Presbyterian Medical Center; Doraid Jarrar, associate clerkship director; Jarrod Predina; and Leonid Emerel.

Gastrointestinal Surgery

The GI division began in 1988 when I appointed Ernie Rosato as its chief. Although Ernie, as a young faculty member, did basic research with members of the Department of Medicine,[13] his attention later became limited largely to his huge practice[14] and the teaching of HUP residents. He continued to participate in academic activity and to contribute to the literature. Because he had the largest practice of general surgery in the Philadelphia region and a reputation as HUP's best teacher, a position as division chief was appropriate. In 1989, Jon Morris, a recruit from a research fellowship at Hopkins, became the first additional member of his division. After sixteen years as division chief, Ernie Rosato stepped aside in 2004, and Jeff Drebin succeeded him. Drebin had a strong research record with a PhD in molecular biology and was also appointed as the department's vice chair of research. In 2009, he became John Rhea Barton Professor and Chairman of Surgery (see Chapter 30).

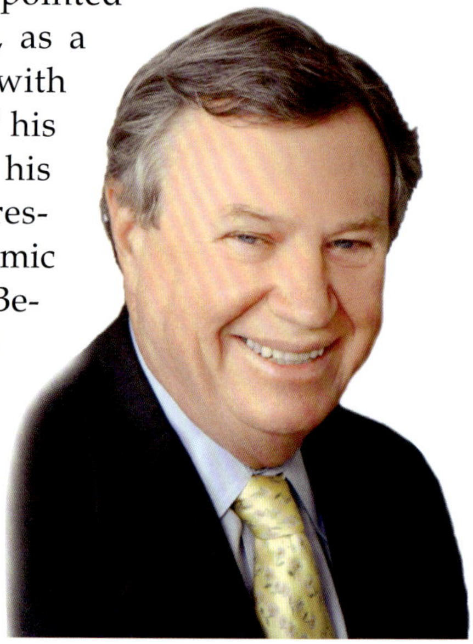

Ernie Rosato

In 2011 Dan Dempsey, Temple's surgery chairman, succeeded Drebin as Penn's GI division chief. He served very effectively in that role up to his retirement from active practice in 2021. Dan is a magna cum laude graduate of Princeton where he majored in the classics, played football, and met his classmate and future wife, Barbara. At the University of Rochester School of Medicine, he won the Class of 1976 Prize. As a surgical resident at HUP, he twice won the surgical scholar award, was elected to AOA, and conducted research in nutrition with Gordon Buzby and Jim Mullen. He then accepted the offer to join his friend and mentor, Wally Ritchie, surgical chairman at Temple. There, his rapid academic advance was marked by multiple teaching awards, appointments as chief of GI surgery, chief of general surgery, and election as president of the medical staff and the medical faculty senate. He became full professor of surgery in 1998.

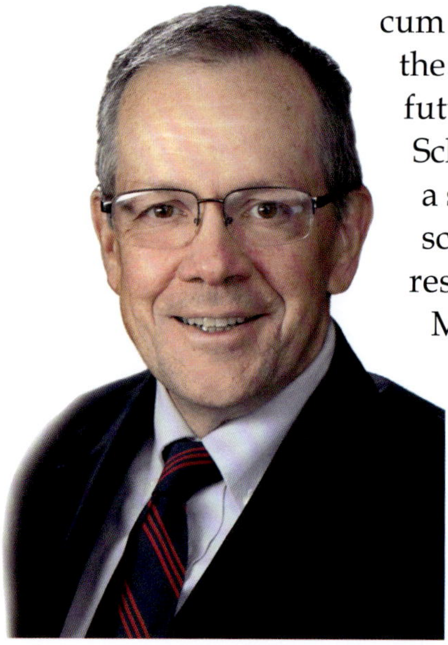

Dan Dempsey

In 1999, Dempsey left Temple, enticed by Penn's recruitment of him as professor and vice chairman of the Department of Surgery and chief of surgery at Pennsylvania Hospital. In 2000, Temple upped the ante to recall him as chairman of the Department of Surgery, a position he held with distinction for twelve years.

In 2011, Dan was welcomed back to Penn as HUP's chief of GI surgery and assistant director of perioperative services. His many contributions to our department as an active clinician,[15,16,17] administrator, and master surgeon are topped only by his selection by the residents as their most important mentor.

In 2019, Dan Dempsey received the prestigious Strittmatter Award of the Philadelphia County Medical Society. This venerable award was first presented in 1923 to America's greatest surgeon of that day, W. W. Keen. Since then, it has been awarded annually to the physician deemed Philadelphia's most deserving by virtue of his or her "advancement of the broad field of medicine through patient care, teaching and leadership." The list of Philadelphia doctor-recipients is impressive. It features Nobel and Lasker award winners and eminent practitioners of all fields of medicine such as Chevalier Jackson, I. S. Ravdin, Jonathan Rhoads, Francis Wood, J. Chalmers DaCosta, Sol Sherry, and others.

When Dempsey took over the GI division, he had already established himself as a prominent surgical leader in Philadelphia and beyond. He was already a member of surgery's premier societies—the University Surgeons and the American Surgical Association. During his ten years as GI Division chief, his consistent performance as a role model and mentor furthered his reputation. During that time, he was elected president of the County Medical Society and was named a member of Penn's Academy of Master Clinicians and the American College of Surgeons Academy of Master Educators. All of this was done while he conducted a large surgical practice and supported his beloved wife, Barbara, through a prolonged, terminal illness. Dan, with the support of the Measey Foundation, has established an endowed professorship in her name. In 2022, Dan elected to step down as GI division chief.

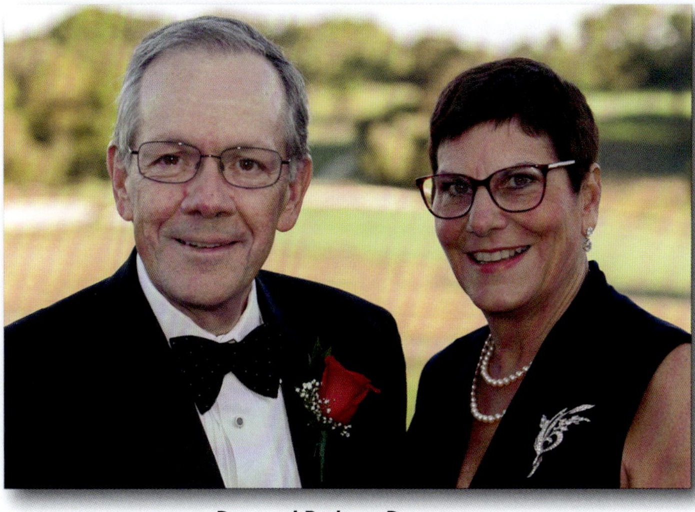

Dan and Barbara Dempsey

After an active search, Charles Vollmer was selected to succeed Dr. Dempsey. Dr. Vollmer is a graduate of Jefferson Medical College and the general surgery residency of Washington University in St. Louis. He then completed a fellowship in hepatobiliary and solid organ transplantation surgery at the University of Toronto. He served on the faculty of

Harvard and Beth Israel Deaconess Medical Center for eight years before moving to Penn in 2011. He was promoted to professor in 2015 and has served as the director of pancreatic surgery and founder and codirector of the Multi-Disciplinary Pancreatic Cyst Program. His primary focus is the pancreas[18] and he has made numerous contributions to clinical outcomes research, particularly regarding postoperative pancreatic fistulas.[19] He has authored over 190 publications, four book chapters, and three books.[20] Dr. Vollmer is well-known internationally and is a member of the editorial boards of the *Annals of Surgery, British Journal of Surgery, Annals of Surgical Oncology, Surgery, Journal of Gastrointestinal Surgery,* and *Journal of Surgical Oncology.* He has been president of the American Hepato-Pancreato-Biliary Association and is a member of the executive committee of the International Hepato-Pancreato-Biliary Association and the National Cancer Care Network Committee on Pancreatic Cancer. He is a member of the American Surgical Association and the Society of Clinical Surgery.

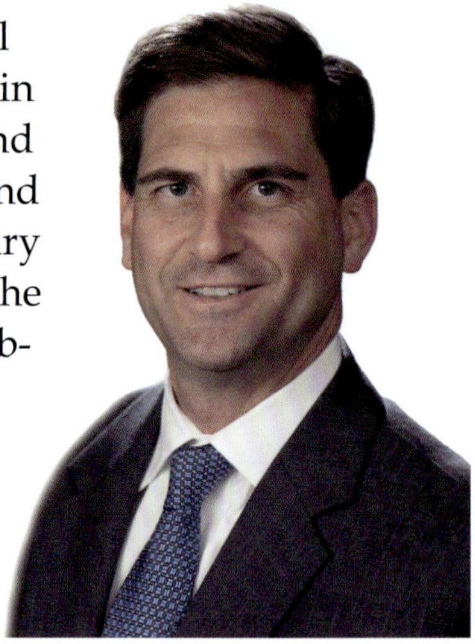

Charles Vollmer

Other faculty members of Dr. Vollmer's division include Kristoffel Dumon, Sean Harbison, Matt Kirkland, Gary Korus, Major Kenneth Lee, Francis E. Rosato, Alan Schuricht, David Wernsing, Noel Williams, Maria Altieri, Victoria Gershuni, Daniel Hashimoto, Jon Morris, Steve Raper, Ron DeMatteo, and Noel Williams who directs the program in bariatric surgery.[21]

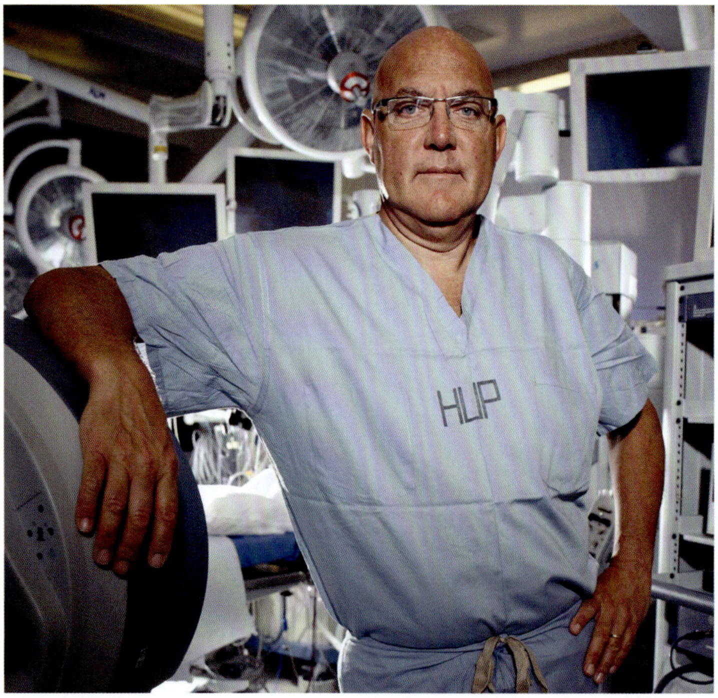

Noel Williams
director, metabolic and bariatric surgery

Cardiovascular Surgery

Although George Muller and I. S. Ravdin performed a few chest operations in the 1930s, this division really began with Julian Johnson in the late 1930s.[22] His training in what was then a new field was limited to a few weeks of watching thoracic operations in Boston, but most of the cardiac procedures that he later performed were self-taught.[23] His pioneering exploits in this field are reviewed in Chapter 18. He also brought open-heart surgery to HUP and was most widely known for a book he coauthored with Charles Kirby on noncardiac surgery of the chest.[24] It became a standard in the field. Johnson trained a number of important surgeons, including Gordon Danielson, who became chief of CT surgery at the Mayo Clinic; John Waldhausen; and William Pierce, a founder of artificial heart and ventricular assist devices (see Chapter 34). Johnson was a member of all the important general surgical societies and also president of the American Association of Thoracic Surgery (AATS) and the Society for Vascular Surgery.

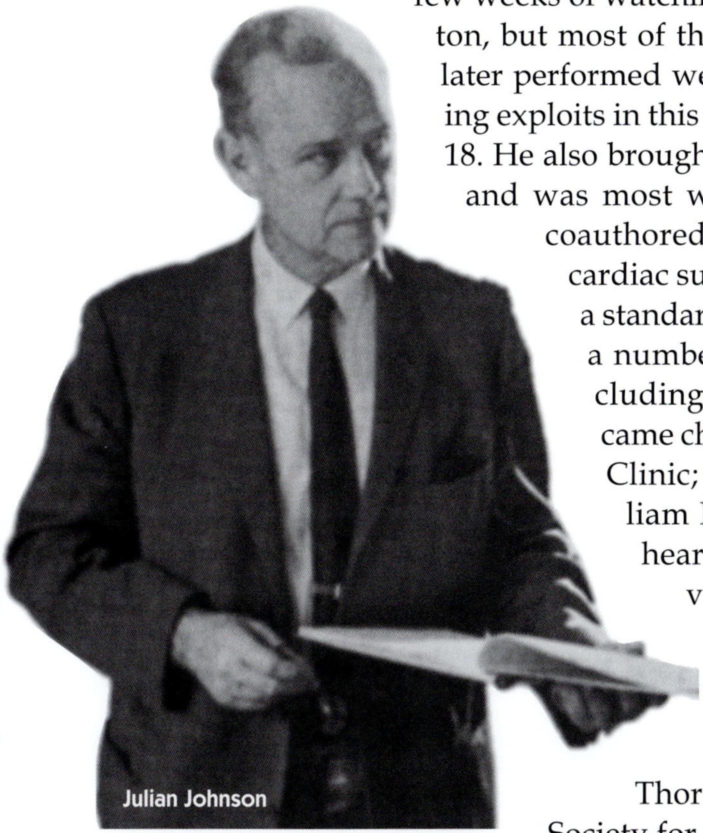
Julian Johnson

After Johnson's understudy, Charles Kirby, died unexpectedly, Dr. Rhoads recruited one of Penn Surgery's most interesting young stars, ostensibly as Johnson's helper. He turned out to be much more.

John Waldhausen was born in New York City in 1929. His parents were German, and as World War II began, they were called home, taking with them their young son. The Waldhausens' aristocratic family background of German military leaders stretched back to generations before either world war. John's privileged childhood was easy until 1944 when he was sent to the Western Front as a noncombatant child, where he was relegated to digging foxholes and tank traps.[25]

When the war ended, he finished high school and passed the Arbitur, which qualified him for university. Determined to return to America, he bartered his prize Märklin electric train set for 900 cigarettes. Their sale to a Polish soldier paid for his passage to New York, where at age seventeen

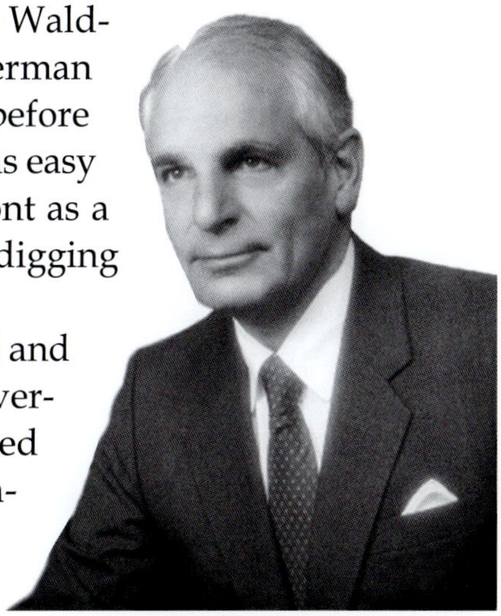
John Waldhausen

he landed, penniless and alone.[26] With the advice and help of an American Army chaplain friend, he secured admittance to a small college in Montana. To support himself, he worked as an orderly in a local hospital and became interested in medicine. He was admitted to medical school at St. Louis University where he was inspired by Hopkins-trained heart surgeon, Rollo Hanlon, who became his lifelong mentor and friend. Hanlon aided his successful application to internship at Hopkins. As a junior resident at Hopkins and fellow at NIH, Waldhausen had an important role in developing Hopkins' first open-heart program. But this was not enough to win him a chief residency in Hopkins' Halsted-style pyramid. To his devastation, he was cut by surgery chairman Blalock. The support of other friends at Hopkins (Frank Spencer, Jim Maloney, and Hank Bahnson) induced Jonathan Rhoads to accept him as a senior resident at HUP. After three years, he was attracted by Harry Shoemaker to Indiana University as chief resident and then in 1962, to the faculty.

After four years at Indiana, Dr. Rhoads brought Waldhausen back to the HUP faculty as associate professor. Chick Koop appointed him chief of pediatric cardiac surgery at CHOP where he developed one of the country's premier programs.[27] He soon emerged as one of American surgery's stars. During his five years at Penn, he was also the most approachable and supportive faculty mentor of young surgeons, including me. He then moved again to become the inaugural chairman of surgery at the new Penn State School of Medicine in Hershey, Pennsylvania. He later also served there as provost and dean. Waldhausen became president of the Society of Clinical Surgery and the American Association for Thoracic Surgery, and editor of the *Journal of Thoracic and Cardiovascular Surgery*. For some years, Waldhausen contended with ischemic heart disease. After surviving two of the country's earliest coronary artery bypass operations and several cardiac arrests reversed successfully by an internal defibrillator, he died in 2012.

After finishing his training under Johnson in 1965, HUP resident Horace MacVaugh joined the faculty. Johnson elected not to initiate coronary artery surgery, so Horace did HUP's first coronary artery bypasses. He was recognized as an exceptionally fine technical surgeon, and by the time Johnson retired in 1973, he had the largest cardiac surgery practice in town. It was assumed that he would be Johnson's successor as division chief. Instead, the new department chairman, Bill Fitts, recruited L. Henry Edmunds to head the CT division. Edmunds was an MGH-trained, seriously dedicated, and versatile academic surgeon with a national reputation based on several productive years on

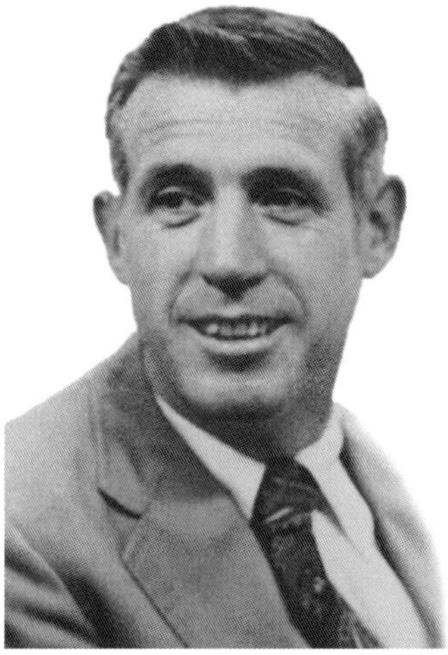

Henry Edmunds

the faculty at UCSF. Fitts assumed that Edmunds's academic approach and research would bolster Penn Surgery's status more than the appointment of a local candidate with a big practice, like MacVaugh. Fitts was right. MacVaugh was disappointed but found solace in taking his practice to a series of other institutions including Jefferson, Lankenau, and Graduate Hospitals.

At Penn, Edmunds became one of the country's foremost leaders in cardiac surgery. I ranked him as the department's best academic surgeon. He was substantially productive in a number of areas. As a scientist, Edmunds made seminal contributions to the understanding of bloodsurface interactions.[28] He was also an important founder of cardiac surgical translational research and the use of large animal models.[29] In 1985, he started HUP's heart transplant program. He was funded by the NIH continuously for over thirty-five years and is also known for a standard textbook of cardiac surgery, illustrated by David Low, a Penn surgeon and artist.[30] Edmunds also headed pediatric cardiac surgery at CHOP after the short tenures of John Waldhausen and Eoin Aberdeen.

Edmunds built one of the best known and most productive heart surgery teams anywhere. He trained or recruited to his faculty a number of important cardiac surgeons including Larry Stephenson, who became chief of cardiothoracic surgery at Wayne State; Dick Edie, who became chief of cardiothoracic surgery at Jefferson; Alden Harken, who became chairman of surgery at the University of Colorado; Paul Addonizio, who became chief of CT surgery at Temple; Verdi DiSesa, who became chief of cardiothoracic surgery at Rush; Chuck Bridges, who became chief of CT surgery at Pennsylvania Hospital; and Rob and Joe Gorman, who made important contributions to the development of heart valves. A review of Edmunds's bibliography indicates that he was an important mentor of multiple generations of the HUP residents and young faculty. To the above list should be added John Macoviak, Joe Bavaria, Mark Ratcliffe, Clark Hargrove, Satoshi Furukawa, Ed Savage, Steve Downey, Ben Jackson, and Larry Kaiser, whom he advised me to recruit in 1992 to start the lung transplant program. Kaiser became chairman of surgery at Penn and later, dean and CEO at Temple.

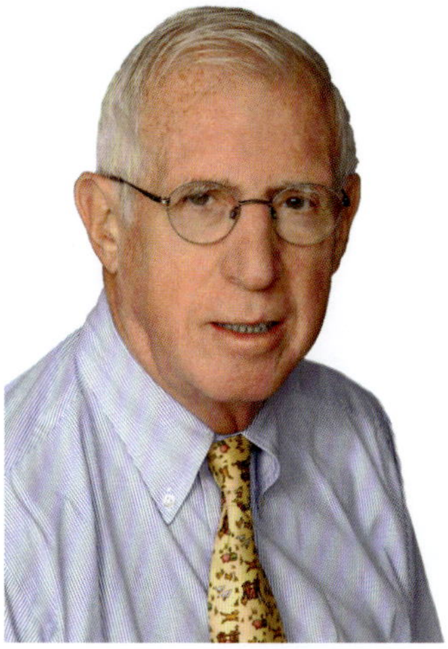
Henry Edmunds

After finishing twenty years as CT division chief, Edmunds turned his attention to an equally important task, becoming editor-in-chief of the *Annals of Thoracic Surgery.* From 2000 to 2015, he greatly increased the journal's quality and reputation, making it the dominant journal in the field.

In 1993, Timothy Gardner was recruited from Johns Hopkins to succeed Edmunds as

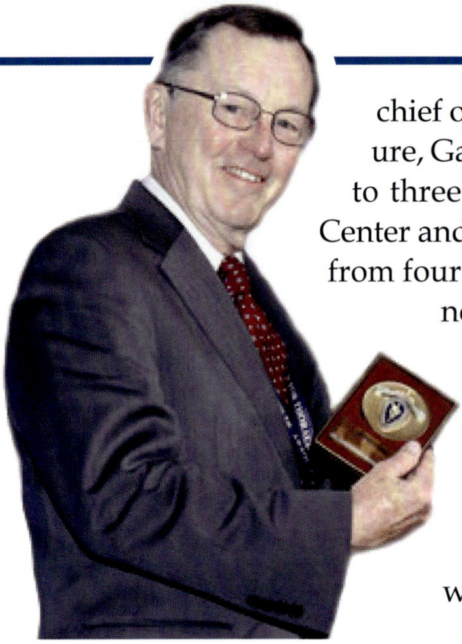

Tim Gardner with AATS Lifetime Achievement Award.

chief of Penn's CT division. During his ten-year tenure, Gardner greatly expanded CT surgery from one to three sites, including Penn Presbyterian Medical Center and Pennsylvania Hospital. The CT faculty grew from four cardiac surgeons to eleven. To CHOP, Gardner recruited Thomas Spray, who became the president of the AATS, and William Gaynor.

Gardner had an important national presence. He served as a councilor, vice president, and then president of the American Association for Thoracic Surgery. He was a director of the American Board of Thoracic Surgery for ten years and served as the board's vice chair and chair from 2001 to 2005. Dr. Gardner also served as an IPA medical officer in the Division of Cardiovascular Diseases at the National Heart, Lung and Blood Institute at National Institutes of Health from 2004 to 2007. He has also been steering committee chair for the Cardiothoracic Surgery Clinical Trials Network sponsored by the National Heart, Lung and Blood Institute. In 2015, Gardner was honored by being named the AATS' Lifetime Achievement Awardee.

Gardner's trainees included Roy Smythe, who became chairman of surgery at Texas A&M; Blair Marshall, who became chief of thoracic surgery at Georgetown; John Kucharczuk, who became chief of general thoracic surgery at HUP; Tom Gleason, who became chief of cardiac surgery at the University of Pittsburgh; Joe Woo, who became chairman of the department of CT surgery at Stanford; and Sloane Guy, chief of CT surgery at Temple and Jefferson.

In 1993 when Gardner came to Penn, he brought with him a former HUP resident whose CT training was at Hopkins, Michael Acker. In 2003, Acker succeeded Gardner as chief of the division. While he was a HUP resident, Acker had done some beautiful experiments with faculty surgeon, Larry Stephenson, showing that electrical pulses could convert fast-twitch skeletal muscle into fatigue-resistant, slow-twitch muscle.[31] In *Science,* they reported that modified skeletal muscles could contract for years and might be used for replacing or augmenting parts of a failing heart.[32] Stephenson continued to work on this model after he became chief of cardiac surgery at Wayne State University.

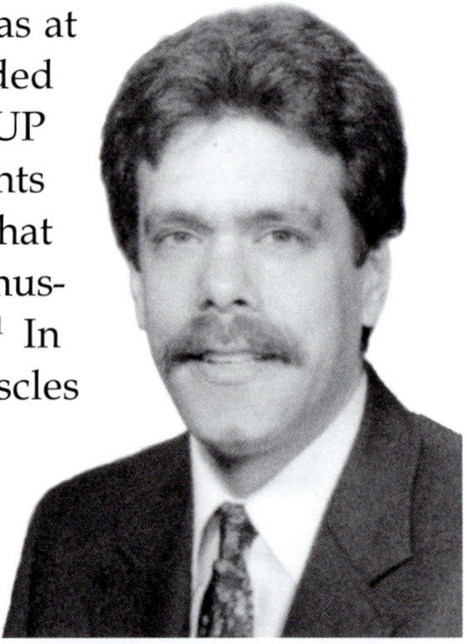

Mike Acker

Acker, who has been president of the AATS, continues to lead Penn's CT surgery. His division has an international reputation for innovation and excellence in complex aortic surgery, ventricular assist devices, transplantation, and minimally invasive valve surgery.[33] Acker is another example of Altemeier's rule. He is not only a virtuoso in clinical heart surgery, but also a professional-level classical guitarist. He often speaks about the parallels between music and surgery in requiring practice, precision, and passion.

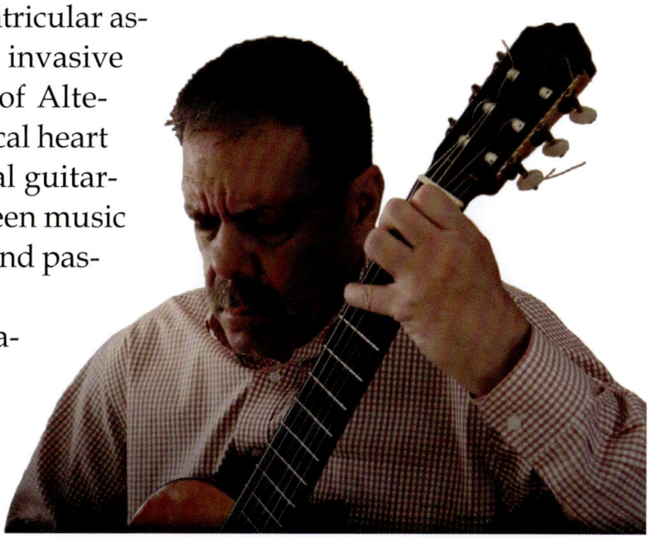
Heart surgeon and classical guitarist, Mike Acker

Vice chief of the CT division is Joseph Bavaria, a national and international leader in the field of endovascular thoracic aortic surgery and transcatheter aortic valve replacement.[34] He is past president of the Society of Thoracic Surgery. Other members of the division are Wilson Szeto, who is chief of CT surgery at Presbyterian as well as director of transcatheter cardioaortic therapy; Satoshi Furukowa, chief of CT surgery at Pennsylvania Hospital; Nimesh Desai, director of thoracic aortic research and codirector of Penn Aorta Center; Pavan Atluri, director of minimally invasive, robotic, cardiac transplantation and mechanical circulatory assist program; Christian Bermudez, director of thoracic transplantation and ECMO; Chase Brown, director of coronary revascularization, Presbyterian Hospital; Marisa Cevasco; Michael Ibrahim, director of mitral and reconstructive valve surgery, Presbyterian Hospital; Jeremy McGarvey; and Clark Hargrove, a master surgeon who is the senior member of the division.

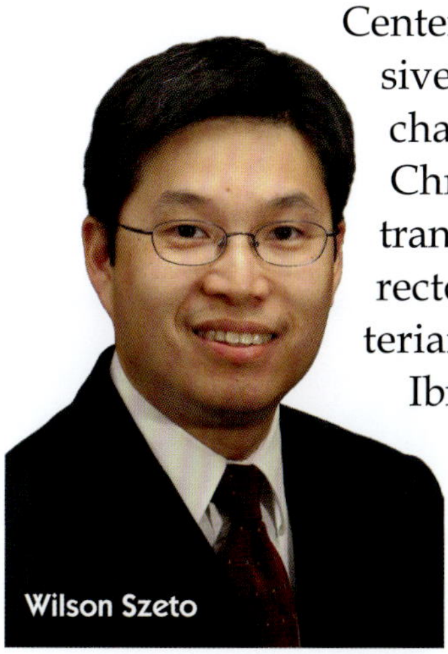
Wilson Szeto

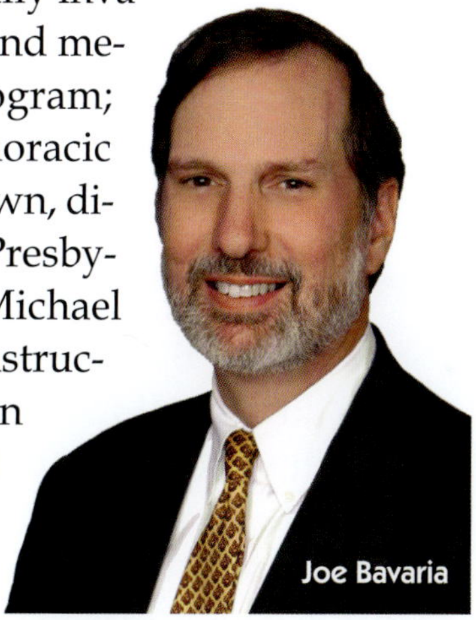
Joe Bavaria

At CHOP, Bill Norwood, Thomas Spray, and William Gaynor have been world-renowned figures in heart surgery for children.

Division of Vascular and Endovascular Surgery

In the late 1930s and early 1940s, Julian Johnson did a few vascular operations, but it was not called a division. A vascular division might well have been started at that time by young HUP faculty surgeon Norman Freeman, who was probably the first US surgeon to devote his attention entirely to vascular disease. At HUP, he started a vascular lab and clinic and did careful physiological studies but few vascular operations. In 1943, Freeman went to India as an important member of Ravdin's 20th General Hospital, but because of a disagreement with

Ravdin, he was not appointed to HUP's postwar faculty. This was too bad because Freeman became a pioneer of the vascular field. In fact, after the war as a faculty member at UCSF, Freeman did several of the world's first vascular procedures, including the first successful resection of an abdominal aortic aneurysm in 1951. His unfortunately lost history is detailed in Chapter 15.

A more familiar version of the origin of Penn's vascular division was Dr. Ravdin's post-World War II choice of his resident, Brooke Roberts, as the faculty member to start that specialty.[35] At first, Brooke's vascular activity was mostly treatment of varicose veins, but by the early 1960s, the prevalence of arterial disease was such that Brooke was kept busy entirely by his practice of vascular operations, such as resection of aneurysms and bypasses of occluded peripheral arteries.

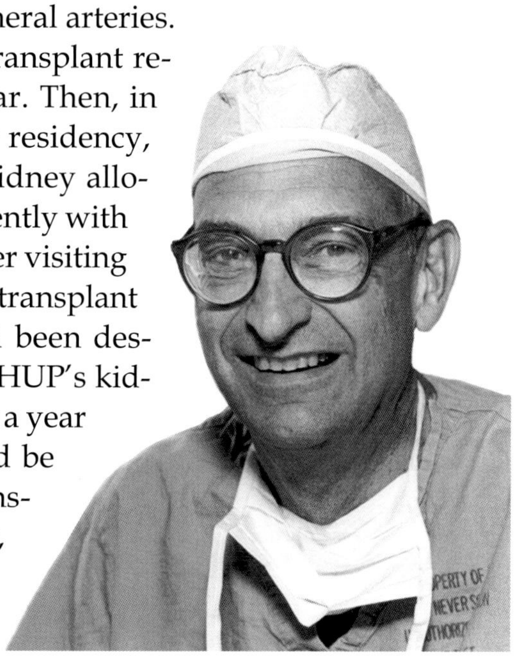
Brooke Roberts

In 1963, only a handful of kidney transplant recipients had survived as long as a year. Then, in 1964, as I finished my general surgery residency, Tom Starzl showed that rejection of kidney allografts could be prevented quite consistently with proper use of immunosuppression. After visiting Starzl in Denver, I decided to become a transplant surgeon. Because Brooke Roberts had been designated as the faculty member to start HUP's kidney transplant program, I signed up for a year as his fellow, anticipating that I would be with him when he did HUP's first transplant. But during my fellowship year, Brooke didn't get a transplant done. Instead, he offered me a job as his junior colleague in what now became a two-man vascular division. Chapter 27 explains how I eventually got to be a transplant surgeon and do HUP's first kidney transplant in 1966.

In addition to his large practice, Brooke established and directed the only vascular fellowship in Philadelphia and one of the first in the United States. I was his second fellow; Harry Nelson was the first. He trained a number of other fellows who went on to populate vascular programs around the country, including Leo Frangipane, Richard Spence, George Volpetti, R. DiGiovanni, Gary Nicholas, Art Baker, Ali Naji, Henry Berkowitz, and Peter McCombs, who later became chief of surgery at Pennsylvania Hospital and the VA Hospital.

In 1971 Henry Berkowitz was recruited as the third of the division's vascular surgeons. Henry built a large practice of vascular surgery and also started one of the first vascular laboratories. Next to join the vascular as well as the transplant division was Leonard Perloff in 1975 (see Chapter 33). Summarized in Chapter 25 are Brooke's substantial accomplishments, including his collaboration with Ernie Ring and other HUP interventional radiologists in balloon dilatation of stenotic arteries.[36] This was actually the beginning of a new field—endovascular surgery.

When Brooke retired in 1982, I succeeded him as head of the vascular division and director of the vascular fellowship. Ron Fairman was my first fellow. A year later, I was named department chairman. I also continued as director of the vascular division until 2001, and during that time trained a number of vascular surgeons and recruited several of them and others to the vascular faculty. These trainees and faculty members included Mike Golden; Jeff Carpenter, now chairman at Rowan University; Ron Fairman, who started the endovascular program and became chief of the division and president of the Society for Vascular Surgery; and Marc Mitchell, who became chairman of surgery at the University of Mississippi.[37]

Ronald Fairman graduated from Muhlenberg College and Jefferson Medical College and had his internship, general, and vascular surgical training at HUP. After spending ten years in very successful private practice at Jeanes Hospital, Ron came back to HUP and started over. Despite being ten years behind in an academic career, he was soon a remarkable success. In 2001, he became chief of the Division of Vascular Surgery and Endovascular Therapy and vice-chairman for clinical affairs at Penn. He performed HUP's first endovascular abdominal aortic aneurysm repairs (EVAR), endovascular thoracic aortic aneurysm repairs (TEVAR), and carotid stents with distal protection to prevent stroke. He developed one of the largest endovascular programs in the country. He has served as a principal investigator (PI) for every FDA-approved EVAR clinical device and as National or Global PI for more than eight pivotal EVAR trials. He has also been the National PI for multiple pivotal TEVAR trials and was PI for the first FDA-approved carotid stent platform with distal protection to prevent stroke. He began the fenestrated aortic stent graft program at Penn in 2005 and

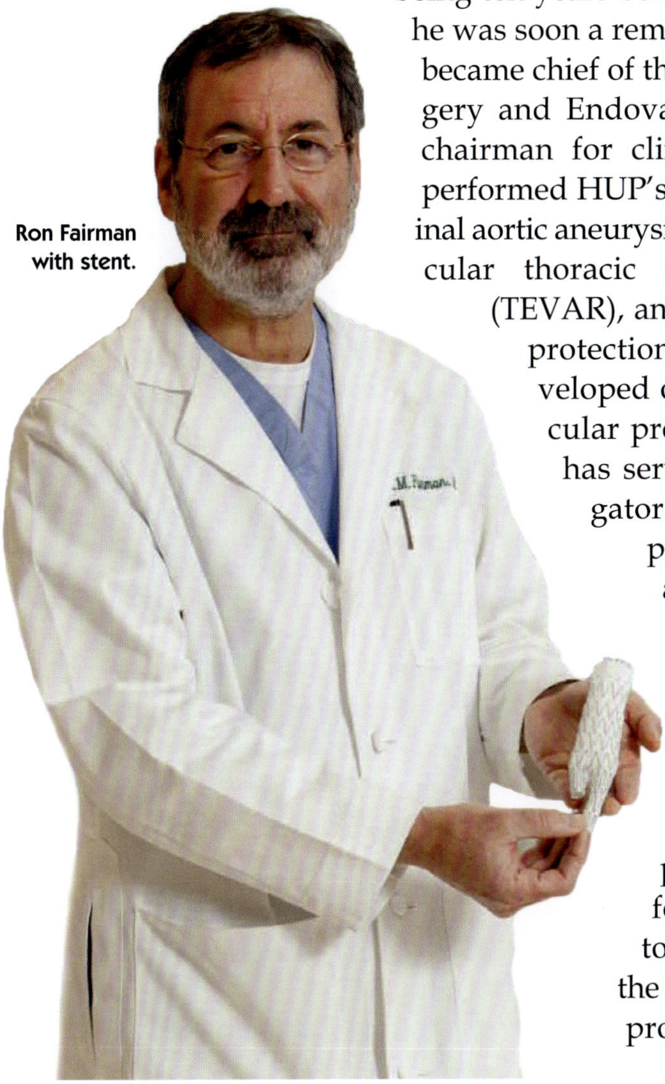

Ron Fairman with stent.

performed the first branched stent graft device at Penn. He has performed well over seventy clinical trials since the mid-1990s and has served as PI for virtually all of them. In 2010, he was named Penn's Luigi Mastroianni Clinical Innovator Awardee. In 2015, he received the University of Pennsylvania Health System Master Clinician Award. Until his retirement in 2019, he maintained a large clinical practice, balancing traditional open and endovascular procedures. His vascular fellowship was highly sought after. In his tenure as division chief, he mentored ten fellows who have become division chiefs or department chairmen at major academic institutions. Ben Jackson was the first to finish his HUP vascular fellowship under Dr. Fairman. He was then recruited to the division's faculty. An exceptional clinician, he also served as the director of the fellowship. In 2022, Dr. Jackson left HUP to become chief of vascular surgery at Lehigh Valley Heart and Vascular Institute.

Dr. Fairman was a frequent invited lecturer at both national and international scientific meetings. In 2017, he served as president of the Society for Vascular Surgery. He is a member of the Halsted Society, the American College of Surgeons, the Society for Clinical Vascular Surgery, and the American Surgical Association. He has published over 250 peer-reviewed manuscripts and over 100 book chapters and reviews. He is on the editorial board of most major vascular surgical and endovascular journals. He is assistant editor for reviews of the *Journal for Vascular Surgery.* In 2008, he became the Barker/Measey endowed professor. In 2016, he was elected to membership in the American Philosophical Society, a rare honor for a physician and surgeon.

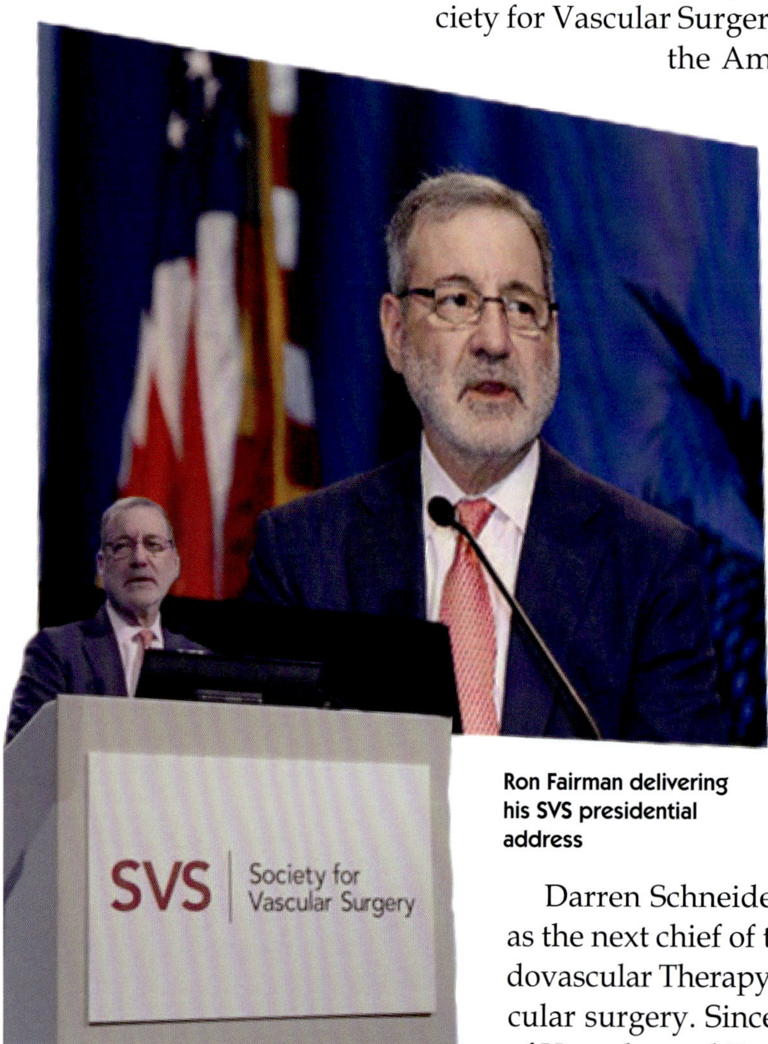

Ron Fairman delivering his SVS presidential address

In 2019, Ron Fairman retired from surgery, though still in full possession of his powers. He chose to reinvent himself again. Since then, he has served the FDA's devices section in evaluating new vascular grafts.

Darren Schneider was recruited to succeed Dr. Fairman as the next chief of the Division of Vascular Surgery and Endovascular Therapy. Dr. Schneider is a national leader in vascular surgery. Since 2010, he had been chief of the Division of Vascular and Endovascular Surgery at New York Presbyterian Hospital and Weill Cornell Medical School.

He attended Stanford University and obtained his medical degree from the University of California, San Diego. He was a resident in

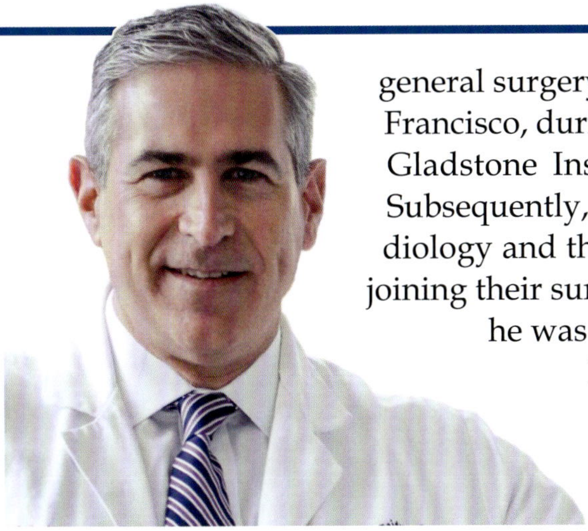
Darren Schneider

general surgery at the University of California, San Francisco, during which he spent three years at the Gladstone Institutes of Cardiovascular Disease. Subsequently, he was a fellow in interventional radiology and then vascular surgery at UCSF before joining their surgery faculty for eight years. In 2010, he was recruited to Cornell.

Dr. Schneider has made numerous contributions to clinical research. He was the national principal investigator for the pivotal, multicenter trial that led to FDA approval of an iliac branch stent graft for iliac artery aneurysms. He is the principal investigator of an ongoing study of endovascular repair of thoracoabdominal aortic aneurysms, using branched and fenestrated stent grafts. He has over 100 publications, twenty-eight chapters/reviews, and over 150 national/international presentations.

Dr. Schneider's numerous leadership roles include presidency of the Northern California Vascular Society and the New York Society for Vascular Surgery. He is on the executive councils of the Eastern Vascular Society and International College of Angiology. He is a distinguished fellow of the Society for Vascular Surgery and is a worthy successor to Dr. Fairman as division chief.

Additional members of Dr. Schneider's division are Venkat Kalapatapu, the division's residency and fellowship director; Grace Wang, director of the vascular lab; Nathan Belkin; Keith Calligaro, chief of vascular surgery, Pennsylvania Hospital; Scott Damrauer, the division's most active basic scientist; Alexander Fairman, in addition to HUP, head of vascular surgery at CHOP; Elizabeth Anne Genevese; Julia Glaser; Shang Loh, chief of vascular surgery at Presbyterian; Douglas Troutman; Mark Mantell, director of vascular access; and Matthew Dougherty.

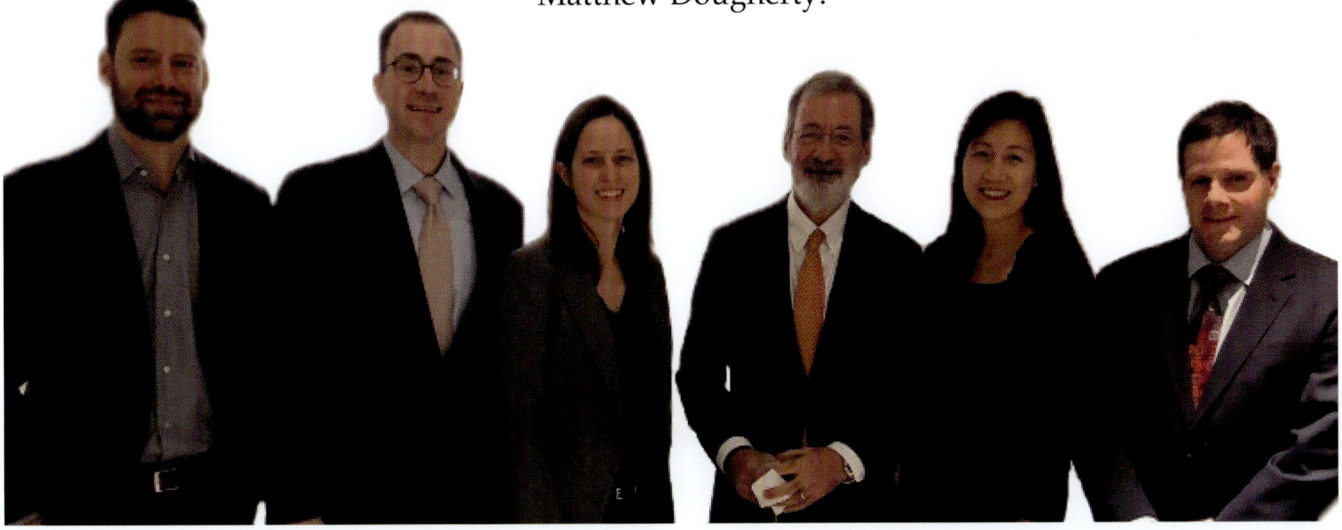
Alex Fairman, Scott Damrauer, Julia Glaser, Ron Fairman, Grace Wang and Ben Jackson

Transplantation Division

Transplantation at HUP began in February 1966 with a kidney transplant. The recipient, Howard Mehl, survived with normal renal function for forty-eight years until he died in his sleep from a myocardial infarction. Since I did the transplant and was the division's director until 2001, much of the division's early history is my story (see Chapter 27). This chapter is mainly devoted to the important contributions of others. For its first ten years, I was the division's only faculty member, but I had the help of a series of remarkable HUP residents who chose to spend their research years in my lab. At the same time as they were doing basic experiments, they worked day, night, and weekends with me as clinical fellows. Listed in order, they were Leonard Perloff, Howard Silberman, Craig Reckard, Mory Ziegler, Steve Bartlett, Ali Naji, Don Dafoe, and Ken Brayman. Remarkably, they all became national leaders in academic transplant surgery at a variety of universities. In 1975, a second faculty member joined the division. This was Len Perloff. He became one of Penn's most accomplished teachers. As the clinical volume continued to grow, Ali Naji and Ken Brayman were added to the division's faculty. Basic research remained a major focus, and the division's national and international reputation grew.

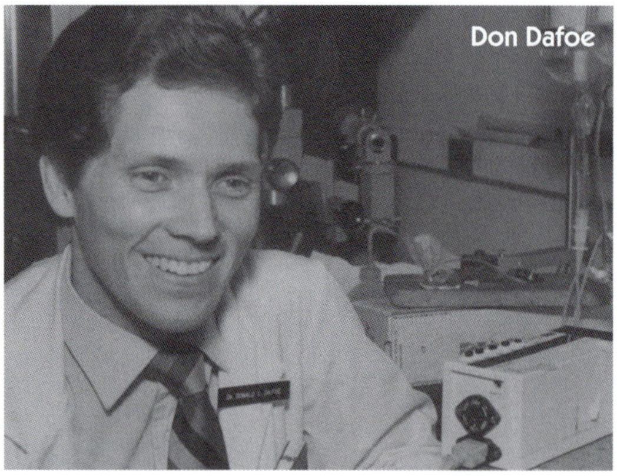
Don Dafoe

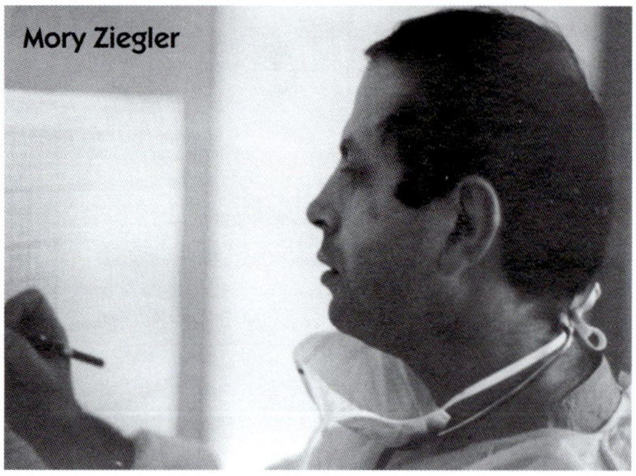
Mory Ziegler

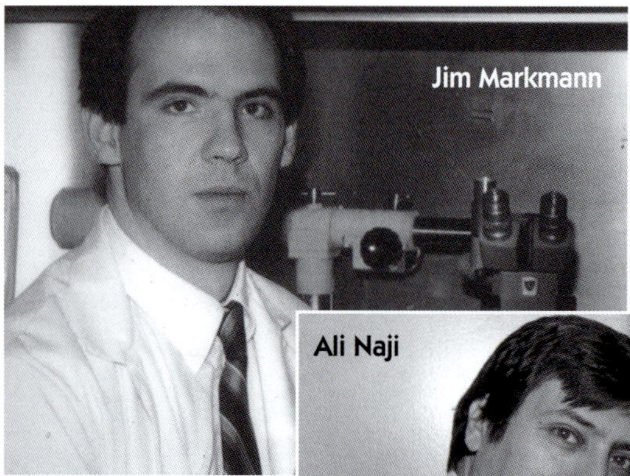
Jim Markmann

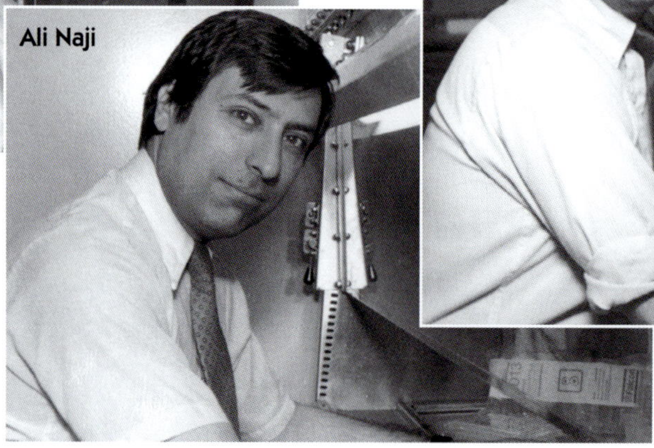
Ali Naji

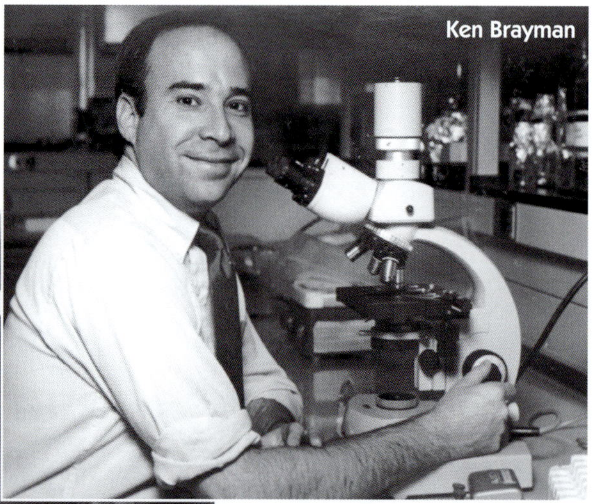
Ken Brayman

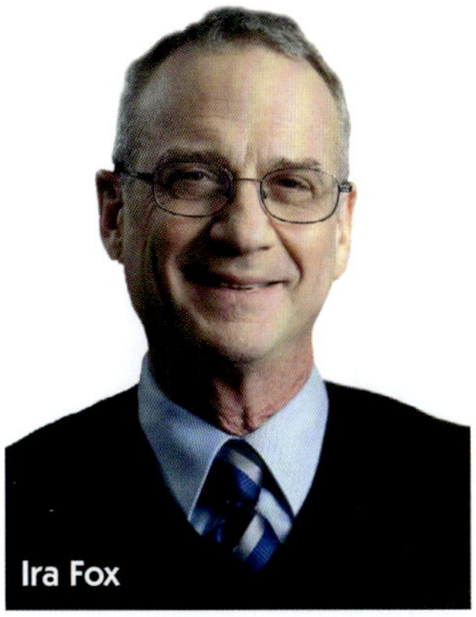

Ira Fox

In 1985, Starzl trainee Ira Fox was recruited to initiate liver transplantation. Over the next ten years, a satisfactory but modest volume program evolved. Don Dafoe was recruited to the faculty from Michigan, and he became the liver transplant leader and briefly the division chief before moving to Stanford in 1998. Mory Ziegler also managed HUP's kidney transplant program for several years while also starting liver transplantation at CHOP.

Remarkably, there were six future university chairs from HUP residents who served part or all of their research fellowships in this division.

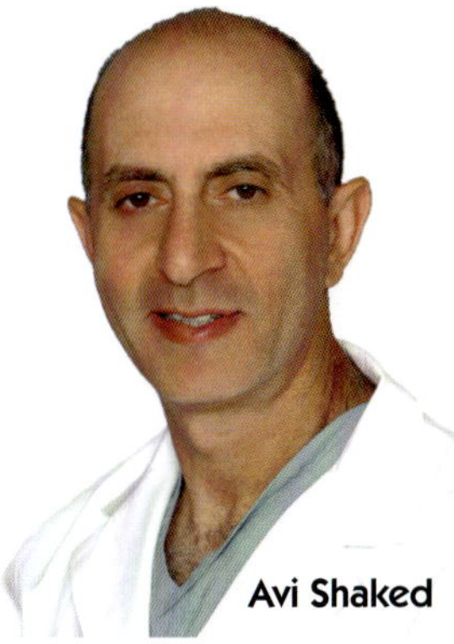

Avi Shaked

In 1985, Avi Shaked and Kim Olthoff were recruited to the faculty, greatly increasing the volume of the liver program.[38] They became leaders in the field and both were elected president of the American Society of Transplant Surgery. In 1998, recruitment of Jim Markmann bolstered the division's liver transplant and research programs.[39] With Ali Naji in 2001, he started a successful human islet transplant program.[40] When I retired as chairman in 2001, Dr. Shaked became the chief of the division and shortly thereafter Director of a new Transplantation Institute. Kim Olthoff then became and remains chief of the division. Since added to the faculty are Peter Abt, who serves as the fellowship program director; Matt Levine, active in basic research as well as a clinician; and Ty Dunn who has special experience in pancreatic transplantation.

Kim Olthoff

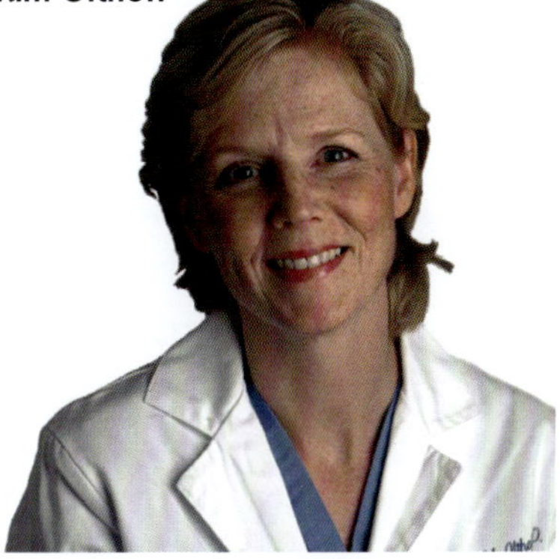

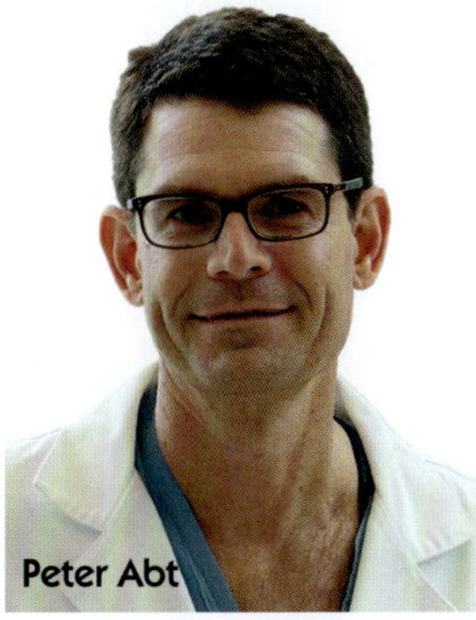

Peter Abt

Page Porrett, Penn PhD, resident, and transplant fellow, performed at HUP the country's third uterus transplant in 2019. After seven years on the Penn faculty, she was recruited in 2020 as Director of Clinical and Translational Research at the University of Alabama.[41] Bob Redman after three years on the faculty,

Matt Levine

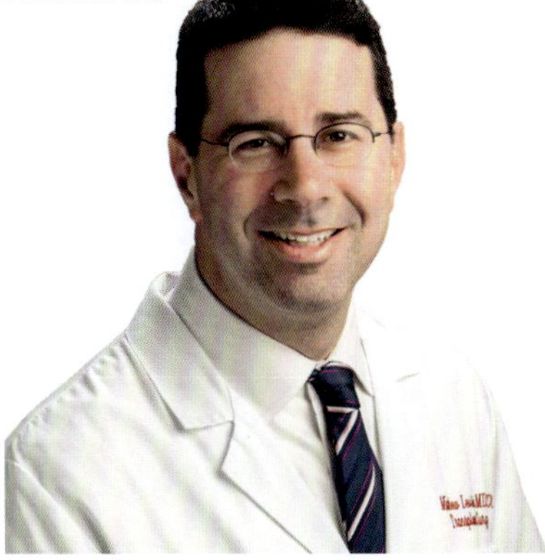

Ty Dunn

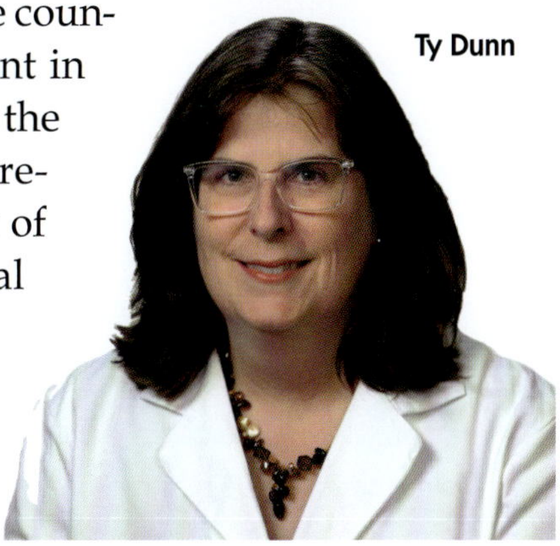

left to become Chief of Transplantation at the University of California, Irvine. All of the current members of this division are members of the American Surgical Association, and all have had NIH research funding. Ali Naji has several times had the most NIH funding of any American surgeon.

Division of Trauma, Critical Care, and Emergency Surgery

Jonathan Rhoads and William Fitts were both considered leading trauma experts. They occupied the top positions in the field as editors of the *Journal of Trauma* and presidents of the field's national societies. However, at HUP, neither had much chance for experience in trauma because there were almost no patients there with traumatic injuries. That changed in 1985 when I was urged by Dean Stemmler to develop a trauma center. The difficulty and eventual success I had in finding a director for the new division of trauma is reviewed in Chapter 32.

Bill Schwab, the inaugural chief of the division, rapidly earned an international reputation in this field. His development of the concept of damage control changed the management of trauma victims worldwide (see chapter 34). In 2005, Dr. Schwab stepped down as chief of the division and after a national search was succeeded by Pat Reilly.

Under Dr. Reilly, the trauma division has continued to thrive. Pat Reilly graduated from Notre Dame and Jefferson Medical College. He was a resident in general surgery at the Medical Center of Delaware and completed a research fellowship at Johns Hopkins. After a fellowship in trauma and critical care at Penn, he joined the faculty in 1995 and was promoted to professor in 2009 and to division chief in 2011. In 2017, he became the C. William Schwab Professor in the Division of Traumatology, Surgical Critical Care, and Emergency Surgery. He has had an illustrious career with over 200 published articles and numerous awards including a Penn Pearl and the Lewis Duhring Outstanding Clinical Specialist Award. He was selected for the inaugural class of Penn's Academy of Master Clinicians and elected to the American Surgical Association.

Dr. Reilly has been President of the Eastern Association for the Surgery of Trauma and in 2023 will be the President of the American Association for the Surgery of Trauma. His division con-

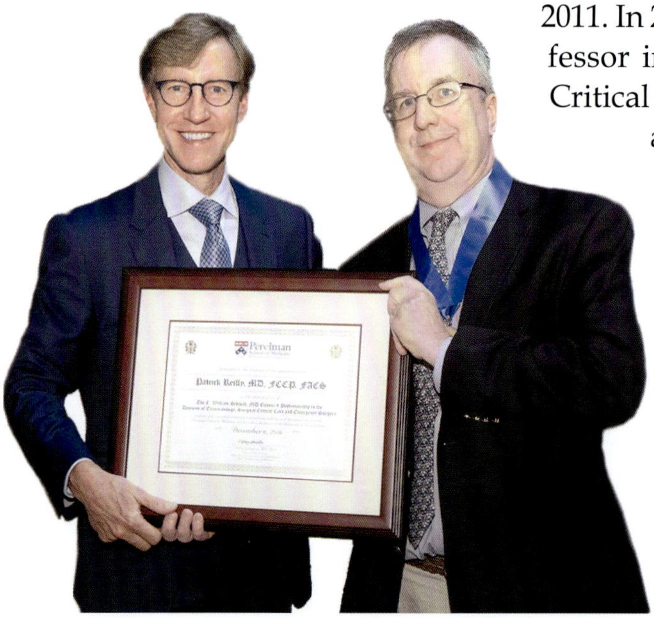

Dean Larry Jameson with Pat Reilly, recipient of the C. William Schwab, MD Endowed Professorship tinues to be a premier group in the country, and he has trained many leaders in the field.

After more than twenty-five years and caring for over 50,000 patients at HUP, Penn's Level 1 Trauma Center relocated to the Penn Presbyterian campus in 2015. A new building was constructed to accommodate this move. Pat Kim, the trauma program medical director, and John Gallagher, the trauma program manager, provided input for the building's design, and Dr. Schwab was the senior consultant.

The new five-story building is truly high tech and state of the art. The first floor houses the John Paul Pryor Shock Trauma and Resuscitation Unit, which has five large trauma bays and two ultrahigh speed CT scanners. The second floor contains a perioperative space and post-anesthesia care units. The third floor is the cardiovascular ICU. The fourth floor is the trauma surgical ICU where injured and other critically ill patients are managed under the leadership of Niels Martin and Jack Gutsche, the comedical directors of the trauma SICU. Finally, a new heavy-duty helipad was built to handle the increasingly larger helicopters used by regional flight programs. The helipad supports the trauma program as well as interhospital transport of patients.

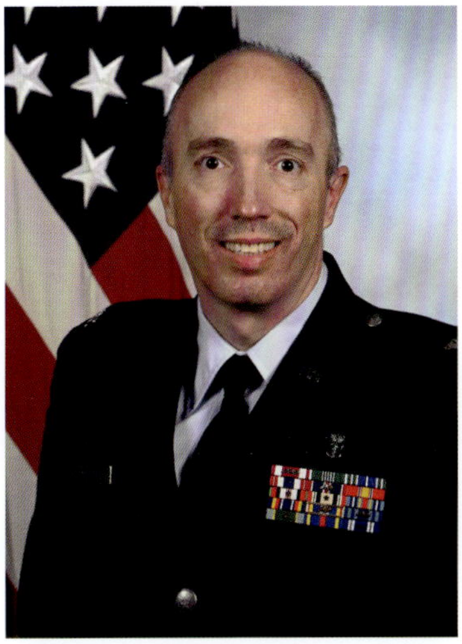

Jeremy Cannon

The Penn Trauma faculty now split their time between the two campuses, with surgical critical care and emergency surgery still functioning at HUP.

At Presbyterian, Jeremy Cannon is medical director and trauma section chief. After graduating from the Air Force Academy and Harvard Medical School, he obtained a master's degree in mechanical engineering from MIT. He then served three tours as an Army trauma surgeon in Afghanistan and Iraq before joining the Penn faculty in 2015. In 2019, he was promoted to colonel in the Air Force Reserves.

Additional faculty members of the trauma division are Gary Bass, Ben Braslow, Elinore Kaufman, Jose Pascual, Shariq Raza, Mark Seamon, Catherine Sharoky, Adam Shiroff, and Lewis Kaplan who is also chief of surgery at the VA Hospital.

Division of Colon and Rectal Surgery

Larry Kaiser started this youngest of the department's divisions in 2002 with the recruitment of Bob Fry as its chief.[42] Trained in surgery at Washington University and in colorectal surgery at Cleveland Clinic, Fry had been a faculty member at Washington University for nine years and division chief at Jefferson for eight years. In 2004, he was president of the American Board of Colon and Rectal Surgery and from 1991 to 1994, president of the Program Directors of Colon and Rectal Surgery.

At Penn from 2002 to 2013, in addition to his role as chief of the Division of Colon and Rectal Surgery, Dr. Fry was chair of surgery at Pennsylvania Hospital. In 2013 while he was still active as a clinical surgeon and division chief, he chose to retire with a plan to become a full-time writer. He had brought Najjia Mahmoud with him from Jefferson to Penn as a junior member of his division. In 2013, she succeeded him as chief of the Division of Colon and Rectal Surgery.

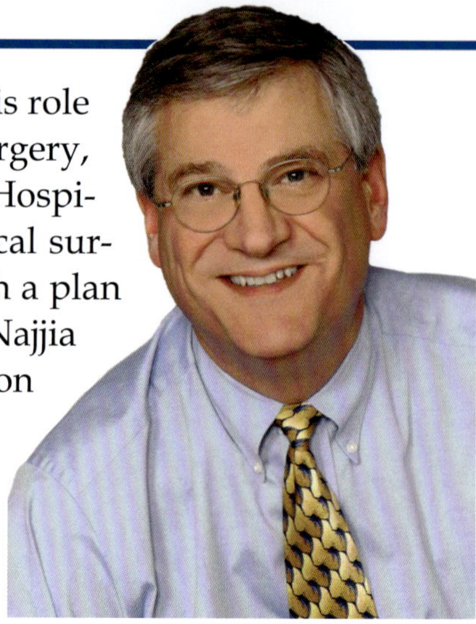

Bob Fry

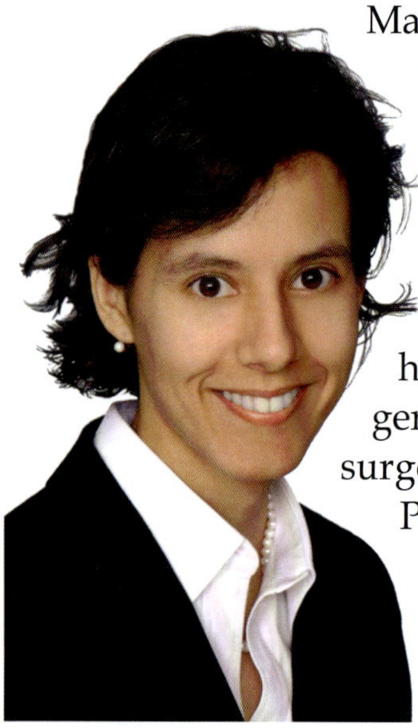

Najjia Mahmoud

Dr. Mahmoud received her MD at Cornell in 1993 and did her residency in surgery at New York Hospital and her fellowship in colorectal surgery at the University of Minnesota before joining the Penn faculty in 2001.[43] Since 2012, she has been the Emilie and Roland T. deHellebranth Professor of Surgery. She is a member of the American Surgical Association and the Halsted Society, and in 2020 was president of the American Board of Colon and Rectal Surgery. During a distinguished career, she has greatly increased the number of surgeons on her division's faculty, which now includes Cary Aarons, Joshua Bleier, Lillias Maguire, Erica Pettke, and Nicole Saur.

A footnote to this division's history is the career of an important Penn surgeon, John Rombeau.[44] As a certified colorectal surgeon, he was one of the department's first specialists. He was recruited to the faculty by Len Miller in 1979, twenty-two years before there was a formal colorectal division. Thus, for his two-decade career at Penn, he was independent.

John Rombeau is a Californian and graduated from Loma Linda Medical School in 1967. After surgical residency at USC (1971–1975), he served a fellowship in colorectal surgery at the Cleveland Clinic. In 1979, he joined the Penn surgery faculty, becoming a full professor in 1994. For twenty-two years, in addition to practicing surgery at HUP, he was a mainstay of the teaching service at the VA and also had a very productive research laboratory. He won multiple teaching awards and mentored in his lab a number of HUP residents, including Ron DeMatteo, Omaida Ve-

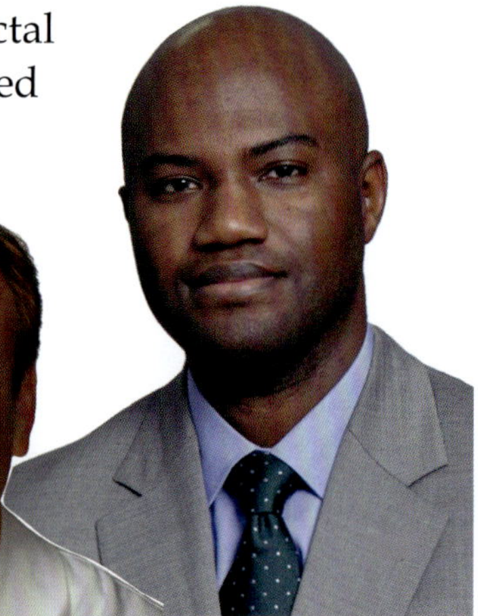

Cary Aarons

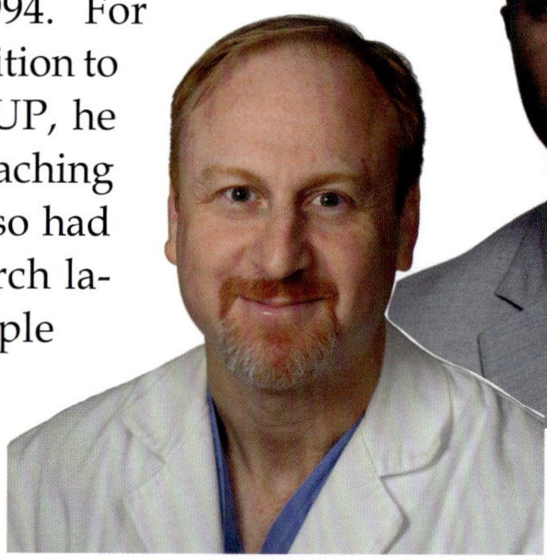

Josh Bleier

lazquez, Danny O. Jacobs, Mark Koruda, Scott Kripke, and Dan Dempsey. His research was largely devoted to metabolism and nutrition. He was a widely recognized authority on enteral and parenteral intravenous nutrition, authoring more than 100 papers and a dozen books on this topic. Additional areas of his research are inflammatory bowel disease and fuels of intestinal cells, including glutamine, pectin, butynate, and short chain fatty acids.

He is a member of the Society of University Surgeons and the American Surgical Association. He was president of the American Society of Parenteral and Enteral Nutrition in 1988, and in 2005 he was president of the Philadelphia Academy of Surgery.

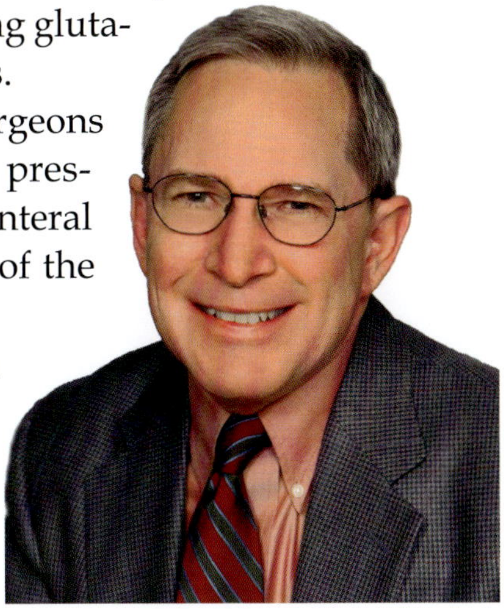

John Rombeau

In 1997, with Donna Muldoon, Jonathan Rhoads's administrative assistant, he wrote a detailed biography of Dr. Rhoads based on extensive interviews with him.[45] In 2002, he was invited by Dan Dempsey to join the Temple faculty where he continued to be active clinically and in research. While at Temple, he wrote a book on surgical mentoring. In 2005, he retired to his native California where he has taught part-time in Stanford's surgical program.

Plastic Surgery

Contributed by Linton Whitaker

The beginning of plastic surgery at the University of Pennsylvania, and in the United States, was in the early 1900s.[46] It was started by Robert H. Ivy, who had graduated from dental school and subsequently medical school at Penn. He was influenced by operations by Sir Harold Gillies in England during World War I in the repair of major posttraumatic defects, as well as those from birth and tumors. Ivy focused on treatment of facial problems and after the war, brought this interest and expertise to Penn. In 1921, he established a preceptorship at the Graduate and Children's Hospitals, one of the first in the US. The American Board of Plastic Surgery was not founded until 1936, and training at Penn in plastic surgery remained a preceptorship until

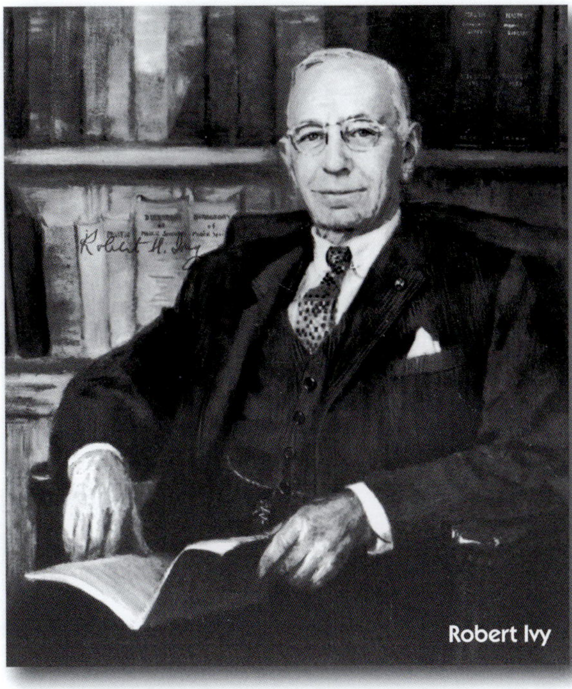

Robert Ivy

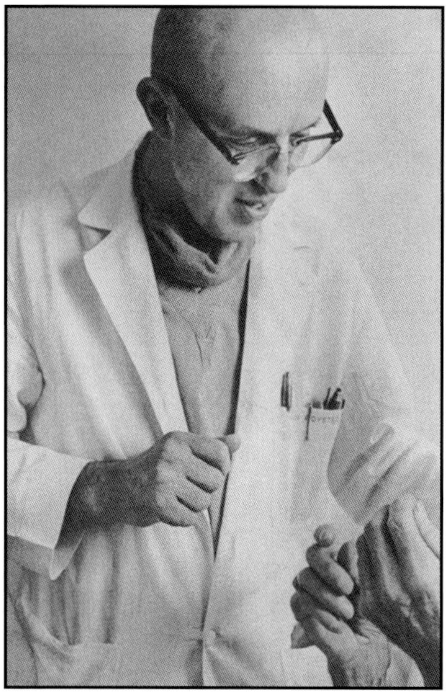

Henry Royster

1957, when it became a certified two-year residency.

Henry P. Royster, after serving in World War II's 20th General Hospital as a general surgeon, became one of I. S. Ravdin's first post-war faculty members at Penn. At Ravdin's suggestion, he founded the plastic surgery training program which became certified by the American Board of Medical Special Specialties in 1957. Royster was chief of the Penn plastic surgery training program from 1957 to 1969, with a focus largely on surgery for head and neck tumors and necessary reconstructive procedures.

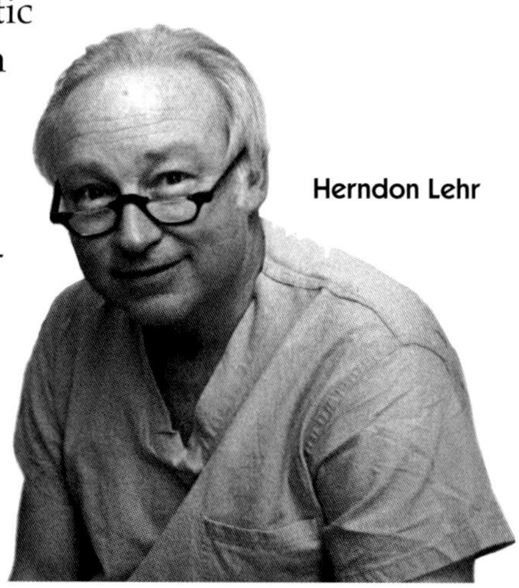

Herndon Lehr

Royster was succeeded in 1970 by Herndon B. Lehr. The two-year plastic residency followed at least three years of general surgery. In addition to his large practice of reconstructive and cosmetic surgery and management of the residency program, Lehr was an active researcher. From cadavers, he collected aortas and other arteries, freeze-dried them, and collaborated with the vascular surgeons in their use as some of the earliest replacements for resected aortic aneurysms and other vascular defects. Lehr also experimented with hypothermia and freezing to preserve animal kidneys and segments of small bowel for experiments in transplantation.

Peter Randall

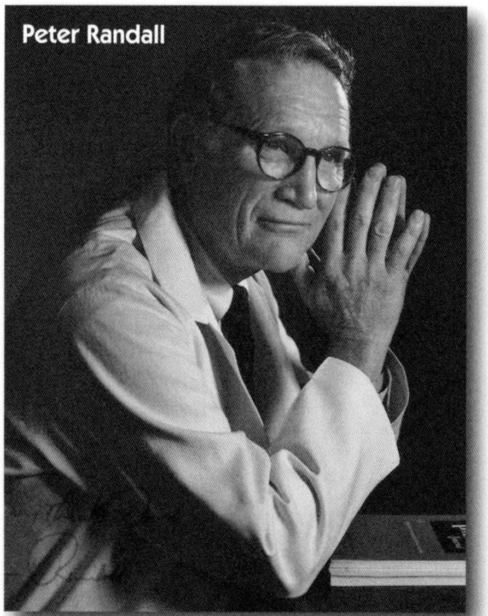

Following Dr. Lehr's unexpected early death, Peter Randall was appointed chief of the division in 1979. He was internationally known for his advances in the treatment of cleft lip and palate. He also became the first chief of plastic surgery at the Children's Hospital of Philadelphia (CHOP) in 1957, resigning that position in 1980 when he became chief at HUP. He eventually trained twenty-six plastic surgery residents.

Upon Dr. Randall's resignation at CHOP, Linton A. Whitaker was appointed chief there (1980–2001) and subsequently as chief at HUP (1987–2005). He trained forty-five residents and thirty craniofacial fellows, the latter in a program that he started in 1975. He was one of the first to bring the field of craniofacial surgery to the United States, broadening it to cosmetic surgery of the bony structure of the face, as well as refining

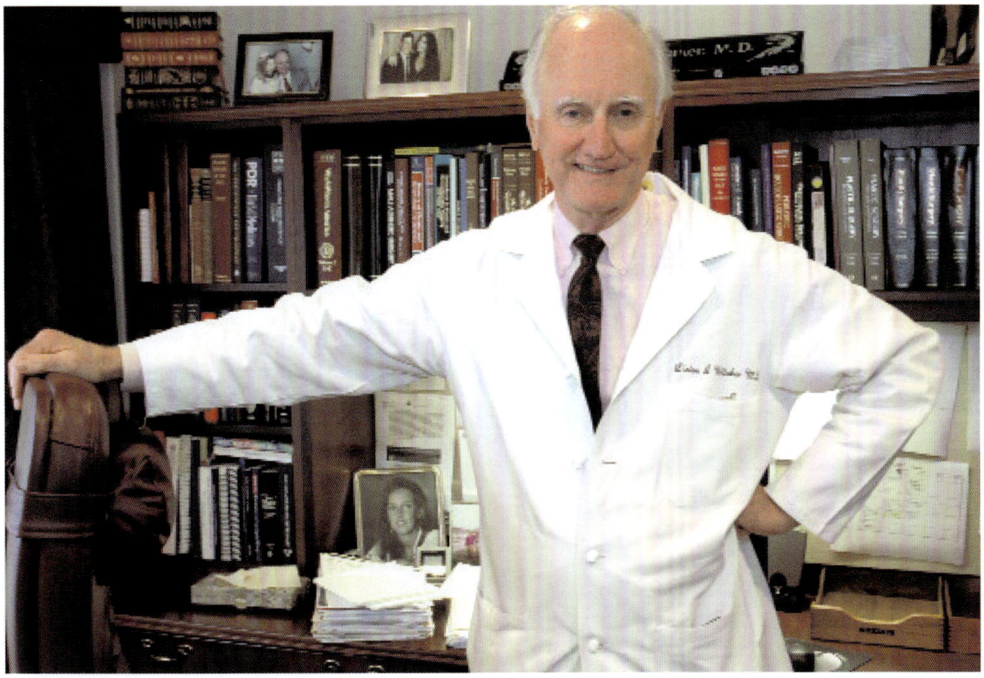

Linton Whitaker

the treatment of posttraumatic, cancer, and birth defects. He was the first to employ these operations in young children. Development of craniofacial surgery was one of the major accomplishments, not only of plastic surgery, but of twentieth-century surgery as a whole. Dr. Whitaker's contribution cannot be overestimated. His trainees have become leaders in this field around the world. Inspired by the excitement of this new field, during the first several decades of Linton's craniofacial program at HUP, more than a third of HUP's graduating general surgery residents elected to take further training in plastic surgery.

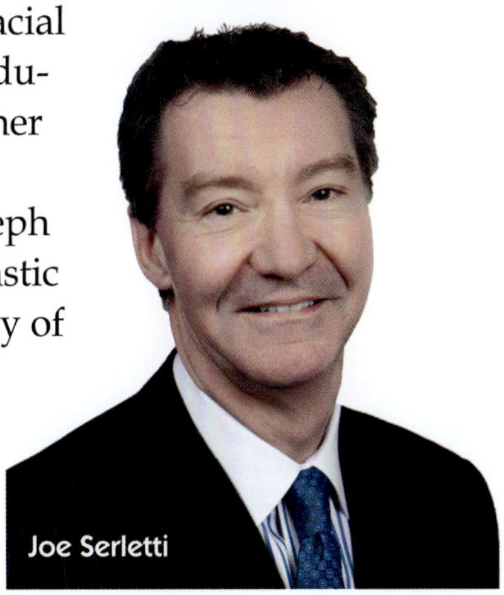

Joe Serletti

When Dr. Whitaker stepped down in 2005, Joseph M. Serletti was appointed chief of the Division of Plastic Surgery at HUP. He had been chief at the University of Rochester before being recruited to Penn and was the first "outsider" to become chief. He is internationally recognized as an expert in microsurgery, transplantation of free flaps, and as an outstanding leader in the world of plastic surgery.

In 2011, another exciting new program began with HUP's first hand transplant. Scott Levin, Penn chairman of orthopedics, professor of plastic surgery, and chairman of the ACS Board of Regents, led this endeavor with the essential participation of Ben Chang, codirector of hand transplantation and associate chief of plastic surgery. This was followed in 2015 with the world's first pediatric bilateral hand transplant in an eight-year-old boy. Both of these patients and another recipient have achieved excellent functional success.

At the inception of the residency in 1957, the faculty at HUP and CHOP consisted of five surgeons. As of 2022, there are twenty-six surgeon faculty members at five hospitals. There are five endowed chairs at CHOP and three at HUP.

The University of Pennsylvania Center for Human Appearance is a unique program. It was founded by Dr. Whitaker in 1987 as the first such center to study and treat all aspects of appearance, and it is now funded in perpetuity by the Edwin and Fannie Gray Hall estate.

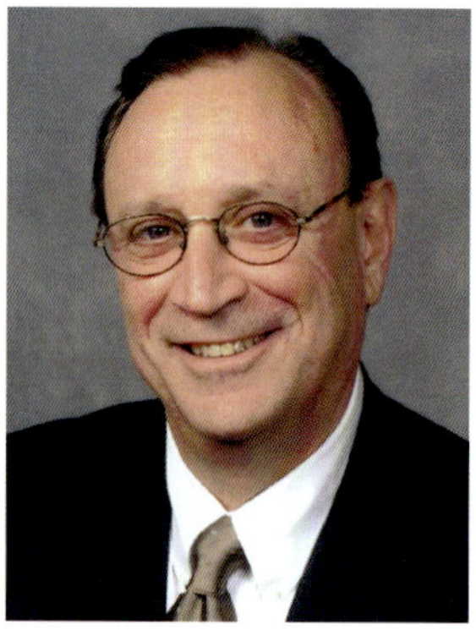

Don LaRossa

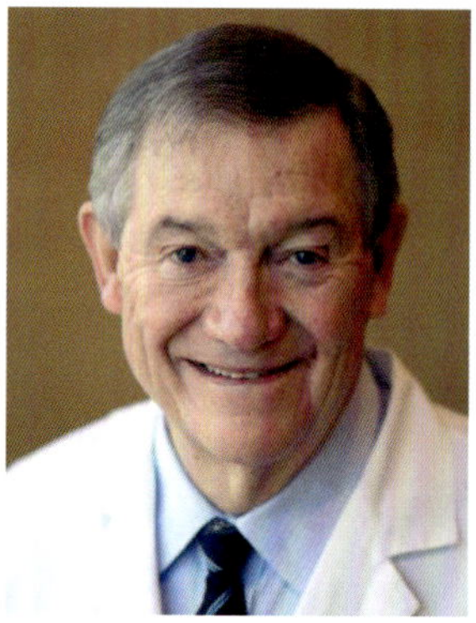

Barry Noone

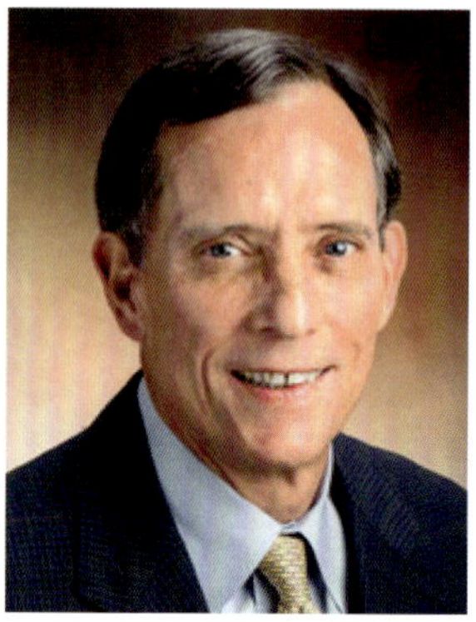

Scott Bartlett

Other major figures in plastic surgery who trained at HUP or were Penn faculty members include Don LaRossa, Barry Noone, Scott Bartlett, Ben Chang, Oksana Jackson, Jesse Taylor, Aron Wahrman, and Scott Levin.

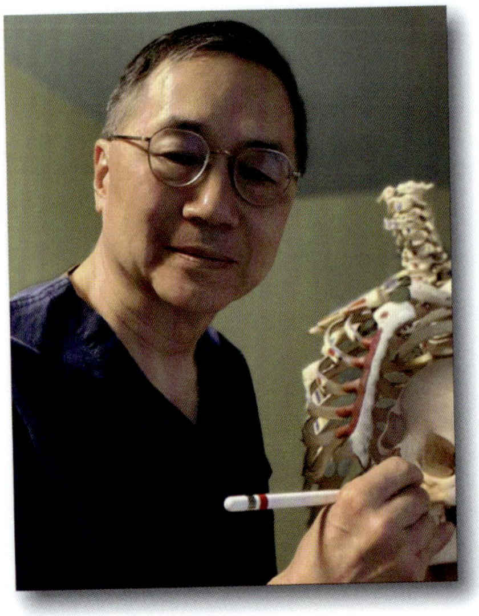

David Low

One of the most accomplished and distinguished of this faculty is David Low, HUP chief resident 1985 to 1986, now professor of surgery at HUP and CHOP. He learned cleft surgery from Don LaRossa and Peter Randall and is now the medical director of a CHOP-based international cleft surgery team, Smiles for Guatemala. In addition to his busy practice, his illustrations appear in many medical journals and textbooks, as well as in the personally illustrated annual Christmas card he sends to his friends.

Division of Urology

Several of the department's early leaders were particularly active in urology. In 1893, J. William White (department chairman, 1900–1910) conducted experiments in dogs showing that castration resulted in shrinkage of the prostate. In 1895, he reported to the American Surgical Association that in 111 patients, castration had alleviated the symptoms caused by enlarged prostates.

Edward Martin (department chair, 1910–1918) was widely known for his treatment of male infertility. He successfully performed a number of operations to treat blocked passages of the vas deferens (see Chapter 10).

Alexander Randall (MD Hopkins 1907, resident in surgery at Philadelphia's German Hospital 1907–1909, resident in urology at Hopkins 1911) was assistant professor to professor at the University of Pennsylvania from 1923 to 1929. He remained on the Penn faculty until 1946. He was a member of the American Surgical Association and the Charaka Club. He was Peter Randall's father.

Boland Hughes was HUP's specialist in urology in the late 1940s and early 1950s. At that time, Paul Lieberman also had an active urology practice.

In 1953, John J. Murphy joined the HUP faculty after completing a surgical residency under Dr. Ravdin and a urology residency at the University of Michigan. He established academic urology at HUP and directed the division of urology from 1953–1980. At HUP, he began transurethral prostatectomy, partial nephrectomy, urodynamic studies in children, and was important in the early renal transplant program. Murphy's NIH-funded training grant allowed initiation of a research program that produced many of the country's next generation of academic urologists. He was widely respected in American urology and as a visiting professor at the Royal College of Surgeons in Ireland and other European centers. He was a member of the Halsted Society and president of the mid-Atlantic section of the American Urological Association. He was a member of the University Surgeons and the American Surgical Association.

In the 1960s, Murphy elected to move from Ravdin's practice group, separating urology from the department financially, though it has remained an important component academically and in research. During this period, Murphy trained the division's future leader, Alan Wein, and mentored several other prominent urologists including Harry Schoenberg, Terry Malloy (later chief at Pennsylvania Hospital), Joe Corriere, Grant Mulholland, Thomas Rohner, and Philip Hanno.

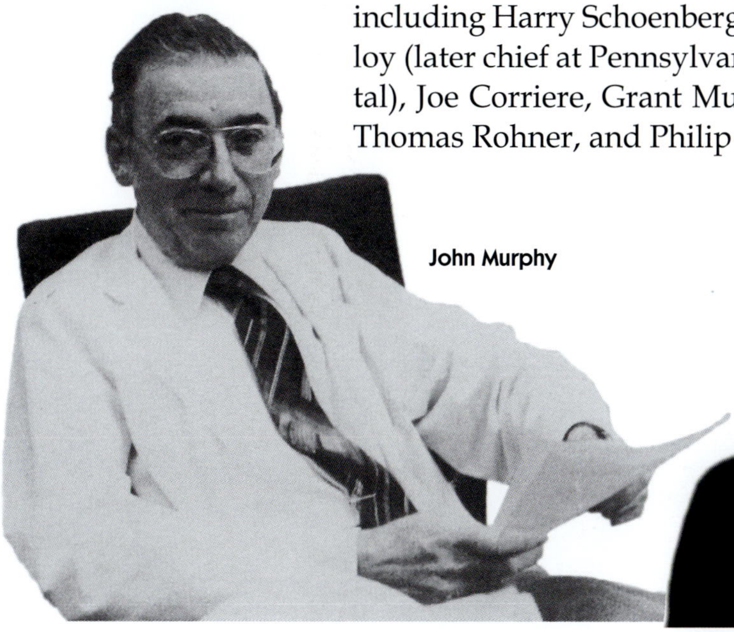

John Murphy

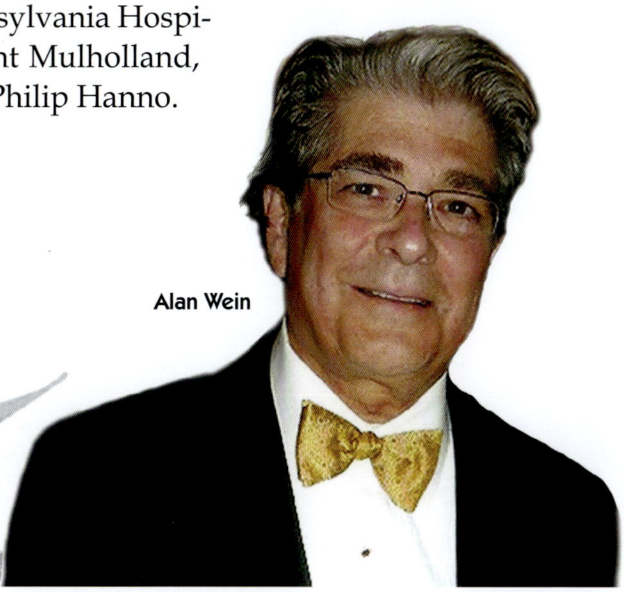

Alan Wein

In 1979, Alan Wein, a graduate of Princeton and Penn Medical School, became acting chief of the division, and in 1981, its official chief. He remained the leader until 2017, a remarkable thirty-six years.[47] During that time, he trained scores of University urologists, including three long-term HUP faculty members—Keith Van Arsdalen in 1982, Bruce Malkowicz in 1986, and his successor, Thomas Guzzo.

Dr. Wein's fields of interest are the evaluation and management of urologic cancer, the physiology and pharmacology of the lower urinary tract, voiding function and dysfunction, including problems related to prostate enlargement, urinary incontinence, and neurologic disease. He has actively pursued research in these areas throughout his career. He has authored more than 800 scientific articles, edited twenty-eight books, and has given over 600 invited lectures. He is editor of the textbook considered to be the standard in urology, *Campbell-Walsh-Wein Urology*.

Dr. Wein is one of the most distinguished and highly decorated members of the University of Pennsylvania faculty. He belongs to all of the scientific societies of urology and, in addition, is a member of the Society of University Surgeons, the American Surgical Association, and the Society of Surgical Oncology. He is a recipient of the Hugh Hampton Young Award from the American Urological Association, the Fernand C. Valentine Award of the New York Academy of Medicine, and the Keyes Medal, which is considered the top citation in urology and is awarded only sparingly. In 2005, he was awarded an honorary PhD by the University of Patras in Greece. In recognition of his remarkable career, in 2014 Penn medical school honored him with its distinguished graduate award.

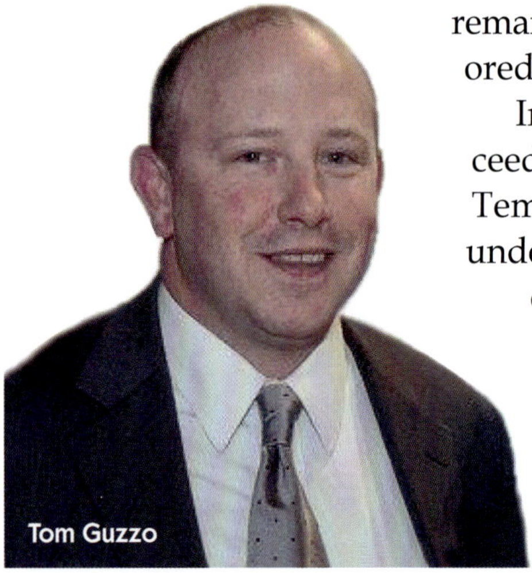
Tom Guzzo

In 2017, Dr. Wein stepped down and was succeeded by Tom Guzzo. Dr. Guzzo is a graduate of Temple School of Medicine. After his residency under Dr. Wein at HUP, he was a fellow in urologic oncology at Johns Hopkins before joining the faculty at Penn. His practice and research is in urological cancer. He is particularly experienced in noninvasive methods of treatment such as laparoscopic and robotic surgery.

Notes

[1] Daly JM. (1986), 10th Anniversary Presidential Address: Parenteral Feeding (1966–1986) Growth and Development of an Individual, a Scientific Discipline and an Organization. *Journal of Parenteral and Enteral Nutrition,* 10: 329–336. https://doi.org/10.1177/014860718601000401.

[2] Copeland EM. John M. Daly, MD: The Wise and Gentleman Surgeon. *Ann Surg Oncol* 29, 2129–2130 (2022). https://doi.org/10.1245/s10434-022-11409-3.

[3] Goldberg, Amy J and Moore, Maureen D. Memoir of John Daly. *Transactions of the American Surgical Association* (2021).

[4] Fraker DL, Harsono H, Lewis R. Minimally invasive parathyroidectomy: benefits and requirements of localization, diagnosis, and intraoperative PTH monitoring. long-term results. *World J Surg* (2009) 33(11):2256–2265. doi:10.1007/s00268-009-0166-4.

[5] Fraker DL, Alexander HR, Andrich M, Rosenberg SA. Treatment of patients with melanoma of the extremity using hyperthermic isolated limb perfusion with melphalan, tumor necrosis factor, and interferon gamma: results of a tumor necrosis factor dose-escalation study. *J Clin Oncol* (1996) 14(2):479–489. doi:10.1200/JCO.1996.14.2.479.

[6] Bartlett DL, Ma G, Alexander HR, Libutti SK, Fraker DL. Isolated limb reperfusion with tumor necrosis factor and melphalan in patients with extremity melanoma after failure of isolated limb perfusion with chemotherapeutics. *Cancer* (1997) 80(11):2084–2090. doi:10.1002/(sici)1097-0142(19971201)80:11<2084::aid-cncr7>3.0.co;2-x.

[7] Canter RJ, Mick R, Kesmodel SB, et al. Intraperitoneal photodynamic therapy causes a capillary-leak syndrome. *Ann Surg Oncol* (2003) 10(5):514–524. doi:10.1245/aso.2003.11.005.

[8] Kaiser LR, Cooper JD, Trulock EP, Pasque MK, Triantafillou A, Haydock D. The evolution of single lung transplantation for emphysema. *Journal of Thoracic & Cardiovascular Surgery*, 102(3): 333–341 (Sept. 1991). Toronto Lung Transplant Group (including Cooper JD). Unilateral lung transplantation for pulmonary fibrosis. *N Engl J Med* (1986) 314(18):1140–1145. doi:10.1056/NEJM198605013141802.

[9] Kaiser LR, Pasque MK, Trulock EP, Dresler CM, Low DE, Cooper JD. Bilateral sequential lung transplantation: The procedure of choice for double-lung replacement. *Annals of Thoracic Surgery*, 52(3): 438–446 (Sept. 1991). Cooper JD. Lung transplantation: a new era. *Ann Thorac Surg* (1987) 44(5):447–448. doi:10.1016/s0003-4975(10)62099-1.

[10] Trulock EP, Cooper JD, Kaiser LR, Pasque MK, Ettinger NA, Dresler CM. The Washington University-Barnes Hospital experience with lung transplantation. Washington University Lung Transplantation Group *Journal of the American Medical Association*, 266(14): 1943–1946 (Oct. 9, 1991).

[11] Smythe WR, Hwang HC, Amin KM, Eck SL, Davidson BL, Wilson JM, Kaiser LR, Albelda SM. Use of recombinant adenovirus to transfer the herpes simplex virus thymidine kinase (HSVtk) gene to thoracic neoplasms: an effective in vitro drug sensitization system. *Cancer research* (1994) 54(8): 2055–2059. Kucharczuk JC, Raper ST, Elshami AA, Amin KM, Sterman DH, Wheeldon EB, Wilson JM, Litzky LA, Kaiser LR, Albelda SM. Safety of intrapleurally administered recombinant adenovirus carrying herpes simplex thymidine kinase cDNA followed by

ganciclovir therapy in non-human primates. *Human Gene Therapy*, 7(18): 2225–2233 (Dec. 1, 1996). Singhal S, Kaiser LR. Cancer chemotherapy using suicide genes. *Surg Oncol Clin N Am* (Jul. 1998) 7(3):505–36. PMID: 9624215.

[12] Bavaria JE, Pochettino A, Kotloff RM, Rosengard BR, Wahl PM, Palevsky HI, Kaiser LR. Effect of volume reduction on lung transplant timing and selection for COPD. *Journal of Thoracic & Cardiovascular Surgery*, 115(1): 9–18 (Jan. 1998).

[13] Rosato EF, Mullen JL, Lanciault G, Rosato FE, Brooks FP. Fasting acid output and plasma gastrin in conscious monkeys. *Proc Soc Exp Biol Med* (1972) 139(3):833–835. doi:10.3181/00379727-139-36247.

[14] Bauer TW, Morris JB, Lowenstein A, Wolferth C, Rosato FE, Rosato EF. The consequences of a major bile duct injury during laparoscopic cholecystectomy. *J Gastrointest Surg* (1998) 2(1):61–66. doi:10.1016/s1091-255x(98)80104-2.

[15] Dempsey DT, Kalan MM, Gerson RS, Parkman HP, Maier WP. Comparison of outcomes following open and laparoscopic esophagomyotomy for achalasia. *Surg Endosc* (1999) 13(8):747–750. doi:10.1007/s004649901091.

[16] Harbison SP, Dempsey DT. Peptic ulcer disease. *Curr Probl Surg* (2005) 42(6):346–454. doi:10.1067/j.cpsurg.2005.02.005.

[17] Wang YR, Richter JE, Dempsey DT. Trends and outcomes of hospitalizations for peptic ulcer disease in the United States, 1993 to 2006. *Ann Surg* (2010) 251(1):51–58. doi:10.1097/SLA.0b013e3181b975b8.

[18] McMillan MT, Malleo G, Bassi C, et al.. Multicenter, Prospective Trial of Selective Drain Management for Pancreatoduodenectomy Using Risk Stratification. *Ann Surg* (2017) 265(6):1209–1218. doi:10.1097/SLA.0000000000001832.

[19] McMillan MT, Zureikat AH, Hogg ME, et al. A Propensity Score-Matched Analysis of Robotic vs Open Pancreatoduodenectomy on Incidence of Pancreatic Fistula. *JAMA Surg* (2017) 152(4):327–335. doi:10.1001/jamasurg.2016.4755.

[20] Hartwig W, Vollmer CM, Fingerhut A, et al. Extended pancreatectomy in pancreatic ductal adenocarcinoma: definition and consensus of the International Study Group for Pancreatic Surgery (ISGPS). *Surgery* (2014) 156(1):1–14. doi:10.1016/j.surg.2014.02.009. Datta J, Vollmer CM Jr. Advances in Surgical Management of Pancreatic Diseases. *Gastroenterol Clin North Am* (2016) 45(1):129–144. doi:10.1016/j.gtc.2015.10.002.

[21] Foster MW, Gershuni VM, Tewksbury CM, et al. Laparoscopic Sleeve Gastrectomy Carries a Lower Perioperative Mortality Including Sudden Cardiac Death over Roux-en-Y Gastric Bypass in Patients with a Prior Cardiac History: An MBSAQIP Analysis. *Obes Surg* (2020) 30(3):812–818. doi:10.1007/s11695-019-04363-9. Neligan PJ, Williams N. Nonsurgical and surgical treatment of obesity. *Anesthesiol Clin North Am* (2005) 23(3):501-vii. doi:10.1016/j.atc.2005.03.008. Neylan CJ, Kannan U, Dempsey DT, Williams NN, Dumon KR. The Surgical Management of Obesity. *Gastroenterol Clin North Am* (2016) 45(4):689–703. doi:10.1016/j.gtc.2016.07.006.

[22] Edmunds LH Jr. In memoriam Julian Johnson (1906–1987). *J Thorac Cardiovasc Surg* (1988) 96(4):515–517.

[23] Johnson J. A Surgeon and Something More. *J Thorac Cardiovasc Surg* (1963) 46:141–149.

[24] Kirby, Charles K and Johnson, Julian. *Surgery of the Chest* (The Year Book Publishers: 1952).

[25] Waldhausen, John. *Finding Home in a World at War* (Baltimore: Gateway Press, 2005).

[26] Heinle JS, Gaynor JW. Historical perspectives of The American Association for

Thoracic Surgery: John Anton Waldhausen (1929–2012). *J Thorac Cardiovasc Surg* (2014) 148(2):381–386. doi:10.1016/j.jtcvs.2014.05.013.

[27] Waldhausen JA, Nahrwold DL. Repair of coarctation of the aorta with a subclavian flap. *J Thorac Cardiovasc Surg.* (1966) 51(4):532–533. Pierce WS, Waldhausen JA, Berman W Jr, Whitman V. Late results of the subclavian flap procedure in infants with coarctation of the thoracic aorta. *Circulation* (1978) 58(3 Pt 2):I78-I82.

[28] Edmunds LH Jr. Blood activation in mechanical circulatory-assist devices. *J Congest Heart Fail Circ Support* 1 (3): 141–147 (2000). Guy TS, Edmunds LH Jr. Hemostasis and Thrombosis. *The Surgical Review: An Integrated Basic and Clinical Study Guide.* D. Kreisel, AS Krupnick, and LR Kaiser (eds.). J.B. Lippincott Inc, Philadelphia, pp. 295–303 (2000).

[29] Edmunds, L, Gorman III, Joseph, Gorman, Robert (2003). Sheep Models of Postinfarction Left Ventricular Remodeling. 10.1007/978-1-4419-9262-8_15.

[30] Edmunds, L. Henry, Norwood, Williams I., Low, David W. *Atlas of Cardiothoracic Surgery* (Philadelphia: Lea & Febinger, 1990).

[31] Acker MA, Hammond RL, Mannion JD, Salmons S, Stephenson LW. An autologous biologic pump motor. *J Thorac Cardiovasc Surg* (1986) 92(4):733–746.

[32] Acker MA, Mannion JD, Brown WE, et al. Canine diaphragm muscle after 1 yr of continuous electrical stimulation: its potential as a myocardial substitute. *J Appl Physiol (1985)* (1987) 62(3):1264–1270. doi:10.1152/jappl.1987.62.3.1264. Acker MA, Hammond RL, Mannion JD, Salmons S, Stephenson LW. Skeletal muscle as the potential power source for a cardiovascular pump: assessment in vivo. *Science* (1987) 236(4799):324–327. doi:10.1126/science.2951849.

[33] Acker MA, Bavaria JE, Barker CF. History and Current Status of Cardiovascular Surgery at the University of Pennsylvania. *Semin Thorac Cardiovasc Surg* (2015) 27(4):370–373. doi:10.1053/j.semtcvs.2015.10.012.

[34] Bavaria, JE, Pechettino, A, Wahl PM, Hall A, Acker M, Gardner TJ. Aortic arch reconstruction with retrograde cerebral perfusion. *Journal of the Pennsylvania Association of Thoracic Surgery* 6:16–25 (1998).

[35] Barker, Clyde F. Memoir of Brooke Roberts. *Transactions of the American Surgical Association* (2003) Vol 121, pp. 372–373.

[36] Spence RK, Freiman DB, Gatenby R, et al. Long-term results of transluminal angioplasty of the iliac and femoral arteries. *Arch Surg* (1981) 116(11):1377–1386. doi:10.1001/archsurg.1981.01380230009002.

[37] Fairman RM. Measuring the worth of a vascular surgeon: Making it personal through a career of service. *J Vasc Surg* (2018) 67(5):1321–1327. doi:10.1016/j.jvs.2018.02.007.

[38] Zamir GA, Olthoff KM, Nunes FA, et al. Liver transplantation at the University of Pennsylvania and the Children's Hospital of Philadelphia. *Clin Transpl* (1999) 223–229.

[39] Abt PL, Mange KC, Olthoff KM, Markmann JF, Reddy KR, Shaked A. Allograft survival following adult-to-adult living donor liver transplantation. *Am J Transplant* (2004) 4(8):1302–1307. doi:10.1111/j.1600-6143.2004.00522.x.

[40] Markmann JF, Deng S, Huang X, et al. Insulin independence following isolated islet transplantation and single islet infusions. *Ann Surg* (2003) 237(6):741–750. doi:10.1097/01.SLA.0000072110.93780.52.

[41] Porrett PM, Nellore A. Immunologic and Infectious Concerns in Uterus

Transplantation. *Clin Obstet Gynecol* (2022) 65(1):37-43. doi:10.1097/GRF.0000000000000686.

[42] Ross HM, Mahmoud N, Fry RD. The current management of rectal cancer. *Curr Probl Surg* (2005) 42(2):72–131. doi:10.1067/j.cpsurg.2004.11.004.

[43] Mahmoud NN, Carothers AM, Grunberger D, et al. Plant phenolics decrease intestinal tumors in an animal model of familial adenomatous polyposis. *Carcinogenesis* (2000) 21(5):921–927. doi:10.1093/carcin/21.5.921. Smith RK, Fry RD, Mahmoud NN, Paulson EC. Surveillance after neoadjuvant therapy in advanced rectal cancer with complete clinical response can have comparable outcomes to total mesorectal excision. *Int J Colorectal Dis* (2015) 30(6):769–774. doi:10.1007/s00384-015-2165-2. Ecker BL, Paulson EC, Datta J, et al. Lymph node identification following neoadjuvant therapy in rectal cancer: A stage-stratified analysis using the surveillance, epidemiology, and end results (SEER)-medicare database. *J Surg Oncol* (2015) 112(4):415–420. doi:10.1002/jso.23991.

[44] Woo EY, Rombeau JL. The Colon Rectum and Anus. In: *The Surgical Review and Integrated Basic and Clinical Science Study Guide*. Philadelphia: Lippincott. Kreisel D, Krupnick AS, Kaiser LR, eds. pp. 235–55 (2001).

[45] Rombeau, John and Muldoon, Donna. *Quaker Sense and Sensibility in the World of Surgery* (Philadelphia: Hanley and Belfus Inc: 1997).

[46] Azoury SC, Kalmar CL, Zimmerman CE, et al. The Linton A. Whitaker Legacy: Cultivating Craniofacial Surgeon Leaders. *Ann Plast Surg* (2021) 86(3):251–256. doi:10.1097/SAP.0000000000002742.

[47] Wein, Alan J. Legends in Urology v27103. *The Canadian Journal of Urology* (June 2020). https://www.canjurol.com/article?ID=3565.

CHAPTER 38

A Time of Change

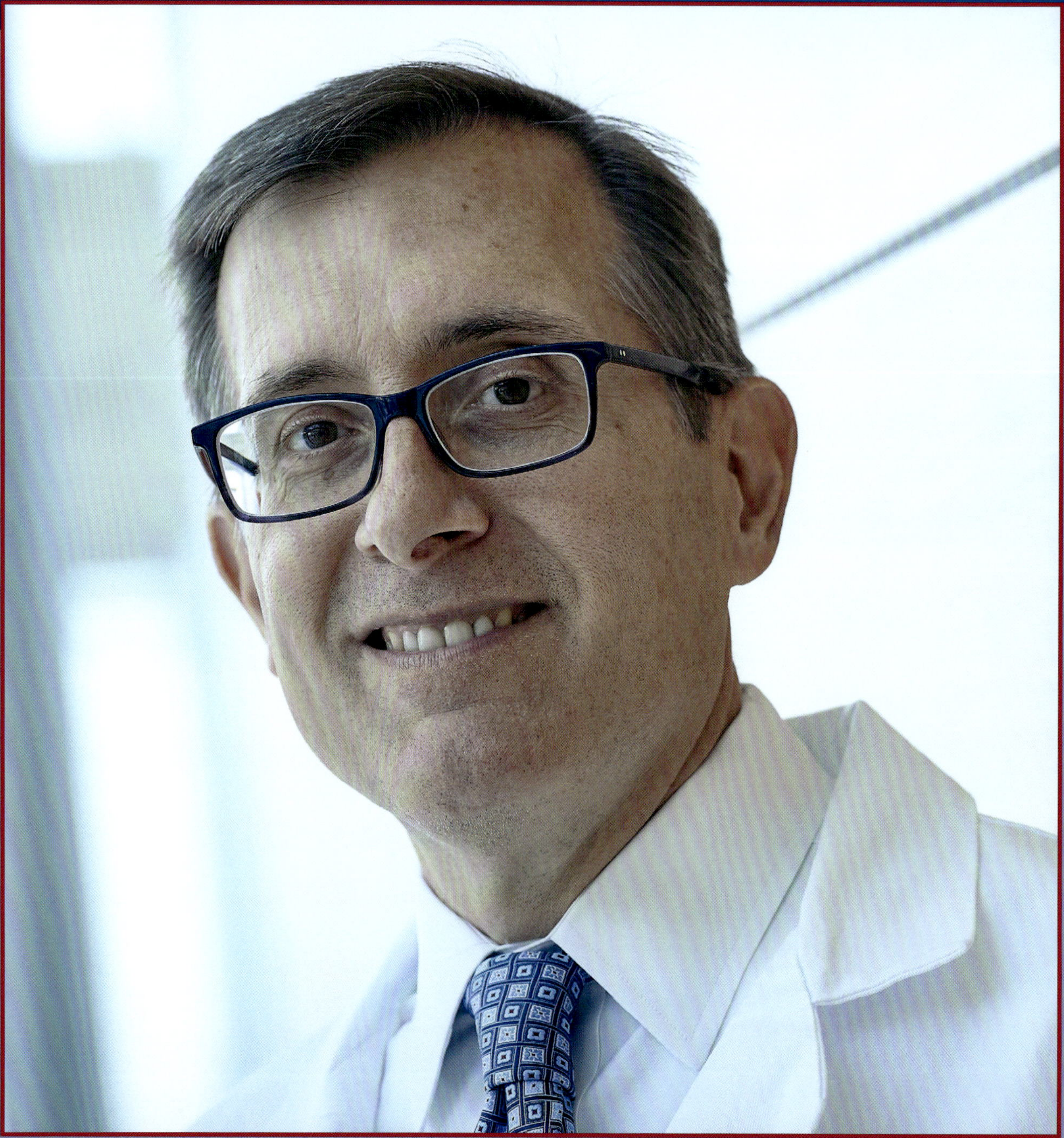

Ronald P. DeMatteo (1965–)

JRB Professor and Chairman of Surgery (2017–present)

Dr. DeMatteo's family story is a classic example of the American dream. His grandparents were immigrants with no money and little education. They landed in Pittsburgh where they lived in an Italian community. His grandfather never learned to speak English. Their son, Ron's father, had an incessant desire for success. He went to college at the University of Pittsburgh and, after several years working at a hospital, went back to school and got an MBA including an internship at Penn. He worked his way up to become CEO of Englewood Hospital in New Jersey. Ron adopted his father's work ethic and has become one of surgery's most accomplished academic figures, an example of a species largely considered to be extinct, a genuine triple threat, an expert clinician, teacher, and basic scientist.

Dr. DeMatteo credits an early interest in biology to his experience with a friend in dissecting a snake. They were helped by his friend's father, a Johns Hopkins pathologist. By the time Ron was in first grade, he had decided to become a surgeon. This decision was reinforced in seventh grade when his dissection of a frog was so good that it was chosen for use in the practical exam for his class.

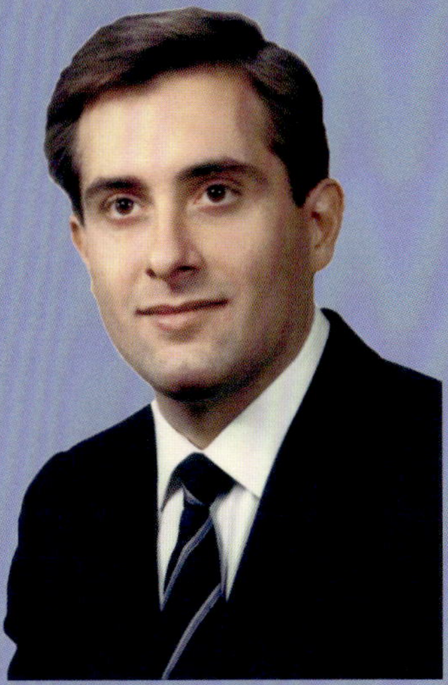

Ron DeMatteo
HUP internship candidate

Later in childhood and through high school and college, he was occupied by other interests: as a caddy at the local golf club observing the basics of the game, designing crossword puzzles well enough to be published by the *New York Times*, playing sports, playing chess, and studying enough to be high school valedictorian.

In college at Johns Hopkins, where he graduated in three years, he played on the golf team, was president of his fraternity and dormitory, and was selected into Phi Beta Kappa. During a summer vacation, his

1990
MD Cornell

1990–1997
Intern and resident at HUP

intent for a surgical career was confirmed when, as a volunteer at Johns Hopkins Hospital, he held retractors for operations by the chief residents, Keith Lillemoe and Charlie Yeo, now department chairs at Mass General and Jefferson.

During medical school in New York City at Cornell, he met Allyson Farmer at a dance. A native of a small town in North Carolina, she was in New York working at a bank while pursuing an MBA at night at New York University. She and Ron married while he was a HUP resident. She worked as an investment banker, eventually becoming one of four managing directors of her firm before retiring to raise their two daughters, Siena and Alessia.

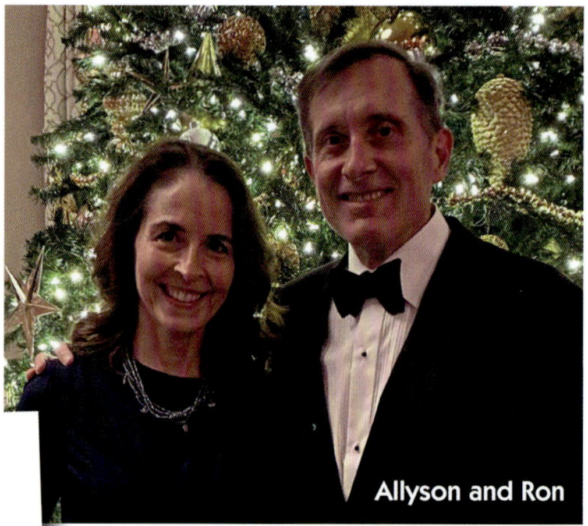
Allyson and Ron

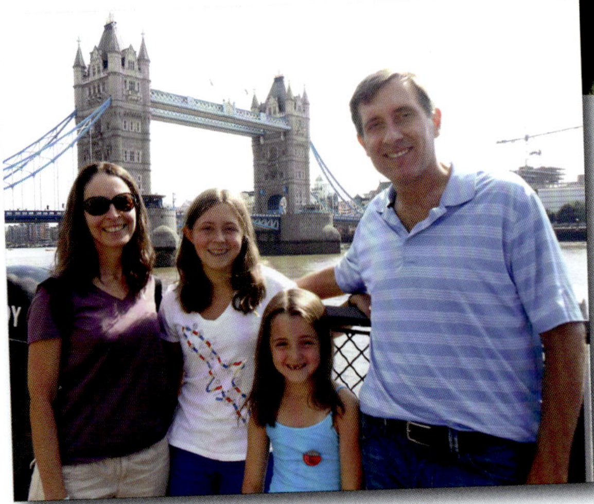
Allyson, Siena, Alessia and Ron

After medical school, where he was president of AOA, he came to Philadelphia where he was an outstanding HUP intern and resident. In addition to his strong performance in technical surgery and patient care, he was the recipient of the Jonathan Rhoads award for research, the Leonard Perloff award for teaching, and the British Journal of Surgery award as the hospital's outstanding surgical resident. In the Christmas skit, he was a hit, impersonating me (as chairman at the time) and making fun of my idiosyncrasies.

Initially, he was not particularly interested in research until his fellow resident Hansell Stedman put him in touch with Steve Raper, a young faculty surgeon about to come from Michigan to Penn with Jim Wilson who had been recruited to start an Institute for Human Gene Therapy. Dr. DeMatteo was overwhelmed by Wilson's large empire, with its rooms full of modern equipment, a dozen postdocs, and several cores. He joined the lab and soon became fascinated with immunology since the immune response was the major limiting factor in using viral vectors for gene therapy. Dr. DeMatteo generously credits me as being a role model of the physician scientist and with inspiring him to pursue research by providing a supportive environment.

For one of his first publications, DeMatteo and colleagues combined gene therapy, virology, modern immunology, and old-fashioned transplantation biology in a paper that was chosen to open the scientific program of the American Surgical Association.[1] Presenting the paper was a heady experience for young DeMatteo since back then, residents were almost never allowed to present papers to this exclusive senior society. He was hooked, addicted to laboratory investigation. By the time he finished his residency, he had published thirteen more research papers with Raper, Wilson, and Markmann in top surgical and basic science journals. Five hundred papers later, as the busy chair of a major department, he still makes time to do his own research.

1997–1999
Fellow in surgical oncology at Memorial Sloan Kettering

While completing his residency, Dr. DeMatteo was torn between careers in transplantation and oncology. Attracted by the variety in Dr. Fraker's extensive tumor practice, he chose surgical oncology and went to New York for Memorial Sloan Kettering's two-year fellowship in this relatively new field and, in addition, a research fellowship with Murray Brennan. His outstanding performance was recognized with the Michael Burt award for clinical excellence. Keeping an eye out for promising research topics, he encountered what turned out to be a lifetime interest—GIST. Ron remembers that "we removed an abdominal tumor and the pathology [report] came back as gastrointestinal stromal tumor (GIST)." He recalls saying that "we did not have that tumor in Philly." In fact, GIST was, at the time, just being recognized as distinct from gastrointestinal leiomyosarcoma. That one case prompted him to summarize MSK's experience of 200 patients with the tumor in a retrospective paper that has been cited over 13,800 times.[2] In New York, there was also time for fun as director of Memorial's holiday video.

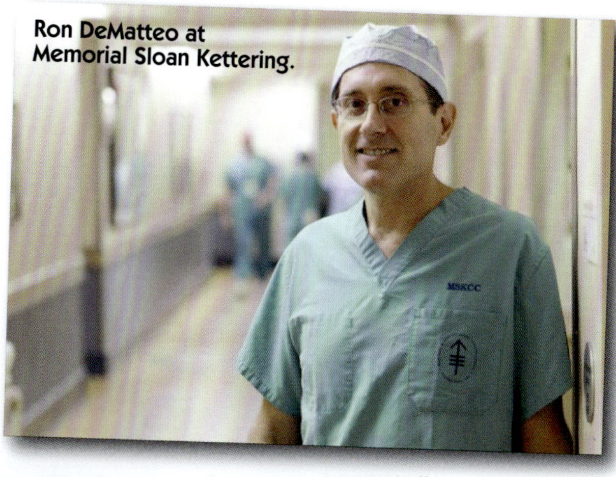

Ron DeMatteo at Memorial Sloan Kettering.

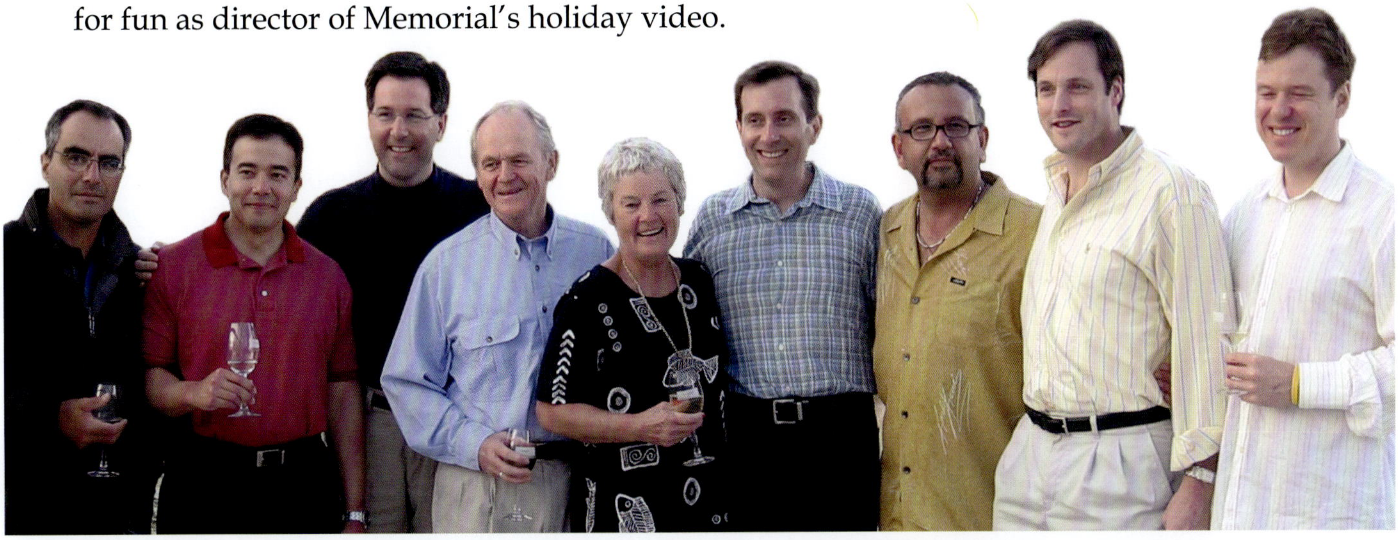
Class of 1999 surgical oncology fellows at MSK from left: Jonathan Koea (international fellow), Richard Schulick (now chair of U Colorado), David Linehan (chair of U Rochester), Murray Brennan and his wife Susie, Ron DeMatteo, Joe Espat (chair of Roger Williams Cancer Center), Steve Hochwald (cancer director of Mt. Sinai Miami), and Andy Smith (CEO of Sunnybrook Hospital Toronto).

2000–2023
Studies of molecular therapy of GI stromal tumors change standard of care

1999–2008
Assistant professor to professor of surgery, Cornell and Memorial Sloan Kettering

2006–2017
Chief of general surgery, Memorial Sloan Kettering

2017
John Rhea Barton Professor and Chairman, Department of Surgery, University of Pennsylvania

Encouraged by this experience, he continued to work on GIST. The drug imatinib was just coming out, and he convinced the NIH to let him run a trial testing placebo versus one year of imatinib after the removal of GISTs. The idea was to try to prevent recurrence. In fact, it did prevent recurrence as long as the patient stayed on the drug. The randomized trial that was running in more than 200 sites in the US and Canada was prematurely stopped by NIH because the imatinib arm did so much better. This resulted in FDA approval of postoperative imatinib and changed the standard of care throughout the world.[3] Because the trial was run through the American College of Surgeons (ACOSOG), he developed connections with Sam Wells and other researchers. Dr. DeMatteo conducted a second national trial on GIST in patients at high risk of postoperative recurrence,[4] and a third establishing that five years of continuous postoperative imatinib results in a very low rate of recurrence.[5]

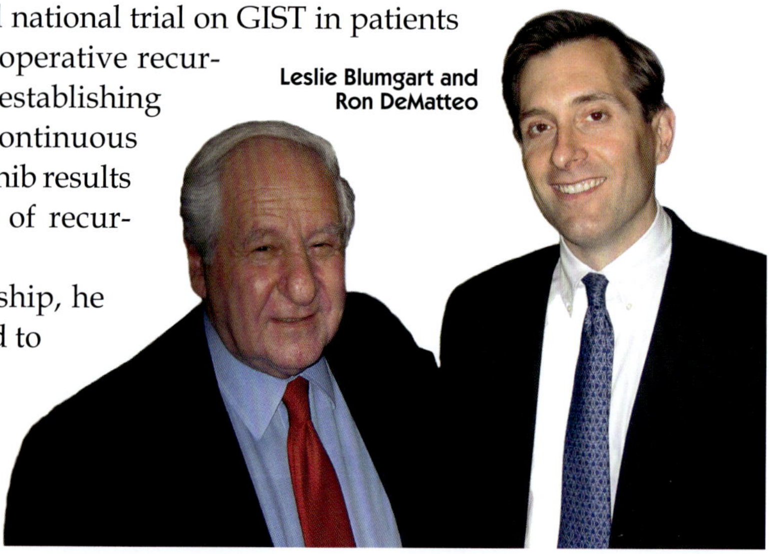
Leslie Blumgart and Ron DeMatteo

After the fellowship, he had initially aspired to return to Penn and work with Dr. Fraker, but instead he came under the strong influence of Leslie Blumgart, a legendary pioneer of liver surgery. Their friendship was a major factor in DeMatteo's acceptance in 1999 of a faculty position at MSK. He soon built a large clinical practice focused on the care of patients with hepatic, biliary, and pancreatic diseases, and with abdominal sarcoma.

After only seven years on the MLK faculty, he became the tenured head of the division of general surgical oncology, vice chair of the Department of Surgery and the inaugural recipient of the Leslie Blumgart Chair of Surgical Oncology. He also held appointments as professor of surgery at Cornell and, though rare for a clinician, he became a member of the Sloan Kettering Institute's Immunology program. From 2012–2017, he represented Memorial Sloan Kettering as associate dean at Weill Cornell Medical College.

Dr. DeMatteo also directed Memorial's primary educational conference for eleven years. He established a model to implant surgeon-scientists in nonsurgeon labs of the institution, doing this with about fifteen surgeons. This helped him to increase the departmental NIH funding by more than 50 percent.

In 2017, Dr. DeMatteo returned to Philadelphia. Despite being the only chairman not simply taken from the Department's current faculty,

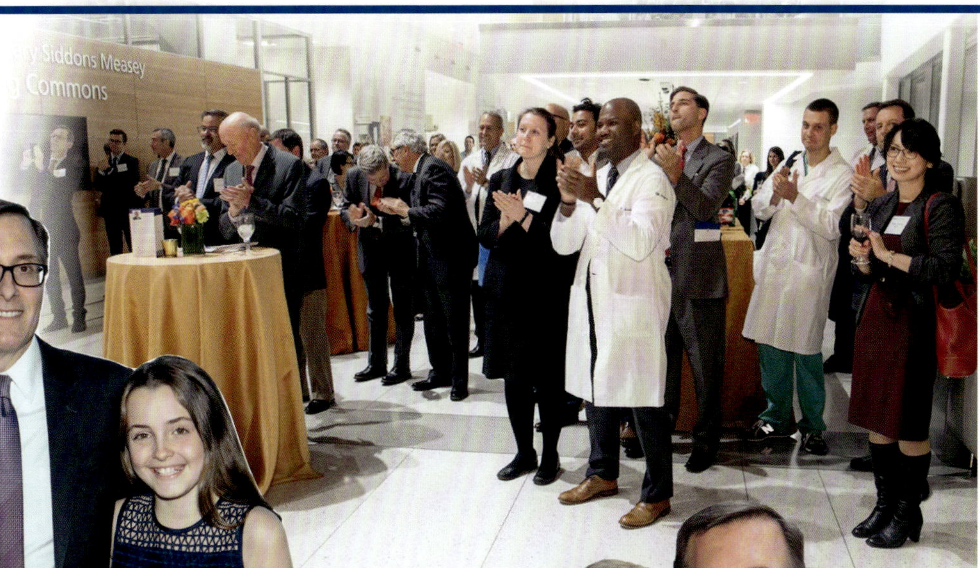

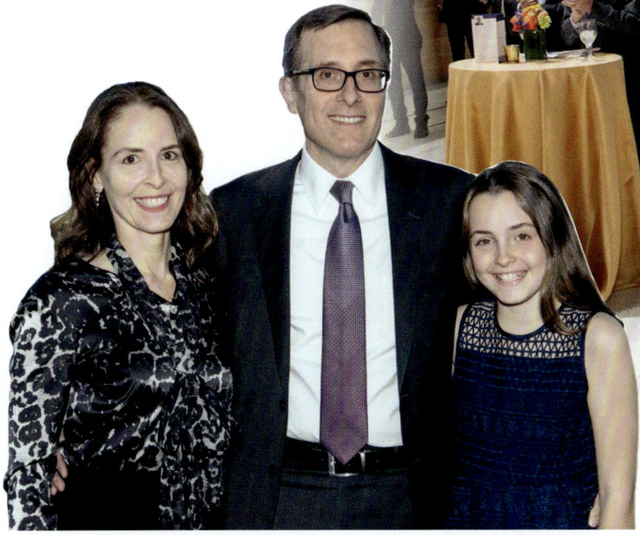

Ron with his wife Allyson and daughter, Alessia

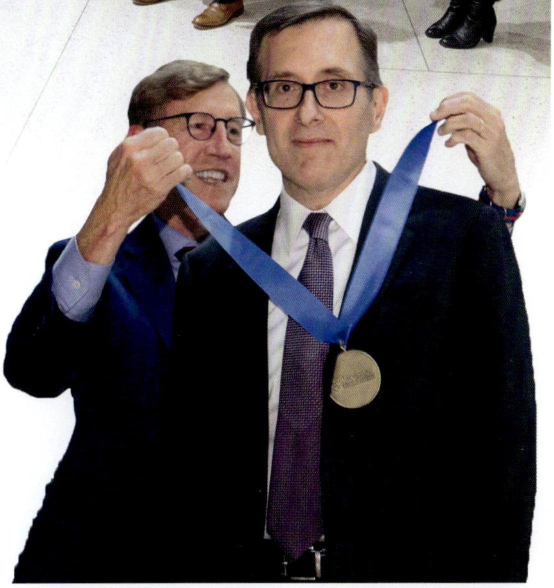

Dean Larry Jameson and Ron DeMatteo

he was a popular choice as the fifteenth John Rhea Barton Professor and the nineteenth Chair of the Department. His many colleagues and friends and family gathered to see Dean Larry Jameson present him with the traditional Penn Chairmanship Medallion.

In addition to his international reputation as a clinical surgeon, Dr. DeMatteo is widely respected for his accomplishments in both basic and clinical research. He is without comparison the best basic scientist of the department's nineteen chairmen. His laboratory investigations have been continuously funded by NIH since 2001. He currently leads a R01 grant of twenty years duration, two other R01s, two R21s, a T32 grant, and is the faculty comentor of a K-12 grant. He has mentored more than forty laboratory fellows, many of whom have since obtained NIH grants and leadership positions at other institutions. He has been chairman of the cancer immunopathology and immunotherapy study section of the NIH. He serves on several guideline committees of the National Comprehensive Cancer Network. He is coeditor of the definitive text of hepatobiliary surgery, *Surgery of the liver, biliary tract and pancreas.* Many of his 500 peer-reviewed publications have appeared in journals such as *Nature Medicine, Lancet, Lancet Oncology, Journal of Clinical Oncology, Journal of Clinical Investigation, Journal of Experimental Medicine,* and *Annals of Surgery.* His H index is a remarkable 120. He is a member of the editorial board of the *Annals of Surgical Oncology,* and for sixteen years, a member of the editorial board of the *Annals of Surgery.*

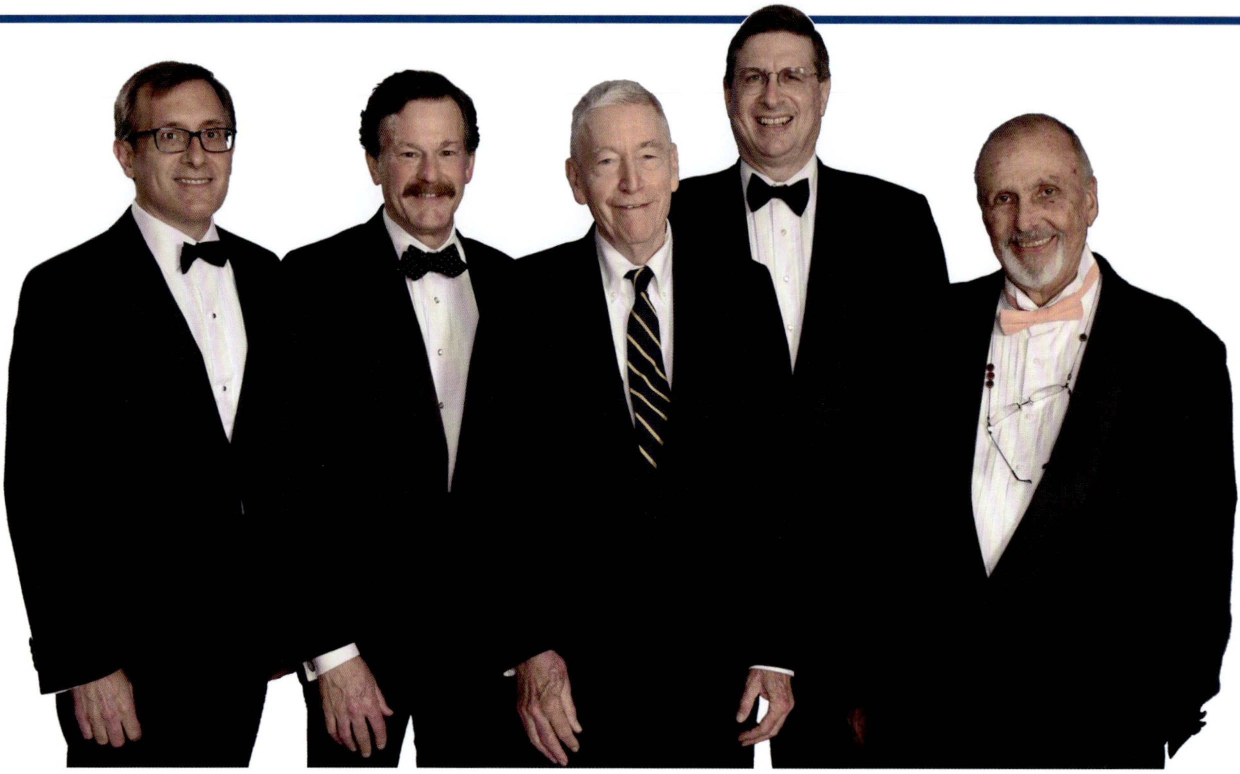

Ron DeMatteo, Larry Kaiser, Clyde Barker, Jeff Drebin and Jim Mullen

After twenty-three years of studying GIST, Dr. DeMatteo in his lab, made up almost entirely of surgical residents, continues to investigate this most common of human sarcomas, employing immunologic, molecular, and clinical approaches. He utilizes genetically engineered mouse models of *Kit*-mutant GIST, studies human GIST[6] in a bio bank of over 500 surgical specimens, and translates his laboratory findings into clinical trials.

Dr. DeMatteo has devoted much effort to surgical education. From 2006 to 2013, he directed Memorial Sloan Kettering's Surgical Oncology Fellowship, mentoring more than 100 clinical fellows in career development, research, and job acquisition. Many of his fellows have assumed leadership positions in academic institutions.

As he had done at MSK, he has established an NIH T32 grant at Penn, the department's first in many years. It supports two years of full-time research under an NIH-sponsored mentor. Taking advantage of support from the Measey Foundation, he has started programs that encourage HUP residents to obtain master's degrees. He requires every resident to write a grant before entering a research lab. Recently, twenty-two HUP residents had nineteen grants. At Penn, as he had done at MSK, he embeds young surgeon scientists into non-surgery labs.

Dr. DeMatteo is the recipient of many honors and awards. He has been elected to the American Society of Clinical Investigation and the Association of American Physicians, both rare honors for a surgeon. He is a member of the American Surgical Association, the Society of Clinical Surgery, the Surgical Biology Club I, the James IV Surgical Association, the Society of University Surgeons, the International Surgical Group, and the Southern Surgical Association, unusual for a Yankee. He is president-elect of the Society of Surgical Oncology, and in 2021, he was elected to membership in the National Academy of Medicine.

Dr. DeMatteo's academic accomplishments and awards compare favorably with those of the department's greatest chairmen, such as Ravdin and Rhoads. He has achieved this while faced with challenges not encountered by other leaders. For starters, there was a worldwide viral epidemic. In the midst of a virtual quarantine, he has maintained the department's first-class performance in clinical activity, education, and research. For NIH funding, it ranks fourth nationally.

During his first six years as chairman, he has dealt with additional circumstances that have changed the world, the school, and social priorities. To succeed, he has needed to make changes in the department greater than those necessary for any earlier department chair.

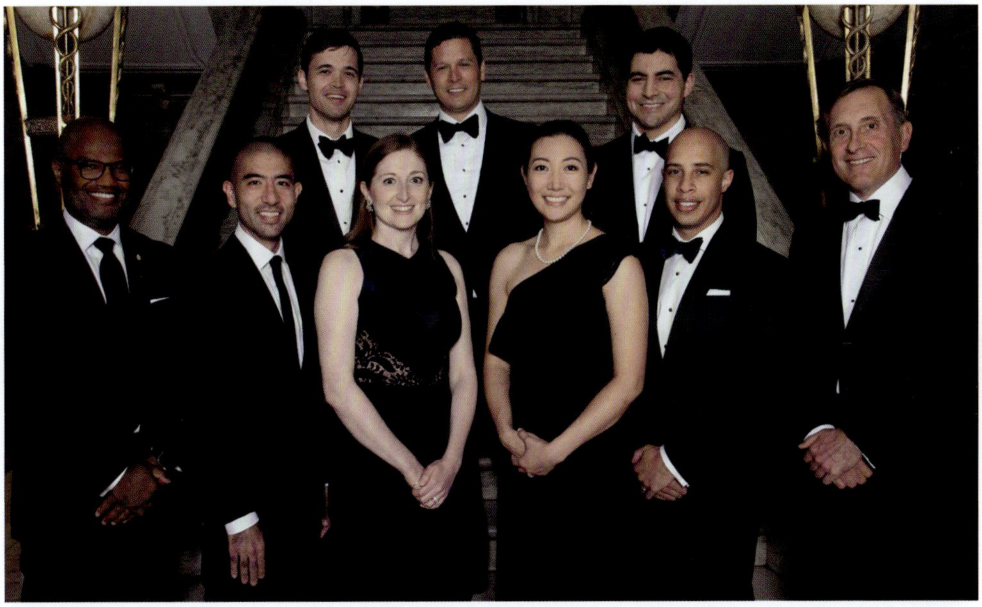

2022 General Surgery Graduates (bottom row L to R) Cary Aarons, Justing Hatchimonji, Lauren Krumeich, Yun Song, Kendall Brooks, Ron DeMatteo, (back row) Mark Etherington, Paul Hernandez and Charlie Vasquez

He has participated in planning the new, 504-bed university hospital, replacing the 139-year-old home of HUP, the nation's first teaching hospital. He has been responsible for the surgical staffing of the new hospital, three newly acquired hospitals, and many new outpatient facilities, some situated in their own large buildings. These additions necessitated a striking increase in the size of the faculty. To accomplish this, he has recruited more than forty-four junior and mid-level faculty, many of them minorities and half of them women. He has also needed to manage turnover of the department's senior leaders, including Drs. Mullen, Fairman, Dempsey, Wein, and Raper.

Dr. DeMatteo's additional changes include new administrative and leadership positions while paying careful attention to the importance of youth, diversity, and fairness in this process. Examples include:

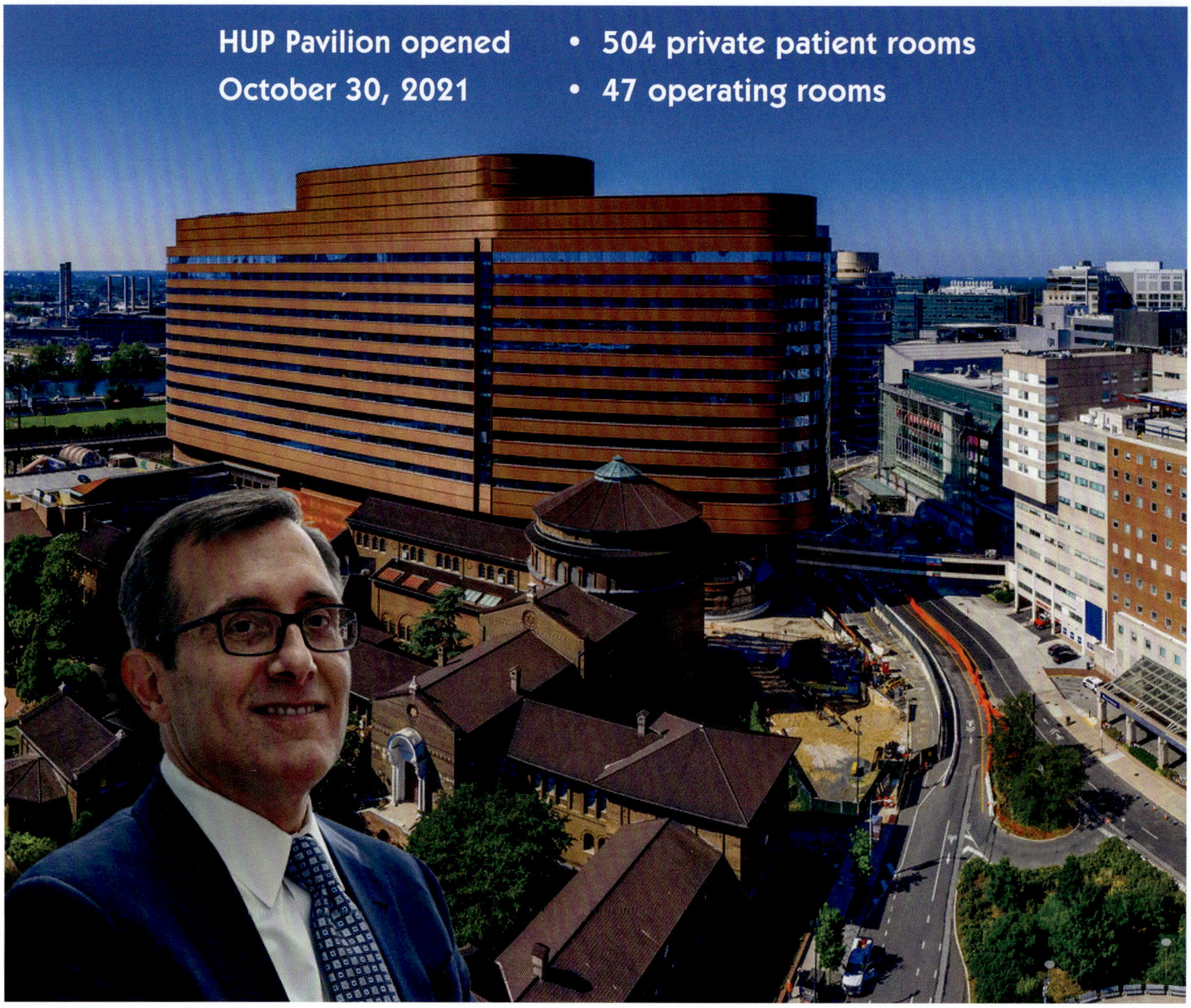
HUP Pavilion opened
October 30, 2021
• 504 private patient rooms
• 47 operating rooms

- Formation of a division of breast surgery with Oluwadamilola Fayanju as chief, the first Black surgeon to lead one of the department's fifteen divisions.

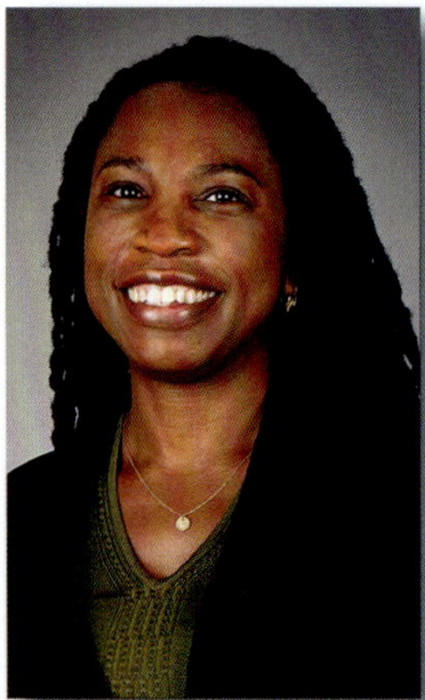

Oluwadamilola Fayanju

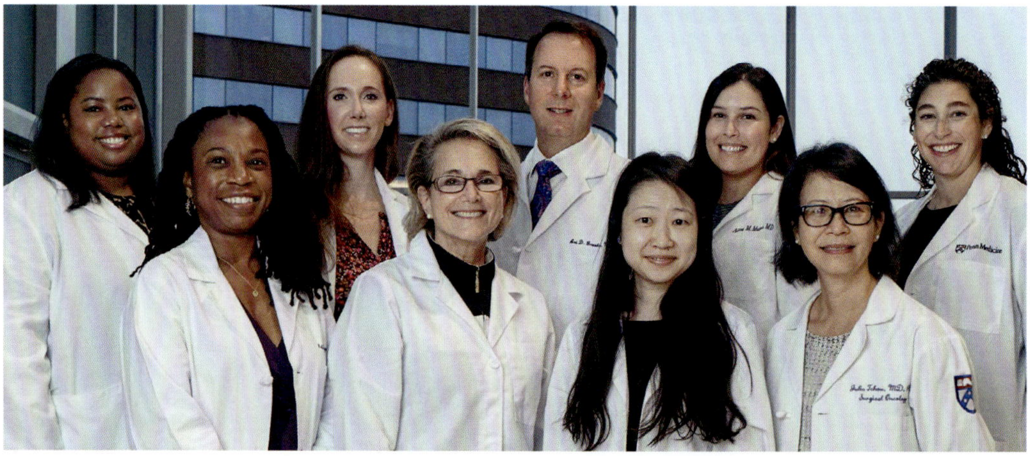

Division of Breast Surgery: (back row) Leisha Elmore, Jami Rothman, Ari Brooks, Alina Mateo, Rebecca Fishman, (front row) Lola Fayanju, Dahlia Sataloff, Jennifer Q. Zhang and Julia Tchou

- Establishment of the new position of executive vice chair of the department with Rachel Kelz as the inaugural chair.

- Establishment of the new position of vice chair for diversity and inclusion with Niels Martin as the inaugural chair.
- Appointment of Cary Aarons and then Ken Lee as successors of Jon Morris after his fourteen years as director of the general surgery residency program.
- Appointment of Sunil Singhal as vice chief for translational research.
- Identifying division chiefs through national searches, previously uncommon for the department.
    - Recruiting Darren Schneider from Cornell to succeed Ron Fairman, who retired after nineteen years as chief of the vascular division.
    - Appointing Charles Vollmer to succeed Dan Dempsey, who retired after ten years as chief of GI surgery.
    - Establishment of a search for a successor to Pat Reilly after his twelve years as chief of the trauma division.
    - Once a national search identifies his successor, Douglas Fraker will step down after twenty-seven years as chief of the surgical oncology division.
    - Initiating a search for Abraham Shaked's successor as director of the transplant institute.
    - Establishment of a search for a successor to Dahlia Sataloff after her ten years as chief of surgery at Pennsylvania Hospital.

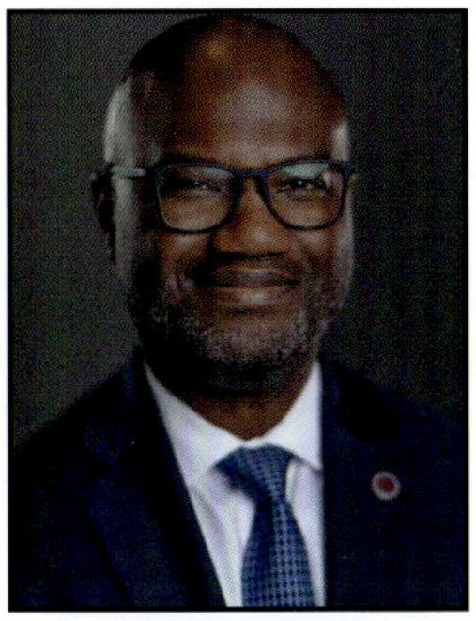

Cary Aarons

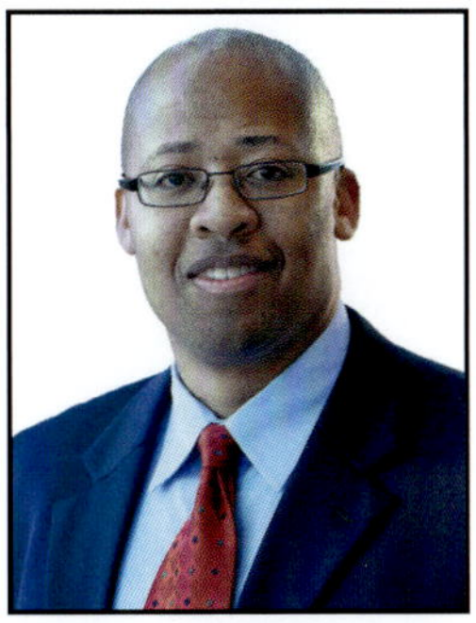

Ken Lee

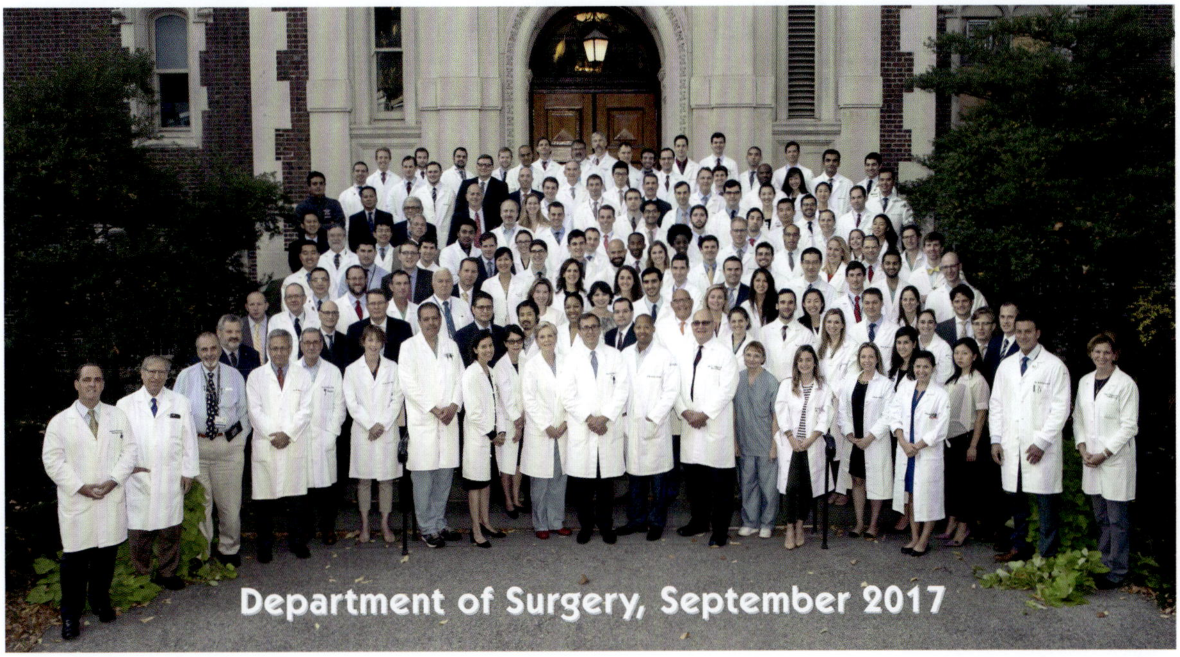

- Increased transparency by including all division chiefs in the department's executive committee.
- Greatly increasing diversity in the residencies and the faculty.
- Half of faculty appointments have been women.
- First HUP-based woman operating cardiac surgeon.
- Growth of the department's endowment by 50 percent.
- Appointments to eleven new endowed professorships.
- Advancing Penn to number 4 nationally in NIH funding.

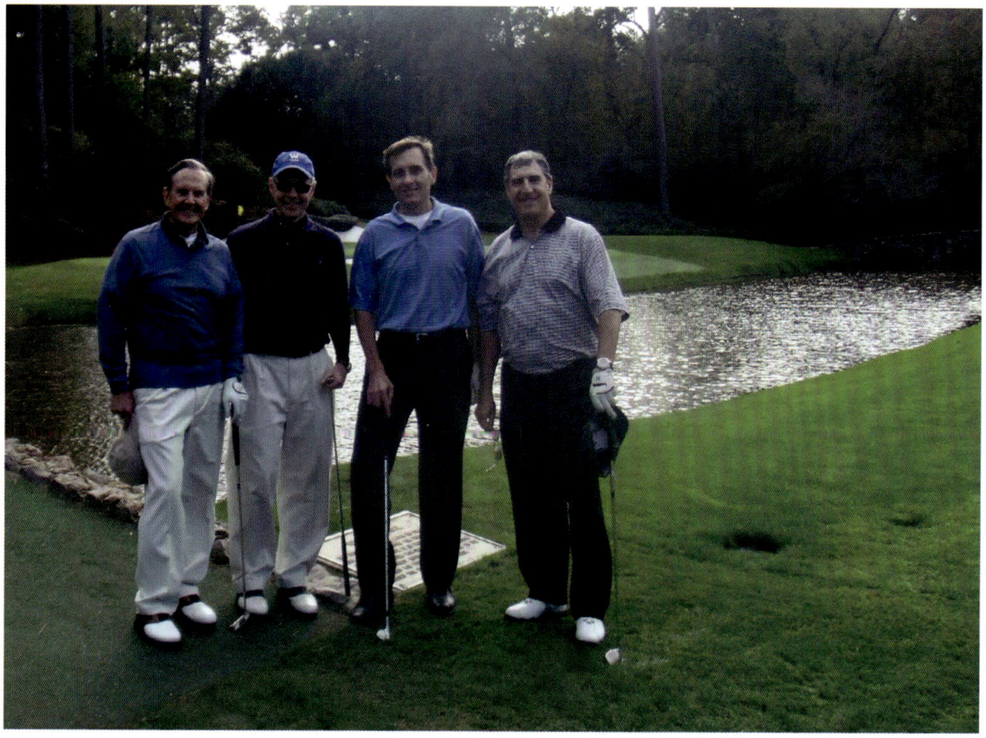

On the Ben Hogan Bridge at Augusta National. From left: Jim Robinson (board member at MSK), Charles Sawyers (scientist), Ron DeMatteo, Peter Scardino (former chair of surgery at MSK).

The move from Manhattan's concrete canyons has allowed Dr. DeMatteo to resume golf. He now has a single-digit handicap and has scored two holes in one on the Philadelphia Country Club's signature par three hole. A good natural athlete, he has also taken up tennis and now plays at a high level in that sport.

Dr. DeMatteo's gifts as a writer are exhibited in his columns for the department's newsletter. These inform alumni and others of changes and progress and in addition, entertain with their insights of wisdom

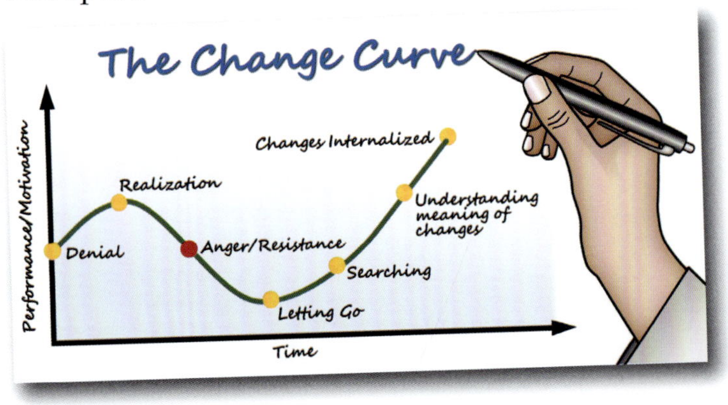

and humor. His column on the stages of change is a thoughtful dissection of the complex evolution the department is going through.

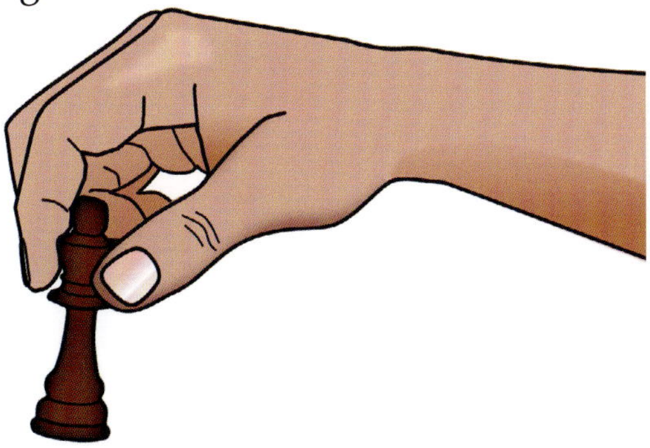

Another of my favorites is his essay on the parallels of surgery and chess. Both require imagination, planning, patience, discipline, and prompt adjustment of strategy if the unexpected is encountered.

It occurs to me that Dr. DeMatteo has had to perform very much like a chess master in adjusting to changes in the academic world. He has been very successful in balancing his responses while maintaining traditional academic values. Fortunately, this has been recognized and applauded by the committee recently charged with reviewing Dr. DeMatteo's first six-year appointment as chairman. He is to be congratulated on the favorable review. I have no doubt that his future terms will be equally productive.

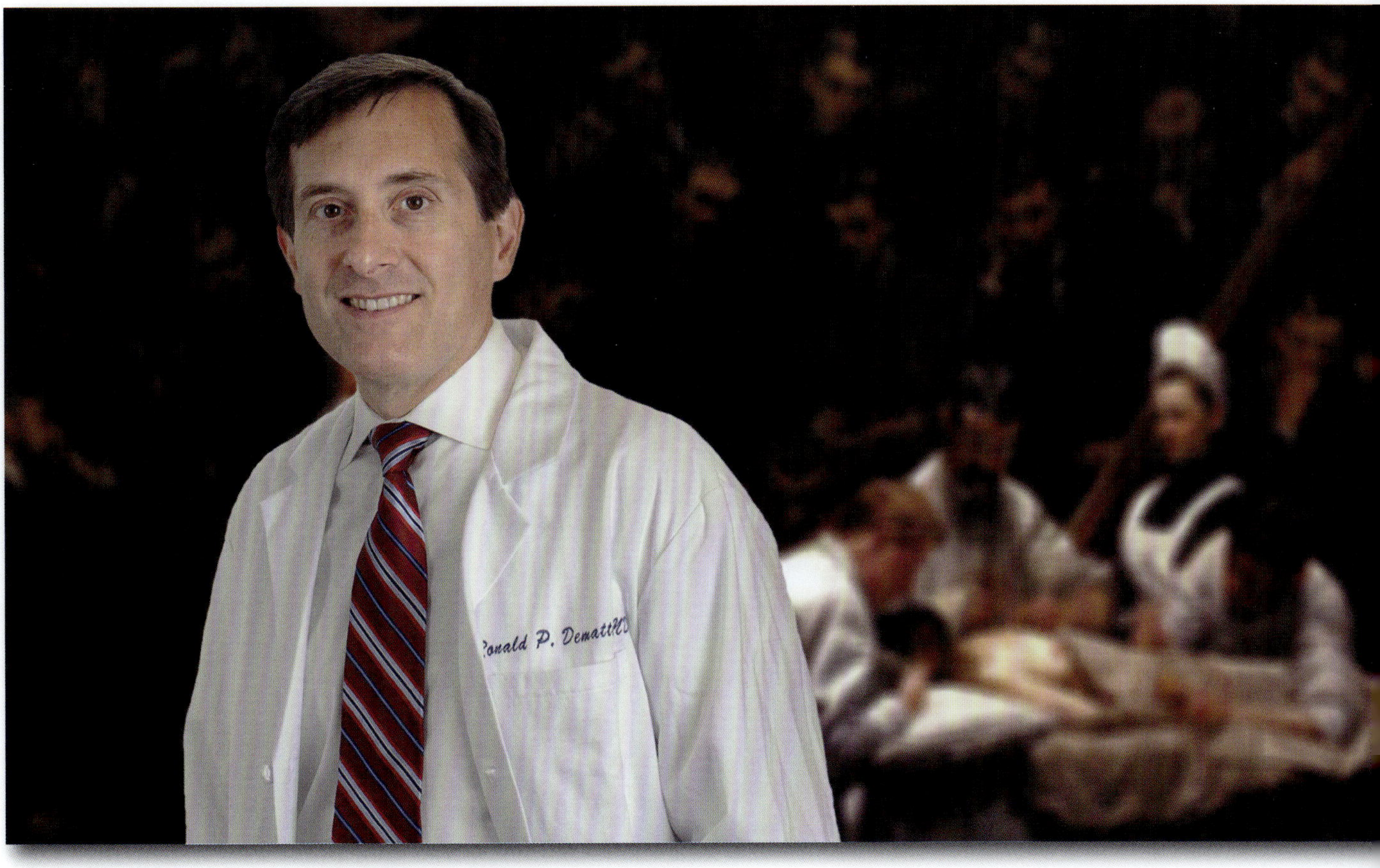

Ronald P. DeMatteo, MD
19th chairman of the Department of Surgery

Notes

[1] DeMatteo RP, Raper SE, Ahn M, Fisher KJ, Burke C, Radu A, Widera G, Claytor BR, Barker CF, Markmann JF. Gene transfer to the thymus: A means of abrogating the immune response to recombinant adenovirus. *Ann Surg* (1995) 222:229–42.

[2] DeMatteo RP, Lewis JJ, Leung D, Mudan SS, Woodruff JL, Brennan MF. Two hundred gastrointestinal stromal tumors—Analysis of recurrence patterns and prognostic factors in survival. *Ann Surg* (2000) 231:51–8.

[3] DeMatteo RP, Ballman KV, Antonescu CR, Maki RG, Pisters PWT, Demetri GD, Blackstein ME, Blanke CD, von Mehren M, Brennan MF, Patel S, McCarter MD, Polikoff JA, Tan BR, Owzar K. ACOSOG Intergroup Adjuvant GIST Study Team. Adjuvant imatinib mesylate after resection of localised, primary gastrointestinal stromal tumour: A randomised, double-blind, placebo-controlled trial. *The Lancet* (2009) 373:1097–104.

[4] DeMatteo RP, Ballman KV, Antonescu CR, Corless C, Kolesnikova V, von Mehren M, McCarter MD, Norton J, Maki RG, Pisters PW, Demetri GD, Brennan MF, Owzar K. American College of Surgeons Oncology Group (ACOSOG) Intergroup Adjuvant GIST Study Team for the Alliance for Clinical Trials in Oncology. Long-term results of adjuvant imatinib mesylate in localized, high-risk, primary gastrointestinal stromal tumor: ACOSOG Z9000 (Alliance) intergroup phase 2 trial. *Ann Surg* (2013) 258:422–9.

[5] Raut CP, Espat NJ, Maki RG, Araujo DM, Trent J, Williams TF, Purkayastha DD, DeMatteo RP. Efficacy and Tolerability of 5-Year Adjuvant Imatinib Treatment for Patients With Resected Intermediate- or High-Risk Primary Gastrointestinal Stromal Tumor: The PERSIST-5 Clinical Trial. *JAMA Oncol* (Dec. 2018) 1;4(12):e184060. doi: 10.1001/jamaoncol.2018.4060. Epub 2018 Dec 13. PMID: 30383140; PMCID: PMC6440723. Cavnar MJ, Seier K, Curtin C, Balachandran VP, Coit DG, Yoon SS, Crago AM, Strong VE, Tap WD, Gönen M, Antonescu CR, Brennan MF, Singer S, and DeMatteo RP. Outcome of 1000 Patients With Gastrointestinal Stromal Tumor (GIST) Treated by Surgery in the Pre- and Post-imatinib Eras. *Annals of surgery* (2021) 273(1), 128–138. https://doi.org/10.1097/SLA.0000000000003277.

[6] Antonescu CR, Besmer P, Guo T, Arkun K, Hom G, Koryotowski B, Leversha MA, Jeffrey PD, Desantis D, Singer S, Brennan MF, Maki RG, DeMatteo RP. Acquired resistance to imatinib in gastrointestinal stromal tumor occurs through secondary gene mutation. *Clin Cancer Res* (2005) 22:4182–90.

Epilogue

If there had been rankings in 1765 when Penn's Department of Surgery began, it would have been ranked as America's best, since it was the first and only one. As we write this some 259 years later, *US News and World Report* ranks it close to the top with only Harvard and Hopkins ahead. Between these times, had there been rankings, Penn might have been placed lower. Early in the twentieth century, it seemed to Provost Edgar Fahs Smith that the University of Pennsylvania (including Surgery) was so far behind the times that it must have been asleep for 100 years. Smith tried to upgrade research in hopes that the impending Flexner Report of 1910 would not expose Penn's deficiencies.

The Flexner Report took it easy on Penn and gave it a pass. Spotting Penn's academic shortcomings required reading between the lines. During the nineteenth and early twentieth centuries, Penn rested on its laurels, and the exalted reputation of its surgical leaders persisted. They remained the most prominent names in the field, despite ignoring research and resident education. After studying Halsted's residency at the new Johns Hopkins medical school, they refused to emulate his methods that were sweeping the country and would soon revolutionize American surgery and medicine. One Penn chairman, world-celebrated John B. Deaver, mistrusted laboratory findings and X-rays, instead relying on his "all-revealing scalpel" and performing a record number of appendectomies, many no doubt lacking appropriate indication. Eldridge Eliason, another nationally-renowned Penn chairman, openly discouraged research by his residents and made fun of those who did it, referring to them as "saltwater surgeons."

In one attempt at reform, Charles Frazier, the school's dean (1903–1909), conspired with his uncle, Provost Charles Custis Harrison, to oust Penn's aging faculty and install in their place young research-based outsiders as the school's leaders. But the old guard, led by surgery chair J. William White, objected, and the newcomers were sent home. Embarrassed by their defeat, the dean and provost resigned. As William Osler observed when leaving Penn for Hopkins, "Nowhere is there more resistance to change than at the University of Pennsylvania."

Finally, in 1945 with the appointment of I. S. Ravdin as chairman, surgery awakened. Ravdin ignored Penn's hidebound traditions, installed Halsted's residency model to train future leaders, and emphasized research, transforming Penn into a modern, academic department. Since then, Jonathan Rhoads and other chairmen have worked to maintain this emphasis.

During its first 100 years, Penn Surgery's professors were the profession's best known and most respected. The smug arrogance of several subsequent surgical leaders allowed the department to fall behind. After a decades-long struggle, Penn Surgery regained a position standing near the top. We have tried to tell this remarkable story with the truth it deserves, without excusing or omitting the bumps on the road. After all, it is the setbacks and recoveries of flawed leaders that enliven a story. We hope you enjoy reading it as much as we did writing it.

While deciding how to finish this account, we were aware that many deserving contemporary Penn surgeons are mentioned only briefly, if at all. We began to list them, but when we had counted more than 100, we realized there wasn't enough time, or room in this book, for everyone. Their essays will have to be written by whoever compiles the next history of this venerable department.

Afterword

Contributed by Ronald P. DeMatteo

When I first asked Dr. Barker to recount the history of Penn Surgery, he responded with a smile and an uncharacteristic mumble. I broached the topic a few more times over the next year, but he pretended not to hear me. There was no other person who could accomplish this feat. Frankly, no one else was qualified. It was now or never. His reluctancy eventually dissipated, and he accepted the Herculean task. To sustain his enthusiasm, I started telling everyone about the project.

Somehow, no one appears to have ever written the history of the oldest Department of Surgery in the country, which was established in 1765. Fortuitously, Dr. Barker has been a self-designated historian for decades. He had already amassed a trove of documents and notes and had delivered innumerable presentations. With his sharpened #2 pencil, he has now stupendously chronicled intriguing details and created captivating anecdotes about Penn Surgery. Of course, "The Book" would not have been possible without his daughter Elizabeth and Robin Noel, who toiled endlessly with drafts and sought permissions for photographs.

Dr. Barker wanted The Book to conclude with how Penn Surgery may evolve farther. This reminded me of the Yogi Berra aphorism, "It's tough to make predictions, especially about the future." As an aside, the physicist Niels Bohr actually derived this statement from a Danish proverb. Anyway, below are some forecasts. Admittedly, some are already in progress.

Faculty: Our faculty size will grow to 225 by the year 2050. Surgeons will largely work in teams and shifts (like transplantation and trauma do now). Robots will replace some of the OR staff, such as scrub technicians and assistant surgeons.

Education: Formal classroom instruction will disappear from medical school, as education will be completely integrated around patient care. The duration of medical school will be reduced to three years. Personal, handheld phones/computers will be allowed during all exams, so memorization will be deemphasized. Virtual reality and simulation will closely approximate real life, which will reduce total surgical training by a few years. Surgeons will be tracked to specialization within one year of general surgery training. Trainee work hours will be reduced to sixty hours per week, mostly as five twelve-hour shifts.

Health care systems: Corporations will take over many hospitals if healthcare is not nationalized. Patient access will be greatly improved by artificial intelligence directing primary care and some advanced care.

Diagnosis/Prevention: Blood analysis in infants will predict many of the diseases that a person is likely to acquire during their lifetime. Blood tests in adulthood will allow for early diagnosis of cancer and other diseases, such as diabetes or dementia. Low-cost, annual imaging will be implemented to screen for diseases. Radiologists and pathologists will be reduced by artificial intelligence diagnostics.

Surgery: Robotic surgery will be widely practiced for nearly all operations, and robots will soon provide excellent haptic feedback. Artificial intelligence will be used routinely in the operating room to guide, if not dictate, intraoperative decision-making. Only a small percentage of operations will require an inpatient stay. Many operations will become obsolete as medical, interventional-guided, and radiation-based therapies improve. Xenotransplantation will be successful in some instances in the second half of the twenty-first century. In the next fifteen years, a new hospital will be built on the main campus as well as the Presbyterian campus. The old HUP ORs will be reopened by 2026 to enable continued growth in Surgery.

Now we just have to hope that someone will want to write Volume II of Penn Surgery. If it takes another 259 years, which would be the year 2283, their great, great, great, great, grandparents have not been born yet. Hopefully, the eccentricity and unique spirit of the Department during the first two-and-a-half centuries will persist and provide sufficient fodder for Volume II.

Endnotes*

Page 2
Unknown, *Dr. William Shippen, Jr.* Oil on canvas, 35.5 × 28.5 in. The Mutter Museum of the College of Physicians of Philadelphia. https://tcpp-emuweb.axiellhosting.com/museum/?record=ecatalogue.138

Page 5
Thom, Robert. *John Hunter: Founder of Scientific Surgery, from " The History of Medicine,"* c. 1952. Oil on canvas. 41 5/16 × 34 in. From the collection of Michigan Medicine, University of Michigan, Gift of Pfizer, Inc., UMHS.20
https://exchange.umma.umich.edu/resources/41231

Zoffany, Johann. *William Hunter lecturing*, 1772. Oil on canvas, 77.4 × 103.5 cm. Royal College of Physicians, London.

Page 6
Lambdin, James Reid. *William Shippen*, n.d. Etching by H. Wright Smith. National Library of Medicine.
http://resource.nlm.nih.gov/101429118

Deroy, Laurent. *State-house*, 1848. Drawn from nature by Aug. Köllner; lith. by Deroy; printed by Cattier. New York; Paris: Published by Goupil, Vibert & Co., [1848]. Lithograph, tinted; 32.8 × 42.3 cm (sheet).

Page 7
Cogswell, William. *John Morgan*, 1852. Oil on canvas. Copy after Angelica Kauffman.
https://pennartcollection.com/collection/art/79/john-morgan-1735-1789/ *Courtesy of the University of Pennsylvania Art Collection, Philadelphia, PA.*

Page 8
John Morgan, 1869. Etching by H. B. Hall. U.S. National Library of Medicine (NLM): Images from the History of Medicine.
http://resource.nlm.nih.gov/101433839

Lambdin, James Reid. *William Shippen*, n.d. Etching by H. Wright Smith. National Library of Medicine.
http://resource.nlm.nih.gov/101429118

Page 9
Duche, Thomas Spence Jr. *John Morgan*, 1784. Oil on canvas, 89.9 × 69.5 cm. Historical Society of Pennsylvania, Philadelphia.

Page 11
Peale, Charles Willson. *William Shippen*, n.d. Oil on canvas.
https://www.med.upenn.edu/psom/william-shippen-md.html
Courtesy of the University of Pennsylvania Art Collection, Philadelphia, PA.

Page 12
Peale, Charles Willson. *Dr. Benjamin Rush*, 1783 and 1786. Oil on canvas, 126.7 × 101.3 cm. Winterthur Museum., Winterthur, DE.
http://museumcollection.winterthur.org/print-record.php?srchfld=irn&name=11281&port=40138&output=HTML

Page 13
Thomas Jefferson, June, Rough Draft of the Declaration of Independence. -06, 1776. Manuscript/Mixed Material. Library of Congress.
https://www.loc.gov/item/mtjbib000156/ With signature of Benjamin Rush superimposed.

Leutze, Emanuel. *Washington Crossing the Delaware*, 1851. Oil on canvas. 149 × 255 in. Metropolitan Museum of Art, New York City.
https://www.metmuseum.org/art/collection/search/11417

Trumbell, John. *The Death of General Mercer at the Battle of Princeton, January 3, 1777*, c. 1789–1831. Oil on canvas. 21 × 30 3/4 in. Yale University Art Gallery, New Haven, CT.
https://artgallery.yale.edu/collections/objects/101

Page 14
Longacre, James Barton. *Patrick Henry*, c. 1835. Watercolor on illustration board. 13.7 × 13.5 cm. National Portrait Gallery, Smithsonian Institution, Washington, DC.
https://npg.si.edu/object/npg_NPG.77.291

Stuart, Gilbert. *Horatio Gates*, c. 1793–94. Oil on canvas. 44 1/4 × 35 7/8 in. The Metropolitan Museum of Art, New York City.
https://www.metmuseum.org/art/collection/search/12667

An ill man being bled by a surgeon. Colored etching by J. Sneyd, 1804, after J. Gillray. Wellcome Collection.
https://wellcomecollection.org/works/htmvf9qp

Page 15
Bates, William. *The MacLise Portrait-Gallery of "Illustrious Literary Characters"*. London: Chatto and Windus, 1883, 333. Illustration of William Cobbett by Daniel Maclise.
https://en.wikisource.org/wiki/The_Maclise_Portrait-Gallery

Stearns, Junius Brutus. *Washington on His Deathbed*, 1851. Oil on canvas, 37 1/4 × 54 1/8 in. Dayton Art Institute.
https://daytonart.emuseum.com/objects/1306/washington-on-his-deathbed

Page 16
Duncan, Louis C. *Benjamin Rush.* "Medical Men in the American Revolution 1775–1783." *The Army Medical Bulletin* 25 (1931). Drawing.
https://medcoeckapwstorprd01.blob.core.usgovcloudapi.net/achh/p176Rush_1726.jpg

Page 23
Gardner, Daniel. *Peggy Shippen and daughter*, c. 1783–89. Oil on canvas, 24.5 × 21.5 in. Atwater Kent Collection at Drexel University, Philadelphia.
https://commons.wikimedia.org/wiki/File:Peggy_Shippen_and_daughter.jpg

Page 24
Sully, Thomas. *Caspar Wistar*, 1830. Copy after Bass Otis. Oil on canvas, 30 × 25 1/8 in. American Philosophical Society, Philadelphia.
https://diglib.amphilsoc.org/islandora/object/graphics%3A4656

Page 25
DiCarlo, Candice. *Nina Long holding model of inner ear by William Rush.* Reprinted from *The Wister Institute Focus*, Spring 2002, 8.

Page 26
Wistar, Caspar. *A System of Anatomy for the Use of Students of Medicine [vol 2.]*. Philadelphia: Thomas Dobson, 1814. Book cover.

Wistar, Caspar. *A System of Anatomy for the Use of Students of Medicine [vol 2.]*. Philadelphia: Thomas Dobson, 1817, Plate XX.

*The APSP has made all reasonable efforts to locate copyright owners and to supply complete and correct credits; if there are errors or omissions, please contact the APSP so that corrections can be addressed in any subsequent edition.

Walcott, Mary Vaux. *American Wisteria (Kraunhia frutescens),* 1925. Watercolor on paper, 10 × 6 7/8 in. Smithsonian American Art Museum, Washington, DC.

Page 27
Leney, William. *John Jones M.D.* Stipple engraving from *The American Medical and Philosophical Register 1813, after p 324.* https://archive.org/details/americanmedicalp31812newy/page/n353/mode/2up

Page 28
Jones, John. *Plain Concise Practical Remarks, on the Treatment of Wounds and Fractures.* Philadelphia: Robert Bell, 1776. Title page.

Page 29
Sharples, Ellen. *Benjamin Rush,* 1805. After James Sharples, Sr. Pastel on paper, 9 × 7 in. Portrait Gallery in the Second Bank of the United States, National Park Service, Philadelphia. https://museum.nps.gov/ParkObjdet.aspx?rID=INDE%20%20%2011871&db=objects&dir=CR%20INDE&osearch=rush&page=1

Page 30
Mosquito. Photograph. http://res.publicdomainfiles.com/pdf_view/41/13519190412587.jpg

Page 31
Rosenthal, Max. *Matthew Clarkson,* 1885. Lithograph. The Miriam and Ira D. Division of Art, Prints and Photographs: Print Collection, The New York Public Library. New York Public Library Digital Collections. https://digitalcollections.nypl.org/items/510d47da-3150-a3d9-e040-e00a18064a99

Hubbard, Elbert. *Little Journeys to the Homes of Great Businessmen, Volume 11.* New York: Wm. M. Wise & Co., 1916. Illustration of Stephen Girard. https://www.gutenberg.org/files/23595/23595-h/23595-h.htm#STEPHEN_GIRARD

McCabe, James. *Great fortunes, and how they were made; on. The struggles and triumphs of our self-made men.* Cincinnati: E. Hannaford & Co., 1871, 62. Illustration of *Girard's Heroism* from original design by G. F. & E. B. Bensell. University of Michigan Library Digital Collections. https://quod.lib.umich.edu/m/moa/ajk6320.0001.001/62

Page 32
Payne, Daniel A. *History of the African Methodist Episcopal Church.* Nashville: A. M. E. Sunday-School Union, 1891. Frontispiece engraving of Richard Allen by John Sartain. https://archive.org/details/historyofafrican00payn/page/n9/mode/2up

Peale, Raphaelle. *Absalom Jones,* 1810. Oil on paper mounted to board, 30 × 25 in. Delaware Art Museum, Wilmington, DE. https://emuseum.delart.org/objects/10348/absalom-jones?ctx=20614c91e32645085d250abb6bf73b17dafbffed&idx=3

Page 38
P. S. Physick M.D. n.d. Lithograph, 1 print. U.S. National Library of Medicine (NLM): Images from the History of Medicine. https://jstor.org/stable/community.28565296

Page 39
Jackson, John. *John Hunter,* 1813. After Sir Joshua Reynolds. Oil on canvas, 55 1/2 × 43 1/4 in. National Portrait Gallery, London. https://www.npg.org.uk/collections/search/portrait/mw03322/John-Hunter

Ramsay, Allan. *William Hunter,* c. 1764–65. Oil on canvas, 37.7 × 29.5 in. Hunterian Museum and Art Gallery, Glasgow. https://www.gla.ac.uk/collections/#/details?irn=36443&catType=C&referrer=/results&q=ramsay

Page 40
St. George's Hospital, Hyde Park Corner: seen from inside Hyde Park. Wood engraving by Greenaway after a print of 1745. 5 5/8 × 8 1/4 in. From "Old and New London: (circa 1878) A Narrative of Its History, Its People, and Its Places. The Western and Northern Studies," by Edward Walford. Cassell, Petter, Galpin & Co., London.

Page 41
Rosenthal, Albert. *Dr. Philip Syng Physick,* 1916. Oil on canvas, 29.25 × 24.25 in. The Mutter Museum of the College of Physicians of Philadelphia. https://tcppemuweb.axiellhosting.com/museum/?record=ecatalogue.220

Sully, Thomas. *Caspar Wistar,* 1830. Copy after Bass Otis. Oil on canvas, 30 × 25 1/8 in. American Philosophical Society, Philadelphia. https://diglib.amphilsoc.org/islandora/object/graphics%3A4656

Dorsey, John Syng. *The Elements of Surgery; for the use of students.* Philadelphia: Edward Parker & Kimbe & Conrad, 1813. Cover and title page.

Conner, J. Del. *Label of Dr. Physick Black Cherry soda.* Photograph. http://drphysick.com/purchasesoda.html *Permission granted by J. Del Conner.*

Page 42
Dodson, R. W., artist. *Philip Syng Physick, c.* 1820. Print: engraving with manuscript annotation, 10 × 6 in. UPX 4, Graphics and portraits Collection, Box 2. University Archives and Records Center, University of Pennsylvania. https://jstor.org/stable/community.22101069

Page 43
Rush, William. *Dr. Philip Syng Physick,* c. 1812–13. Painted Plaster, 26 × 16 × 10 in. High Museum of Art, Atlanta, GA. https://high.org/collection/dr-philip-syng-physick/

Page 44
Goodman, Charles and Piggot, Robert. *John Sing Dorsey, M.D.,* 1819. After Thomas Sully. Engraving in black on wove paper, 4 13/16 × 3 7/8 in. Corcoran Collection, National Gallery of Art, Washington, DC. https://www.nga.gov/collection/art-object-page.197331.html

Page 45
Dorsey, John Syng. *The Elements of Surgery, 2nd ed.* Philadelphia: E. & R. Parker & Benjamin Warner, 1818. Plates after pp. 52 and 188. https://archive.org/details/2552014RX1.nlm.nih.gov/mode/2up

Page 46
Wood, Joseph. *William Gibson,* 1819. Oil on wood, 8.375 × 6.375 in. The Mutter Museum of the College of Physicians of Philadelphia. https://tcpp-emuweb.axiellhosting.com/museum/?record=ecatalogue.79

Page 50
Baker, I.H., photographer. *William Gibson, c.* 1847. Print: engraving, 7.9 × 5.6 in. UPF 1.9 AR, Alumni Records Collection. University Archives and Records Center, University of Pennsylvania. https://jstor.org/stable/community.22106883

Page 52
Wood, Joseph. *William Gibson,* 1819. Oil on wood, 8.375 × 6.375 in. The Mutter Museum of the College of Physicians of Philadelphia. https://tcpp-emuweb.axiellhosting.com/museum/?record=ecatalogue.79

Sadler, William. *The Battle of Waterloo,* 1815 June. Oil on canvas, 31.8 × 69.6 in. Private Collection. https://commons.wikimedia.org/wiki/File:Battle_of_Waterloo_1815.PNG

Page 53
O'Brien, R. *Crawford W. Long, M.D. Discoverer of anaesthesia demonstrated on James M. Venables by the use of sulphuric ether at Jefferson, Jackson Co., Georgia, March 30th, 1842,* c. 1877. Engraving. Boston Medical Library. https://collections.countway.harvard.edu/onview/items/show/18110

Gibson, William. *The Institutes and Practice of Surgery, Vol II, 4th ed.* Philadelphia: Carey, Lea & Blanchard, 1835. Illustration.

Gibson, William. *The Institutes and Practices of Surgery.* (Philadelphia: Carey, Lea & Blanchard, 1824). Book cover, title page.

Page 54
Neagle, John B. *William Gibson*, 1855. Oil on canvas. 126.6cm × 101.2cm. https://npg.si.edu/object/npg_PA330047 Courtesy of the University of Pennsylvania Art Collection, Philadelphia, PA.

Page 58
Neagle, John B. *William Horner*, c. 1836. Oil on canvas. https://www.med.upenn.edu/psom/william-edmonds-horner-md.html Courtesy of the University of Pennsylvania Art Collection, Philadelphia, PA.

Page 59
Welch and Walters, photographer. *William Edmund Horner*, 1846. Print: engraving with manuscript annotation, 8.9 × 5.8 in. UPX 4, Graphics and portraits Collection, Box 1. University Archives and Records Center, University of Pennsylvania. https://jstor.org/stable/community.22104910

Page 60
Illustration of tensor tarsi muscle from *Philadelphia Journal of the Medical and Physical Sciences*, Vol. 8, (1824), 70–80. Historical Collections, College of Physicians of Philadelphia.

Page 61
Horner, William E. *A Treatise on Pathological Anatomy*. Philadelphia: Carey, Lea & Carey, 1829. Title page. https://wellcomecollection.org/works/dmhf6qwt

Sully, Thomas. *William Edmonds Horner*, 1836. Oil on wood, 19 11/16 × 16 3/4 in. Wistar Institute, Philadelphia. https://npg.si.edu/object/npg_PA330341

Edouart, Auguste. *William Horner and William Gibson*, 1843. Ink wash, chalk, and cut paper on paper, 11 1/16 × 8 3/4 in. National Portrait Gallery, Smithsonian Institution, Washington, DC. https://npg.si.edu/object/npg_S_NPG.91.126.70.B

Page 64
Waugh, Samuel Bell. *Henry Hollingsworth Smith*, 1871. Oil on canvas. https://www.med.upenn.edu/psom/henry-hollingsworth-smith-md.html Courtesy of the University of Pennsylvania Art Collection, Philadelphia, PA.

Page 65
Taylor, William Curtis. *Portrait of Henry Hollingsworth Smith, M.D.*, Albumin print, 20 × 17 cm. Free Library of Philadelphia. https://libwww.freelibrary.org/digital/item/2346

Page 66
Smith, Henry Hollingsworth. *A System of Operative Surgery: Based Upon the Practice of Surgeons in the United States*. Philadelphia: Lippincott, Grambo & Co., 1852. Title page. https://www.google.com/books/edition/A_System_of_Operative_Surgery/Zhw6AQAAMAAJ?hl=en&gbpv=0

Smith, Henry Hollingsworth. *A System of Operative Surgery: Based Upon the Practice of Surgeons in the United States*. Philadelphia: Lippincott, Grambo & Co., 1852. Plate VIII following p. 76.

Page 67
Adams, J. Howe. *History of the Life of D. Hayes Agnew*. Philadelphia and London: The F. A. Davis Company, 1892. Photo of D. Hayes Agnew facing p. 108.

Magnus, Charles. *Satterlee U.S.A. General Hospital, West Philadelphia*, c. 1864. Published by James D. Gay. Hand-colored chromolithograph. The Library Company of Philadelphia. https://digital.librarycompany.org/islandora/object/digitool%3A65951

Page 68
Henry Hollingsworth Smith, c. 1865. Photograph, 4 × 4 in. UPF 1.9 AR, Alumni Records Collection, Box 2527. University Archives and Records Center, University of Pennsylvania. https://jstor.org/stable/community.22109125

Page 72
D. Hayes (David Hayes) Agnew, 1892. Photograph, 6.0 × 3.5 in. UPF 1.9 AR, Alumni Records Collection. University Archives and Records Center, University of Pennsylvania. https://jstor.org/stable/community.22103519

Eakins, Thomas. *Agnew Clinic*, 1889. Oil on canvas, 74 1/2 × 130 1/2 in. University of Pennsylvania. School of Medicine. https://jstor.org/stable/community.14623616 Courtesy of the University of Pennsylvania Art Collection, Philadelphia, PA.

Page 73
Uhle, Bernard. *David Hayes Agnew*, 1889. Oil on canvas, 51.5 × 37.5 in. The Mutter Museum of the College of Physicians of Philadelphia. https://tcppemuweb.axiellhosting.com/museum/?record=ecatalogue.193

Dimino, T. *Dr. Samuel David Gross*, 1909. Oil on canvas, 35.25 × 28.25 in. The Mutter Museum of the College of Physicians of Philadelphia. https://tcppemuweb.axiellhosting.com/museum/?record=ecatalogue.196

Circle of Eakins, *Thomas Eakins leaning against building*, c. 1870–76. Photograph, 4 × 3 1/4 in. Pennsylvania Academy of Fine Arts, Philadelphia. https://www.pafa.org/museum/collection/item/thomas-eakins-leaning-against-building-0

Page 74
Adams, J. Howe. *History of the Life of D. Hayes Agnew*. Philadelphia and London: The F. A. Davis Company, 1892. Agnew coat of arms facing p. 18.

Page 75
Adams, J. Howe. *History of the Life of D. Hayes Agnew*. Philadelphia and London: The F. A. Davis Company, 1892. Photo of Philadelphia School of Anatomy facing p.78.

Pelham, Camden. *The Chronicles of Crime*. London: T. Miles & Co., 1887. Engraving by Hablot Knight Browne of *Resurrectionists*, 1887, from original drawing by "Phiz." https://archive.org/details/chroniclesofcri01pelh/page/n317/mode/2up?view=theater

Page 76
Adams, J. Howe. *History of the Life of D. Hayes Agnew*. Philadelphia and London: The F. A. Davis Company, 1892. Photo of D. Hayes Agnew facing p.108.

P.S. Duval & Son, Printer, and James Fuller Queen. *Mower U.S.A. General Hostital [sic], Chestnut Hill, Philadelphia/J. Queen, del.; P.S. Duval & Son, lith.*, ca. 1865. Philadelphia: P.S. Duval & Son. Hand-colored lithograph. https://www.loc.gov/item/2003655784/

Waugh, Samuel Bell. *Henry Hollingsworth Smith*, 1871. Oil on canvas. https://www.med.upenn.edu/psom/henry-hollingsworth-smith-md.html Courtesy of the University of Pennsylvania Art Collection, Philadelphia, PA.

Page 77
Agnew, D. Hayes. *The Principals and Practice of Surgery, Vol II, 2nd ed.* Philadelphia: J. B. Lippincott Co., 1889, 671. Figure 1406. https://www.google.com/books/edition/The_Principles_and_practice_of_surgery_v/wn1fmg-7xEIC?hl=en&gbpv=1

Agnew, D. Hayes. *The Principals and Practice of Surgery, Vol II, 2nd ed.* Philadelphia: J. B. Lippincott Co., 1889, 672. Figure 1408. https://www.google.com/books/edition/The_Principles_and_practice_of_surgery_v/wn1fmg-7xEIC?hl=en&gbpv=1

Page 78
Agnew, D. Hayes. *The Principals and Practice of Surgery Vol I–III.* Photo courtesy of Clyde Barker.

Dimino, T. *Dr. Samuel David Gross*, 1909. Oil on canvas, 35.25 × 28.25 in. The Mutter Museum of the College of Physicians of Philadelphia. https://tcppemuweb.axiellhosting.com/museum/?record=ecatalogue.196

Pres. James Garfield, 1881. Photograph. Library of Congress. https://hdl.loc.gov/loc.pnp/cwpbh.03744

Washington, D.C.–The attack on the President's life–Scene in the ladies' room of the Baltimore and Ohio Railroad depot–The arrest of the assassin/from sketches by our special artist's [sic] A. Berghaus and C. Upham Illus. in: *Frank Leslie's illustrated newspaper,* 1881 July 16, pp. 332–333. Library of Congress, Washington, DC. https://www.loc.gov/pictures/item/96521930/

Page 79
The Wounded President: Ascertaining the location of the bullet. Harper's Weekly, August 13, 1881. From a sketch by W. Shinkle. https://archive.org/details/sim_harpers-weekly_1881-08-13_25_1286/page/n11/mode/2up

Rogers, William Allen. *The President's Room [Pres. Garfield on his death bed],* 1881. Wood engraving on paper, 13 11/16 × 19 3/4 in. Clark Art Institute. https://www.clarkart.edu/artpiece/detail/The-President-s-Room-Pres-Garfield-on-his-deat-(1)

Bickersteth, R. A. *Joseph Lister,* (n.d.) Photograph. U.S. National Library of Medicine (NLM): Images from the History of Medicine. http://resource.nlm.nih.gov/101421935.

Page 80
Eakins, Thomas. *Portrait of Samuel D. Gross (The Gross Clinic),* 1875. Oil on canvas, 8 feet × 6 feet 6 inches. Philadelphia Museum of Art. https://philamuseum.org/collection/object/299524

Page 81
Chambers, George, photographer. *Agnew Clinic, Interior, Surgery Demonstration.* 1886 March 30. Photograph, 6 × 8 in. UPX 12, University Photograph Collection, Box 59, folder 1. University Archives and Records Center, University of Pennsylvania. https://jstor.org/stable/community.22109289

Page 82
Eakins, Thomas. *Agnew Clinic,* 1889. Oil on canvas, 74 1/2 × 130 1/2 inches. University of Pennsylvania. School of Medicine. https://jstor.org/stable/community.14623616 Courtesy of the University of Pennsylvania Art Collection, Philadelphia, PA.

Page 83
Closeup of *Agnew Clinic.*

Page 90
Phillips, H. C. *John Ashhurst.* U.S. National Library of Medicine (NLM): Images from the History of Medicine. http://resource.nlm.nih.gov/101409530

Page 92
Ashhurst Jr., John. *The Principals and Practice of Surgery.* Photo by Elizabeth Barker.

Ashhurst Jr., John. *The Principals and Practice of Surgery, 2nd ed.* Philadelphia: Henry C. Lea, 1878, 117. Figures 53–54. https://www.biblio.com/book/principles-practice-surgery-john-ashhurst-jr/d/1295227317#gallery-3

Page 93
Borie, Adolph. *Dr. John Ashhurst, Jr.,* 1910–12. Oil on canvas, 71 × 46 in. The Mutter Museum of the College of Physicians of Philadelphia. https://tcpp-emuweb.axiellhosting.com/museum/?record=ecatalogue.178

Flanders, Lowell, photographer. *Ashhurst Room, College of Physicians* of *Philadelphia,* 2024.

Page 98
Gray, photographer. *J. William (James William) White, c.* 1880. Photograph, 6 .9 × 4.8 in. UPF 1.9 AR, Alumni Records Collection. University Archives and Records Center, University of Pennsylvania. https://jstor.org/stable/community.22103536

Page 99
Portrait of Louis Agassiz. In this photo he is seen demonstrating his theory of jelly-fish, corals and starfish, 1872. Photograph. The Miriam and Ira D. Wallach Division of Art, Prints and Photographs: Photography Collection, The New York Public Library. https://digitalcollections.nypl.org/items/510d47d9-4028-a3d9-e040-e00a18064a99

USC&GSS Ferdinand R. Hassler, 1893. Photograph. National Oceanic and Atmospheric Administration. https://photolib.noaa.gov/Collections/Sailing-For-Science/Nineteenth-Century-Ships/emodule/586/eitem/9884

Page 100
Map of J. William White's swim from Newport to Narragansett. Graphic courtesy of Robin Noel.

Rittenhouse, Rex. "City's Last Duel Not Even Romantic." *Philadelphia Record,* December 19, 1944.

Page 101
Closeup of *Agnew Clinic.*

Eakins, Thomas. *Agnew Clinic,* 1889. Oil on canvas, 74 1/2 × 130 1/2 inches. University of Pennsylvania. School of Medicine. https://jstor.org/stable/community.14623616 Courtesy of the University of Pennsylvania Art Collection, Philadelphia, PA.

Collage of newspaper clippings from July 8, 1883. "Making Business for His Profession," *Sunday World.* "Slugged by a Surgeon," *The Times,* and [...], The *Sunday Item.*

Page 102
Burnett, Charles H. [and others]. *An American Textbook of Surgery: for practitioners and students.* ed. William W. Keen and J. William White. Philadelphia: W. B. Saunders, 1892. https://wellcomecollection.org/works/vtbap4jc

White, J. William. "The Use of Skiagraphy for the Detection and Location of Foreign Bodies Impacted in the Œsophagus." *Annals of Surgery* 24, no. 2 (1896 Aug): 238–242.

White, J. William. "The Results of Double Castration in Hypertrophy of the Prostate." *Annals of Surgery* 22 (1895 Jul): 1–80.

Page 103
Sargent, John Singer. *J. William White,* c. 1909. Oil on canvas. https://www.med.upenn.edu/psom/james-william-white-md-phd.html Courtesy of the University of Pennsylvania Art Collection, Philadelphia, PA.

Page 108
Rittenberg, Henry R. *Edward Martin,* c. 1913. Oil on canvas. https://www.med.upenn.edu/psom/edward-martin-md-facs.html Courtesy of the University of Pennsylvania Art Collection, Philadelphia, PA.

Page 109
Jequier, Anne M. "Edward Martin (1859–1938). The founding father of modern clinical andrology." *International Journal of Andrology,* 14 (1991): 1–10. https://onlinelibrary.wiley.com/doi/epdf/10.1111/j.1365-2605.1991.tb01057.x

Fig. 2 of preceding article—*A drawing of the operation of epididymo-vasostomy as carried out by Edward Martin.*

Page 110
History of United States Army Base Hospital No. 20: Organized at the University of Pennsylvania. Philadelphia: E.A. Wright, 1920, 8. Photograph of Col. Edward Martin M.C. http://books.google.com/books?id=J0ASAQAAMAAJ

Spanish-American War, Nurses from the University of Pennsylvania Tending Ill Soldiers on Hospital Train. 1898. Photograph, 4 × 6 in. UPX 12, University Photograph Collection, Box 59, folder 16. University Archives and Records Center, University of Pennsylvania. https://jstor.org/stable/community.22102371

Page 111
Clinedinst, Barnett McFee. *Franklin W. Martin,* Washington, DC, "Portrait of Franklin H. Martin, MD, FACS, 1857–1935," The American College of Surgeons Archives. Photograph. https://www.facs.org/about-acs/archives/past-

highlights/martinhighlight/ *Image courtesy of the Archives of the American College of Surgeons.*

Page 112
Edward Martin. American College of Surgeons, Photograph. *Image courtesy of the Archives of the American College of Surgeons.*

Edward Martin. "Edward Martin, MD, FACS, 1859–1938," The American College of Surgeons Archives. Photograph. https://www.facs.org/about-acs/archives/past-highlights/edwardmartinhighlight/ *Image courtesy of the Archives of the American College of Surgeons.*

Franklin Martin. American College of Surgeons. Photograph. *Image courtesy of the Archives of the American College of Surgeons*

Page 114
"Dr. Edward Martin, Surgeon, Using Golf Stick, Will Try to Amputate $100,000 from C. H. Geist's Pocket," *Evening Ledger–Philadelphia*, May 29, 1883. Cartoon by Carl Zeisberg. https://chroniclingamerica.loc.gov/lccn/sn83045211/1915-05-27/ed-1/seq-3/

Barker, Clyde, photographer. *Inkwell with hole,* c. 2000. Hospital of the University of Pennsylvania.

Page 118
Borie, Adolph. *John B. Deaver*, 1920. Oil on canvas. https://www.med.upenn.edu/psom/john-b-deaver-md.html Courtesy of the University of Pennsylvania Art Collection, Philadelphia, Pennsylvania.

Page 119
Four of John B. Deaver's textbooks. (Volumes 1–3 of *Surgical Anatomy* and *A Treatise on Appendicitis.*) Photograph.

John B. Deaver, M.D. n.d. Halftone, 1 photomechanical reproduction. U.S. National Library of Medicine (NLM): Images from the History of Medicine. https://jstor.org/stable/community.28562501

U.S. National Library of Medicine (NLM): Images from the History of Medicine. https://library.artstor.org/asset/28562501.

Page 120
John B. Deaver. Photograph.

Gray, photographer. *J. William White,* c. 1880. Portrait Photograph, 6 .9 × 4.8 in. UPF 1.9 AR, Alumni Records Collection. University Archives and Records Center, University of Pennsylvania. https://jstor.org/stable/community.22103536.

Cade, J. Jarvis, artist., and Phillips, Photographer. *John B. Deaver.* Engraving. U.S. National Library of Medicine (NLM): Images from the History of Medicine. https://jstor.org/stable/community.28545347

U.S. National Library of Medicine (NLM): Images from the History of Medicine. https://library.artstor.org/asset/28545347

Page 121
Frese, Carl. *A Short History and Description of the German Hospital, Philadelphia, PA.* Philadelphia: Girard Printing House, 1895, 3. Photograph of German Hospital. https://archive.org/details/68120450R.nlm.nih.gov/page/n7/mode/2up

Page 122
Deaver, John Blair. *A Treatise on Appendicitis, 2nd ed.* Philadelphia: P. Blakeston's Son & Co., 1900. https://books.google.com/books/about/A_Treatise_on_Appendicitis.html?id=2SrOE-YqCXAC

Sterner, Albert. Deaver's *surgical clinic,* c. 1929. Lankenau Hospital, Wynnewood, Pennsylvania.

Page 123
Gutekunst, Frederick, photographer. *Charles Harrison Frazier,* c. 1910. Portrait Photograph, 5.5 × 4 in. UPF 1.9 AR, Alumni Records Collection, Box 819. University Archives and Records Center, University of Pennsylvania. https://jstor.org/stable/community.22101310

Page 124
Robinson, Danforth. *John B. Deaver. Imago Chirurgii, 1913–1963* (Ethicon: Somerville, NJ, 1963), 16. Drawing. ©Ethicon, Inc. (2024). Reproduced with permission.

Page 130
Gutekunst, Frederick, photographer. *Charles Harrison Frazier,* c. 1910. Portrait Photograph, 5.5 × 4 in. UPF 1.9 AR, Alumni Records Collection, Box 819. University Archives and Records Center, University of Pennsylvania. https://jstor.org/stable/community.22101310

Page 131
Charles Frazier. Prabook. Photograph. https://prabook.com/web/charles.frazier/3759146#gallery

Page 132
The World's Work, Volume XX, May to October 1910, A History of Our Time. Photograph of Abraham Flexner taken by Hollinger, NY. https://archive.org/stream/worldswork20gard#page/13100/mode/2up

Flexner, Abraham. *Medical Education in the United States and Canada: A Report to The Carnegie Foundation for the Advancement of Teaching.* 1910. https://en.wikipedia.org/wiki/File:Carnegie_Flexner_Report.djvu

Page 133
Charles Curtis Harrison, c. 1900. Portrait Photograph, 6 × 9 in. UPF 1.9 AR, Alumni Records Collection, Box 1066. University Archives and Records Center, University of Pennsylvania. https://jstor.org/stable/community.22109248

David Linn Edsall, 1904?. Photograph. Countway Library of Medicine, Harvard University. https://digitalcollections.library.harvard.edu/catalog/med00049c00118

Vonnoh, Robert William. *Dr. Silas Weir Mitchell,* 1918. Oil on canvas, 29 × 36 in. Pennsylvania Academy of Fine Arts, Philadelphia. https://www.pafa.org/museum/collection/item/dr-silas-weir-mitchell

Page 134
The modification of the Hartley-Krause subtemporal approach performed by Spiller and Frazier. Dandy WE. The brain. *Walters W, Ellis FH Jr Lewis-Walters practice of surgery*, vol. XII. (WF Prior Co, Hagerstown, MD, 1963). Illustration. https://www.researchgate.net/figure/The-modification-of-the-Hartley-Krause-subtemporal-approach-performed-by-Spiller-and_fig2_342064804

Page 135
Charles H. Frazier, 1921. Box 4, Ser. 4. MSS 2/0288-01. Courtesy of the College of Physicians of Philadelphia.

Page 136
Roscher, Frederick. *Charles Harrison Frazier*, 1930. Oil on canvas. https://www.med.upenn.edu/psom/charles-harrison-frazier-md.html Courtesy of the University of Pennsylvania Art Collection, Philadelphia, Pennsylvania.

L. Kraeer Ferguson. Photograph.

Page 137
Faber, Erwin F. *Charles Frazier,* (n.d.). Etching. U.S. National Library of Medicine (NLM): Images from the History of Medicine. http://resource.nlm.nih.gov/101415402

Page 144
Eldridge Eliason. University of Pennsylvania School of Medicine, *Scope* (Philadelphia, 1944/45), 26. University Archives and Records Center, University of Pennsylvania.

Page 145
Yale University Gymnastics Team, 1901. Yale Athletics Photographs (RU 691). Yale University Library, New Haven, Connecticut. https://collections.library.yale.edu/catalog/10010594

Yale University Baseball Team, 1901. Yale Athletics Photographs (RU 691). Yale University Library, New Haven, Connecticut. https://collections.library.yale.edu/catalog/10010593

Page 146
Eliason in scrubs. University of Pennsylvania School of Medicine, *Scope* (Philadelphia, 1944/45), 28. University Archives and Records Center, University of Pennsylvania.

Eliason in car. University of Pennsylvania School of Medicine, *Scope* (Philadelphia, 1944/45), 28. University Archives and Records Center, University of Pennsylvania.

Page 147
Eliason with nurse. University of Pennsylvania School of Medicine, *Scope* (Philadelphia, 1944/45), 28. University Archives and Records Center, University of Pennsylvania.

Page 148
Eliason standing. University of Pennsylvania School of Medicine, *Scope* (Philadelphia, 1944/45), 28. University Archives and Records Center, University of Pennsylvania.

Page 149
Eliason service team. Photograph.

Page 150
John Paul North. University of Pennsylvania School of Medicine, *Scope* (Philadelphia, 1942), 27. University Archives and Records Center, University of Pennsylvania.

Page 151
William H. M. Erb, Sr. University of Pennsylvania School of Medicine, *Scope* (Philadelphia, 1968), 133. University Archives and Records Center, University of Pennsylvania.

Charles W. McLaughlin Jr. DigitalCommons@UNMC, University of Nebraska Medical Center. Photograph. https://digitalcommons.unmc.edu/oral_hist/12/. *Permission granted by DiAnna Hemsath, Robert S. Wigton Department of Special Collections and Archives*

Page 152
Julian Johnson. University of Pennsylvania School of Medicine, *Scope* (Philadelphia, 1962), 82. University Archives and Records Center, University of Pennsylvania.

Cap. Charles Bittinger. *Rear Admiral Robert B. Brown, USN MC.* Naval History and Heritage Command (1964). Photograph. https://www.history.navy.mil/content/history/nhhc/our-collections/photography/numerical-list-of-images/nhhc-series/nh-series/NH-56000/NH-56262-KN.html

Page 153
Lloyd Stevens. University of Pennsylvania School of Medicine, *Scope* (Philadelphia, 1968), 136. University Archives and Records Center, University of Pennsylvania.

Bob Welty. University of Pennsylvania School of Medicine, *Scope* (Philadelphia, 1944/45), 24. University Archives and Records Center, University of Pennsylvania.

Page 158
Caniff, Milton. *I. S. Ravdin,* March 21, 1958. 4th Floor of Silverstein Building, Hospital of the University of Pennsylvania. With permission from Anne Ravdin.

Page 159
I. S. Ravdin as child with family. Photograph. UPT 50 R252, box 188, ff 1. University Archives and Records Center, University of Pennsylvania.

Page 160
Private Ravdin with National Guardsmen, 1916. Photograph. UPT 50 R252, box 182, ff 32. University Archives and Records Center, University of Pennsylvania.

Detail of Private Ravdin with National Guardsmen, 1916. Photograph. UPT 50 R252, box 182, ff 32. University Archives and Records Center, University of Pennsylvania.

Brig. Gen. John J. "Black Jack" Pershing crossing the Rio Grande into Mexico with the Western Column at the beginning of the Punitive Expedition, 1916. Photograph. U.S. Army Military History Institute. https://history.army.mil/html/books/077/77-1/cmhPub_077-1.pdf

The World's Work, Volume XXVII. Garden City New York: Doubleday, Page & Co., 1914, 274. Photograph of Pancho Villa. https://archive.org/details/worldswork28gard/page/274/mode/2up?view=theater

Page 161
I. S. Ravdin as intern. Photograph. With permission from Anne Ravdin.

I. S. Ravdin with wife, Elizabeth. Photograph. UPT 50 R252, box 185, scrapbook 1. University Archives and Records Center, University of Pennsylvania.

Gutekunst, Frederick, photographer. *Charles Harrison Frazier,* c. 1910. Portrait Photograph, 5.5 × 4 in. UPF 1.9 AR, Alumni Records Collection, Box 819. University Archives and Records Center, University of Pennsylvania. https://jstor.org/stable/community.22101310

Robinson, Danforth. *George P. Muller. Imago Chirurgii, 1913–1963* (Ethicon: Somerville, NJ, 1963), 52. Drawing. ©*Ethicon, Inc. (2024). Reproduced with permission.*

Cade, J. Jarvis, artist., and Phillips, Photographer. *John B. Deaver.* Engraving. U.S. National Library of Medicine (NLM): Images from the History of Medicine. https://jstor.org/stable/community.28545347

U.S. National Library of Medicine (NLM): Images from the History of Medicine. https://library.artstor.org/asset/28545347

Page 162
I. S. Ravdin. Photograph. UPT 50 R252, box 185, scrapbook 5. University Archives and Records Center, University of PA.

John H. Gibbon, Jr. (double portrait), 1963. Photograph, 5 × 7 in. Courtesy of Siegman Archives at Thomas Jefferson University, Philadelphia. https://jdc.jefferson.edu/historical_photos/1202/

Portrait of Henry Hallett Dale, head and shoulders. Wellcome Collection. Attribution 4.0 International (CC BY 4.0). https://wellcomecollection.org/works/t9xsyps6

Sir Edward Albert Sharpey-Schafer. Photograph by J. Russell & Sons. Wellcome Collection. https://wellcomecollection.org/works/fk2j9yyh

Page 163
John Berton Carnett. UPF 1.9AR, box #360 (negative). University Archives and Records Center, University of Pennsylvania.

George Leib Harrison. UPF 1.9AR, box #1067 (negative). University Archives and Records Center, University of Pennsylvania.

I. S. Ravdin and Jonathan Rhoads. Reprinted from *Jonathan E. Rhoads 80th Birthday Symposium,* ed. Clyde F. Barker and John M. Daly. Philadelphia: J. B. Lippincott Co., 1989, xiv.

Eliason service team. Photograph.

Ravdin, IS, Harry M. Vars, Elizabeth Thorogood, Julius Schultz, and Julian Johnson. The Liver Glycogen and Lipid Concentrations Following Intravenous Administration and Diet in the Dog and Man in the Presence of Liver Damage. *Annals of Surgery* 114, no. 6 (1941 Dec): 1018–1025, https://www.ncbi.nlm.nih.gov/pmc/articles/PMC1385840/

Page 164
Jonathan Rhoads. Photograph. *With permission from George Rhoads.*

Eldridge Eliason. Photograph. UPF 1.9AR, box #680. University Archives and Records Center, University of Pennsylvania.

Ravdin, Isidore S. 1942. *A Philadelphia Doctor's Story of Pearl Harbor; an Informal Talk Delivered at a Meeting Called by Blackwell Newhall,*

Chairman Southeastern Pennsylvania Chapter of the American Red Cross, February 9, 1942. With permission from Anne Ravdin.

Doctor Flies Drugs to Hawaii, 1941. Newspaper clipping. *With permission from Anne Ravdin.*

Dr. I. S. Ravdin, Prominent Surgeon, Goes to Honolulu, 1941. Newspaper clipping. *With permission from Anne Ravdin.*

Allen Oldfather Whipple. Photograph. Courtesy of the College of Physicians of Philadelphia.

Page 165
20th General Hospital, Main Entrance, c. 1944. Photograph, 4 × 6.75 in. UPT 50 R252, I.S. Ravdin Papers, Box 167, folder 5. University Archives and Records Center, University of Pennsylvania. https://jstor.org/stable/community.22101220

20th General Hospital Team. University of Pennsylvania School of Medicine, *Scope* (Philadelphia, 1943), 136–137. University Archives and Records Center, University of Pennsylvania.

Operating Theater at 20th General Hospital, Ledo, Assam, India during World War II, c. 1944. Photo courtesy of the US Army Office of Medical History. https://www.armyheritage.org/soldier-stories-information/mud-and-mustard-gas-sweat-and-bugs-the-20th-general-hospital/

Map of route of Merrill's Marauders. Graphic courtesy of Robin Noel.

The Quebec Conference, Canada, August 1943 (William Lyon Mackenzie King, Franklin Roosevelt, Winston Churchill, and the Earl of Athlone). Photograph. Imperial War Museum, London. https://www.iwm.org.uk/collections/item/object/205123909

Page 166
General Stillwell and I. S. Ravdin making rounds. Photograph. https://www.cbi-theater.com/hospitals/_cbi_hospitals_pictures.html *With permission from Anne Ravdin.*

General Lewis A. Pick presents Ravdin with Legion of Merit. Photograph. https://archives.upenn.edu/exhibits/penn-history/base-hospitals/ *With permission from Anne Ravdin.*

General Frank Merrill. "MG Frank D. Merrill, Commander 5307th Composite Unit." US Army Special Operations Command. Photograph. https://arsof-history.org/icons/merrill.html

Page 167
United States Mint. *Merrill's Marauders Bronze Medal,* 1.5 in. *Photo by Elizabeth Barker.*

Reis, Lieut R. *I. S. Ravdin with General Merrill,* June 12, 1944. Photograph. http://www.cbi-theater.com/csdavis_archive_5/csdavis_photos.html

Lord Mountbatten with bandaged eye. Photograph. *With permission from Anne Ravdin.*

Certificate of thanks from Lord Mountbatten to Ravdin, March 18, 1944. UPT 50 R252, OS 7. University Archives and Records Center, University of Pennsylvania.

Dr. Ravdin and Mountbatten. Photograph. UPT 50 R252, box 185, scrapbook 3. University Archives and Records Center, University of Pennsylvania.

A C-47 transport aircraft drops supplies by parachute to Allied troops in action against Japanese forces; a common event during the fighting in Burma and India during 1944. European Center of Military History. Photograph. https://eucmh.com/2020/05/05/5307-galahad-cbi-feb-may-1944/#google_vignette

Clasen, Jonnie Melillo. *Merrill's Marauders crossing bridge.* "'Expendable' WWII Merrill's Marauders survive into their 100s." US Army. Photograph. https://www.army.mil/article/173880/expendable_wwii_merrills_marauders_survive_into_their_100s

Marauders move to the front, via the Ledo Road. 1944 February. "Merrill's Marauders Photographs, 1944 and 1945." Government photos in the Sam Wilson Papers that document the Burma Campaign of 1944. Photograph. https://generalsamvwilson.wordpress.com/2020/09/07/merrills-marauders-photographs-1944/

Page 168
I.S. Ravdin, Lt. Anderson, Major Baggs, in India. 1945 July. Photograph, 10 × 8 in. UPT 50 R252, I.S. Ravdin Papers, Box 182, folder 33. University Archives and Records Center, University of Pennsylvania. https://jstor.org/stable/community.22108767

Welcome home celebration. Photograph. *With permission from Anne Ravdin.*

Dr. Ravdin, faculty and residents at dinner. Photograph. UPT 50 R252, box 182, ff 2. University Archives and Records Center, University of Pennsylvania.

I. S. Ravdin discussing President Eisenhower operation. Photograph. *With permission from Anne Ravdin.*

Ravdin at desk with flag. Photograph. UPT 50 R252, box 185, scrapbook 5. University Archives and Records Center, University of Pennsylvania.

Page 169
Ravdin disciplines assistant. Photograph. UPT 50 R252, box 185, scrapbook 1. University Archives and Records Center, University of Pennsylvania.

Page 170
I.S. Ravdin, Dwight D. Eisenhower, and Leon J. Obermeyer. 1964 May 26. Photograph, 10 × 8 in. UPT 50 R252, I.S. Ravdin Papers, Box 182, folder 13. University Archives and Records Center, University of Pennsylvania. https://jstor.org/stable/community.22108766

Dr. Ravdin and Gregory Peck. Photograph. UPT 50 R252, box 185, scrapbook 2. University Archives and Records Center, University of Pennsylvania.

President Eisenhower and Dr. Ravdin. Photograph. UPT 50 R252, box 185, scrapbook 6. University Archives and Records Center, University of Pennsylvania.

Dr. Ravdin, President Johnson and Lady Bird Johnson. Photograph. UPT 50 R252, box 185, scrapbook 2. University Archives and Records Center, University of Pennsylvania.

Ravdin and Pope Pius XII. Photograph. *With permission from Anne Ravdin.*

Page 171
Ravdin in long red underwear. Photograph. UPT 50 R252, box 185, scrapbook 3. University Archives and Records Center, University of Pennsylvania.

Ravdin, deep-sea fishing. Photograph. UPT 50 R252, box 185, scrapbook 1. University Archives and Records Center, University of Pennsylvania.

Dr. Ravdin at Christmas party for nurses. Photograph. UPT 50 R252, box 185, scrapbook 1. University Archives and Records Center, University of Pennsylvania.

Dr. Ravdin and Brooke Roberts in long scrub dresses. Photograph. UPT 50, R252, box 182, ff 72. University Archives and Records Center, University of Pennsylvania.

Caniff, Milton, artist. *Steve Canyon Comic Strip, Featuring Dr. I.S. Ravdin.* https://www.pennmedicine.org/news/publications-and-special-projects/penn-medicine-magazine/archived-issues/2015/summer-2015/ravdin *Courtesy of the Milton Caniff Estate. © 2024 CLASSIC COOL - Milton Caniff Estate - All rights reserved.*

Caniff, Milton, artist. *Steve Canyon Comic Strip, 13 October 1957, Featuring Dr. I.S. Ravdin.* 1957 October 13. Comics: color, 7.5 in × 14 in. UPT 50 R252, I.S. Ravdin Papers, Box OS 4. https://jstor.org/stable/community.22101526 *Courtesy of the Milton Caniff Estate. © 2024 CLASSIC COOL - Milton Caniff Estate - All rights reserved.*

Page 172
Ravdin walking down hallway. University of Pennsylvania School of Medicine, *Scope* (Philadelphia, 1966), 87. University Archives and Records Center, University of Pennsylvania.

Jim Robinson. University of Pennsylvania School of Medicine, *Scope* (Philadelphia, 1958), 103. University Archives and Records Center, University of Pennsylvania.

Page 173
Dr. Ravdin with building models. Photograph. UPT 50 R252, box 188, ff 1. University Archives and Records Center, University of Pennsylvania.

Ravdin looking up at building. University of Pennsylvania School of Medicine, *Scope* (Philadelphia, 1963), 73. University Archives and Records Center, University of Pennsylvania.

Dr. Ravdin in hardhat. Photograph. UPT 50 R252, box 185, ff 2. University Archives and Records Center, University of Pennsylvania.

Dr. Ravdin at his portrait unveiling. Photograph. UPF 1.9AR, box #2176. University Archives and Records Center, University of Pennsylvania.

Ravdin looking through window. University of Pennsylvania School of Medicine, *Scope* (Philadelphia, 1962), 75. University Archives and Records Center, University of Pennsylvania.

Page 174
I.S. Ravdin, c. 1940. Photograph: with manuscript annotation, 9.9 × 7.4 in. UPF 1.9 AR, Alumni Records Collection. University Archives and Records Center, University of Pennsylvania. https://jstor.org/stable/community.22106935

Page 175
William Stewart Halsted, c. 1880. Photograph. Alan Mason Chesney Archives of the Johns Hopkins Medical Institution, Baltimore, Maryland.

William T. Fitts, Jr. University of Pennsylvania School of Medicine, *Scope* (Philadelphia, 1950), "Medicine" section. University Archives and Records Center, University of Pennsylvania.

Page 176
C. Everett Koop. Photograph.

Charles K. Kirby. University of Pennsylvania School of Medicine, *Scope* (Philadelphia, 1950), p. immediately after "Surgery". University Archives and Records Center, University of Pennsylvania.

Cletus Schwegman. University of Pennsylvania School of Medicine, *Scope* (Philadelphia, 1966), 89. University Archives and Records Center, University of Pennsylvania.

Page 177
James D. Hardy. University of Pennsylvania School of Medicine, *Scope* (Philadelphia, 1942), 40. University Archives and Records Center, University of Pennsylvania.

Fletcher, Archibald G. *Archibald Fletcher, 1946. To India and Beyond, Memoirs of a Missionary Surgeon* (Xlibris, March 11, 2005): 69. Photograph. *Permission granted by John Fletcher.*

Page 178
Dr. Ravdin and John Howard. Photograph. UPT 50 R252, box 185, scrapbook 3. University Archives and Records Center, University of Pennsylvania.

William Dyson. University of Pennsylvania School of Medicine, *Scope* (Philadelphia, 1975), 22. University Archives and Records Center, University of Pennsylvania.

Brooke Roberts. University of Pennsylvania School of Medicine, *Scope* (Philadelphia, 1965), 160. University Archives and Records Center, University of Pennsylvania.

Page 179
Harold Barker. University of Pennsylvania School of Medicine, *Scope* (Philadelphia, 1943), 35. University Archives and Records Center, University of Pennsylvania.

William Blakemore. Photograph.

Barker, Clyde, J. Daly, editors. *Nicholas Gimble.* Jonathan E. Rhoads Eightieth Birthday Symposium (Philadelphia: J.B. Lippincott, 1989). Photograph.

Page 180
Robert Ravdin. University of Pennsylvania School of Medicine, *Scope* (Philadelphia, 1957), 50. University Archives and Records Center, University of Pennsylvania.

William Stainback, 1951 June 29. Photograph.

Julius Mackie. University of Pennsylvania School of Medicine, *Scope* (Philadelphia, 1974), 46. University Archives and Records Center, University of Pennsylvania.

William DeMuth Jr. "Dr.William Demuth, early member of the Department of Surgery, passes away." (September 17, 2015). Photograph. https://www.psu.edu/news/medicine/story/dr-william-demuth-early-member-department-surgery-passes-away/ *Permission granted by Tessa Marie Commercial.*

Page 181
Henry Moss, 1951 June 29. Photograph.

Gerald Peskin. Photograph.

Marshall Orloff. Photograph. *With permission from Lisa Ann Orloff.*

Page 182
James H. Robinson, c. 1975. Photograph. Courtesy of Siegman Archives at Thomas Jefferson University, Philadelphia.

James C. Thompson. "Legends, 2006." The Lundquist Institute. Photograph. https://lundquist.org/legends

Page 183
Harold Zintel. University of Pennsylvania School of Medicine, *Scope* (Philadelphia, 1950), 3 pages after "Surgery". University Archives and Records Center, University of Pennsylvania.

Page 184
John Thomas, 1951 June 29. Photograph.

Dorothy Bender. Photograph. https://www.findagrave.com/memorial/96898926/doris-harriet-maxwell

Page 193
Ewing, Harris A. *Walter Freeman and James W. Watts looking at X-ray.* "Turning the Mind Inside Out." *Saturday Evening Post* (May 24, 1941), 18–19. Photograph. https://commons.wikimedia.org/wiki/File:Turning_the_Mind_Inside_Out_Saturday_Evening_Post_24_May_1941_a_detail_1.jpg

Freeman, Walter and James W. Watts. *Transorbital lobotomy instrument. Treatment of Mental Disorders and Intractable Pain* (Spingfield, IL: C. C. Thomas, 1950). Illustration. https://nihrecord.nih.gov/2019/11/01/when-faces-made-case-lobotomy

Page 194
Norman Freeman. University of Pennsylvania School of Medicine, *Scope* (Philadelphia, 1943), 20. University Archives and Records Center, University of Pennsylvania.

Page 195
Connolly, John E. *Norman Freeman in uniform.* "Norman Freeman: The 'first' American specialist in vascular surgery." *The Society for Vascular Surgery and International Society for Cardiovascular Surgery,* 22, no. 1 (1995): 188–94. Photograph. https://core.ac.uk/download/pdf/82521792.pdf

Page 196
Freeman, NE and FH Leeds. *Femorofemoral bypass, Fig. 4.* "Operations on large arteries. *Western Journal of Medicine,* October, no. 77 (1952), 229–33 https://pubmed.ncbi.nlm.nih.gov/13009464/ *Permission granted by Elsevier.*

Freeman, NE and FH Leeds. *Bypass of ligated abdomial aortic aneurysm, Fig. 5.* "Operations on large arteries. *Western Journal of Medicine,* October, no. 77 (1952), 229–33 https://pubmed.ncbi.nlm.nih.gov/13009464/ *Permission granted by Elsevier.*

Page 201
Bernard Fisher M.D. and his brother Edwin R. Fisher M.D. in the Laboratory of Experimental Surgery at the University Of Pittsburgh, 1957. PITTMED (University of Pittsburgh, Winter 2018). Photograph. https://www.pittmed.health.pitt.edu/story/against-tide *From the collection of Bernard Fisher, MD. Permission courtesy of Beth Fisher, MD.*

Page 202
Fisher, Bernard, Robert G. Ravdin, Robert K. Ausman, Nelson H. Slack, George E. Moore, and Rudolf J. "Surgical Adjuvant Chemotherapy in Cancer of the Breast." *Annals of Surgery* 168, no. 3 (September 1968): 337–356, https://www.ncbi.nlm.nih.gov/pmc/articles/PMC1387335/

Page 204
Bernard Fisher. Wikimedia Commons. Photograph. https://commons.wikimedia.org/wiki/File:Nci-vol-8226-300_bernard_fisher.jpg

Page 205
Bernard Fisher. "Bernard Fisher, a pioneer in breast cancer research, dies at 101." Pittwire. University of Pittsburgh (October 21, 2019). Photograph. https://www.pitt.edu/pittwire/features-articles/bernard-fisher-md-pioneer-breast-cancer-research-dies-101.

Page 209
Ian Folkert and Hilary Bollman. Photograph. *With permission from Ian Folkert.*

Anna Garcia. Photograph. *With permission from Anna Garcia.*

Page 210
Shanks, Nelson. *Julian Johnson*, c. 1965–1975. Oil on canvas. https://www.jtcvs.org/cms/attachment/4ba37ee7-473d-43c3-9f4a-3d2a54125a53/gr2.jpg *Courtesy of the University of Pennsylvania Art Collection, Philadelphia, Pennsylvania.*

Page 212
Julian Johnson operating. "The American Doctor." *Saturday Evening Post* (June 15, 1963). Cover photograph. https://www.coverbrowser.com/covers/saturday-evening-post/44#i2151

Page 215
Julian Johnson in blood-soaked gown. University of Pennsylvania School of Medicine, *Scope* (Philadelphia, 1960), 58. University Archives and Records Center, University of Pennsylvania.

Page 219
Julian Johnson. University of Pennsylvania School of Medicine, *Scope* (Philadelphia, 1962), 82. University Archives and Records Center, University of Pennsylvania.

Page 222
Karsh, Yousuf. *Jonathan Rhoads,* 1983 Nov 21. Photograph. *Courtesy of the Estate of Yousuf Karsh.*

Page 223
Jonathan Rhoads. Photograph. *With permission from George Rhoads.*

Jonathan Rhoads with feet up, laughing. Photograph.

Rombeau, John L. and Donna Muldoon. *Jonathan Rhoads (pole vaulting). Jonathan Rhoads, MD: Quaker Sense and Sensibility in the World of Surgery* (Philadelphia: Hanley & Belfus, 1997), 51. Photograph.

Page 224
Eldridge Eliason. Photograph. UPF 1.9AR, box #680. University Archives and Records Center, University of Pennsylvania.

Jonathan Rhoads at desk. University of Pennsylvania School of Medicine, *Scope* (Philadelphia, 1962), 75. University Archives and Records Center, University of Pennsylvania.

Barker, Clyde. *Jonathan Rhoads. Jonathan E. Rhoads Eightieth Birthday Symposium.* (Philadelphia: Lippincott Williams & Wilkins, 1989), 257. Photograph.

Shumacker, Harris B. *Allen Whipple. History of the Society of Clinical Surgery* (London: Benham Press, 1977), 59. Photograph.

Page 225
Barker, Clyde. *Rhoads family. Jonathan E. Rhoads Eightieth Birthday Symposium.* (Philadelphia: Lippincott Williams & Wilkins, 1989), 257. Photograph.

Rombeau, John L. and Donna Muldoon. *Jonathan and Kitty (on stilts) Rhoads. Jonathan Rhoads, MD: Quaker Sense and* Sensibility *in the World of Surgery* (Philadelphia: Hanley & Belfus, 1997), 257. Photograph.

Page 226
Barker, Clyde. *University of Pennsylvania provosts. Jonathan E. Rhoads Eightieth Birthday Symposium.* (Philadelphia: Lippincott Williams & Wilkins, 1989), 259. Photograph.

Rombeau, John L. and Donna Muldoon. *Henry Vars, Stan Dudrick, Jonathan Rhoads.* Jonathan *Rhoads, MD: Quaker Sense and Sensibility in the World of Surgery* (Philadelphia: Hanley & Belfus, 1997), 259. Photograph.

Page 227
Stan Dudrick with puppy. Reprinted from cover of *Journal of Parenteral and Enteral Nutrition* vol. 44, no. 2 (February 2020).

Dudrick SJ, DW Wilmore, HM Vars, JE Rhoads. *Puppies from IV nutrition study.* "Long-term parenteral nutrition with growth development and positive nitrogen." *Surgery,* 64 (1968). 134–142. *Permission granted by Elsevier.*

Page 228
Barker, Clyde. *President Ronald Reagan and Jonathan Rhoads. Jonathan E. Rhoads Eightieth Birthday Symposium.* (Philadelphia: Lippincott Williams & Wilkins, 1989), 259. Photograph.

Page 229
The speakers at the Jonathan E. Rhoads Birthday Symposium. Reprinted from *Jonathan E. Rhoads 80th Birthday Symposium,* ed. Clyde F. Barker and John M. Daly. Philadelphia: J. B. Lippincott Co., 1989, xiv.

Page 230
Jonathan and Kitty Rhoads. Photograph. *With permission from George Rhoads.*

Page 231
Rombeau, John L. and Donna Muldoon. *Jonathan Rhoads at podium. Jonathan Rhoads, MD: Quaker Sense and Sensibility in the World of Surgery* (Philadelphia: Hanley & Belfus, 1997), 251.

Jonathan Rhoads, standing in front of Rhoads Pavilion. Photograph. *With permission from George Rhoads.*

Robert D. Lynn Associates, architects. *Rhoads Pavilion,* c. 1994. Architectural rendering. *With permission from EwingCole.*

Page 232
Shanks, Nelson. *Jonathan E. Rhoads,* 1980. Oil on canvas, 39 1/2 × 35 1/2 in. https://npg.si.edu/object/npg_PA330124 Courtesy of the University of Pennsylvania Art Collection, Philadelphia, Pennsylvania.

Page 250
Shanks, Nelson. *William Fitts.* Oil on canvas. Courtesy of the University of Pennsylvania Art Collection, Philadelphia, Pennsylvania.

Page 251
William Fitts as officer. Photograph. *Courtesy of Michael A. Fitts.*

Page 252
William Fitts in scrubs sitting. University of Pennsylvania School of Medicine, *Scope* (Philadelphia, 1972), 75. University Archives and Records Center, University of Pennsylvania.

Page 253
William Fitts laughing. University of Pennsylvania School of Medicine, Scope (Philadelphia, 1970), 110. University Archives and Records Center, University of Pennsylvania.

Page 255
William Fitts on teaching rounds. University of Pennsylvania School of Medicine, Scope (Philadelphia, 1976), 174. University Archives and Records Center, University of Pennsylvania.

Page 256
William Fitts on phone. University of Pennsylvania School of Medicine, *Scope* (Philadelphia, 1981), 30. University Archives and Records Center, University of Pennsylvania.

Page 258
Karsh, Yousuf. *Leonard Miller,* 1991 Mar 22. Photograph. *Courtesy of the Estate of Yousuf Karsh.*

Page 259
Leonard Miller. Photograph.

Page 261
Leonard Miller, teaching at bedside, 1972. Photograph.

Page 262
Leonard Miller. University of Pennsylvania School of Medicine, *Scope* (Philadelphia, 1972), 18. University Archives and Records Center, University of Pennsylvania.

Page 263
Leonard Miller, in front of his portrait. Photograph.

Page 266
Alfred Gellhorn. University of Pennsylvania School of Medicine, *Scope* (Philadelphia, 1974), 7. University Archives and Records Center, University of Pennsylvania.

Page 268
Edward J. Stemmler, c. 1975. Portrait Photograph, 9.5 × 7.2 in. UPT 50 S825, Edward J. Stemmler Papers, Box 7, folder 15. University Archives and Records Center, University of Pennsylvania. https://jstor.org/stable/community.22106790.

Page 270
Bill Kelley with University President Rodin and Ben Franklin statue. Photograph. *With permission from Bill Kelley.*

Bill Kelley (in color). Photograph. *With permission from Bill Kelley.*

Bill Kelley with hand at chin. Photograph. *With permission from Bill Kelley.*

Bill Kelley holding Penn flag. Photograph. *With permission from Bill Kelley.*

Bill Kelley at microphone. Photograph. *With permission from Bill Kelley.*

Bill Kelley talking with hands. Photograph. *With permission from Bill Kelley.*

Bill Kelley standing looking up. Photograph. With *permission from Bill Kelley.*

Page 274
Karsh, Yousuf. *Brooke Roberts,* 1983 Aug 30. Photograph. *Courtesy of the Estate of* Yousuf *Karsh.*

Page 275
Brooke Roberts. University of Pennsylvania School of Medicine, *Scope* (Philadelphia, 1965), 160. University Archives and Records Center, University of Pennsylvania.

Page 276
Barker, Clyde, photographer. *Brooke Roberts.*

Page 277
Shanks, Nelson. *Brooke Roberts,* 1983. Oil on canvas. https://www.med.upenn.edu/psom/brooke-roberts-md.html Courtesy of the University of Pennsylvania Art Collection, Philadelphia, PA.

Page 290
Karsh, Yousuf. *Clyde Barker,* 1987 Jan 16. Photograph. Courtesy of the Estate of Yousuf Karsh.

Page 291
Tom Starzl and Clyde Barker. Photograph courtesy of Clyde Barker.

Page 292
Earl, Roland, Clyde and Hal Barker. Photograph by Kathleen Barker.

Page 293
Clyde and Dode Barker. Photograph by Robert Davis.

1954 Cornell tennis team. Photograph.

Page 294
Clyde Barker playing tennis at the U.S. Open, Forest Hills. Photograph by Fred G. Barker.

Clyde Barker as intern, 1959. Photograph by Dorothy Barker.

Page 295
Shanks, Nelson. *Julian Johnson*, c. 1965–1975. Oil on canvas. https://www.jtcvs.org/cms/attachment/4ba37ee7-473d-43c3-9f4a-3d2a54125a53/gr2.jpg Courtesy of the University of Pennsylvania Art Collection, Philadelphia, PA.

Davidson, Lauren. *Thomas E. Starzl.* "Dr. Thomas E. Starzl's Legacy." *Pittsburgh Magazine* (April 26, 2017). Photograph. https://www.pittsburghmagazine.com/dr-thomas-e-starzls-legacy/

Page 296
Max the dog. Photograph by Fred G. Barker.

Barker family. Photograph courtesy of Clyde Barker.

Karsh, Yousuf. *Brooke Roberts,* 1983 Aug 30. Photograph. *Courtesy of the Estate of Yousuf Karsh.*

Barker, Clyde, photographer. *Rupert Billingham.*

Clyde Barker at microscope. Photograph by Leonard Perloff.

Page 297
Critchlow, Bob, photographer. *Clyde Barker operating.*

Barker, Clyde F. and RE Billingham. "The role of afferent lymphatics in the rejection of skin homografts," *Journal of Experimental* Medicine 128, no. 1 (July 1, 1968): 197–221. https://www.ncbi.nlm.nih.gov/pmc/articles/PMC2138504/

Page 298
Joe Mehl, Howard Mehl and Clyde Barker. Photograph. *With permission from Howard Nathan.*

Low, David. *Reconstruction of renal artery with aneurysm.* Drawing. *With permission from David Low.*

Clyde Barker and Omaida Velázquez operating. Private photograph.

Page 299
Barker, Clyde, photographer. *Craig Reckard.*

Barker, Clyde, photographer. *Mory Ziegler.*

Reckard CR, Ziegler MM, Barker CF. "Physiological and immunological consequences of transplanting isolated pancreatic islets." *Surgery* 74, no. 6 (1973 Jul):91–9. Graphs. https://pubmed.ncbi.nlm.nih.gov/4146046/

Page 300
Clyde Barker and Howard Nathan, with Gift of Life logo. Photograph. With permission from Howard Nathan.

Ron Fairman and Clyde Barker. Photograph courtesy of Clyde Barker.

Marc Mitchell. Photograph. *With permission from Marc Mitchell.*

Page 301
Clyde Barker, Brooke Roberts, Leonard Miller, and Jonathan Rhoads. Photograph courtesy of Clyde Barker.

Burke, Daniel, photographer. *Jim Mullen and Clyde Barker. Courtesy of Daniel Burke Photography.*

Page 302
John Daly. Photograph.

Page 303
Linton Whitaker. Photograph. *With permission from Linton Whitaker.*

William Fitts on phone. University of Pennsylvania School of Medicine, *Scope* (Philadelphia, 1981), 30. University Archives and Records Center, University of Pennsylvania.

Bill Schwab. Photograph. *With permission from Bill Schwab.*

Mike Rotondo. Photograph. *With permission from Mike Rotondo.*

Mike Nance. Photograph. *With permission from Mike Nance.*

Pat Reilly. Photograph. *With permission from Pat Reilly.*

Ernie Rosato. Photograph. *With permission from Geraldine Rosato.*

Page 304
Clyde Barker and Bill Kelley, 1998. Photograph. *With permission from Bill Kelley.*

HUP Department Heads. Photograph courtesy of Clyde Barker.

Barker, Clyde, photographer. *Andy Posselt.*

Barker, Clyde, photographer. *Ali Naji.*

Barker, Clyde, photographer. *Jim Markman.*

Barker, Clyde, photographer. *Michael Choti.*

Tomaszewski, John E., photographer. *Cover of Science. Science,* 249, no. 4974 (September 14, 1990). Photograph. https://www.science.org/toc/science/249/4974

Page 305
Andy Posselt, Clyde Barker and Ali Naji. Photograph courtesy of Clyde Barker.

Posselt, Andrew M., Clyde F. Barker, John E. Tomaszewski, James F. Markmann, Michael A. Choti, and Alina Ji. "Induction of Donor-Specific Unresponsiveness by Intrathymic Islet Transplantation." *Science* 249, no. 4974 (September 14, 1990), 1293–1295. Figures. https://www.science.org/doi/10.1126/science.2119056 *Reprinted with permission from AAAS.*

Page 306
Henry Edmunds. University of Pennsylvania School of Medicine, *Scope* (Philadelphia, 1975), 22. University Archives and Records Center, University of Pennsylvania.

Tim Gardner. Photograph. *With permission from Tim Gardner.*

Mike Acker. Photograph. *With permission from Mike Acker.*

Joe Bavaria. Photograph. *With permission from Joe Bavaria.*

Avi Shaked. Photograph. *With permission from Avi Shaked.*

Kim Olthoff. Photograph. *With permission from Kim Olthoff.*

Jim Markmann and Clyde Barker. Photograph. *With permission from Jim Markmann.*

Page 307
Wall of Fame, 4 Maloney. Photograph courtesy of Dan Dempsey.

Page 308
Barker, Clyde, photographer. *Dode Barker.*

Page 309
Logo for Cultural Partnerships, Mid-Day Arts Series.

Cover of Philadelphia Antiques Show Catalogue, 1993. UPG 28.1 University Archives and Records Center, University of Pennsylvania.

Barker, Clyde, photographer. *Dode Barker with Eiffel Tower.*

Page 310
Clyde Barker, APS President. Photograph. American Philosophical Society, Philadelphia, PA.

Tom Starzl and Clyde Barker, 2009. *Photograph courtesy of Clyde Barker.*

Clyde Barker accepting the Medawar Prize, 2010. *Photograph courtesy of Ali Naji.*

Medawar Prize medal. Photo by Elizabeth Barker.

Page 311
Robert Vinoly Architects, *Clyde F. Barker Transplant House.* Photo by Elizabeth Barker.

Page 312
Friedman, Jon. *Clyde Barker,* 2001. Oil on canvas. https://jonrfriedman.com/Portraits/Public%20Commissions/Clyde%20Barker/#images-2 *Courtesy of the University of Pennsylvania Art Collection, Philadelphia, PA.*

Pages 316–333
All photographs with permission of the subjects, when possible. Many thanks to Kelly & Massa Photography for the later year photographs.

Page 334
Larry Kaiser. Photograph courtesy of Lien Nibauer Photography.

Page 335
Larry Kaiser. Photograph. *With permission from Larry Kaiser.*

Page 336
Joe Shrager. Photograph. *With permission from Joe Shrager.*

Joe Friedberg. Photograph. *With permission from Joe Friedberg.*

Jo Buyske. Photograph. *With permission from Joe Buyske.*

Roy Smythe and Larry Kaiser. Photograph. *With permission from Roy Smythe.*

Page 337
Bob Fry. Photograph. With permission from Bob Fry.

Burke, Daniel, photographer. *Jon Morris and Larry Kaiser. Courtesy of Daniel Burke Photography.*

Dr. Larry Kaiser and Lindy Snider. Main Line Today (March 20, 2017). Photograph. https://mainlinetoday.com/life-style/dr-larry-kaiser-and-lindy-snider/ *Permission granted by Main Line News.*

Page 338
Larry Kaiser and Joel Cooper. Photograph. *With permission from Larry Kaiser.*

Larry Kaiser, Lindy Snider, Ed Snider, Philadelphia Flyers fundraiser. Mainline Media News (February 7, 2013). Photograph. https://www.mainlinemedianews.com/2013/02/07/flyers-fundraiser-brings-in-funds-for-less-fortunate/ *Permission granted by Main Line News.*

Page 339
Friedman, Jon. *Larry Kaiser,* 2008. Oil on canvas. With permission from the artist. https://jonrfriedman.com/Portraits/Public%20Commissions/larry-kaiser/#images-2

Page 342
Jeff Drebin. Photograph. *With permission from Jeff Drebin.*

Page 343
Jeff Drebin. Photograph. *With permission from Jeff Drebin.*

Burke, Daniel, photographer. *Jeff Drebin and Mark Greene. Courtesy of Daniel Burke Photography.*

Page 344
Burke, Daniel, photographer. *Ralph Muller, Larry Jameson, Jeff Drebin, Clyde Barker, Mark Greene. Courtesy of Daniel Burke Photography.*

Jeff Drebin, in scrubs. Photograph. *With permission from Jeff Drebin.*

Page 345
Drebin, Jeffrey A., Victoria C. Link, David F. Stern, Robert A. Weinberg, Mark I. Greene. "Down-modulation of an oncogene protein product and reversion of the transformed phenotype by monoclonal antibodies." *Cell* 41, no. 3 (July 1985): 695–706. https://www.cell.com/cell/abstract/S0092-8674(85)80050-7

Page 346
Jeff Drebin and Jeff Gordon. Photograph. *With permission from Jeff Drebin.*

Jeff Drebin with 2016 Chief Residents. Photograph. *With permission from Jeff Drebin.*

Page 347
Burke, Daniel, photographer. *Harrison, Linda, Jeff, and Lizzie Drebin. Courtesy of Daniel Burke Photography.*

Page 348
Burke, Daniel, photographer. *Ron DeMatteo, Jeff Drebin, and Jon Friedman (artist) in front of portrait of Dr. Drebin. Courtesy of Daniel Burke Photography.*

Page 350
C. Everett Koop. Photograph.

Page 351
William E. Ladd. Boston Children's Hospital Archives. Photograph.

Burke, Larry and Anna Stredulinsky. *Halifax Explosion 100th Anniversary Stamp.* Canada Post. Image. https://www.canadapost-postescanada.ca/cpc/en/personal/collectibles/stamp-stories/2017-11-09-halifax-explosion-100th-anniversary Canada Post © 2017.

Page 352
Moore, Francis D. and Judah Folkman. *Robert Gross. Robert Edward Gross, 1905–1988, A Biographical Memoir.* National Academy of Sciences (Washington, DC: National Academies Press, 1995). Photograph. http://www.nasonline.org/publications/biographical-memoirs/memoir-pdfs/gross-robert.pdf *Permission granted by the National Academies Press.*

Donahoe, Patricia K. *Judah Folkman. Judah Folkman, 1933–2008. Biographical Memoirs.* National Academy of Sciences (2014). Photograph. http://www.nasonline.org/publications/biographical-memoirs/memoir-pdfs/folkman-judah.pdf *Permission granted by the Harvard News Office.*

Page 353
Barker, Clyde, photographer. *Moritz Ziegler.*

Steven Fishman. Boston Children's Hospital. Photograph. https://www.childrenshospital.org/about-us/our-leadership/steven-j-fishman *Reprinted by permission of Dr. Steven J. Fishman.*

Page 354
C. Everett Koop. University of Pennsylvania School of Medicine, *Scope* (Philadelphia, 1981), 69. University Archives and Records Center, University of Pennsylvania.

Page 355
C. Everett Koop in NICU. University of Pennsylvania School of Medicine, *Scope* (Philadelphia, 1974), 44. University Archives and Records Center, University of Pennsylvania.

Page 356
C. Everett Koop holding separated conjoined twins. University of Pennsylvania School of Medicine, *Scope* (Philadelphia, 1975), 34. University Archives and Records Center, University of Pennsylvania.

Page 357
C. Everett Koop, with flag. "C. Everett Koop." The C. Everett Koop Papers. National Library of Medicine. Photograph. https://profiles.nlm.nih.gov/spotlight/qq/catalog/nlm:nlmuid-101584930X741-img

Page 358
The White House. *C. Everett Koop with President Ronald Reagan.* The C. Everett Koop Papers. National Library of Medicine (1980s). Photograph. https://profiles.nlm.nih.gov/spotlight/qq/catalog/nlm:nlmuid-101584930X52-img

Page 359
Cole, Jim. *Former U.S. Surgeon General Dr. C. Everett Koop.* 2002. *The Christian Science Monitor*, February 25, 2013. Photograph. https://www.csmonitor.com/USA/Latest-News-Wires/2013/0225/C.-Everett-Koop-Reagan-s-revolutionary-surgeon-general-dies

Page 360
James A. O'Neill. "Dr. James O'Neill Jr. to Present Canizaro Visiting Professor Lecture." Weill Cornell Medicine (November 22, 2002). Photograph. https://news.weill.cornell.edu/news/2002/11/dr-james-oneill-jr-to-present-canizaro-visiting-professor-lecture *Permission granted by James A. O'Neill.*

Page 362
Barker, Clyde, photographer. *Moritz Ziegler.*

Page 363
Scott Adzick. Photograph. *With permission from Scott Adzick.*

Page 365
Mike Nance. Photograph. *With permission from Mike Nance.*

Holly Hedrick. Photograph. *With permission from Holly Hedrick.*

Page 366
Alan Flake. Photograph. *With permission from Alan Flake.*

Page 368
Leney, William. *John Jones M.D.* Stipple engraving from *The American Medical and Philosophical Register 1813,* after p. 324. https://archive.org/details/americanmedicalp31812newy/page/n353/mode/2up

John Morgan, c. 1780. Autographed Portrait Print from Original Painting, 10.5 × 8.5 in. UPX 4, Graphics and portraits Collection, Box 2. University Archives and Records Center, University of Pennsylvania. https://jstor.org/stable/community.22101009

Unknown, *Dr. William Shippen, Jr.* Oil on canvas, 35.5 × 28.5 in. The Mutter Museum of the College of Physicians of Philadelphia. https://tcpp-emuweb.axiellhosting.com/museum/?record=ecatalogue.138

Peale, Charles Willson. *Dr. Benjamin Rush,* 1783 and 1786. Oil on canvas, 126.7 × 101.3 cm. Winterthur Museum., Winterthur, Delaware. http://museumcollection.winterthur.org/print-record.php?srchfld=irn&name=11281&port=40138&output=HTML

Page 369
Jackman, W. G., artist. *Caspar Wistar,* c. 1800. Print: engraving with manuscript annotation, 7 × 5 in. UPX 4, Graphics and portraits Collection, Box 2. University Archives and Records Center, University of Pennsylvania. https://jstor.org/stable/community.22101076

Admission Ticket, Lectures on Anatomy, Surgery and Midwifery by William Shippen and Caspar Wistar. 1801 Nov 2. Text: with manuscript annotation, 2.5 × 3.7 in. UPT 50 D992, Benjamin Woolsey Dwight and Francis E. Dwight Papers, Box 1, folder 1. University Archives and Records Center, University of Pennsylvania. https://jstor.org/stable/community.22106827

Engraving by James Akin, published in Caspar Wistar's "A Description of the Bones Deposited, by the President, in the Museum of the Society, and Represented in the Annexed Plates." *Transactions of the American Philosophical Society* 4 (1799): 526–31. https://doi.org/10.2307/1005128

Andre, Major John. *Self-portrait,* 1780 Oct 1. Pen and brown ink, 4 × 5 1/8 in. Yale University Art Gallery, New Haven, Connecticut. https://artgallery.yale.edu/collections/objects/47

Page 370
Andre, John. *Mrs. Margaret [Peggy] Shippen Arnold.* Watercolor copy of pencil sketch, 13.6 × 20.8 cm. Historical Society of Pennsylvania, Philadelphia. https://digitallibrary.hsp.org/index.php/Detail/objects/2819

Hart, Thomas. *Benedict Arnold,* 1776. Color mezzotint, 35.4 × 25.1 cm. Brown University Library. https://library.brown.edu/cds/repository2/repoman.php?verb=render&id=1194635475812500&view=showmods

Page 371
Welch and Walters, photographer. *William Edmund Horner,* 1846. Print: engraving with manuscript annotation, 8.9 × 5.8 in. UPX 4, Graphics and portraits Collection, Box 1. University Archives and Records Center, University of Pennsylvania. https://jstor.org/stable/community.22104910

Page 372
Henry Hollingsworth Smith, c. 1865. Photograph, 4 × 4 in. UPF 1.9 AR, Alumni Records Collection, Box 2527. University Archives and Records Center, University of Pennsylvania. https://jstor.org/stable/community.22109125

Dr. D. Hayes Agnew, 1863–65. Albumin. U.S. National Library of Medicine (NLM): Images from the History of Medicine. http://resource.nlm.nih.gov/101425687

Phillips, H. C. *John Ashhurst.* U.S. National Library of Medicine (NLM): Images from the History of Medicine. http://resource.nlm.nih.gov/101409530

John Shaw Billings, c. 1862. Photograph, 3 9/16 × 2 3/16 in. National Portrait Gallery, Smithsonian Institution, Washington, DC. https://npg.si.edu/object/npg_NPG.77.191

P.S. Duval & Son, Printer, and James Fuller Queen. *Mower U.S.A. General Hostital [sic], Chestnut Hill, Philadelphia/J. Queen, del.; P.S. Duval & Son, lith.,* ca. 1865. Philadelphia: P.S. Duval & Son. Hand-colored lithograph. https://www.loc.gov/item/2003655784/

Page 373
John Shaw Billings. Photograph. U.S. National Library of Medicine (NLM): Images from the History of Medicine. http://resource.nlm.nih.gov/101408952

Surgeon Gen. Barnes, c. 1865–80. Photograph. Brady-Handy photograph collection, Library of Congress, Prints and Photographs Division. https://www.loc.gov/pictures/collection/brhc/item/2017894281/

John S. Billings and Thomas W. Wise in Library Hall, 1887. Photograph, 17 × 21 cm. U.S. National Library of Medicine (NLM): Images from the History of Medicine. http://resource.nlm.nih.gov/101445634

Page 374
Detroit Publishing Co., publisher. *Baltimore, Md., Johns Hopkins Hospital, main building,* 1890–1910. Photograph. Library of Congress Prints and Photographs Division. https://www.loc.gov/pictures/item/2016795386/

Page 375
Penn's Hygiene Building. Photograph. Popular Science Monthly Volume 49 (August 1896). https://en.wikisource.org/wiki/Popular_Science_Monthly/Volume_49/August_1896/Science_at_the_University_of_Pennsylvania

John Shaw Billings. Photograph. U.S. National Library of Medicine (NLM): Images from the History of Medicine. http://resource.nlm.nih.gov/101408957

Beaux, Cecelia. *John Shaw Billings, M.D.,* 1895. Oil on canvas. National Library of Medicine. https://www.nlm.nih.gov/exhibition/tour/portraits1.html

Page 376
Detroit Publishing Co., Publisher. *New York Public Library,* ca. 1908. Photograph. Library of Congress. https://www.loc.gov/item/2016816376/

Remember the Maine pin, c. 1898. Robert Bowen Collection, National Park Service. https://www.nps.gov/prsf/learn/historyculture/spanish-american-war-a-splendid-little-war.htm

Page 377
Remington, Frederic. *Charge of the Rough Riders at San Juan Hill,* 1898. Oil on canvas.

History of United States Army Base Hospital No. 20: Organized at the University of Pennsylvania. Philadelphia: E.A. Wright, 1920, 8. Photograph of Col. Edward Martin M.C. http://books.google.com/books?id=J0ASAQAAMAAJ

Page 378
Base Hospital No. 20, officers, 1919. Photograph. https://archives.upenn.edu/exhibits/penn-history/base-hospitals/

History of United States Army Base Hospital No. 20: Organized at the University of Pennsylvania. Philadelphia: E.A. Wright, 1920, 147. Photograph of Lieutenant-Nurses of Base Hospital 20, November 1918. http://books.google.com/books?id=J0ASAQAAMAAJ

Pin, "U of P" "U.S. Army Base Hospital No. 20." 1918. Three-dimensional artifact, 1.6 × 1.9 in. MEM, University Memorabilia Collection, Box 59, folder 461. University Archives and Records Center, University of Pennsylvania. https://jstor.org/stable/community.22103423

U.S. Army Signal Corps. *First aid station located in the basement of a shattered house,* c. 1914–18. Photograph. National Library of Medicine. https://collections.nlm.nih.gov/catalog/nlm:nlmuid-101447558-img

Page 379
Who's Who in Philadelphia Wartime. Philadelphia: Stafford's National News Service, 1920, 34. Photograph of Dr. John Berton Carnett. https://archive.org/details/whoswhoinphilade00phil/page/34/mode/2up?ref=ol&view=theater&q=carnett

Liberty Loan Parade at Philadelphia, Pennsylvania, 28 September 1918. Photograph. Naval History and Heritage Command. https://www.history.navy.mil/content/history/nhhc/our-collections/photography/numerical-list-of-images/nhhc-series/nh-series/NH-41000/NH-41730.html

Page 380
George Leib Harrison. UPF 1.9AR, box #1067 (negative). University Archives and Records Center, University of Pennsylvania.

Haeseler, photographer. *J. William White.* c. 1910. Photograph, 9 .5 × 7.5 in. UPF 1.9 AR, Alumni Records Collection. University Archives and Records Center, University of Pennsylvania. https://jstor.org/stable/community.22103537

American Ambulance Hospital, Paris, c. 1914–1917. Photograph. Weill Cornell Medicine Samuel J. Wood Library, New York, NY. https://library.weill.cornell.edu/archives-blog/we-heard-call-american-ambulance-hospital

Page 381
"Dr. I. S. Ravdin, Prominent Surgeon, Goes to Honolulu," 1941. *With permission from Anne Ravdin.*

Seeley, Dave. *Bombing of Pearl Harbor.* Kate Marks. "Attack on Pearl Harbor!" Junior Scholastic (November 20, 2017). Illustration. https://junior.scholastic.com/issues/2017-18/112017/attack-on-pearl-harbor.html

Ravdin, Isidore S. *Program cover.* "A Philadelphia doctor's story of Pearl Harbor." Southeastern Pennsylvania Chapter of the American Red Cross (February 9, 1942). https://www.worldcat.org/title/19753031

Page 382
Francis Wood. Photograph.

Julian Johnson. Photograph.

Cletus Schwegman. Photograph.

John Mitchell Dean. Photograph. UPT 50 R252, box 182, ff 33. University Archives and Records Center, University of Pennsylvania.

Harold Scheie. Photograph. UPT 50 R252, box 185, scrapbook 8. University Archives and Records Center, University of Pennsylvania.

Robert Groff. University of Pennsylvania School of Medicine, *Scope* (Philadelphia, 1943), 138. University Archives and Records Center, University of Pennsylvania.

Dietz, James. *Of Their Own Accord,* Merrill's Marauders Rangers in Burma, 16¾" × 22", The Art of James Dietz, Historical Military Artist. Print. https://www.jamesdietz.com/store/prints/world-war-ii/of-their-own-accord/ *Reprinted by permission of James Dietz.*

Lancswolf. *Merrill's Marauder's badge.* Wikimedia Commons. Drawing. https://commons.wikimedia.org/wiki/File:Merrills_Marauders.svg

Page 383
John H. Gibbon, Jr. (double portrait), 1963. Photograph, 5 × 7 in. Courtesy of Siegman Archives at Thomas Jefferson University, Philadelphia. https://jdc.jefferson.edu/historical_photos/1202/

Shumaker, Harris B. *John Gibbon (in uniform). A Dream of the Heart* (Fithian Press, January 1, 1999), 146. Photograph.

Page 384
Shumaker, Harris B. *John Gibbon and officer. A Dream of the Heart* (Fithian Press, January 1, 1999), 136. Photograph.

Page 385
Hal Barker. Photograph courtesy of Clyde Barker.

Fletcher, Archibald G. *Archibald Fletcher, 1946. To India and Beyond, Memoirs of a Missionary Surgeon* (Xlibris, March 11, 2005): 69. Photograph. *Permission granted by John Fletcher.*

Jim Hardy. Hardy family photo. Photograph. *Permission granted by Dr. Katherine Hardy Little.*

US Army Signal Corps. *General George Patton.* Library of Congress (March 30, 1943). Photograph. https://www.loc.gov/item/2004672054/

Patton prayer card. "Patton's Prayer." *Nothing & Easting.* Photograph. https://oldtopographer.net/2016/12/24/pattons-prayer/

Page 386
L. Kraeer Ferguson. Photograph.

Penn Navy Team. University of Pennsylvania School of Medicine, *Scope* (Philadelphia, 1943), 133. University Archives and Records Center, University of Pennsylvania.

Duffy, Kelly. *USS Solace (AH-5) in Hawaii, ca. 1941.* "Navy Nurses: The Heroines of Pearl Harbor." National Museum of the American Sailor (December 2, 2020). Photograph. https://sailorsattic.wordpress.com/2020/12/02/navy-nurses-the-heroines-of-pearl-harbor/.

Robert Bruce Brown. Photograph. Navy Memorial. https://navylog.navymemorial.org/brown-robert-102

Page 387
Frogman using gear. "Photos: What Happened to Catalina Island During WWII?" Catalina Island Museum. Photograph. https://laist.com/podcasts/off-ramp/photos-what-happened-to-catalina-island-during-wwii *Reprinted by permission of Catalina Museum for Art and History.*

Finlayson, Kenneth. *Christian Lambertsen (in swimsuit, standing).* "Key West: Home of ARSOF Underwater Operations." *Veritas* 3, no. 1 (2007). Photograph. https://arsof-history.org/articles/v3n1_key_west_page_1.html

Page 388
Hevesi, Dennis. Lambertsen, inventor of the scuba gear. "Christian Lambertsen, Inventor of Scuba Precursor, Dies at 93." *The New York Times* (Feb. 25, 2011). Photograph. https://www.nytimes.com/2011/02/26/us/26lambertsen.html.

Sacquety, Troy J. *Aquatic Pioneer: Dr. Christian Lambertsen.* "Operation Boston, An OSS Combined Operation in the Indian Ocean. General ARSOF History. Photograph. https://arsof-history.org/articles/v5n1_operation_boston_page_1.html#lambertsen

Page 389
Sacquety, Troy J. *A MU swimmer wearing a Model 10 LARU, training to breach anti-submarine nets at Guantanamo Bay, Cuba, in 1944.* "Operation Boston, An OSS Combined Operation in the Indian Ocean. General ARSOF History. Photograph. https://arsof-history.org/articles/v5n1_operation_boston_page_1.html#lambertsen

Page 390
Professor Christian Lambertson. University of Pennsylvania School of Medicine, *Scope* (Philadelphia, 1960), 35. University Archives and Records Center, University of Pennsylvania.

Mason, Frank. *Christian Lambertson.* Oil on canvas. https://www.med.upenn.edu/psom/christian-j-lambertsen-md.html Courtesy of the University of Pennsylvania Art Collection, Philadelphia, PA.

Page 391
Biddle, Charles John. *The way of the eagle.* New York: Charles Scribeners Sons, 1919. Frontispiece photo of *Charles John Biddle.* https://archive.org/details/wayofeagle00biddrich/page/n5/mode/2up

The John Scott Award. Board of Directors of City Trusts of Philadelphia. Photograph. https://thejohnscottaward.github.io/jsc/index.html

Page 392
Henry Keep, rowing team picture. Henry B. Keep, 1941. Princeton Rowing. Princeton University. Photograph. https://rowing.princeton.edu/people/henry-b-keep-1941/

DVD cover of *A Bridge Too Far.* Metro-Goldwyn-Mayer Studios Inc. All Rights Reserved.

Page 393
Henry Blair Keep Jr. Photograph. https://www.findagrave.com/memorial/192763819/henry-blair-keep

Noon, Steve. *Crossing the Waal, September 20, 1944.* "Campaign 270, Operation Market Garden 1944." Osprey Publishing. Watercolor and gouache. https://www.steve-noon.co.uk/contactform.html *Artwork by Steve Noon © Osprey Publishing.*

Page 394
Davis, Richard. *Yours, D3.* Acorn Alliance (2000). Book cover. *Permission granted by Anne Davis Peterson.*

Henry Keep's citation for a Bronze Star. Facebook. Photograph. https://scontent-lga3-1.xx.fbcdn.net/v/t1.6435-9/36667431_2043759169030489_2898630147684958208_n.jpg?_nc_cat=100&ccb=1-5&_nc_sid=730e14

Page 395
Anadalusia stone façade. https://www.findagrave.com/memorial/192763819/henry-blair-keep

Andalusia House. "Andalusia Historic House, Gardens and Arboretum." Visit Bucks County, Pennsylvania. Photograph. https://www.visitbuckscounty.com/listing/andalusia-historic-house-gardens-and-arboretum/164/ *Permission granted by Andalusia Historic House, Gardens & Arboretum. Permission granted by Connie S. Griffith Houchins, photographer.*

Dr. Ravdin and John Howard. Photograph. UPT 50 R252, box 185, scrapbook 3. University Archives and Records Center, University of Pennsylvania.

Page 396
Hussain, S. Amjad, Justin A. Julian, Jonathan H. Demeter, Joseph J. Sferra, F. Charles Brunicardi. *John Howard, smiling in glasses.* "John M. Howard: A pioneer in vascular, trauma, and pancreatic surgery." *Bulletin of the American College of Surgeons* (May 2019). Photograph. https://bulletin.facs.org/2019/05/john-m-howard-a-pioneer-in-vascular-trauma-and-pancreatic-surgery/.

Hussain, S. Amjad, Justin A. Julian, Jonathan H. Demeter, Joseph J. Sferra, F. Charles Brunicardi. *John Howard in Korea.* "John M. Howard: A pioneer in vascular, trauma, and pancreatic surgery." *Bulletin of the American College of Surgeons* (May 2019). Photograph. https://bulletin.facs.org/2019/05/john-m-howard-a-pioneer-in-vascular-trauma-and-pancreatic-surgery/

A U.S. Air Force Sikorsky H-5 of the 3rd Air Rescue Squadron lands in Korea to evacuate wounded, 1 July 1951. Photograph. https://commons.wikimedia.org/wiki/File:Sikorsky_H-5_of_3rd_ARS_lands_to_recover_wounded_1951.JPEG

Page 397
Finnegan, James. *Jim Finnegan in scrubs.* "My War–Dr. James Finnegan" (9.12, 2011). Historynet. Photograph. https://www.historynet.com/my-war-dr-james-o-finnegan/ *Permission granted by Linda Finnegan.*

Finnegan, James O. *In the Company of Marines: A Surgeon Remembers Vietnam* (lulu.com, September 8, 2010). Cover photograph. https://www.amazon.com/Company-Marines-Surgeon-Remembers-Vietnam/dp/0557066395 *Permission granted by Linda Finnegan.*

Page 398
James Finnegan. Photograph. *With permission from Linda Finnegan.*

Ron Fairman, operating. Photograph. *With permission from Ron Fairman.*

Page 399
Sloane Guy. Photograph. *With permission from Sloane Guy.*

John Pryor. Photograph. *With permission from Carmela Calvo.*

John P. Pryor, MD 1966–2008 ribbon logo. With permission from Carmela Calvo.

Page 400
Pryor, Richard J. *Alright, Let's Call It a Draw.* Lanxnal (June 18, 2012). Kelly Fahey, cover design; Ryan Donnell, cover photograph. Book cover photograph. https://www.amazon.com/Alright-Lets-Call-Draw-Pryor/dp/0985755008 *Permission granted by Richard J. Pryor.*

Page 401
Jonathan Rhoads. Photograph. *With permission from George Rhoads.*

William Fitts on phone. University of Pennsylvania School of Medicine, *Scope* (Philadelphia, 1981), 30. University Archives and Records Center, University of Pennsylvania.

Bill Schwab. Photograph. With permission from Bill Schwab.

Larry Stephenson. University of Pennsylvania School of Medicine, *Scope* (Philadelphia, 1983), 78. University Archives and Records Center, University of Pennsylvania.

Page 402
PennSTAR helipad. Photograph. *With permission from Bill Schwab.*

Page 403
Mike Rotondo. Photograph. *With permission from Mike Rotondo.*

Don Kauder. Photograph. *With permission from Don Kauder.*

Pat Reilly. Photograph. *With permission from Pat Reilly.*

Mike Nance. Photograph. *With permission from Mike Nance.*

Page 404
John Pryor and Bill Schwab. Photograph. *With permission from Bill Schwab.*

John Paul Pryor Shock Trauma and Resuscitation Unit in the Trauma Center at Penn Presbyterian Medical Center (outside). Photograph. https://www.uphs.upenn.edu/pastoral/cpe/trauma_description_for_CPE.html *With permission from Bill Schwab.*

John Paul Pryor Shock Trauma and Resuscitation Unit in the Trauma Center at Penn Presbyterian Medical Center (inside). Photograph. *Courtesy of Halkin Mason Photography.*

Page 408
Bill Inouye. Photograph.

Tule Lake Segregation Center, 1946. "Tule Lake Segregation Center Pamphlet." National Park Service. Photograph. https://www.nps.gov/tule/planyourvisit/tule-lake-segregation-center-pamphlet.htm

Page 409
Coil dialyzer. Home Dialysis Central. Photograph. https://homedialysis.org/home-dialysis-basics/machines-and-supplies/dialysis-museum *Permission is granted by the Medical Education Institute and Jim Curtis, photographer.*

Page 411
Karsh, Yousuf. *Leonard Miller,* 1991 Mar 22. Photograph. *Courtesy of the Estate of Yousuf Karsh.*

Page 412
Jack Mackie. Photograph.

Page 414
Barker, Clyde, photographer. *Jack and Joan Mackie.*

Page 415
Alden Harken. University of Pennsylvania School of Medicine, *Scope* (Philadelphia, 1966), 15. University Archives and Records Center, University of Pennsylvania.

Page 416
Leonard Perloff. University of Pennsylvania School of Medicine, *Scope* (Philadelphia, 1978), 32. University Archives and Records Center, University of Pennsylvania.

Page 418
Gordon Buzby. Photograph. *With permission from Karen Buzby.*

Davis, Jason, photographer. *Buzby Award. With permission from Jason Davis.*

Page 419
Alejandro, Carlos, photographer. *Jim Mullen. © Carlos Alejandro Photography.*

Page 421
Jon Morris. Photograph. *With permission from Jon Morris.*

Page 422
Ernie Rosato. Photograph. *With permission from Geraldine Rosato.*

Page 424
Ernie and Gerry Rosato. Photograph. *With permission from Geraldine Rosato.*

Page 425
Doug Fraker. Photograph. *With permission from Doug Fraker.*

Page 426
Cunicelli, Ed, photographer. *Robert Roses. Courtesy of Ed Cunicelli.*

Cornwell, Dean. *Osler at Old Blockley.* (Philadelphia: John Wyeth and Brother, Inc., date unknown). National Library of Medicine. Photograph. https://collections.nlm.nih.gov/catalog/nlm:nlmuid-101651378-img

Page 427
DeBalko, David, photographer. *Sean Harbison. Courtesy of DeBalko Photography LLC.*

Sean Harbison operating on a gorilla. Philadelphia Zoo. Photograph. https://dixon.philly.com/wp-content/uploads/2017/08/681829_283002c4d26d028.jpg *Permission granted by the Philadelphia Zoo.*

Page 432
John H. Gibbon, Jr. (double portrait), 1963. Photograph, 5 × 7 in. Courtesy of Siegman Archives at Thomas Jefferson University, Philadelphia. https://jdc.jefferson.edu/historical_photos/1202/

Page 434
Norman Freeman. University of Pennsylvania School of Medicine, *Scope* (Philadelphia, 1943), 20. University Archives and Records Center, University of Pennsylvania.

William Inouye. University of Pennsylvania School of Medicine, *Scope* (Philadelphia, 1971), 21. University Archives and Records Center, University of Pennsylvania.

Coil dialyzer. Home Dialysis Central. Photograph. https://homedialysis.org/home-dialysis-basics/machines-and-supplies/dialysis-museum *Permission is granted by the Medical Education Institute and Jim Curtis, photographer.*

Freeman, NE and FH Leeds. *Whole blood injected into closed aneurysmal wall at pressure equal to one-half that of systolic blood pressure to buttress vein graft, Fig. 10.* "Operations on large arteries. *Western Journal of Medicine*, October, no. 77 (1952), 229–33 https://pubmed.ncbi.nlm.nih.gov/13009464/ *Permission granted by Elsevier.*

Page 435
James Hardy. The University of Mississippi Medical Center. Photograph. https://twitter.com/UMMCnews/status/1403435860670881796/photo/2 *Permission granted by the University of Mississippi Medical Center and Dr. Katherine Hardy Little.*

Page 436
William Pierce with heart pump. Lehigh University (1958). Photograph. https://www1.lehigh.edu/about/timeline/1940-1969

Page 438
Barker, Clyde F. and RE Billingham. *Mouse.* "The role of afferent lymphatics in the rejection of skin homografts," *Journal of Experimental Medicine* 128, no. 1 (July 1, 1968): 197–221. Drawing. https://www.ncbi.nlm.nih.gov/pmc/articles/PMC2138504/

Barker, Clyde F. and RE Billingham. *Showing a freshly prepared isolated skin flap with its vascular umbilical cord and inlaid skin homograft.* "The role of afferent lymphatics in the rejection of skin homografts." *Journal of Experimental Medicine*, 128, no. 1 (July 1, 1968): 197–221. Drawing. https://www.ncbi.nlm.nih.gov/pmc/articles/PMC2138504/

Page 439
Stan Dudrick with puppy. Reprinted from cover of *Journal of Parenteral and Enteral Nutrition* vol. 44, no. 2 (February 2020).

Infant at [...] completion of 44 days of nutrition administered exclusively by vein. Reprinted from Wilmore DW, Dudrick SJ. "Growth and Development of an Infant Receiving All Nutrients Exclusively by Vein." *JAMA.* 203, no. 10 (1968 March 4):862. https://pubmed.ncbi.nlm.nih.gov/4965871/

Douglas Wilmore. Brigham and Women's Hospital (Harvard). Photograph. https://surgery.bwh.harvard.edu/history/ *Permission granted by Douglas Wilmore.*

Page 440
ASA Medallion for Scientific Achievement. Photo by Elizabeth Barker.

Page 442
Bernard Fisher. "Bernard Fisher, a pioneer in breast cancer research, dies at 101." Pittwire. University of Pittsburgh (October 21, 2019). Photograph. https://www.pitt.edu/pittwire/features-articles/bernard-fisher-md-pioneer-breast-cancer-research-dies-101

Rombeau, John L. and Donna Muldoon. *Harry Vars. Jonathan Rhoads, MD: Quaker Sense and Sensibility in the World of Surgery* (Philadelphia: Hanley & Belfus, 1997): 177. Photograph.

Page 443
Patel, Smruit, Christopher Markosian, Osamah J. Choudhry, Jeffrey Thomas Keller. *Portrait of neurosurgeon Peter J. Jannetta (1932–2016).* "The historical evolution of microvascular decompression for trigeminal neuralgia: from Dandy's discovery to Jannetta's legacy." *Acta Neurochirugica,* 162, no. 17 (November 2020). Photograph. https://www.researchgate.net/figure/Portrait-of-neurosurgeon-Peter-J-Jannetta-1932-2016-Permission-courtesy-of-Raymond-F_fig8_342064804 *Reprinted by permission of Raymond F. Sekula Jr.*

Page 444
Ali Naji. Photograph. *With permission from Ali Naji.*

Page 445
Divyansh Agarwal, Ali Naji, and Chengyang Liu. *Cover of Nature Metabolism. Nature Metabolism*, 21, no. 10 (October 2020). Photograph. https://www.nature.com/natmetab/volumes/2/issues/10

Page 446
Joel Cooper and Tom Hall, 1983. Photograph. *With permission from Joel Cooper.*

Page 447
PennSTAR helipad. Photograph. *With permission from Bill Schwab.*

Page 449
Bill Schwab. Photograph. *With permission from Bill Schwab.*

Mike Rotondo. Photograph. *With permission from Mike Rotondo.*

Page 450
Brian Czerniecki. Photograph. *With permission from Brian Czerniecki.*

Ben Chang. Photograph. *With permission from Ben Chang.*

Scott Levin. Photograph. *With permission from Scott Levin.*

Zion Harvey, with football. Photograph. *With permission from Ben Chang.*

Page 451
DeBalko, David, photographer. *Steven Raper. Courtesy of DeBalko Photography LLC.*

Omaida Velazquez. The University of Miami Miller School of Medicine. Photograph. https://med.miami.edu/faculty/omaida-c-velazquez-md-facs *Permission granted by Omaida C. Velázquez, MD, PhD, professor of surgery with tenure, David Kimmelman Endowed Chair of Vascular and Endovascular Surgery, University of Miami.*

Page 452
Hansell Stedman. Photograph. *With permission from Hansell Stedman.*

Page 454
Rachel Kelz. Photograph. *With permission from Rachel Kelz.*

Page 455
Cunicelli, Ed, photographer. *Sunil SInghal. Courtesy of Ed Cunicelli.*

Glowing tumors. Photograph. With permission from Sunil Singhal. https://www.pennmedicine.org/news/news-releases/2021/november/fda-approves-glowing-tumor-imaging-drug-to-better-identify-ovarian-cancer-cells

Page 465
R. Scott Jones. Society of Clinical Surgery. Photograph. https://societyofclinicalsurgery.com/senior-members/jones/ *Permission granted by the Society of Clinical Surgery.*

Edward M. Copeland. "Southern Surgical Association honors Copeland, UF surgeons present at association meeting." Department of Surgery. University of Florida (January 23, 2014).

Photograph. https://surgery.med.ufl.edu/2014/01/23/southern-surgical-association-honors-copeland-uf-surgeons-present-at-association-meeting/ *Permission granted by Edward M. Copeland III.*

James C. Thompson. "Legends, 2006." The Lundquist Institute. Photograph. https://lundquist.org/legends

James D. Hardy. "History of Cardiac Surgery." Eskind Biomedical Library. Vanderbilt University. Photograph. https://www.library.vanderbilt.edu/specialcollections/history-of-medicine/exhibits/cardiac_surgery/ *Permission granted by Dr. Katherine Hardy Little.*

Page 466
Stanley J. Dudrick. Photograph.

Barker, Clyde, photographer. *Moritz Ziegler.*

C. Everett Koop. Photograph.

Page 467
Cunicelli, Ed, photographer. *Ronald DeMatteo. Courtesy of Ed Cunicelli.*

Page 468
Stephen Bartlett. Photograph. *With permission from Stephen Bartlett.*

Danny O. Jacobs. Photograph. Personal image of Danny Jacobs previously shared with HUP Surgery. *With permission from Danny Jacobs.*

Page 469
W. Roy Smythe. SomaLogic. Photograph. https://somalogic.com/wp-content/uploads/2022/07/Roy-Smythe-Bio-Jul2022.pdf. *Permission granted by W. Roy Smythe*

Page 470
James D. Luketich. University of Pittsburgh Medical Center Medical Media. Photograph. *Permission granted by James D. Luketich.*

Page 471
Michael Choti, MD. *Banner Health.* 2024. Photograph. *Permission granted by Michael Choti.*

Page 472
Howard A. Reber. Hirschberg Foundation for Pancreatic Cancer Research. Photograph. *Permission granted by Monica Campos, Ex. Dir., the Hirschberg Foundation.*

Page 474
Omaida Velazquez. "Faculty Profiles." Miller School of Medicine. University of Miami. Photograph. https://med.miami.edu/graduate-studies/doctoral-programs/executive-ph,-d-,d,-d-,-in-biochemistry-and-molecular-biology/faculty-profiles *Permission granted by Omaida C. Velázquez, MD, PhD, professor of surgery with tenure, David Kimmelman Endowed Chair of Vascular and Endovascular Surgery, University of Miami.*

Page 475
James F. Markmann. Society of Clinical Surgery. Photograph. *Permission granted by the Society of Clinical Surgery.*

Page 477
Ken Brayman. Photograph. *With permission from Ken Brayman.*

Page 478
Steven Fishman. Boston Children's Hospital. Photograph. *Reprinted by permission of Dr. Steven J. Fishman.*

Page 479
Mark Fairies. Cedars-Sinai Medical Center. Photograph. *Permission granted by Mark Fairies.*

Joseph Woo. Stanford Medicine. Photograph. *Reprinted by permission of Joseph Woo.*

Page 480
Isabelle Bedrosian. The University of Texas MD Anderson Cancer Center. Photograph. *Copyright held by, and used with permission of, The Board of Regents of the University of Texas System through The University of Texas MD Anderson Cancer Center.*

Page 481
Heung Bae Kim. Boston Children's Hospital. Photograph. *Reprinted by permission of Dr. Heung Bae Kim.*

Page 485
D. Hayes (David Hayes) Agnew, 1892. Photograph, 6.0 × 3.5 in. UPF 1.9 AR, Alumni Records Collection. University Archives and Records Center, University of Pennsylvania. https://jstor.org/stable/community.22103519

Page 486
Shanks, Nelson. *Julian Johnson,* c. 1965-1975. Oil on canvas. https://www.jtcvs.org/cms/attachment/4ba37ee7-473d-43c3-9f4a-3d2a54125a53/gr2.jpg Courtesy of the University of Pennsylvania Art Collection, Philadelphia, Pennsylvania.

Page 487
Robert Ravdin. University of Pennsylvania School of Medicine, *Scope* (Philadelphia, 1972), 35. University Archives and Records Center, University of Pennsylvania.

Page 488
Julius A. Mackie. Photograph.

Page 489
Gordon Buzby. Photograph. *With permission from Karen Buzby.*

Linton Whitaker. Photograph. *With permission from Linton Whitaker.*

Page 490
John P. Pryor, M.D., aboard a military plane in Iraq, December 2008. Photograph. *With permission from Carmela Calvo.*

Ernie Rosato. Photograph. *With permission from Geraldine Rosato.*

Page 491
Barker, Clyde, photographer. *Dan and Barbara Dempsey.*

Page 492
Robinson, Danforth. *I. S. Ravdin. Imago Chirurgii, 1913–1963* (Ethicon: Somerville, NJ, 1963), 88. Drawing. *©Ethicon, Inc. (2024). Reproduced with permission.*

Page 493
William Fitts laughing. University of Pennsylvania School of Medicine, *Scope* (Philadelphia, 1970), 110. University Archives and Records Center, University of Pennsylvania.

Page 494
Jonathan Rhoads. Photograph. *With permission from George Rhoads.*

Page 497
Jonathan Rhoads and John Daly. Photograph. *With permission from George Rhoads.*

John Daly. Photograph.

Page 499
DeBalko, David, photographer. *Doug Fraker. Courtesy of DeBalko Photography LLC.*

Page 500
Larry Kaiser. Photograph. *With permission from Larry Kaiser.*

Joel Cooper. Photograph. *With permission from Joel Cooper.*

Page 501
John Kucharczuk. Photograph. *With permission from John Kucharczuk.*

Cunicelli, Ed, photographer. *Sunil SInghal. Courtesy of Ed Cunicelli.*

Page 502
Ernie Rosato. Photograph. *With permission from Geraldine Rosato.*

Dan Dempsey. Photograph. *With permission from Dan Dempsey.*

Page 503
Barker, Clyde, photographer. *Dan and Barbara Dempsey.*

Page 504
Charles Vollmer. Photograph. *With permission from Charles Vollmer.*

Noel Williams. Photograph. *With permission from Noel Williams.*

Page 505
Julian Johnson. University of Pennsylvania School of Medicine, *Scope* (Philadelphia, 1962), 82. University Archives and Records Center, University of Pennsylvania.

Heinle, Jeffrey S. and J. William Gaynor. *John Waldhausen.* "Historical perspectives of the American Association for thoracic surgery: John Anton Waldhausen (1929–2012)." *The Journal of Thoracic and Cardiovascular Surgery* 148, no. 2 (August 2014): 381–86. Photograph.
https://www.jtcvs.org/article/S0022-5223(14)00534-0/fulltext

Page 506
Henry Edmunds. University of Pennsylvania School of Medicine, *Scope* (Philadelphia, 1975), 22. University Archives and Records Center, University of Pennsylvania.

Page 507
Henry Edmunds. Photograph. *With permission from Henry Edmunds.*

Page 508
Mike Acker. Photograph. *With permission from Mike Acker.*

Allred, Martin J. *Timothy J. Gardner.* Nationwide Photographers. Christian Care News (July 2, 2015). Photograph.
https://news.christianacare.org/2015/07/timothy-j-gardner-m-d-receives-aats-lifetime-achievement-award/ *Reprinted by permission of Martin J. Allred, Nationwide Photographers.*

Page 509
Mike Acker, with guitar. Video still.
https://www.youtube.com/watch?v=DQ4j4z0SaLI&t=8s
With permission from Mike Acker.

Joe Bavaria. Photograph. *With permission from Joe Bavaria.*

Wilson Szeto. Photograph. *With permission from Wilson Szeto.*

Page 510
Barker, Clyde, photographer. *Brooke Roberts.*

Page 511
DeBalko, David, photographer. *Ron Fairman, with stent. Courtesy of DeBalko Photography LLC.*

Page 512
Ron Fairman as president of SVS. Photograph. *With permission from Ron Fairman.*

Page 513
Darren Schneider. Photograph. *With permission from Darren Schneider.*

Alex Fairman, Scott Damrauer, Julia Glaser, Ron Fairman, Grace Wang, Ben Jackson. Photograph. *With permission from Ron Fairman.*

Page 514
Barker, Clyde, photographer. *Don DaFoe.*

Barker, Clyde, photographer. *Moritz Ziegler.*

Barker, Clyde, photographer. *Jim Markmann.*

Barker, Clyde, photographer. *Ken Brayman.*

Barker, Clyde, photographer. *Ali Naji.*

Page 515
Kim Olthoff. Photograph. *With permission from Kim Olthoff.*

Avi Shaked. Photograph. *With permission from Avi Shaked.*

Cunicelli, Ed, photographer. *Peter Abt. Courtesy of Ed Cunicelli.*

Crane, Paul, photographer. *Matt Levine. Courtesy of Crane Photography, Inc.*

DeBalko, David, photographer. *Ty Dunn. Courtesy of DeBalko Photography LLC.*

Ira Fox. University of Pittsburgh Medical Center. Photograph. *Permission granted by Ira J. Fox.*

Page 516
Burke, Daniel, photographer. *Larry Jameson and Pat Reilly. Courtesy of Daniel Burke Photography.*

Page 517
Jeremy Cannon. Photograph. *Permission granted by Dr. Jeremy Cannon.*

Page 518
Bob Fry. Photograph, *With permission from Bob Fry.*

Najjia Mahmoud. Photograph. *With permission from Najjia Mahmoud.*

Cary Aarons. Photograph. *With permission from Cary Aarons.*

DeBalko, David, photographer. *Josh Bleier. Courtesy of DeBalko Photography LLC.*

Page 519
John Rombeau. Photograph. *With permission from John Rombeau.*

Allen, Agnew. *Robert Ivy.* Oil on canvas. *Courtesy of the University of Pennsylvania Art Collection, Philadelphia, PA.*

Page 520
Phillips, Robert, photographer. *The Pennsylvania Gazette* (May 1968), cover photo of Henry Royster. *Courtesy of The Pennsylvania Gazette.*

Herndon Lehr. Photograph.

Karsh, Yousuf. *Peter Randall,* 1989 Jan 20. Photograph. *Courtesy of the Estate of Yousuf Karsh.*

Page 521
Linton Whitaker. Photograph. *With permission from Linton Whitaker.*

Burke, Daniel, photographer. *Joe Serletti. Courtesy of Daniel Burke Photography.*

Page 522
Don LaRossa. Photograph.

Barry Noone. Photograph. *With permission from Barry Noone.*

Scott Bartlett. Photograph. *With permission from Scott Bartlett.*

David W. Low. Plural Publishing Inc. Photograph.
https://www.pluralpublishing.com/author/david-w-low
Permission granted by Dr. David W. Low.

Page 523
Alan Wein. Photograph. *With permission from Alan Wein.*

John Murphy. University of Pennsylvania School of Medicine, *Scope* (Philadelphia, 1978), 31. University Archives and Records Center, University of Pennsylvania.

Page 524
Burke, Daniel, photographer. *Tom Guzzo. Courtesy of Daniel Burke Photography.*

Page 530
Cunicelli, Ed, photographer. *Ronald DeMatteo. Courtesy of Ed Cunicelli.*

Page 531
Ron DeMatteo. Photograph. *Courtesy of Ron DeMatteo.*

Page 532
Ron and Allyson DeMatteo. Photograph. *Courtesy of Ron DeMatteo.*

Allyson, Siena, Aleesia and Ron DeMatteo. Photograph. *Courtesy of Ron DeMatteo.*

Page 533
Class of 1999 Surgical Oncology Fellows at MSK. Photograph. *Courtesy of Ron DeMatteo.*

Ron DeMatteo. Memorial Sloan Kettering Cancer Center. Photograph. *Permission granted by Dr. Ron DeMatteo.*

Page 534
Leslie Blumgart and Ron DeMatteo. Photograph. *Courtesy of Ron DeMatteo.*

Page 535
Burke, Daniel, photographer. *Allyson, Ron and Alessia DeMatteo. Courtesy of Daniel Burke Photography.*

Burke, Daniel, photographer. *Crowd at DeMatteo welcoming ceremony. Courtesy of Daniel Burke Photography.*

Burke, Daniel, photographer. *Dean Larry Jameson and Ron DeMatteo. Courtesy of Daniel Burke Photography.*

Page 536
Ron DeMatteo, Larry Kaiser, Clyde Barker, Jeff Drebin, Jim Mullen. Photograph.

Page 537
Ron DeMatteo with 2022 General Surgery Graduates. Photograph. *With permission from Ron DeMatteo.*

Page 538
HUP Pavilion. Photograph.

Cunicelli, Ed, photographer. *Ron DeMatteo. Courtesy of Ed Cunicelli.*

Division of Breast Surgery. Photograph. *With permission from Oluwadamilola Fayanju.*

DeBalko, David, photographer. *Oluwadamilola Fayanju. Courtesy of DeBalko Photography LLC.*

Page 539
Cary Aarons. Photograph. *With permission from Cary Aarons.*

Cunicelli, Ed, photographer. *Major Kenneth Lee. Courtesy of Ed Cunicelli.*

Department of Surgery, September 2017. Photograph. *With permission from Ron DeMatteo.*

Page 540
Jim Robinson, Charles Sawyers, Ron DeMatteo and Peter Scardino. Photograph. *Courtesy of Ron DeMatteo.*

The Change Curve. Graphic courtesy of Robin Noel.

Page 541
Hand and chess piece. Graphic courtesy of Robin Noel.

Ron DeMatteo. Photograph. *With permission from Ron DeMatteo.*

Eakins, Thomas. *Agnew Clinic,* 1889. Oil on canvas, 74 1/2 × 130 1/2 inches. University of Pennsylvania. School of Medicine. https://jstor.org/stable/community.14623616 Courtesy of the University of Pennsylvania Art Collection, Philadelphia, PA.

Thank you to Vince Massa, David DeBalko, and Daniel Burke and the photographers of *Scope* for their valuable contributions.

Index

All pages with images are set in *italic*.

B

C

D

E

F

G

H

I

J

K

L

M

R

S

Y

Z